KINESIOLOGY

Twelfth Edition

KINESIOLOGY

Scientific Basis of Human Motion

Nancy Hamilton, Ph.D.
University of Northern Iowa

Wendi Weimar, Ph.D.
Auburn University

Kathryn Luttgens, Ph.D.
Professor Emerita, Northeastern University

Mc Graw Hill
Connect Learn Succeed™

The McGraw-Hill Companies

KINESIOLOGY: SCIENTIFIC BASIS OF HUMAN MOTION, TWELFTH EDITION

Published by McGraw-Hill, a business unit of The McGraw-Hill Companies, Inc., 1221 Avenue of the Americas, New York, NY 10020.

This book is printed on acid-free paper.

6 7 8 9 10 11 QVS/QVS 22 21 20 19 18

ISBN 978-0-07-802254-8
MHID 0-07-802254-1

Vice President & Editor-in-Chief: *Michael Ryan*
Vice President EDP/Central Publishing Services: *Kimberly Meriwether David*
Publisher: *William Glass*
Editorial Coordinator: *Marley Magaziner*
Executive Marketing Manager: *Pamela S. Cooper*
Senior Project Manager: *Joyce Watters*
Buyer: *Nicole Baumgartner*
Design Coordinator: *Brenda A. Rolwes*
Senior Photo Editor: *Natalia Peschiera*
Media Project Manager: *Sridevi Palani*
Compositor: *Glyph International*
Typeface: *10/12 Times Roman*
Printer: *Quad/Graphics*

Library of Congress Cataloging-in-Publication Data

Hamilton, Nancy (Nancy Patricia), 1946-
Kinesiology : scientific basis of human motion.—12th ed. / Nancy Hamilton, Wendi Weimar, Kathryn Luttgens.
p. cm.
Luttgens' name appears first on the earlier editions.
Includes bibliographical references and index.
ISBN 978-0-07-802254-8 (alk. paper)
1. Kinesiology—Textbooks. I. Weimar, Wendi. II. Luttgens, Kathryn, 1926- III. Title.
QP303.L87 2011
612.7'6—dc22

2010049595

www.mhhe.com

Brief Contents

CONTENTS

Preface to the Twelfth Edition

Since the publication of the first edition of this text, courses in kinesiology have undergone many changes in both content and emphasis. Each subsequent edition has reflected these changes, and the twelfth edition is no exception. The primary goals of this revision have been to update and expand the material where appropriate and to strengthen the textbook as a pedagogical tool. Several chapters have been condensed or rewritten to focus on the most critical points. The resultant content makes this a book ideally suited to help students achieve an understanding of the integrated nature of kinesiology as an area of study that includes both anatomical and biomechanical components.

AUDIENCE

In the twenty-first century, the traditional course often titled kinesiology has been separated into courses in anatomy and biomechanics. This text attempts to integrate the anatomy of human movement with the mechanics of human movement. It is neither an anatomy text nor a biomechanics text, but is an integrated kinesiology text. The textbook is designed as a basic source to introduce the undergraduate student to the fundamentals of kinesiology. Because the fundamentals are presented without compromising basic theory, this book may be used as an introductory text. The book presents the subject in a fashion that presupposes some background in anatomy and a little in physics. The text does not shy away from presenting material that requires some theoretical foundations in these areas. Whatever background is needed to understand the various applications is supplied, and numerous examples and exercises are provided. There is extensive discussion of both anatomical and biomechanical fundamentals of human motion and the application of these fundamentals to the analysis of a wide variety of motor skills. For these reasons, the text is especially appropriate for use in courses with these objectives:

1. To afford students the opportunity to learn a systematic approach to the analysis of human motion
2. To provide information that will help students obtain an understanding of the anatomical and biomechanical fundamentals of human motion
3. To provide the types of experiences that ask students to apply anatomical and biomechanical analysis to the learning and improvement of a broad spectrum of movement activities

The introduction to each section includes the assumptions about student preparation and sources for review to meet those assumed levels of readiness.

ORGANIZATION

The **Introduction to the Study of Kinesiology** is a single chapter that sets the stage by presenting a kinesiological analysis model. This chapter is intended to lay the foundation for the remainder of the text. It is here that the student will learn to organize the thought process involved in understanding human movement. It is critical that the study of kinesiology begin here—with a systematic approach to learning.

Part I, Anatomical and Physiological Fundamentals of Human Motion, consists of eight chapters, each beginning with a discussion of the anatomical background essential for understanding human movement followed by the presentation of a systematic approach to kinesiological analysis. The emphasis throughout is on the *relation of anatomical structure to function,* not on anatomy as such. It is assumed throughout this section that the student has acquired a basic knowledge of static anatomy as applied to stationary models, skeletons, and cadavers. The emphasis in this text is the dynamic anatomy of the moving body. Applications of the knowledge of structure to the analysis of human motion are introduced in these early chapters so that the student can begin to put theory into practice immediately, rather than wait until the knowledge base is more complete. Additional laboratory experiences have been added to assist with this practice.

Part II, Fundamentals of Biomechanics, presents the fundamentals of biomechanics as they apply to human movement analysis. The first chapter introduces the student to terminology and to the units of measure used when motion and the forces that cause it are studied. This chapter is followed by chapters in which motion and the forces that cause and modify it are described. The section concludes with a chapter on the center of gravity and stability.

Part II provides an elementary approach to the material without oversimplifying to the point where misconceptions could occur. In many instances the student is shown the "proof" of a principle through experimental examples or mathematical derivation. This approach is used in the belief that greater understanding will result. The reward will be greater comprehension of the reasons "why" optimum movement patterns occur as they do. It should be remembered, however, that the emphasis in a first undergraduate course in kinesiology should be on the development of the qualitative method of analysis. The introduction of the quantitative method, if used, should be limited to understanding fundamental concepts and not for extensive application to analysis of movement patterns.

Part III, Motor Skills, utilizes the kinesiological analysis system that has been developed in concert with the anatomical and mechanical concepts that have been presented. This analysis model forms the basis for the organization of the eight chapters in Part III. In each of these chapters the basic principles of anatomy and mechanics are identified and applied to specific motor skills. Sample analyses are also included.

PEDAGOGICAL FEATURES

Helpful pedagogical tools in every chapter successfully assist the learning process. These include chapter outlines, objectives, laboratory experiences, and references and selected readings.

Eight comprehensive appendices have been updated to provide material that supplements the basic concepts presented in the text:

A. Classification of Joints and Their Movements
B. Joint Range of Motion
C. Muscular Attachments and Nerve Supply
D. Mathematics Review
E. Table of Trigonometric Functions
F. U.S.–Metric Equivalents
G. Exercises for Kinesiological Analysis
H. Answers to Problems in Part II

Additionally, an online lab manual is available at the text's website at **www.mhhe.com/hamilton 12e.** This downloadable manual takes many of the laboratory experiences from the text and guides the student through the process of using an experiential approach whether it be experimentation, problem solving, observation, or analysis.

NEW TO THIS EDITION

Once again the text has been revised in response to feedback from instructors and students, and includes new information as well as more thorough discussions and appropriate applications throughout:

- Chapter 1 has been reorganized and rewritten around the SEE principle—safety, effectiveness, and efficiency—with the focus shifted toward identifying critical elements for analysis. Students should be encouraged to think about those elements that have the greatest effect on the motion being studied.
- Chapter 14, **The Center of Gravity and Stability,** now includes information on posture in order to emphasize postural adaptations to support movement and balance. The posture section includes new explanations of anticipatory and compensatory postural adjustments.
- The chapter on fitness and exercise, Chapter 15, has been rewritten to emphasize the mechanics of strength training. Attention is given to core strengthening, upper body strengthening, and lower body strengthening, including an analysis of the back squat.
- A new discussion of wheelchair propulsion and wheelchair modification is included in Chapter 18, **Locomotion: Solid Surface.** This chapter also includes updated scholarship on obesity's effect on walking gait.
- Chapter 22, **Instrumentation for Motion Analysis,** includes new information on the sampling theorem (Nyquist sampling theorem), optoelectric systems, and electromagnetic systems
- A number of mechanical relationships have been presented in chart form in several chapters to increase student understanding of these relationships.
- References and selected readings have been updated and new evidence-based information has been integrated throughout the text. This includes new data on bone growth, spine stability, swimming research, and others.
- Updated figures, including new core exercises and sport exercises, have been added to **Appendix G.**

ANCILLARIES

Online Learning Center (www.mhhe.com/hamilton12e)

This comprehensive website offers a number of resources to students and instructors and is available free to users of the text. Features for instructors include downloadable ancillaries, such as an Instructor's Manual, sample tests, and PowerPoint presentations to accompany each chapter. Additional resources include laboratory notes to be used in conjunction with the lab experiences in the text, a sample term project, and links to online professional resources.

Student resources include a comprehensive laboratory manual that reinforces the concepts in the text.

CourseSmart eTextbooks

This text is available as an eTextbook from CourseSmart, a new way for faculty to find and review eTextbooks. It's also a great option for students who are interested in accessing their course materials digitally and saving money. CourseSmart offers thousands of the most eommonly adopted textbooks across hundreds of courses from a wide variety of higher education publishers. It is the only place for faculty to review and compare the full text of a textbook online, providing immediate access without the environmental impact of requesting a print exam copy. At CourseSmart, students can save up to 50% off the cost of a print book, reduce their impact on the environment, and gain access to powerful web tools for learning including full text search, notes and highlighting, and email tools for sharing notes between classmates. For further details contact your sales representative or go to www.coursesmart.com.

McGraw-Hill Create www.mcgrawhillcreate.com

Craft your teaching resources to match the way you teach! With McGraw-Hill Create you can easily rearrange chapters, combine material from other content sources, and quickly upload content you have written like your course syllabus or teaching notes. Find the content you need in Create by searching through thousands of leading McGraw-Hill textbooks. Arrange your book to fit your teaching style. Create even allows you to personalize your book's appearance by selecting the cover and adding your name, school, and course information. Order a Create book and you'll receive a complimentary print review copy in 3–5 business days or a complimentary electronic review copy (eComp) via email in about one hour. Go to www.mcgrawhillcreate.com today and register. Experience how McGraw-Hill Create empowers you to teach *your* students *your* way.

Anatomy & Physiology Revealed CD-ROM #1: Skeletal and Muscular System (ISBN 0-07-297299-8)

Developed by the Medical College of Ohio, this is the ultimate interactive cadaver dissection experience. This state-of-the-art tutorial uses cadaver photos combined with a layering technique that allows the student to peel away layers of the human body to reveal structures beneath the surface. *Anatomy & Physiology Revealed* offers animations, radiologic imaging, audio pronunciations, and a comprehensive quizzing tool. This tutorial is available as a stand-alone or can be combined with any of McGraw-Hill's textbooks. Contact your sales representative for more information.

ACKNOWLEDGMENTS

Our thanks to the following individuals who served as reviewers for this edition for their helpful comments and suggestions in revising the text:

Greg Farnell, University of Central Oklahoma
John C. Garner, University of Mississippi
Amy Gyorkos, Western Michigan University
Kevin McCurdy, Texas State University
Susan Muller, Salisbury University

Appreciation is also expressed to the authors and publishers who graciously gave permission to quote passages and reproduce illustrations from their publications. We also acknowledge our indebtedness to the generations of students whose stimulus has been a vital reason for the existence of this book. Finally, we are sincerely grateful to the editorial and production staffs of McGraw-Hill for their helpfulness throughout the preparation of this edition.

Nancy Hamilton, *Cedar Falls, Iowa*
Wendi Weimar, *Auburn, Alabama*
Kathryn Luttgens, *Wellesley, Massachusetts*

Preface to the First Edition—1950

This book is intended as a kinesiology text both for the teacher and for the student. It is believed that there is enough material to use it as a text for a full year's course yet, at the same time, by judicious selection of the subject matter, by omission of the supplementary material, and by the substitution of classroom demonstrations for some of the laboratory exercises, the book should serve equally well as a text for a one-semester course in kinesiology. It is left to the discretion of the instructor to select the material that meets his particular needs.

In its original form this textbook was an unpublished handbook–laboratory manual. It was used by the author in her kinesiology classes for three years before it was expanded to its present form. The original manual did not serve as an independent textbook. It was intended to be used as a companion book to a kinesiology or anatomy text. Since this limited its usefulness, however, it was decided to expand it to what is intended as a complete and independent textbook. For those who like to use a single textbook for a course it should suffice. To help the student (and the instructor) in collateral reading, most chapters in this text contain a comprehensive bibliography. In many cases there is also a list of readings which are particularly recommended. These bibliographies and reading lists provide a rich source of information for the inquiring student.

In regard to the value of laboratory exercises and projects as a means of learning, James B. Stroud, in his book *Psychology in Education,* points out that "Effectiveness of instruction is not determined so much by what the teacher does, as by what he leads the pupils to do. . . ." Again, "Perhaps one of the most successful procedures for infusing learning with significance has been the [educational method known as] constructive activities. . . . The activity is thus a means of making learning meaningful and of giving it a purpose." In accord with this point of view numerous laboratory exercises are suggested. In conformity to the same principle, only a few complete analyses of skills are presented, for it is the writer's contention that the students will gain far more from making one complete analysis himself or herself than from reading a dozen or more ready-made analyses.

As a further means of enriching the kinesiology course a number of the chapters include supplementary material in the form of brief descriptions of research projects in the field of anatomy and kinesiology. A few of these were carried out by the author, but the majority were conducted by other investigators and reported in professional journals. The purpose of including this material is to broaden the instructor's background and to provide supplementary reading assignments for advanced students.

It has been the intention of the author to write simply and to use nontechnical terminology whenever this conveyed the meaning as clearly and specifically as technical terms. The latter have been used, however, whenever they served to avoid ambiguity. While it is desirable for the kinesiology students to enlarge their scientific vocabulary, a text which confronts him with a stagering list of new and strange words defeats its purpose. Textbooks should stimulate the curiosity of their readers, not frighten them with a forbidding vocabulary.

The author acknowledges her indebtedness to many individuals without whose help it is doubtful if this book could have been written. She wishes to express her grateful appreciation particularly to Professor C. H. McCloy of the State University of Iowa for his continued guidance, encouragement, and criticism, also for his generous permission to use material from his course in The Mechanical Analysis of Motor Skills, and to the students in her kinesiology classes of the last three years who served patiently as "guinea pigs" and who made many constructive suggestions concerning the laboratory exercises.

For the illustrations, which add immeasurably to the usefulness of the text, grateful acknowledgment is made to Miss Mildred Codding, who made the anatomic drawings.

The author is under obligation to a number of individuals for the use of photographs and to several publishers for permission to reproduce copyrighted materials. To all writers and teachers from whom the author, either wittingly or unwittingly, has derived ideas which have provided the necessary background for the writing of this book she humbly acknowledges her indebtedness.

Katharine F. Wells
1950

We continue to dedicate this text to the memory of Katharine F. Wells, pioneer author and originator of the original version of this book. This twelfth edition carries on a proud contribution to the professional literature of human motion study started by Dr. Wells in 1950, and continued with her active participation through the seventh edition. Although much of the content of the current text has changed since that first edition, there remains a significant heritage that can be traced back to her original work. Through her influence, she helped define and structure the teaching and study of kinesiology for many generations of students. The authors of this twelfth edition are honored to be the current stewards for this classic text.

CHAPTER 1

Introduction to the Study of Kinesiology

OUTLINE

- ***The Nature of Kinesiology***
  - The SEE Principle
  - Methods of Study
- ***Components of a Kinesiological Analysis***
  - Description of the Motor Skill
  - Anatomical Analysis
  - Mechanical Analysis
  - Prescription for Improvement of Performance
- ***Laboratory Experiences***

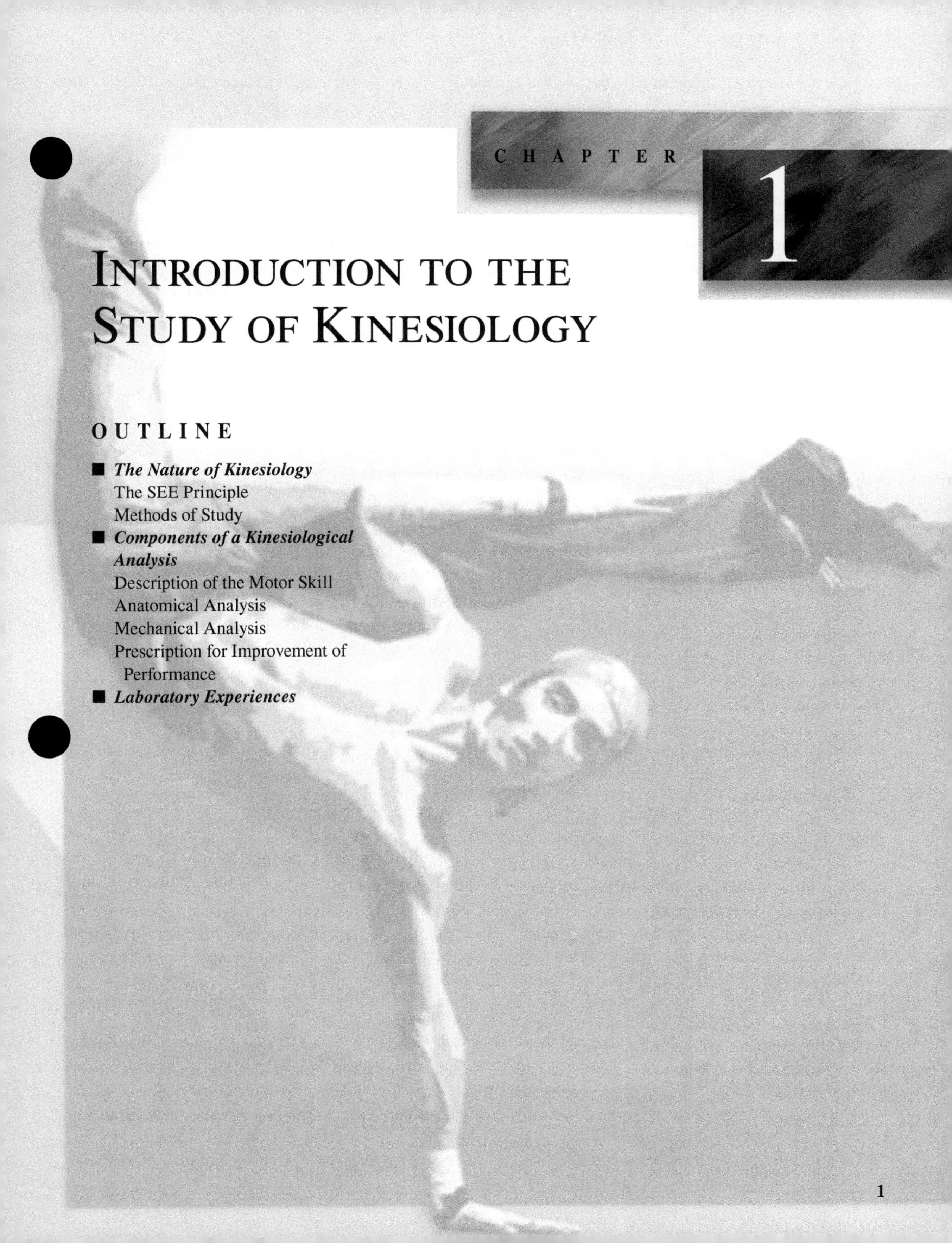

OBJECTIVES

At the conclusion of this chapter, the student should be able to:

1. Define *kinesiology* and explain its importance to the student of human motion.
2. Describe the major components of a kinesiological analysis.
3. Prepare a description of a selected motor skill, breaking it down into component phases and identifying starting and ending points.
4. Determine the simultaneous-sequential nature of a variety of movement skills.
5. Classify motor skills using the classification system presented.
6. State the mechanical purpose of a variety of movement skills.

THE NATURE OF KINESIOLOGY

Kinesiology, as it is known in physical education, athletic training, physical therapy, orthopedics, and physical medicine, is the study of human movement from the point of view of the physical sciences. The study of the human body as a machine for the performance of work has its foundations in three major areas of study—namely, mechanics, anatomy, and physiology; more specifically, biomechanics, musculoskeletal anatomy, and neuromuscular physiology. The accumulated knowledge of these three fields forms the foundation for the study of human movement.

Some authorities refer to kinesiology as a science in its own right; others claim that it should be called a study rather than a true science because the principles on which it is based are derived from basic sciences such as anatomy, physiology, and physics. In any event, its unique contribution is that it selects from many sciences those principles that are pertinent to human motion and systematizes their application. However it may be categorized, to the inquiring student it is a door opening into a whole new world of discovery and appreciation. Human motion, which most of us have taken for granted all our lives, is seen through new eyes. One who gives it any thought whatever cannot help being impressed not only by the beauty of human motion but also by its apparently infinite possibilities, its meaningfulness, its orderliness, its adaptability to the surrounding environment. Nothing is haphazard; nothing is left to chance. Every structure that participates in the movements of the body does so according to physical and physiological principles. The student of kinesiology, like the student of anatomy, physiology, psychology, genetics, and other biological sciences, can only look with wonder at the intricate mechanism of the body.

The SEE Principle

Kinesiology is not studied merely to incite our interest in a fascinating and mysterious subject. It has a useful purpose. We study kinesiology to improve performance by learning how to analyze the movements of the human body and to discover their underlying principles. The study of kinesiology is an essential part of the educational experience of students of physical education, dance, sport, and physical medicine. Knowledge of kinesiology has a threefold purpose for practitioners in any of these fields. It should enable them to help their students or clients perform with optimum *safety, effectiveness,* and *efficiency* (*SEE*). Safety is becoming a greater concern of all movement professionals. It is imperative to structure the movements of students or clients to avoid doing harm to the body. At the same time, both the educator and the therapist set goals for effective performance. We judge the effectiveness of a performance by success or failure in meeting those goals. And in producing an effective performance, the movement specialist also strives with the student or client to achieve the movement goal with the least amount of effort, as efficiently as possible. *Safety, effectiveness,* and *efficiency,* then, are the underlying aims in all of our uses of kinesiology for the analysis and modification of human movement.

Kinesiology helps prepare physical educators, coaches, and fitness professionals to teach effective performance in both fundamental and specialized motor skills. Furthermore, it enables them to evaluate exercises and activities from the point of view of their effect on the human structure. The human body improves with use (within limits), *provided it is used in accordance with the principles of efficient human motion*. The function of kinesiology in physical education, therefore, is to contribute not only to *successful participation* in various physical activities but also to the *improvement* of the human structure through the intelligent selection of activities and the efficient use of the body.

The physical or occupational therapist and the athletic trainer are primarily concerned with the effect that exercises and other techniques of physical medicine have on the body. He or she is concerned particularly with the restoration of impaired function and with methods of compensating for lost function. Although effective performance remains a primary goal, to the therapist "effective performance" refers not so much to *skillful* performance in athletic activities as to *adequate* performance in the activities associated with daily living. Whereas the educator applies knowledge of kinesiology chiefly to the movements of the normal body, the therapist is concerned with the movements of a body that has suffered an impairment in function.

Methods of Study

Once the study of kinesiology is begun, one of the most satisfactory ways of proceeding is by supplementing book study with laboratory experimentation. It is a truism that we learn best by doing. Laboratory experiences should include two types of activity. The first type consists of experiments performed under controlled conditions. Activities in this category are selected to help the student gain insight into and understand the nature and complexity of human motion. Although the emphasis is primarily on qualitative analysis in beginning study, some quantification of data is appropriate, as is the use of "laboratory type" instruments. Especially helpful is the video recorder, whose use enables the careful and prolonged study of a very small moment in the performance of a technique and permits the observation of detail unavailable to the naked eye. In more advanced study, the use of advanced measurement methodology and more advanced electronic equipment such as electromyography, force-sensing instruments, and computer simulation are common. As these technologies become more sophisticated, so does our ability to use them to increase the depth of our knowledge and understanding of human motion.

The second type of laboratory experience should consist of practice in analysis under the conditions that exist every day in the gymnasium or clinic. Only through practice under these conditions will the student learn how to apply a knowledge of kinesiology and develop the qualitative skills necessary for accurate observation, diagnosis, and treatment of faulty motor performance.

Whatever method of teaching or study is employed, the student should keep in mind the aims of kinesiology study and the intended applications for what will be learned. The analysis of motion is not an end in itself but rather a means of learning new movement patterns and improving the safety, effectiveness, and efficiency of old ones. This is as true for the physical therapist teaching amputees and paraplegics to walk again as it is for the physical educator teaching a sport technique. Finally, it must be remembered that the skill itself is of less importance than the one who practices it. Kinesiology serves only half its purpose when it provides information of value for learning or teaching motor skills. It must also serve to lay the foundation for perfecting, repairing, and keeping in good condition that incomparable mechanism—the human body.

Components of a Kinesiological Analysis

In any formal field of study, the task of analysis must proceed along a logical and structured plan. This plan must be constructed so that it is both appropriate to the activity and can be readily applied by the practitioner. The teacher, therapist, trainer, athlete, and coach all benefit from knowing how to conduct a kinesiological analysis of a motor skill. The teaching of motor skills, whether it takes place in the clinic, in the fitness facility, or on the playing field, consists of presenting a skill and knowing what points to emphasize. It also largely consists of diagnosing difficulties, correcting errors, and eliminating actions that limit performance. The specialist in motor skills must also be aware of the types of injuries that are likely to occur during a particular activity and how to prevent them. To accurately prescribe the movements necessary for rehabilitation, the therapist or trainer must know joint structure and exercise tolerances. An athlete in training must understand the kinesiological factors involved in performance to optimize training effects while guarding against deleterious actions. These tasks that, on the surface, may seem simple can indeed be quite complex, if for no other reason than that motor skills themselves are complex. An effective aid in helping one understand the basic elements and requirements of a motor skill is a systematic kinesiological analysis.

The tools needed for the execution of a detailed kinesiological analysis are introduced in subsequent chapters. The anatomical components of human movements—the bones, joints, muscles, and related portions of the nervous system—and the mechanical bases for human motion are presented. The basic movements of the body segments are described, and it is shown how the observation of both anatomical and mechanical principles contributes to the efficient use of the body in the performance of motor skills. A kinesiological analysis is the application of this information to assessing the effectiveness of a given motor performance. It consists of

1. *describing* a skill in a logical and systematic fashion by breaking it down into its constituent elements;
2. *evaluating* the performance of the skill by determining whether and how the related anatomical and mechanical principles have been violated; and
3. *prescribing* corrections based on an appropriate identification of the cause or causes.

The basic components for the kinesiological analysis of a motor skill are outlined in Table 1.1. In this type of analysis the emphasis is on a qualitative assessment of the performance, which may be conducted with the assistance of videotapes, digital images, or the naked eye. In any case, the analyst must use a systematic approach in the observation of the performance. Have someone demonstrate the movement to be analyzed both before and at frequent intervals throughout the analysis. In lieu of this, a video or digital recording is an excellent substitute. If this is not available, a series of still shots or even a single photograph or sketch is helpful. In the initial stages of learning analysis procedures, movement may appear rapid and confusing. With the aid of recording equipment and with much practice, the analyst will gain the skills required for an accurate and systematic approach to observation.

Description of the Motor Skill

The description of the motor skill being analyzed consists of four elements that together help the analyst focus on the essential nature of the skill.

Primary Purpose of a Motor Skill

The first step in the description phase of the analysis is to identify the primary purpose of the movement. Without a clear understanding of why the movement is being performed, it is

TABLE 1.1 Outline for a Kinesiological Analysis

A. Description of the motor skill performance
   1. Primary purpose of the skill
   2. Movement phases
   3. Classification of the skill
   4. Simultaneous-sequential nature of the motion
B. Anatomical analysis
   1. Joint actions and segment motions
   2. Muscle participation and form of contraction
   3. Neuromuscular considerations
   4. Anatomical principles related to effective and safe performance
C. Mechanical analysis
   1. Underlying mechanics objective(s)
   2. Nature of forces causing or impeding motion
   3. Identify the critical elements
   4. Mechanical principles that apply concerning
      a. safety
      b. effectiveness
      c. efficiency
   5. Identification of errors
      a. What are the errors?
      b. What are the sources of error?
D. Prescriptions for improvement of performance indicate how the performance should be changed so that the principles are no longer violated.

virtually impossible to evaluate its effectiveness. In this statement of purpose, applicable references to speed, accuracy, form, and distance should be included. For example, the purpose of the 50-meter backstroke is to cover the course in the shortest amount of time. Speed is a major factor. The purpose of swinging an ax is to split a piece of wood. Both speed and accuracy are critical elements if the wood is to be safely split into kindling. The purpose of the springboard dive is to execute the motion according to a prescribed form. Neither speed nor accuracy is stressed; success is measured on appearance alone. The purpose of putting in golf is to sink the ball into the cup from a relatively short distance away. The prime determinant of success in putting is accuracy (Figure 1.1).

Movement Phases

It is often beneficial to break down a motion into separate parts, or "phases." Often these phases are fairly obvious, based on the motion. For example, a throw has a windup phase, a throwing phase where the arm comes forward, and a follow-through phase after release (Figure 1.2). In some skills, the phases are not as obvious; but to make the analysis manageable, some sort of division should be made.

It is critical that the appropriate starting and ending points for each phase be identified. Two primary factors must be considered in the choice of starting point. The first factor is to consider *when* in the motion the analysis should begin. Many movement skills are discrete; that is, they have a very definite beginning and ending. In such movements the starting point for analysis is fairly obvious—at the beginning of the first phase—as in a throwing skill, which starts with the windup. Other skills are more continuous in nature, either because they are done in a repetitive manner or because one movement flows immediately into the next. Walking is a good example of a cyclical skill, whereas many team sports include movements that change constantly. In a continuous movement situation, the analyst must carefully choose a starting point that will give adequate information about the movement of interest while not ignoring the resultant effects of the previous movement. In walking, many analysts start the first phase of the analysis as the toe leaves the ground and end the last phase when that same toe is about to leave the ground in the next step cycle; others start the phase as the heel strikes the floor and end with the subsequent heel strike.

Classification of the Motor Skills

Motor skills take many forms and are used for many purposes. The therapist is interested in

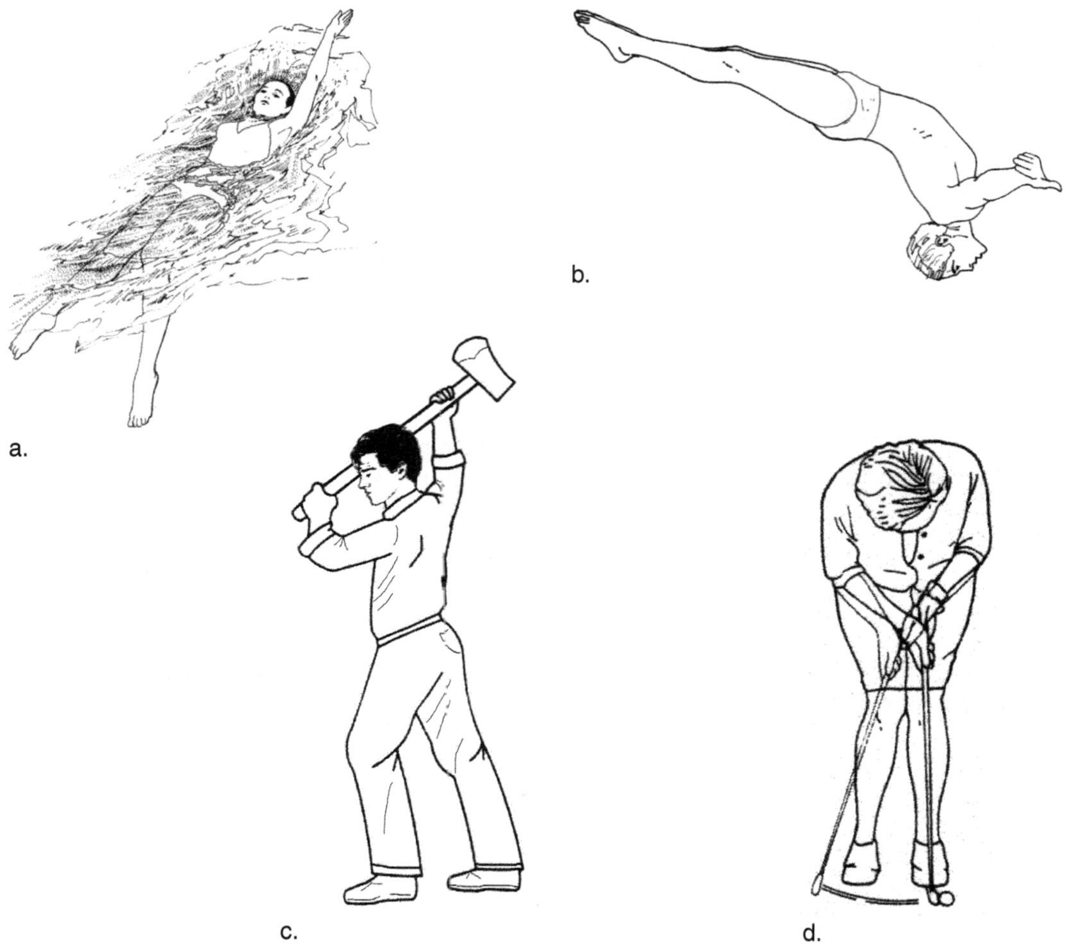

Figure 1.1 Examples of the primary purpose of a motion: (a) maximum speed; (b) following a prescribed pattern; (c) optimum speed and accuracy; (d) maximum accuracy.

using physical skills and exercise to rehabilitate individuals for independent living or work; the teacher uses motor skills for health, learning, and play; the athlete and coach strive to produce near-perfect performance. Each practitioner requires an understanding of the body and mechanical laws that govern motion. A classification scheme is important because it permits the variety of potential movement skills to be organized into a manageable grouping. This manner of organization facilitates the recognition of commonalities across movements. It also fosters increased understanding by enabling one to focus on either differences or similarities in movement patterns, as the situation demands. Classification of movement patterns and skills provides further clues as to the nature of both the anatomical and mechanical requirements of a particular group of skills.

The following system for classifying motor skills takes into account the objective of the skill, the medium in which the skill occurs, and the nature of the motion.

Classification of Motor Skill Patterns

I. Maintaining erect posture
II. Movement for exercise and fitness

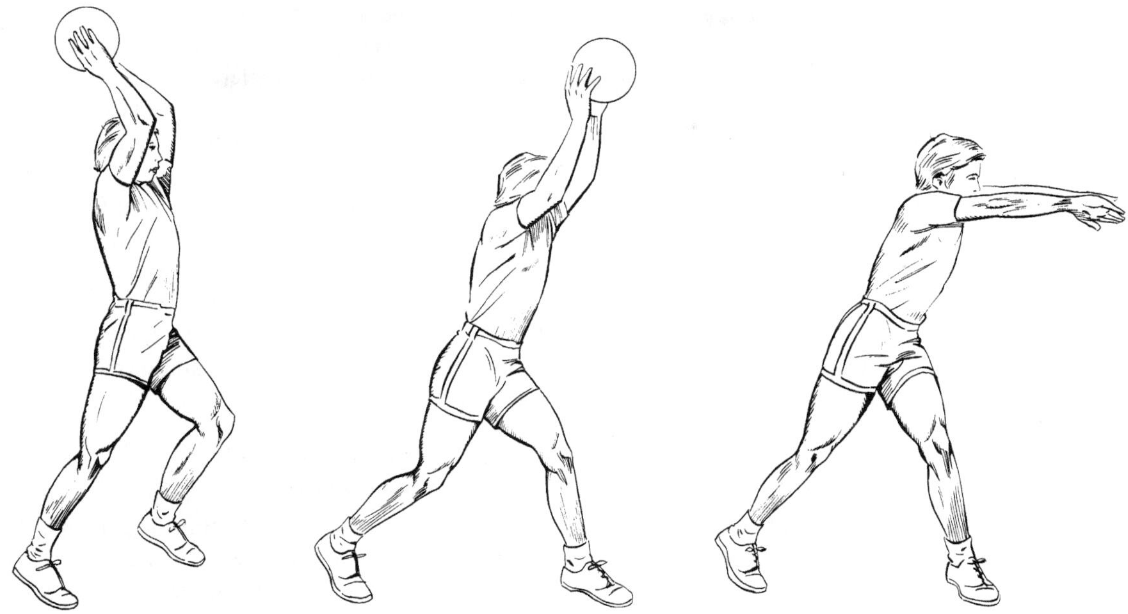

Figure 1.2 The soccer throw-in can be divided into three phases: (a) windup (preparatory) phase; (b) throwing (propulsion) phase; (c) follow-through phase.

III. Giving motion
    A. To external objects
        1. Pushing and pulling
            a. Lifting and carrying
            b. Punching
        2. Throwing, striking, and kicking
    B. To one's own body
        1. Supported by the ground or other resistant surface
            a. Locomotion on foot
            b. Locomotion on wheels, blades, and runners
            c. Rotary locomotion
        2. Suspended and free of support
            a. Swinging activities on trapeze, flying rings, or similar equipment
            b. Hand traveling on traveling rings or horizontal ladder
            c. Unsupported (i.e., projected into or falling through the air)
            d. Weightlessness
        3. Supported by water
            a. Swimming
            b. Aquatic stunts
            c. Boating
IV. Receiving impact
    A. From one's own body in landing from a jump or fall
    B. From external objects in catching, trapping, spotting, or intercepting

The four major headings in this outline are maintaining erect posture, movement for exercise and fitness, giving motion, and receiving impact. Some may question the reason for treating the maintenance of erect posture as a major category instead of including it under giving motion to one's own body. The rationale for this decision is that the emphasis here is on adjusting to the immediate environment rather than on making a movement in the sense that one usually interprets this concept. With one exception, the adjustments are made from a stationary position, the exception being a shift in stance necessitated by standing on a moving base. This action does not involve moving from one place to another but only widening the stance and facing in a different direction to maintain balance. The erect posture then becomes the foundation and starting point for subsequent dynamic postures and motions.

The initial step in the classification of movement is to determine in which major category the skill belongs, and then in which secondary, and possibly tertiary, category. A forehand drive in tennis, for instance, belongs in the primary category of giving motion to an external object and in the secondary one of striking. Turning a cartwheel is a form of giving motion to one's own body while it is supported by the ground and is classified further as rotary locomotion.

In addition to pinpointing the exact categories to which the skill belongs, a number of other factors should be considered. Many skills consist of a series of phases that cut across different categories, and these must be considered separately. The tennis serve, like the forehand drive, is a form of striking; but it also involves tossing the ball, a push pattern skill that should not be overlooked. Vaults over a gymnasium box or horse consist of the approach, the placement of the hands, the momentary support by the hands, and the push-off from the box. This phase is followed by the projection of the body, together with the necessary adjustments of the bodily segments, and finally by the landing, which involves movements of the upper extremities and trunk as well as of the lower extremities. In pole vaulting and rock climbing, there is a smooth transition from pulling to pushing. In hurdling, repeated alternation occurs between the run and the hurdles without any break in rhythm. In many basketball shots for the basket, the shot is accompanied by a jump. All phases of the skill should be included in the analysis.

In many skills, especially those involving either the giving or the receiving of a force of appreciable magnitude, the ability to maintain balance is an all-important feature. Maintaining balance effectively means observing the principles of balance and posture adjustment as well as those relating to the specific form of giving motion or receiving impact. Lifting a heavy weight from the floor or down from a shelf is a good example of a motion-giving activity whose effectiveness depends largely on the maintenance of a posture that favors lifting.

The standing long jump shown in Figure 1.3 is a skill that belongs in the major category of giving motion to one's own body. The initial phases before the takeoff, landing, and recovery phases belong in the secondary category of movement on a solid base, whereas the flight phase is an activity of the unsupported category.

Simultaneous-Sequential Nature of the Motion

Because it is comprised of joints and levers, the body can move in a wonderful variety of ways. To simplify the complexities of such a wide range of possibilities, it is important to understand that when motions are combined, bodily movements may be classified as occurring on a continuum ranging from the *simultaneous* to the *sequential* use of the body segments. The simultaneous use of the body segments, where the various segments move as one, is exemplified by motions such as pushing, pulling, or lifting objects. In a simultaneous movement pattern, all of the movement is directed along a straight line. Simultaneous use of body segments is the only way it is anatomically possible to move the hand or foot in a straight line. This straight-line application of force by the hand or foot is the most advantageous method to use when overcoming heavy or large objects or external forces such as those encountered in pushing file cabinets and lifting weights. In addition, when accuracy is important, such as in putting in golf, lunging in fencing (movement of the arm and weapon), and punching, it is more effective to involve the segments in a simultaneous fashion.

When it is important to have maximum speed at impact or release, a sequential use of the body segments is appropriate. The use of the segments in an orderly sequence so that subsequent segments are accelerated at the appropriate time

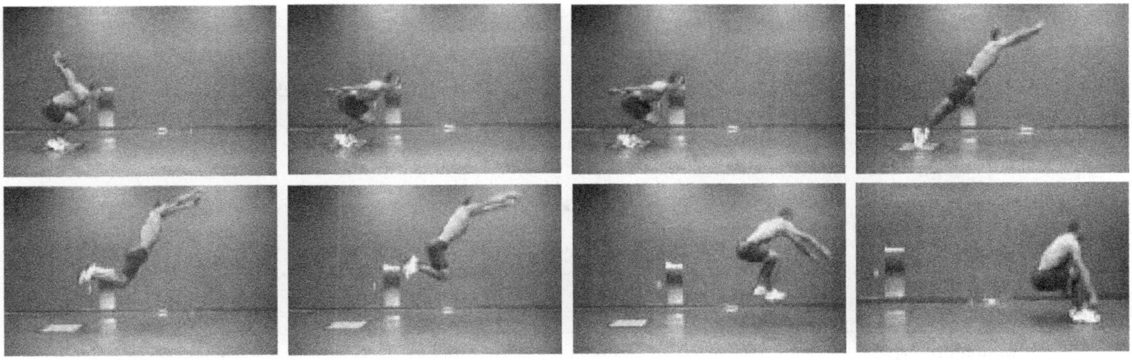

a.

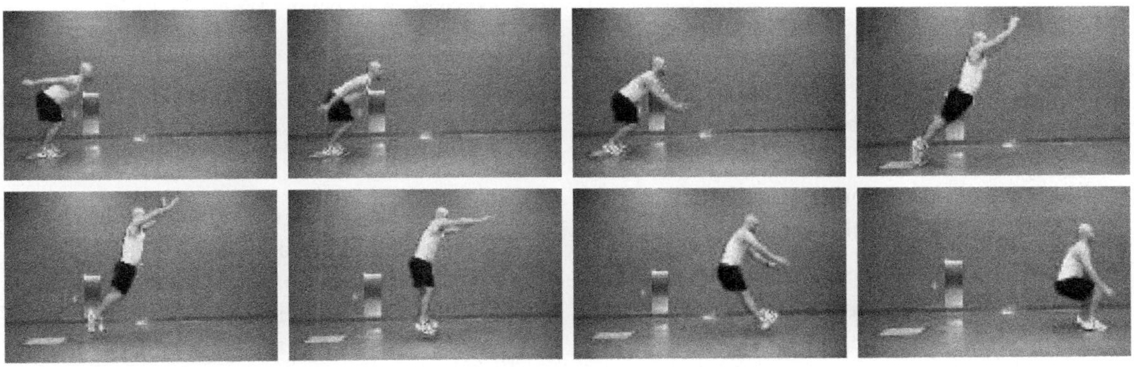

b.

Figure 1.3 Standing long jump: (a) better technique; (b) poorer technique.

to create the highest possible speed is critical in activities exemplified by throwing, striking movements such as batting or the golf drive, and kicking. Sequential movements produce forces applied so that the final segment moves along a curved path. The farther this curved path is from the center of the motion, the greater will be the speed of the throwing, striking, or kicking segment.

Motions may occur anywhere along this simultaneous-sequential continuum, or they may combine the two basic forms (Figure 1.4). The skill of putting the shot, for example, involves the sequential use of the lower extremities and trunk followed by the simultaneous use of the upper extremity to safely move the relatively large weight of the shot. For our purposes, simultaneous motions and those combination motions that occur at the simultaneous end of the continuum are classified as push-pull motions, and those at the other end, the sequential end, are classified as throwing, striking, and kicking patterns.

To clarify the nature of the motion at any given point in the performance, it is desirable to break down the total movement into phases for analysis. Using the standing long jump (see Figure 1.3) as an example, an analysis of the nature of the motion might be as follows:

1. Preparatory phase—simultaneous motion of the joints of the lower extremity, into a semi-squat position
2. Execution (force) phase—simultaneous extension of the segments in a forward-upward direction

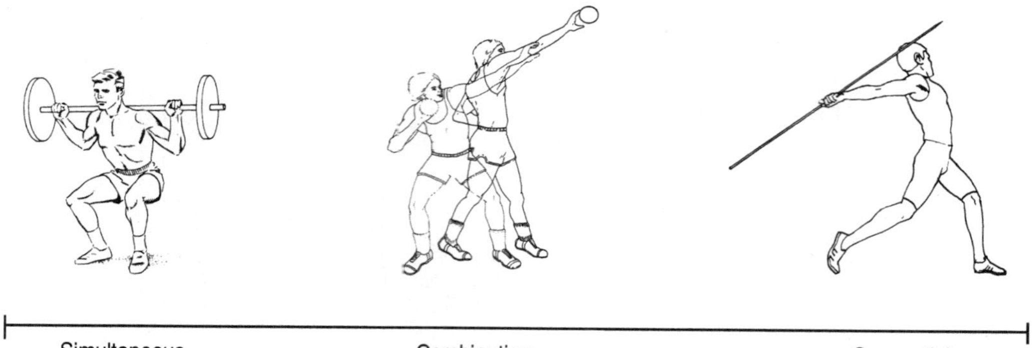

Figure 1.4 Examples of skills on the simultaneous to sequential continuum.

3. Flight (unsupported) phase—sequential motion of the lower body to "whip" the legs forward
4. Landing phase—simultaneous flexion of the lower extremity to take up the shock of the landing forces

Having now described the motor skill by clarifying the primary purpose, classifying the skill, and establishing the simultaneous-sequential nature of the skill, *analysis* of the performance is the next, and critical, step. In evaluating the motion from the starting point, the analyst must then consider to what extent the performer conforms to the anatomical and mechanical requirements necessary to achieve the stated purpose of the motion. Failure to perform in accordance with the principles that govern motion will produce a less than optimal performance. For this reason, the analyst should be conversant with the anatomical and mechanical principles that are critical for the movement skill in question.

Anatomical Analysis

The anatomical analysis of a movement should include an examination of the skeletal joint action, a description of segment motion, an account of the muscle participation, and an identification of the neuromuscular mechanisms involved. Anatomical analysis involves analysis of a process rather than a product. That is, it is a review of how the body accomplishes the task rather than an in-depth examination of the results. It should attempt to give specific answers to the following questions:

1. Which joints are involved, and what are their exact movements in the motor skill?

   For each phase of the technique and for each joint participating in the phase, the precise joint action and segment being moved should be identified and recorded, as was done for the sample analysis of the force phase of the standing long jump shown in Table 1.2.
2. Are any of the joints used to the limit of their range of motion?
3. Which muscles are responsible for the joint actions, and what is the nature of their contraction?

   The muscular action is identified for each joint movement and recorded next to the joint actions in Table 1.2. This implies identifying not only the muscles that are contracting but also their precise function in the movement and the kind of contraction they are undergoing. Identification of the force causing the motion facilitates the subsequent identification of the muscle and type of contraction involved.
4. Which neuromuscular mechanisms are likely to help or hinder the action, and what is the nature of their involvement?

TABLE 1.2 Chart for Anatomical Analysis of a Motor Skill

Skill being analyzed: Standing long jump (see Figure 1.3)
Phase being analyzed: Force phase

Name of Joint	Starting Position	Observed Joint Action	Segment Being Moved	Force for Movement	Main Muscle Groups Active	Kind of Contraction
Metatarso-phalangeal	Extended	Hyperextension/flexion	Foot	Muscle	Extensors/flexors	Concentric
Ankle	Dorsiflexed	Plantar flexion	Lower leg	Muscle	Plantar flexors	Concentric
Knee	Flexed	Extension	Thighs	Muscle	Extensors	Concentric
Hip	Flexed	Extension	Pelvis	Muscle	Extensors	Concentric
Pelvis	Decreased tilt	Increased tilt	Trunk	Muscle	Spinal extensors	Concentric
Lumbar spine	Flexion	Extension	Trunk	Muscle	Spinal extensors	Concentric
Thoracic spine	Slight flexion	Extension	Trunk	Muscle	Spinal extensors	Concentric
Cervical spine	Hyperextended	Flexion	Neck	Muscle	Spinal flexors	Concentric
Shoulder girdle	Upward tilt	Upward rotation, abduction	Shoulder girdle	Muscle	Upward rotators	Concentric
					Abductors	Concentric
Shoulder joint	Hyperextension,	Flexion	Upper extremity	Muscle	Flexors	Concentric
	medial rotation	—	—	—	—	—
Elbow	Extended	—	—	—	Extensors	Static
Radioulnar	Pronated	—	—	—	—	—
Wrist	Extended	—	—	—	Extensors	Static
Phalanges	Extended	—	—	—	Extensors	Static

Source: Patterned after format presented in *Kinesiology and Applied Anatomy* (6th ed., pp. 339–347), by P. I. Rasch & R. K. Burke. Copyright © 1978 Lea & Febiger, Malvern, PA. Reprinted by permission. This form for recording an anatomical analysis may be reproduced for class use without specific permission.

The muscle-response patterns of well-learned motor skills involve the integrated action of many reflexes and the inhibition of others. After repeated viewing of the performance "live" or on a recording, the student should name and discuss the reflexes that could be acting at various points in each phase.

5. Which anatomical principles contribute to maximal efficiency and accuracy in the performance of the motor skill?
6. Which principles are directly related to the avoidance of injury?

   In any analysis, a set of anatomical principles governing the safe and effective performance of the movement skill must be considered. These principles take into account the structure and function of the human body, human tolerance of both internal and external stresses, and the efficiency of movement patterns. Hudson (1995) has also suggested that it is critical to examine such core concepts as range of motion, the number of body parts involved, the nature of the body parts involved, and the coordination of the movement. In addition, it is important to look at the alignment of the body and the reflexes that might be utilized. Anatomical principles of motion then stipulate the way in which each of these core concepts apply to a specific movement. In particular, anatomical principles speak to the qualities associated with each of these concepts.

Mechanical Analysis

In performing a mechanical analysis of a motor skill, the human body is often viewed as a "machine," subject to the same laws and mechanical principles that govern the actions of any other machine. The mechanical analysis of human performance involves the identification of laws and principles that help explain the most appropriate form for the execution of the activity and identify the mechanical reasons for success or failure. To assess the mechanical nature of a technique and use this information in helping performers choose movements that will result in skillful motion, the analyzer should attempt to identify those principles and laws that verify the actions as desirable. Once the movement is classified according to an outline such as that on pages 6–7, the analyst should determine exactly how and when the movements of the performance do or do not satisfy the standards of good performance as explained by the laws and principles of mechanics. Once this process is accomplished, a greater depth of understanding of the skill is achieved, and the basis for making change is founded on sound knowledge and understanding of the reasons "why."

Underlying Mechanics Objective

To explain the mechanical factors that contribute most to performance, it is first necessary to define clearly the purpose or objective of the motion involved. The focus of the statement of mechanical objective will be on the desired outcome of the motion, which is necessary to measure effectiveness. Several systems have been proposed for the classification of mechanical objectives of human movement. A synthesis of many of those systems is presented here as a simplified set of objectives.

The underlying objective of a motion may be

1. Balance
   a. Regain stability
   b. Attain mobility
2. Locomotion
   a. Travel from point to point
   b. Travel a prescribed distance
   c. Travel a prescribed pattern
3. Projection
   a. For maximum height
   b. For maximum range
   c. For maximum accuracy
   d. For optimum speed and accuracy
4. Manipulation
   a. Of objects
   b. To reproduce a pattern
   c. Of a resistance

5. Maximum effort
   a. Maximum speed
   b. Maximum power
   c. Maximum force

Each of these underlying mechanical objectives requires consideration of different but overlapping sets of mechanical factors. The standing long jump, for instance, has the underlying mechanical objective of projection of the body for maximum range (distance). The question now becomes one of determining what must be done in mechanical terms to produce the maximum distance. Because the distance traveled is in the air, the body becomes a projectile, and those factors that cause the projectile to travel the farthest are those that must be considered.

Nature of the Forces Causing or Impeding Motion

To accurately analyze the efficiency with which a motor skill is performed, the analyst must be aware of the kind of motion being performed (classification and simultaneous-sequential nature) and the forces that are acting to cause, modify, or prevent that motion. Pushing and pulling forces, weight and resistance, and twisting and turning forces must all be identified and their effects noted. Muscle force applied through the joints' range of motion to propel the body through the air for maximum distance is a force-causing motion. A force-resisting motion is the resistance force offered by the weight of the jumper. Impact with the ground at the end of the jump will produce a force-stopping motion. Other impeding forces might be produced by lack of strength or limited range of motion.

Identification of Critical Elements

Knowing what to examine and what to measure is an important part of any kinesiological analysis. In every motor skill, there is a set of *critical elements.* The elements of the movement that contribute most to safety, effectiveness, and efficiency need to be identified so that appropriate attention may be given to them. The critical elements of a motor skill are very dependent upon the mechanical purpose of the motion. As an example, in the overhand throw the mechanical purpose may be projection for maximum distance. The initial critical element, therefore, would be the velocity of the ball at release. As we learn later in this text, velocity includes both the speed of the ball at release and the angle at which it is thrown. These two factors determine where the ball goes. Once this primary critical element has been identified, the analyst must then determine what is critical in developing this primary element. In the throw example, we should recognize that the push off the ground, the rotation of the left hip, the speed of arm motion, the range of motion used, and the adequate transfer of momentum are all critical elements of the performance.

Mechanical Principles

Identification of the mechanical principles related to the execution of the skill is the next step in establishing causes of error in the performance of the skill. Safety, effectiveness, and efficiency should be dealt with at this point. It is important that the student recognize how the application of forces affects each aspect of the SEE principle. Which forces are likely to produce injury if applied incorrectly? How much or how little force in what direction will produce the desired result? What must be done to ensure that there is no wasted motion?

The critical elements identified in the previous step will help determine the mechanical principles that apply to a given motor skill. In fact, critical elements and mechanical principles are highly interdependent and should be examined together. Focusing on these principles and how they relate to the skill suggests the potential sources of error. Each movement phase must be considered in turn. The core concepts from which these principles are derived include considerations of the speed of the movement, the forces involved in the movement, balance, direction, and timing, and the pressure of air or water. If the motion involves projecting something into the air, the concepts of extension at release (or contact), path of the object, and spin must also be considered. Once again, the primary concern is the quality of each of these factors that is required for an optimum performance. In deriving mechanical principles, one might discuss how much speed or how much force, as well as the direction of the force. It might become important to know how much air pressure is acting or what angle produces the best path of a thrown object.

Identification of Errors

Diagnosing the cause of an error is difficult because the cause may be far removed from the observed effect. The purpose in identifying the mechanical principles is to locate potential sources for error. Given the purpose of the skill, which of the principles, if violated, has the greatest potential for limiting performance? How? These are the most troublesome questions to answer. Without quantitative data, it is difficult to make any selection with certainty. And even with the support of such data, which indeed can provide us with much useful information, we still cannot be certain. At this time, no general method is available to identify and establish the order of importance for those factors that limit performance. One must rely primarily on knowledge of the technique and the principles of mechanics that apply.

As a general rule, it is probably most beneficial to start seeking sources of error at that point where the initial force is applied. In most movements on land, this point is where the feet are in contact with the ground. To produce a motion, it is usually necessary to push against the ground. This initial push contributes greatly to the force developed in the motion. It is wise to focus the attention here first rather than at the end point of the sum total of all the segmental movements that are taking place.

Again, using the example of the standing long jump, we know that *speed* and *direction* are the two most important factors in performance. The direction is governed by the direction of the jumper's takeoff. It appears, then, that this takeoff might be the best place to start. The speed and direction of the jump depend on the speed, force, and direction of the push against the ground. The faster the legs can move, the greater will be the push off the ground.

Prescription for Improvement of Performance

After the performance has been described in anatomical and mechanical detail and the causes for error have been identified, the analyst must decide on the appropriate strategy for effecting change in the performance so that it conforms to the anatomical and mechanical ideal. Now the analyst becomes an instructor who must decide not only what must be done, but how best to communicate that information to the performer in a manner that makes sense. The task is like that of a physician who uses vast medical knowledge to prescribe bed rest as the best cure for an ailment. The cure may be simple, but the complexities attached to knowing what to do, and why, and then making that information understandable to the patient are far from simple. The instructor of motor skills needs to develop ability as a prescriber as well as an analyst. Both talents will improve with practice. As more systematic analyses are performed, the analyst becomes aware of characteristics common to groups of skills. Common errors and their causes will emerge for related skills as well as similar or common prescriptions appropriate for correcting the errors. The important thing to remember is to concentrate on the causes of errors, not on the resultant symptoms. Before the physician can prescribe for a limping gait, the cause must be known and the viable options for treatment identified. Before an instructor of motor skills can prescribe for improvement of a standing long jump or any other motor performance, the cause(s) for the error must be known and the valid options for correction determined.

References and Selected Readings

Clarys, J. P., and Alewaeters, K. (2003). Science and sports: A brief history of muscle, motion and ad hoc organizations. *Journal of Sports Sciences,* 21(9), 669–677.

Elliott, B. (1999). Biomechanics: An integral part of sport science and sport medicine. *Journal of Science and Medicine in Sport,* 2(4), 299–310.

Hudson, J. L. (1995). Core concepts in kinesiology. *Journal of Physical Education, Recreation and Dance,* 66(5), 54–56.

Hughes, M. D., & Bartlett, R. M. (2002). The use of performance indicators in performance analysis. *Journal of Sports Sciences,* 20(10), 739–754.

Knudson, D. (2007). Qualitative biomechanical principles for application in coaching. *Sports Biomechanics,* 6(1), 109–118.

Lees, A. (2002). Technique analysis in sports: A critical review. *Journal of Sports Sciences,* 20(10), 813–828.

Laboratory Experiences

1. Select three motor skills from different sections of Appendix G. Identify the underlying mechanics objective for each skill, and classify each according to the outline for classification of motor skills.
2. Using a simple skill of the student's choosing, prepare a qualitative description of a motor skill. Include a statement of purpose, nature of the motion, and a description of how the motion is broken into phases.
3. Using the skill from Experience 2, utilize observation to identify the joints and basic muscle groups involved in the motion.

PART

I

Anatomical and Physiological Fundamentals of Human Motion

Introduction to Part I

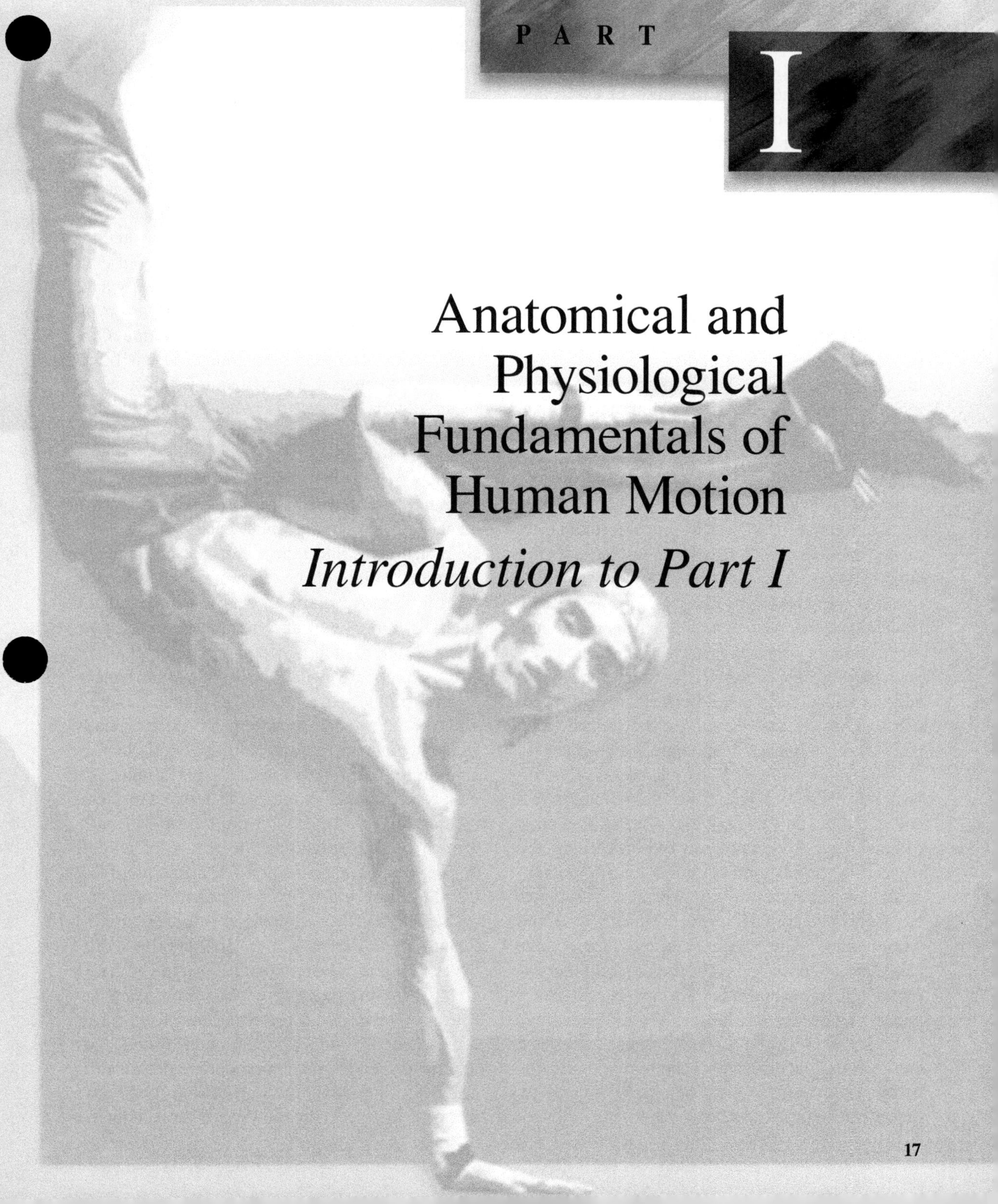

Where does anatomy end and biomechanics begin? In truth, there is no answer because the question itself is not valid. One might as well ask, "Where does the study of words end and the writing of compositions (or articles, or books) begin?" or "Where does the study of building materials end and the designing and erecting of buildings begin?" Just as words are the elements used in all writing, whether creative, factual, or expository, and just as bricks, wood, cement, metal, and glass are some of the elements used in building, so bones, joints, muscles, connective tissue, blood vessels, and nerves are the vital elements of human motion. They are the essential elements used in batting a baseball, passing and carrying a football, shooting a basketball into the basket—in fact, in all running, walking, jumping, throwing, striking, catching, and swimming; likewise, one finds them in keyboarding, manual labor, painting, sewing, knitting, and so forth, almost without end.

One aim of Part I is to prepare students of human motion, whether they are in physical education, athletic training, physical therapy, occupational therapy, exercise science, or other related professions, to systematically analyze human movements in terms of muscles, joints, and nervous system integration and to apply the knowledge provided to improve performance in motor skills. This section should not be looked upon merely as a review of anatomy but as the very foundation for analysis of human motion. It demonstrates the close relationships between anatomical structure and function, and it provides a body of knowledge that can be utilized in learning and perfecting various motor skills. It aims to demonstrate how the bones, joints, and muscles serve as elements in anatomical levers, which act in accord with the laws of mechanics. It also strives to make clear the influences of gravitational and other external forces on muscular actions. For instance, under certain circumstances, these forces may cause an action to be the exact opposite of what one would expect in view of the movement that is being performed. It should be obvious, therefore, that memorizing the actions of muscles will not prepare the student to make accurate analyses. Rather, a true understanding of all the conditions that influence the functions of the muscles is necessary.

Part I contains eight chapters—two on the musculoskeletal system and its movements, one on the neuromuscular aspects of motion, and five on the anatomy and fundamental movements of specific segments of the body. The order in which these chapters are studied is entirely optional. Students who use this text may differ widely in their educational backgrounds. Some may already have completed courses in anatomy, possibly even including the experience of human dissection. Others may have had only brief courses and will feel the need to receive more detailed information. In an attempt to meet the needs of all students, whatever their backgrounds, in Part I we have presented fairly complete coverage of the aspects of anatomy that relate to movement and, at the same time, have omitted details whose relation to movement seem less significant. Hence, specific muscle attachments and innervation are not included in the main body of the text but may be found in chart form in Appendix C. On the other hand, the muscle's line of pull and its relation to the joint at which the motion is occurring are emphasized because these are essential elements of movement.

To provide the student of human motion with the knowledge necessary for systematically analyzing human motion and applying such an analysis to the improvement of performance in motor skills—and to equip the instructor, therapist, coach, or trainer with the anatomical background for understanding the nature of athletic injuries and their prevention—it might seem that the student should wait until the entire anatomical section has been completed before attempting to analyze movement. On the contrary, the earlier the application of knowledge begins, the better. In fact, attempting to analyze basic movements according to the model presented in Chapter 1 as soon as possible serves as a stimulus to the study of anatomy. Following the procedure described in Chapter 1 throughout the study of Part I will pave the way for the later analysis of more complex movements. Procedural steps for analyzing fitness exercises, sport skills, and other physical activities are presented in Chapter 1 (p. 4). For the present, however, it is suggested that the student make simple joint, muscle, and neuromuscular analyses until the process is thoroughly familiar.

In the following chapters, the reader may notice several references that may seem dated. Because of their continued timeliness, however, these classic works are still in use today. The seminal work by Basmajian and DeLuca, for instance, was done in 1985, but it stands today as a classic in the study of muscles and is still cited as a primary reference in current research.

Assumption

- Students have had a course in musculoskeletal anatomy.

Review

- Any basic anatomy text.
- Muscle attachment sites are listed in Appendix C.

National Association for Sport and Physical Education. 2003. Guidelines for undergraduate biomechanics. AAHPERD. www.aahperd.org/naspe/publications/teachingTools/guidance.cfm

CHAPTER

2 THE MUSCULOSKELETAL SYSTEM

The Skeletal Framework and Its Movements

OUTLINE

- ***The Bones***
  - Skeletal Changes
  - Types of Bones
  - Mechanical Axis of a Bone
- ***Articulations***
  - Structural Classification
  - Suggestions for Studying Joint Structure
  - Joint Stability
  - Factors Affecting the Range of Motion
  - Methods of Assessing a Joint's Range of Motion
  - Average Ranges of Joint Motion
- ***Orientation of the Body***
  - The Center of Gravity
  - The Line of Gravity
  - Orientation Planes of the Body and Axes of Motion
  - Standard Starting Positions
- ***Fundamental Movements of the Major Body Segments***
  - Movements in the Sagittal Plane about a Bilateral Axis
  - Movements in the Frontal Plane about an Anteroposterior Axis
  - Movements in the Transverse Plane about a Vertical Axis
  - Movements in a Combination of Planes
  - Naming Joint Actions in Complex Movements
  - Nonaxial Movements
- ***Analyzing Joint Motions***
- ***Laboratory Experiences***

OBJECTIVES

At the conclusion of this chapter, the student should be able to:

1. Classify joints according to structure and explain the relationship between a joint structure and its capacity for movement.
2. Explain how the schedule of ossification of epiphyseal cartilage is related to the nature of activities suitable for different age groups.
3. Name the factors that contribute to joint range of motion and stability and explain the relationship that exists between range of motion and stability.
4. Assess a joint's range of motion, evaluate the range, and describe desirable procedures for changing it when indicated.
5. Name and define the orientation positions and planes of the body and the axes of motion.
6. Demonstrate and name fundamental movement patterns using correct movement terminology.
7. Isolate and name single joint actions that are part of complex movements.
8. Perform an anatomical analysis of the joint actions and planes of motion for a selected motor skill.

It is customary—especially for students of human movement and exercise—to begin the study of anatomy with a detailed study of the bones, then to proceed to the joints, and then to the muscles. This path of investigation sometimes dampens the enthusiasm of students, whose chief focus of interest is movement. Therefore, this chapter and the next emphasize the concept of the total musculoskeletal system as a mechanism for motion. It is hoped that by using this concept the student will find the study of the structural elements of this system more meaningful.

As the phrase implies, the musculoskeletal framework is an arrangement of bones and muscles. Adjacent bones are attached to one another by joints, which provide for the motion of the articulating bones, and the muscles that span the joints provide the force for moving the bones to which they are attached. Mechanically, the total bone–joint–muscle structure is an intricate combination of levers that makes possible a great number of coordinated movements, ranging from the small hand and finger motions used in assembling a television set or playing the piano to the total body movements of a swimmer or a pole vaulter. Any single one of the levers involved in such movements is relatively simple.

In physics we are taught that a lever is defined as a rigid bar that turns about a fulcrum (fixed axis or pivot) when force is applied to it at some specific point. An anatomical lever, therefore, is simply a bone that engages in an angular or turning type of movement when a force is applied to it. This force may be the contracting force of a muscle attached to the bone, or it may be an external force such as gravity or an external weight. If the force is muscle, it is always a pulling force, because muscles, being flexible, are unable to push; they can only pull. If the force is external, such as when a weight is too heavy to be maintained, the muscle force controls the rate at which the lever is allowed to move.

THE BONES

Although anatomy texts give the number of bones in the human skeleton as 206, only 177 of them engage in voluntary movement. The skeleton consists of two major parts, the axial skeleton and the appendicular skeleton (Figure 2.1). The axial section comprises the skull, spinal column, sternum, and ribs, and the appendicular section includes the bones of the upper and lower extremities. The bones of the upper extremity include the

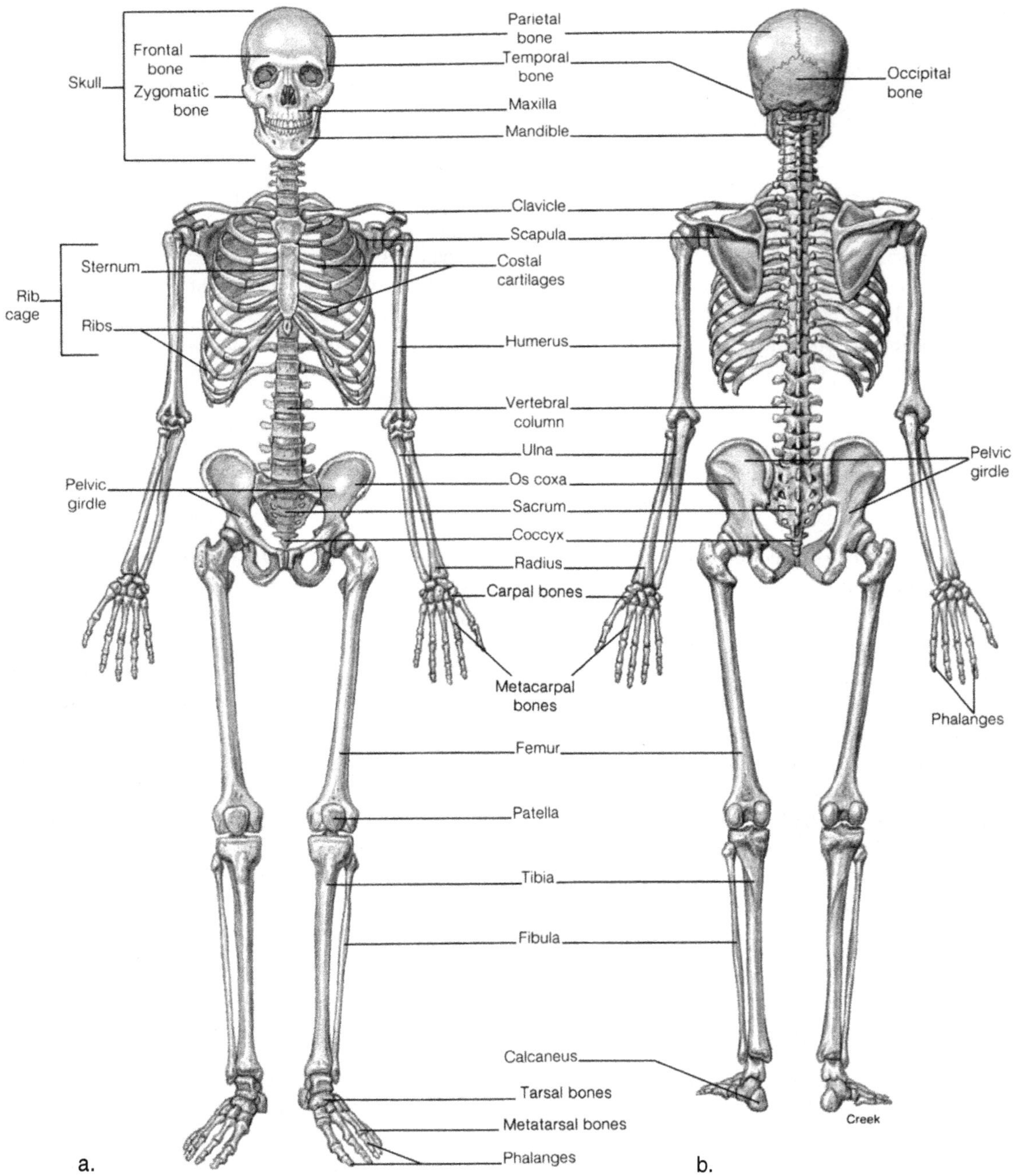

Figure 2.1 Skeleton. (a) Anterior view. (b) Posterior view. From Kent M. Van De Graaff and Stuart Ira Fox, *Concepts of Human Anatomy and Physiology,* 4th ed. Copyright © 1995 Wm C. Brown Communications, Inc., Dubuque, IA. Reprinted by permission of Times Mirror Higher Education Group, Inc., Dubuque, IA. All Rights Reserved.

scapula, clavicle, humerus, ulna, radius, carpal bones, metacarpals, and phalanges, and those of the lower extremity include the three fused bones of the pelvis, the femur, tibia, fibula, tarsal bones, metatarsals, and phalanges. Although the pelvis may be classified with either the axial or the appendicular skeleton, it is actually a link between the axial skeleton and the lower extremity branch of the appendicular skeleton and is functionally as important to one as to the other. The skeleton serves to support weight, as a place for muscles to attach, and to protect critical structures such as the spinal cord, brain, and various organs.

The process of bone development, referred to as *osteogenesis,* begins with the formation of chondrocytes. These cells lay down a matrix upon which osteoblasts form bone. Osteogenesis is a complex process that continues throughout the life span to some degree. Bone is resorbed by osteoclast action and reformed by osteoblasts. Bone growth takes place at the growth plates, or epiphyses, where cartilage calcifies and is converted into bone. Bone growth is regulated by several factors, including genetics, growth hormones, and mechanical loading. Dynamic mechanical loading from a variety of physical activities has been found to have an effect on growth (Villemure & Stokes, 2009). Growth peaks after puberty, but bone regeneration continues in response to muscle activity, stress, injury, and aging. Bone growth, or demineralization, also occurs in response to the levels of a number of hormones, including, but not limited to, estrogen and testosterone. Exercise is one of the best ways to ensure bone growth and strengthening.

Bone develops into two primary types. Compact (or cortical) bone is the dense layer of bone that makes up the outer layer of bone, especially in the long bones. Cancellous (or trabecular) bone has a more open, spongy appearance. This type of bone allows for a relatively high strength-to-weight ratio. As can be seen in Figure 2.2, cancellous bone forms a series of trusses that are aligned to tolerate compressive stress. Cancellous bone is found throughout the body but is especially prevalent in the condyles and epicondyles of the long bones and in the vertebral bodies of the spine.

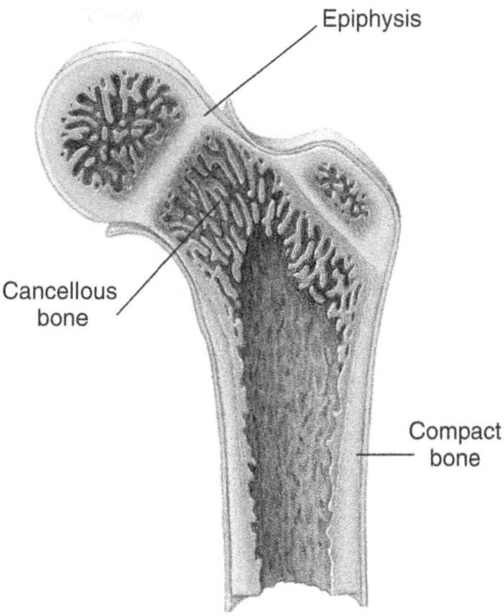

Figure 2.2 Compact and cancellous bone.

Skeletal Changes

Growth

An *epiphysis* is a part of a bone separated from the main bone by a layer of cartilage whose presence in the bone is an indication that the bone has not completed its growth. In the long bones the shaft is separated from the ends and from articulating knobs by epiphyseal cartilages. This is where growth occurs. As growth ceases, the cartilages gradually become ossified (replaced by bone) and, when closure is complete, no more growth can occur (Tables 2.1 & 2.2). Surprisingly, several epiphyses do not completely ossify until the twentieth, or even the twenty-fifth, year of life. Hence, most high school students and many college men are engaging in vigorous sports before their bones are fully matured. Physical education instructors, trainers, and coaches need to be aware of this fact. Although this is not usually harmful in the case of noncontact sports, in violent contact sports like football and boxing the consequences may be extremely serious. An interesting review by Caine, DiFiori, and Maffulli (2006) points out the frequency of sport involvement in epiphyseal injuries in children. They have determined that approximately 30% of such injuries are due to sport involvement. Contact

TABLE 2.1 Approximate Ages of Epiphyseal Closures*

	Age
SPINAL COLUMN	
Vertebrae and sacrum	25
THORAX	
Sternum	25
Ribs	25
UPPER EXTREMITY	
Clavicle	25
Scapula	15–17
Humerus	
Head fused with shaft	20
Lateral epicondyle	16–17
Medial epicondyle	18
Ulna	
Olecranon	16
Lower end	20
Radius	
Head and shaft	18–19
Lower end to shaft	20
LOWER EXTREMITY	
Pelvic bone	
Inferior rami of pubis and ischium (almost complete)	7–8
Acetabulum	20–25
Femur	
Greater and lesser trochanters	18
Head	18
Lower end	20
Tibia	
Upper end	20
Lower end	18
Fibula	
Upper end	25
Lower end	20

*Listed by body section.

Source: Data from Goss (1980).

sports such as American football and high-repetition activities such as gymnastics seem to produce the most frequent injuries. Additional concerns are running, overhead activities, and activities that involve upper extremity weight bearing.

Practitioners must remember that until growth ends at maturation, the epiphyseal plates are quite vulnerable. Care should be taken to encourage a variety of activities. Indications of pain should not ignored or dismissed. Young performers should be monitored for growth spurt activity, as the epiphyseal region is more susceptible to injury at this time. The practitioner should emphasize slow, progressive building of strength, with an emphasis on quality rather than quantity.

TABLE 2.2 Approximate Ages of Epiphyseal Closures*

Approximate Age
7–8
Inferior rami of pubis and ischium almost complete
15–17
Upper extremity: scapula, lateral epicondyle of humerus, olecranon process of ulna
18–19
Upper extremity: medial epicondyle of humerus, head and shaft of radius
Lower extremity: femoral head and greater and lesser trochanters, lower end of tibia
About 20
Upper extremity: humeral head, lower ends of radius and ulna
Lower extremity: lower ends of femur and fibula, upper end of tibia
20–25
Lower extremity: acetabulum in pelvis
25
Spine: vertebrae and sacrum
Upper extremity: clavicle
Lower extremity: upper end of fibula
Thorax: sternum and ribs

*Listed by age.

Source: Data from Goss (1980).

Degeneration

Consideration also must be given to the other end of the age spectrum, the elderly, and the concern for osteoporosis. *Osteoporosis* is the loss of calcium, other minerals, and the matrix from the bones, which causes the bones to become porous and brittle. Some of this loss is natural, resulting from the aging process. With aging, the production of the bone-building *osteoblasts* declines, while there is an increase in the production of bone-eroding *osteoclasts*. The basis for this change has been linked to hormonal changes that occur with age, primarily in women. Other factors may include vitamin deficiencies, inactivity, or poor nutrition. In serious cases, bones subjected to weight bearing and muscle pull may collapse. In some situations, falling may be the result of bones breaking from their brittleness. At best, osteoporosis negatively affects a person's ability to move. Current research indicates that the negative effects may be reduced through good nutrition and regular exercise throughout life. Moreover, nutrition, hormone regulation, and regular exercise begun late in life also tend to control some of the adverse effects of osteoporosis.

Types of Bones

In spite of the great variety of shapes and sizes of bones, there are only four major bone categories: long, short, flat, and irregular.

Long Bones

Characterized by a cylindrical shaft with relatively broad, knobby ends. The shaft or body has thick walls of compact bone and contains a central cavity known as a medullary canal. The bones belonging in this category are the clavicle, humerus, ulna, radius, metacarpals, and phalanges of the upper extremity, and the femur, tibia, fibula, metatarsals, and phalanges of the lower extremity.

Short Bones

Relatively small, chunky, solid bones. The carpals and tarsals (wrist and ankle bones) belong to this category.

Flat Bones

Flat, platelike bones. The sternum, scapulae, ribs, and pelvic bones are examples.

Irregular Bones

The bones of the spinal column. The twenty-four vertebrae, the sacrum, and the coccyx are found in this category.

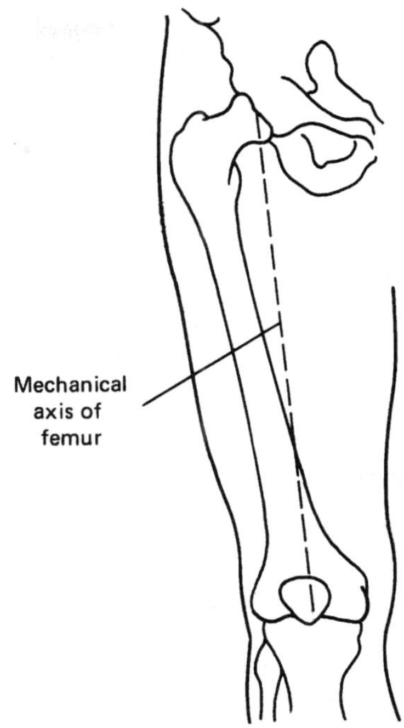

Figure 2.3 Mechanical axis of femur.

Mechanical Axis of a Bone

It has already been stated that bones serve as levers. When muscular action is analyzed mechanically, one must know what is meant by the *mechanical axis* of the bone, or the body segment, that is serving as the lever. The student will find it advantageous, therefore, to learn what this term is now while studying the bones. *The mechanical axis of a bone or segment is a straight line that connects the midpoint of the joint at one end with the midpoint of the joint at the other end or, in the case of a terminal segment, with the midpoint of its distal end.* This axis does not necessarily pass lengthwise through the shaft of the bony lever. If the shaft is curved or if the articulating process projects at an angle from the shaft, the greater part of the axis may lie outside the shaft, as in the case of the femur (Figure 2.3).

ARTICULATIONS

The structure and function of joints are so interrelated that it is difficult to discuss them separately. Hence, in the discussion of structure, there is much that relates to function and, conversely, much that relates to structure when function is discussed. Careful inspection of the joints depicted in Figure 2.4 shows the relationship between the shape of the joint and the movements it permits. In much the same way that railroad tracks determine the route available to the train, the configuration of the bones that form an articulation, together with the reinforcing ligaments, determine and limit the movements that the involved segment can make.

Structural Classification

There are many different patterns of joint structure, and these form the basis for their classification. The classification found in most anatomy texts is based on the presence or absence of a joint cavity—that is, a space between the articulating surfaces of the bones. Each type of joint is further classified either according to shape or according to the nature of the tissues that connect the bones. These classifications, with their subdivisions, may be grasped more readily in outline form and in Figure 2.4:

I. Diarthrosis (from the Greek, meaning a joint in which there is a separation or articular cavity) (Figures 2.5 and 2.6)
   A. Characteristics
      1. An articular cavity is present.
      2. The joint is encased within a sleevelike, ligamentous capsule.
      3. The capsule is lined with synovial membrane that secretes synovial fluid for lubricating the joint.
      4. The articular surfaces are smooth.
      5. The articular surfaces are covered with cartilage, usually hyaline, but occasionally fibrocartilage.
   B. Classification
      1. Irregular (arthrodial; plane). The joint surfaces are irregularly shaped, usually flat or slightly curved. The only movement permitted is of a gliding nature; hence, it is nonaxial.
      2. Hinge (ginglymus). One surface is spool-like; the other is concave. The concave surface fits over the spool-like process and glides partially around it in a hinge type of movement. This constitutes movement in one plane about a single axis of motion; hence, it is uniaxial. The movements that occur are flexion and extension.
      3. Pivot (trochoid; screw). This kind of joint may be characterized by a peglike pivot, as in the joint between atlas and axis, or by two long bones fitting against each other near each end in such a way that one bone can roll around the other one, as do the radius and ulna of the forearm. In the latter type, a small concave notch on one bone fits against the rounded surface of the other. The rounded surface may be either the edge of a disc (like the head of the radius) or a rounded knob (like the head of the ulna). The only movement permitted in either kind of pivot joint is rotation. It is a movement in one plane about a single axis; hence, the joint is uniaxial.
      4. Condyloid (ovoid; ellipsoidal). An oval or egg-shaped convex surface fits into a reciprocally shaped concave surface. Movement can occur in two planes, forward and backward, and from side to side. The former movement is flexion and extension, and the latter abduction and adduction or lateral flexion. The joint is biaxial. When these movements are performed sequentially, they constitute circumduction.
      5. Saddle (sellar; reciprocal reception). This may be thought of as a modification of a condyloid joint. Both ends of the convex surface are tipped up, making the surface

	Nonaxial (0 axes)	**Uniaxial (1 axis)**	**Biaxial (2 axes)**	**Triaxial (3 axes)**
	Plane joint	*Hinge joint*	*Condyloid joint*	*Ball and socket joint*
	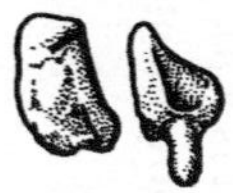	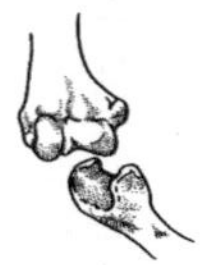	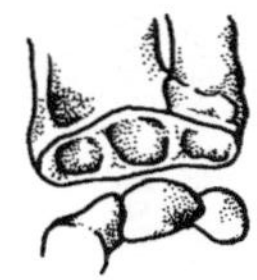	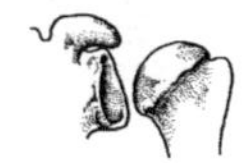
	Carpal joints	Elbow	Metacarpophalangeal joints	Hip
		Pivot joint	*Saddle joint*	
		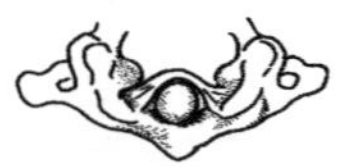	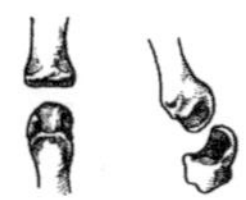	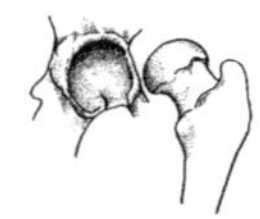
		Atlantoaxial joint	Thumb	Shoulder
Planes of motion	None	Sagittal OR Transverse	Sagittal AND Frontal	Sagittal Frontal Transverse
Primary axes	None	Bilateral OR Longitudinal	Bilateral AND Anteroposterior	Bilateral Anteroposterior Longitudinal
Movements	Sliding or gliding	Flexion/Extension OR Rotation Pronation/Supination	Flexion/Extension Abduction/Adduction	Flexion/Extension Abduction/Adduction Rotation

Figure 2.4 Joint classifications.

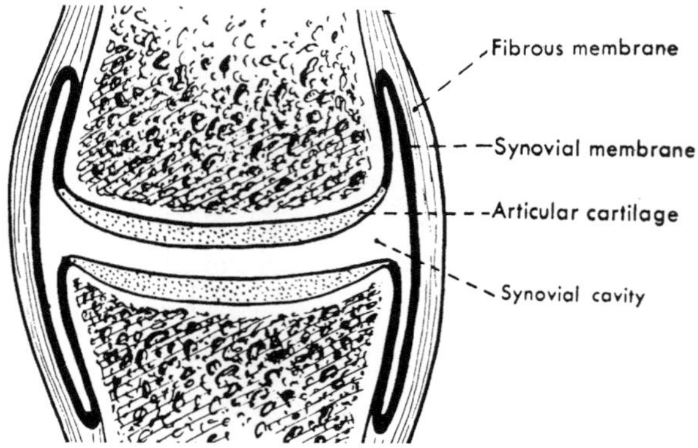

Figure 2.5 Frontal section of a diarthrodial joint. From W. H. Hollinshead and D. B. Jenkins, *Functional Anatomy of the Limbs and Back,* 5th ed. Copyright © 1981 W. B. Saunders, Orlando, FL. Reprinted by permission.

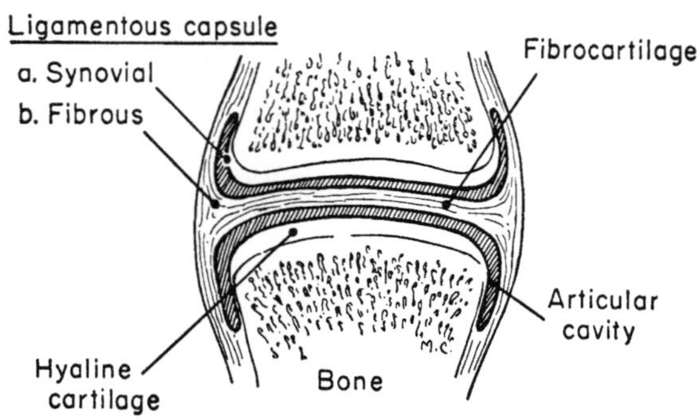

Figure 2.6 Frontal section of a diarthrodial joint having fibrocartilage.

concave in the other direction, like a western saddle. Fitting over this is a reciprocally concave-convex surface. This is a biaxial joint, permitting flexion and extension, abduction and adduction, and circumduction. The saddle joint has greater freedom of motion than the condyloid joint.

6. Ball-and-socket (spheroidal; enarthrodial). In this type of joint the spherical head of one bone fits into the cup or saucerlike cavity of the other bone (see Figures 5.7, 5.8, 7.8, and 7.9). It is much like the swivel joint on a trailer hitch. It permits flexion and extension, abduction and adduction, circumduction (the sequential combination of the preceding four motions), horizontal adduction and abductions, and rotation. It is a triaxial joint because it permits movements about three axes.

(See Appendix B for a more complete chart of diarthrodial joints and their motions.)

II. Synarthrosis (from the Greek, meaning literally "with joint" or, according to our usage, a joint in which there is no separation or articular cavity)
   A. Characteristics
      1. In two of the types (cartilaginous and fibrous), the two bones are united by

means of an intervening substance, such as cartilage or fibrous tissue, which is continuous with the joint surfaces.

2. The third type (ligamentous) is not a true joint but is a ligamentous connection between two bones, which may or may not be contiguous.
3. There is no articular cavity, hence no capsule, synovial membrane, or synovial fluid.

B. Classification

1. Cartilaginous. Only the joints that are united by fibrocartilage permit motion of a bending and twisting nature. Example of fibrocartilaginous type: articulations between the bodies of the vertebrae (see Figure 9.2). Those united by hyaline cartilage permit only a slight compression. Example of hyaline type: epiphyseal unions.
2. Fibrous. The edges of bone are united by means of a thin layer of fibrous tissue that is continuous with the periosteum. No movements are permitted. Only example: the sutures of the skull.
3. Ligamentous. Two bodies, which may be adjacent or may be quite widely separated, are tied together by one or more ligaments. These ligaments may be in the form of cords, bands, or flat sheets. The movement that occurs is usually limited and of no specific type. Examples: coracoacromial union (Figure 5.9); midunion of radius and ulna (see Figures 6.2 and 6.3).

C. Summary

The synarthrodial joints of greatest concern to the kinesiologist are those of the vertebral bodies. The thickness of the intervertebral discs permits a moderate amount of motion simulating that of ball-and-socket joints. The movements are flexion and extension, lateral flexion, circumduction, and rotation.

Suggestions for Studying Joint Structure

To understand thoroughly the structure of a joint and especially the relation of structure to function, the student should supplement book study with firsthand study of a skeleton or of the disarticulated bones that enter into the formation of each major joint.

The movements of each joint should be studied both on the skeleton and on the living subject. When using the latter method, it is important to consider all the joints involved in the movement in question. For instance, in studying the movements of the elbow joint, the articulation between the humerus and radius must not be overlooked. The close relationship that exists between certain joints should be noted, for example, the relationship between the elbow joint and proximal radioulnar articulation. The tilting of the pelvis that accompanies many movements of the lower extremity and lumbar spine should be recognized, as should the movements of the shoulder girdle that accompany those of the shoulder joint. A particular pitfall awaits those who study the movements of the shoulder joint only by observing the living subject. If not forewarned, students may overlook the part played by the shoulder girdle. Its movements may be detected by palpating the scapula and clavicle in all movements of the upper arm. To follow the movements of the scapula, the thumb should be placed at the inferior angle, one finger on the root of the scapular spine and another on the acromion process. Firm contact should be maintained as the scapula moves.

A student of movement must always be observant of motion possibilities in all the joints and not limit attention to just one joint. Only through the cooperative involvement of various parts can the total range of movement potential be experienced and understood. Therefore, focusing on one joint would be misleading and would result in misinterpretations of what was being observed.

Joint Stability

The function of the joints is obviously to provide the bones with a means of moving or, rather, of being moved. But because such provisions bring with them a threat of instability, the joints have what might be called a secondary function of providing for stability without interfering with the desired motions.

All the joints of the body do not have the same degree of strength or stability. Some, such as the hip or elbow, are fairly stable. Others, such as the shoulder or knee, are less stable and therefore more easily injured. The strength or degree of freedom of joints follows Emerson's law: "For everything that is given, something is taken." In the shoulder, movement is gained at the expense of stability, whereas in the hip, movement is sacrificed for stability.

By *joint stability* we mean resistance to displacement. Some widely accepted factors in joint stability are the joint ligaments such as the lateral ligaments of hinge joints, the shape of the bony structure, muscle tension (see stabilizing components of muscular force), fascia, and atmospheric pressure. The latter is particularly effective at the hip joint. Proprioception and neuromuscular control are also important considerations in stability.

Shape of Bony Structure

Shape may refer to the kind of joint, such as hinge, condyloid, or ball-and-socket, but it is even more likely to refer to specific characteristics of the particular joint. Both the shoulder and the hip joints, for instance, are ball-and-socket joints, yet they differ markedly in their stability. The depth of the cuplike acetabulum of the hip joint, in contrast to the small size and shallowness of the glenoid fossa of the shoulder joint, is a case in point. The bony structure of the hip joint obviously gives greater protection against displacement. This difference is reflective of the weight-bearing function of the lower extremity and manipulation function of the upper extremity.

Ligamentous Arrangements

Ligaments are strong, flexible, stress-resistant, somewhat elastic, fibrous tissues that may be in the form of straplike bands or round cords. They attach the ends of the bones that form a movable joint and help maintain them in the right relationship to each other. They also check the movement when it reaches its normal limits, and they resist movements for which the joint is not constructed. For instance, the collateral ligaments of the knee help prevent any tendency there might be for this joint to abduct or adduct. Likewise, the ulnar and radial collateral ligaments of the elbow prevent abduction and adduction. The ligaments do not always succeed in preventing abnormal or excessive movements, because collisions and violent motions may cause them to tear. Also, if they are subject to prolonged periods of stress (a force that deforms), they become abnormally stretched. Because they are not very elastic (i.e., they do not have the capability to return quickly to normal shape) following deformation, ligaments take a long time to recover from a stretch. If overstretched, they may never regain their normal length. Ligaments stretched and damaged in joint injuries should be given plenty of time to heal before being subjected to strenuous activity and strain (deformation). As long as the ligaments remain undamaged, they are an important factor in contributing to joint stability, but once stretched, their usefulness is permanently affected and joint stability is diminished.

Muscular Arrangement

The muscles and muscle tendons that span the joint also play a part in the stability of joints, especially in those joints whose bony structure contributes little to stability. The shoulder joint is a notable example, getting its greatest strength from the shoulder and arm muscles that cross it. (See Chapter 5 for an in-depth discussion of the stability of the shoulder joint.)

Of the muscles that act on the shoulder joint, four of them, known as the rotator cuff (subscapularis, supraspinatus, infraspinatus, and teres minor), are particularly important as stabilizers of this joint. One of their chief functions is protection of the shoulder joint and prevention of displacement of the humeral head. Figure 5.13 shows that all four of these muscles have a strong inward pull on the humeral head toward the glenoid fossa. Likewise, the knee joint depends greatly on the tendons of the quadriceps femoris and hamstring muscles for its strength. A most important defense against joint injury is an increase in the strength of the muscles that support the joint. The role of muscles as stabilizers, as opposed to that of movers or neutralizers, is included in greater detail in Chapter 3.

Fascia and Skin

Fasciae consist of fibrous connective tissue that forms sheaths for individual muscles, partitions that lie between muscles, and smaller partitions that separate bundles of muscle fibers within a single muscle. According to their location and function, they may vary in structure from thin membranes to tough, fibrous sheets. In composition they are similar to ligaments in that they are flexible and elastic, within limits, but are susceptible to permanent stretch if subjected to stress that is too intense or too prolonged. The iliotibial tract of the fascia lata and the thick skin covering the knee joint are examples of fascia and skin serving to help stabilize a joint.

Atmospheric Pressure

Atmospheric pressure plays a key role in stability of both the hip and the shoulder (glenohumeral) joints. The slight negative pressure that exists within the joint capsules forms a vacuum that holds the head of the long bone into the socket. This pressure has been found to serve a role in joint stability that may be equal to that of muscle. The absence of this vacuum, as might happen in an injury, may disrupt joint mechanics (Habermeyer et al. 1992; Wingstrand et al. 1990).

Factors Affecting the Range of Motion

The simplest way to limit motion is to put an obstacle in the path of the moving object. An obstacle limiting joint motion may be of soft or rigid tissue or both. Consequently, all joints in the same individual do not have the same amount of movement, and the same joints in different individuals do not have the same amount or range of motion (ROM). The ROM depends on several factors. Three factors that affect the stability of a joint are also related to its range of motion. These are the shape of the articular surfaces, the restraining effect of the ligaments, and the controlling action of the muscles.

Muscles and their tendons are undoubtedly the single most important factor in maintaining both the stability and degree of movement in joints. The tightness of the hamstring tendons (behind the knees) is often felt when someone attempts to touch the toes without bending the knees. Many have also discovered that continued practice will stretch these tendons and improve the joint's range of motion appreciably. It is important to remember that flexibility should not exceed the muscles' ability to maintain the integrity of the joints. Exercising the muscles on all sides of a joint can contribute to both flexibility and strength. The apposition of bulky tissue also affects the degree of movement in a joint. Well-developed musculature or excessive fatty tissue will restrict motion. Bulky arm muscles restrict flexion of the forearm at the elbow, and large deposits of abdominal fat limit trunk flexion. Additional factors in the range of motion include gender, body build, heredity (in addition to body build), occupation, personal exercise habits, state of physical fitness, injury, and age.

Any conditions or diseases resulting in a decrease in range of motion may limit one's ability in activities of daily living or participation in physical activity. Reduction in range of motion may result in loss of ability to withstand normal stresses and may result in pain. Therefore, movement opportunities are avoided, resulting in further decreases in joint mobility. This negative cycle often typifies joint disease and injury. One such condition is arthritis, which can affect a person of any age. Regardless of age, maintaining range of movement without pain must be a goal in order to control for other complications. Exercises done in water have been found to be beneficial, as have exercises using elastic bands and other light resistance devices.

Methods of Assessing a Joint's Range of Motion

The usual way to assess a joint's range of motion is to measure the number of degrees from the starting position of the segment to its position at the end of its maximal movement. This is the way to measure flexion; extension is usually measured as the return movement from flexion. If the movement continues beyond the starting position, that constitutes hyperextension. Abduction and adduction are measured separately from the starting position or, if desired, the total range from maximal abduction to maximal adduction is measured.

Measuring ROM can be done in various ways, depending on the joint that is measured. The instrument most commonly used is the double-armed goniometer, with one arm stationary and the other movable (Figure 2.7). The pin or axis of the movable arm is placed directly over the center of the joint at which the motion occurs. The stationary arm is held in line with the stationary segment, and the movable arm is either held against the segment as it moves or placed in line with the segment after its limit of motion has been reached. At the completion of the movement, the indicator shows the number of degrees through which the segment has moved. When the anatomical landmarks are well defined, and the examiner has identified the joint center properly, the use of the goniometer may be considered accurate, but when the bony landmarks are not well defined because of excess soft tissue coverage or other causes, or the goniometer axis is not properly placed over the joint axis, the goniometer may provide inaccurate information. For enhanced accuracy of the joint being measured, all other joints and segments should be stabilized. Digital methods of measuring joint angles are often used in laboratory settings and will be discussed more completely in Chapter 22.

A more recent method makes use of videotape. Before filming the subject, joint centers are marked so as to be visible in the projected image. Joint angles can then be obtained from the projected images. The range of motion is the difference between the joint angles of two images, one at the start of the movement and the other at its completion (Figure 2.8). When this method is used, the segment action must occur in the picture plane (i.e., at a right angle to the camera).

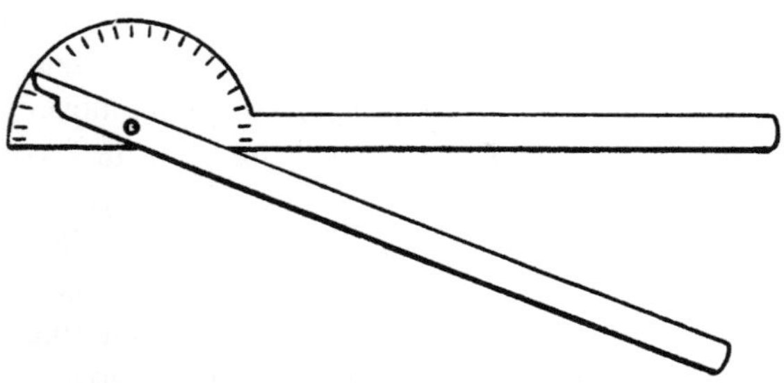

Figure 2.7 Double-armed goniometer.

Average Ranges of Joint Motion

Because of the many factors that affect range of motion, including differences in measuring techniques, ranges vary and it is difficult to establish norms. Age, gender, body build, and level of activity may all be factors. Where the extremities are concerned, the individual's opposite is perhaps the best norm. Some averages that may be used as a guide are presented in Table 2.3. Illustrations showing joint range of motion for most fundamental movements are found in Appendix B.

ORIENTATION OF THE BODY

In preparation for defining the fundamental movements of the major segments of the body and for the analysis of these movements, certain orientation concepts and points of reference need to be established. The essential ones are the center of gravity, the line of gravity, the orientation planes of the body and axes of motion, and the standard starting positions from which the fundamental movements are made.

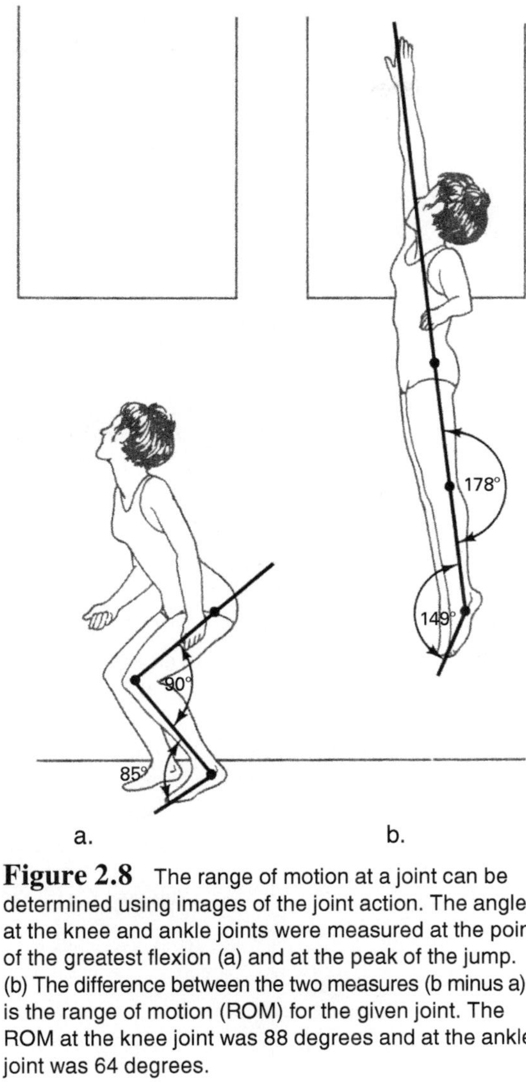

Figure 2.8 The range of motion at a joint can be determined using images of the joint action. The angles at the knee and ankle joints were measured at the point of the greatest flexion (a) and at the peak of the jump. (b) The difference between the two measures (b minus a) is the range of motion (ROM) for the given joint. The ROM at the knee joint was 88 degrees and at the ankle joint was 64 degrees.

The Center of Gravity

The *center of gravity* is defined as a point representing the weight center of an object; it is also "that point in a body about which all the parts exactly balance each other" and can be viewed as "the point at which the entire weight of the body may be considered concentrated." In a perfect sphere or cube, the weight center coincides with the geometric center. Its precise location in the human body depends on the individual's anatomical structure, habitual standing posture, current position, and whether external weights are being supported. In a person of average build, standing erect with the arms hanging at the sides, the center of gravity is located in the pelvis in front of the upper part of the sacrum. It is usually lower in women than in men because of women's heavier pelvises and thighs and shorter legs. (See Chapter 14 for a more detailed discussion of the center of gravity and related concepts.)

The Line of Gravity

The **line of gravity** is a vertical line that, by definition, passes through the center of gravity. Hence, its location depends on the position of the center of gravity, which changes with every shift of the body's position.

Orientation Planes of the Body and Axes of Motion

Three traditional planes correspond to the three dimensions of space. Each plane is perpendicular to each of the other two. There are likewise three axes of motion, each perpendicular to the plane in which the motion occurs. The planes and axes of the body are defined as follows.

1. The **sagittal,** or median, **plane** is a vertical plane passing through the body from front to back, dividing it into right and left halves (Figure 2.9a)
2. The **frontal,** or coronal, **plane** is a vertical plane passing through the body from side to side, dividing it into anterior and posterior halves (Figure 2.9b)
3. The **transverse,** or horizontal, **plane** is a plane that passes horizontally through the body, dividing it into upper and lower halves (Figure 2.9c)

Because each plane *bisects* the body, it follows that each plane must pass through the center of gravity. Hence, the center of gravity may be defined as the point at which the three planes of the

TABLE 2.3 Average Ranges of Joint Motion

Joint	Sources 1	2	3	4
Elbow				
Flexion	140	145	145	145
Hyperextension	0	0	0	0–10
Forearm				
Pronation	80	90	90	80
Supination	80	85	90	90
Wrist				
Extension	60	70	70	50
Flexion	60	90		60
Radial flexion	20	20	20	20
Ulnar flexion	30	30	35	30
Shoulder				
Flexion	180	170	130	180
Hyperextension	50	30	80	60
Abduction	180	170	180	180
Adduction	50			
Horizontal flexion				135
Horizontal extension				45
Shoulder				
Rotation (arm in abduction)				
Inward	90	90	70	60–90
Outward	90	90	70	90
Hip				
Flexion	100	120	125	120
Hyperextension	30	10	10	30
Abduction	40	45	45	45
Adduction	20		10	0–25
Rotation (in extension)				
Inward	40	35	45	40–45
Outward	50	45	45	45
Knee				
Flexion	150	120	140	130
Ankle				
Plantar flexion	20	45	45	50
Dorsiflexion	30	15	20	20
Spine (cervical)				
Flexion	60			40
Hyperextension	75			40
Lateral flexion	45			45
Rotation	80			50
Spine (thoracic and lumbar)				
Flexion	45–50			45
Hyperextension	25			20–35
Lateral flexion	25			30
Rotation	30			45

Sources: Data from (1) *Guide to the Evaluation of Permanent Impairment* (3rd ed. rev.), 1990, Chicago: American Medical Association. (2) *Brunnstrom's Clinical Kinesiology* (4th ed.), by L. K. Smith & L. D. Lehmkuhl, 1983, Philadelphia: F. A. Davis., (3) *Muscles: Testing and Function* (2nd ed.), by H. O. Kendall et al., 1971, Baltimore, MD: Williams & Wilkins. (4) *International SFTR Method of Measuring and Recording Joint Motion*, by J. J. Gerhardt & O. A. Russe, 1975, Bern, Switzerland: Hans Huber Publishers.

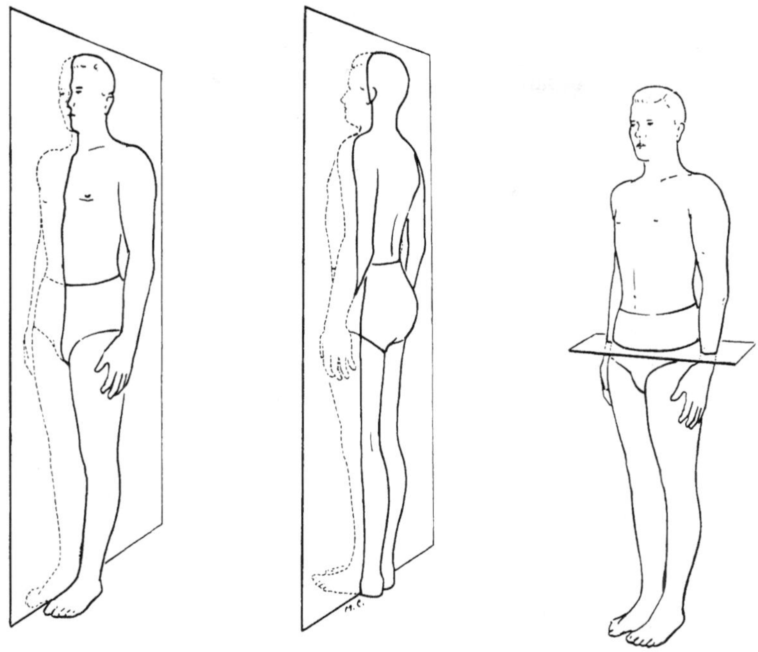

a. b. c.

Figure 2.9 The planes of the body: (a) sagittal, or median, plane; (b) frontal, or coronal, plane; (c) transverse, or horizontal, plane.

body intersect one another, and the line of gravity as the vertical line at which the two vertical planes intersect each other. When describing a movement in terms of a plane, such as "a movement of the forearm in the sagittal plane," we mean that the movement occurs in a plane parallel to the sagittal plane. It does not necessarily imply that the movement occurs in a plane passing through the center of gravity. If the latter is intended, the term *cardinal plane* is used. Therefore, it may be concluded that there are only three cardinal planes but an infinite number of vertical and horizontal planes parallel to the cardinal planes. Thus, nodding the head is a movement occurring in the cardinal sagittal plane, but movement of either leg or arm forward-upward is movement occurring in the sagittal plane.

Axes

1. The **bilateral axis** (mediolateral) passes horizontally from side to side.
2. The **anteroposterior** or **AP axis** passes horizontally from front to back.
3. The **vertical** (longitudinal) **axis** is perpendicular to the ground.

A rotary movement of a segment of the body occurs *in* a plane and *around* an axis. The axis around which the movement takes place is always at right angles to the plane in which it occurs. One may consider the axis to be an imaginary rod placed in such a position (perpendicular to each plane) so that the segment is permitted to move about this axis. Forward lifting of the leg (flexion) occurs in the sagittal plane about a bilateral axis, sideward raising of the arm (abduction) occurs in the frontal plane about an anteroposterior axis, and turning the head to the side (lateral rotation) is movement in the transverse plane about a vertical axis.

An understanding of planes and axes may guide the observer into the best position to observe or record a motion. Movement in a transverse plane is observed most easily from above or below. Movement within a sagittal plane is best observed from the side. These positions are parallel to the axis about which the movements are occurring.

Standard Starting Positions

Fundamental Standing Position

In this position the individual stands erect with the feet slightly separated and parallel, the arms hanging easily at the sides with palms facing the body (Figure 2.10a). This is the position usually accepted as the point of reference for analyzing all the movements of the body's segments, *except those of the forearm.*

Anatomical Standing Position

This is the position usually depicted in anatomy textbooks. The individual is erect, with the elbows fully extended and the palms facing forward. The legs and feet are the same as for the fundamental standing position (Figure 2.10b). It is usually accepted as the point of reference for the movements of the forearm, hand, and fingers.

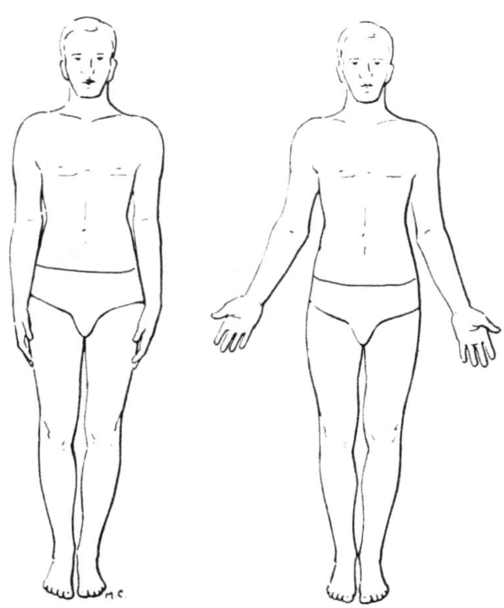

Figure 2.10 Standing positions: (a) fundamental standing position; (b) anatomical standing position.

FUNDAMENTAL MOVEMENTS OF THE MAJOR BODY SEGMENTS

Being a multijointed structure, the human body consists of many movable segments. When we watch skillful acrobats, dancers, or basketball players, it might seem like a hopeless task to try to organize their movements into a single, meaningful classification. The task is greatly simplified, however, when we consider one segment at a time and visualize each movement as though it were performed from the *anatomical standing position.* This may take a bit of imagination, but knowing ahead of time the movements of which each joint in the body is capable is nine-tenths of the battle. These movements are described in Chapters 4 through 9 in the systematic discussions of the regions of the body. The following information is basic to an understanding of the movements of specific joints and segments.

Movements in the Sagittal Plane about a Bilateral Axis (Figure 2.11a)

Flexion

The angle at the joint diminishes. Examples include the following:

1. Tipping the head forward.
2. Lifting the foot and leg backward from the knee.
3. Raising the entire lower extremity forward-upward as though kicking.
4. With the upper arm remaining at the side, raising the forearm straight forward (Figure 2.11a).
5. With the elbow straight, raising the entire upper extremity forward-upward. The "diminishing angle" is hard to see in this movement until one views the raising of the arm from the shoulder in the same way that the raising of the thigh from the hip joint is viewed. In the latter, one automatically notices the angle that appears between the top of the thigh and the trunk. Similarly, when raising the arm, the angle to look for is the angle between the top of the arm and the neck–head

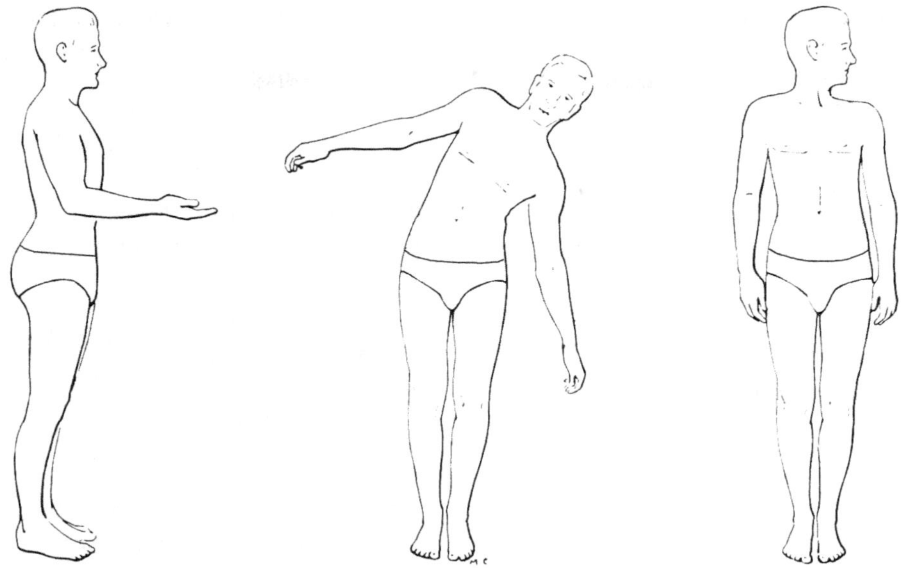

a. b. c.

Figure 2.11 Movements of the body in three planes: (a) movement of the forearm in the sagittal plane around a bilateral axis; (b) movement of the trunk in the frontal plane around an anteroposterior axis; (c) movement of the head in the transverse plane around a vertical axis.

segment, not the angle between the underside of the raised arm and the trunk. One must view the sagittal plane movements of the arm at the shoulder as being similar to those of the thigh at the hip joint.

For general purposes the upper arm may be considered fully flexed when it has reached the overhead vertical position. Later, when the role of the shoulder girdle in arm movements has been studied, it will be seen that the elevation of the arm does not occur solely at the shoulder joint. The movements of the scapula and clavicle are an important part of the total arm movement. Strictly speaking, the shoulder joint is in a fully flexed position when the humerus is raised until it is parallel with the long axis of the scapula (i.e., when it is in the same plane as the scapula). For the present, however, the upper arm will be considered fully flexed when it has been raised forward-upward until it has reached the vertical position and hyperflexed when it passes beyond this.

Extension

The return movement from flexion.

Hyperflexion

This term refers only to the movement of the upper arm. When the arm is flexed beyond the vertical, it is considered to be hyperflexed. In other joints of the body, flexion is terminated by contact of the moving segment with another part of the body—for example, the forearm against the upper arm, the lower leg against the thigh, or by structural limitations of the joints themselves (e.g., flexion of the thoracic and lumbar spine).

Hyperextension

The continuation of extension beyond the starting position or beyond the straight line. Examples include the following:

1. Hyperextension of the upper arm is said to occur when the arm is extended backward beyond the body.

2. The forearm is considered to be hyperextended when the angle at the elbow joint has exceeded 180 degrees.

Reduction of Hyperextension

Return movement from hyperextension. This movement could also be called flexion to the starting position—that is, the fundamental or the anatomical starting position, as the case may be.

Movements in the Frontal Plane about an Anteroposterior Axis (Figure 2.11b)

Viewed from the front or back.

Abduction

Sideward movement away from the midline or sagittal plane or, in the case of the fingers, away from the midline of the hand. This term is used most commonly for sideward movements of the upper arm away from the trunk—in other words, sideward elevation of the arm—and for sideward elevation of the lower extremity. The jumping-jack exercise involves both of these.

Adduction

The return movement from abduction.

Lateral Flexion

This term refers to the lateral bending of the head or trunk. It may also be used for sideward movements of the middle finger, but the more specific terms *radial* or *ulnar* flexion are usually used for these.

Hyperabduction

Like hyperflexion, this term usually refers to the upper arm when the latter is abducted beyond the vertical, as seen from the front or back.

Hyperadduction

The trunk blocks hyperadduction of the upper extremity, and the presence of the supporting lower extremity blocks hyperadduction of the other lower extremity. By combining slight flexion with hyperadduction, the upper extremities can move across the front of the body, and one lower extremity can move across in front of the supporting one.

Reduction of Hyperadduction

The return movement from hyperadduction.

Reduction of Lateral Flexion

The return movement from lateral flexion.

Movements in the Transverse Plane about a Vertical Axis (Figure 2.11c)

Viewed or visualized from overhead or from directly beneath, as through a glass platform. The point of reference for all rotations of the upper extremities is the midposition as in the fundamental (not anatomical) standing position.

Rotation Left and Right

Applies to rotation of the head, neck, or pelvis in such a way that the anterior aspect turns, respectively, to the left or right.

Outward (External) and Inward (Internal) Rotation

Applies to rotation of the thigh, the upper arm, or the upper or lower extremity as a whole in such a way that the anterior aspect of the segment turns laterally or medially.

Supination and Pronation

Apply, respectively, to outward (lateral) and inward (medial) rotation of the forearm.

Reduction of Outward Rotation, Inward Rotation, Supination, or Pronation

Rotation of the segment back to the midposition.

Movements in a Combination of Planes

Circumduction

An orderly sequence of the movements that occur in the sagittal, frontal, and intermediate oblique planes so that the segment as a whole describes a cone is known as *circumduction*. It consists of an axial movement that may occur in any plane. The movement may occur at biaxial or triaxial joints. Arm circling and trunk circling are examples of circumduction.

Naming Joint Actions in Complex Movements

It is important to note that although all movements do not begin from the anatomical standing position, the joint actions are still named as if they were occurring in the anatomical standing position; however, the plane and axis are identified as those in which the movement actually occurs. An example is flexion and extension of the forearm at the elbow joint. Beginning from the anatomical standing position, this joint action occurs within the sagittal plane about a bilateral axis. If, however, the elbow movement is preceded by 90 degrees of flexion and inward rotation of the arm at the shoulder joint, elbow flexion and extension are described as occurring within the horizontal plane about a longitudinal axis.

Nonaxial Movements

Movements permitted at any diarthrodial joint except the arthrodial or plane joints are rotary movements and occur in a plane about an axis. Movements in plane joints are nonaxial. An example is the gliding movement that occurs between the articular facets of the spinal column. Nonaxial movements of body segments may occur when they are moved as the result of rotary action of adjacent segments. In a pushing action, the hand moves linearly forward in the sagittal plane because of the axial movements of the arm segments at the shoulder, elbow, and wrist joints. Similarly, in a deep knee bend, the trunk and head move linearly because of the rotary actions of the leg segments.

ANALYZING JOINT MOTIONS

The first four columns of the anatomical analysis model presented in Table 1.2 deal primarily with the orientation of the body segments and the patterns of joint motion. For each phase of the technique and for each joint participating in the phase, the precise joint action and segment being moved should be identified and recorded. The plane of motion for each joint should be stipulated, along with the axis of joint motion. If it seems desirable to measure the range of motion in a given joint, this can be done from sequential motion pictures.

Once the information used in the anatomical model has been collected and examined, the analyst can begin to evaluate the performance in terms of joint motions. This evaluation should take into account some basic anatomical principles. Returning to the long jump example, several joint action principles apply.

Alignment

The proper alignment of segments may differ from movement to movement. The optimum segmental alignment for any skill should be determined based on efficiency, effectiveness, and safety. In the standing long jump example, the joints of the lower extremity need to be fully extended at takeoff to impart maximum jumping force. Because this is a jump for horizontal distance, the joints should be aligned in such a way as to ensure that the center of gravity is in front of the feet at the moment of takeoff.

Range of Motion

Each joint in the body has a limit to its range of motion. The range of motion limitations of the body and the range of motion demands of the activity must be compatible to avoid injury while still producing an effective performance. A limited range of motion in the standing long jump will shorten the amount of extension possible and thereby decrease the length of time over which the push-off force will be applied.

Flexibility

Flexibility reduces the internal resistance to motion. The maintenance of normal flexibility is an important consideration for all. In the jump example, flexibility in the joints of the lower extremity will allow for optimum flexion in the lower extremities while reducing the risk of injury.

REFERENCES AND SELECTED READINGS

Caine, D., DiFiori, J., & Maffulli, N. (2006). Physeal injuries in children's and youth sports: Reasons for concern? *British Journal of Sports Medicine,* 40(9), 749–760.

Downey, P. A., & Siegel, M. I. (2006). Bone biology and the clinical implications for osteoporosis. *Physical Therapy,* 86(1), 77–91.

Goss, C. M. (Ed.). (1980). *Gray's anatomy of the human body* (36th ed.). Philadelphia: Lea & Febiger.

Habermeyer, P., Schuller, U., & Wiedemann, E. (1992). The intra-articular pressure of the shoulder: An experimental study on the role of the glenoid labrum in stabilizing the joint. *Arthroscopy,* 8(2), 166–172.

Lindberg, M. K., Vandenput, L., Moverare Skrtic, S., Vanderschueren, D., Boonen, S., Bouillon, R. R., et al. (2005). Androgens and the skeleton. *Minerva Endocrinologica,* 30(1), 15–25.

Mackie, E. J. (2003). Osteoblasts: Novel roles in orchestration of skeletal architecture. *International Journal of Biochemistry & Cell Biology,* 35(9): 1301–1305.

Olsen, B. R., Reginato, A. M., & Wang, W. (2000). Bone development. *Annual Review of Cell and Developmental Biology,* 16, 191–220.

Pietschmann, P., Rauner, M., Sipos, W., & Kerschan-Schindl, K. (2009). Osteoporosis: An age-related and gender-specific disease—A mini-review. *Gerontology,* 55, 3–12.

Reimann, B. L., & Lephart, S. M. (2002a). The sensorimotor system. Part I. The physiologic basis of functional joint stability. *Journal of Athletic Training,* 37(1), 71–79.

Riemann, B. L., & Lephart, S. M. (2002b). The sensorimotor system. Part II. The role of proprioception in motor control and functional joint stability. *Journal of Athletic Training,* 37(1), 80–84.

Skerry, T. M. (2008). The response of bone to mechanical loading and disuse: Fundamental principles and influences on osteoblast/osteocyte homeostasis. *Archives of Biochemistry and Biophysics,* 473, 117–123.

Talts, J. F., Pfeifer, A., Hofmann, F., Hunziker, E. B., Zhou, X. H., Aszodi, A., et al. (1998). Endochondral ossification is dependent on the mechanical properties of cartilage tissue and on intracellular signals in chondrocytes. *Annals of the New York Academy of Science,* 23(857), 74–85.

Turner, C. H., & Robling, A. G. (2005). Exercises for improving bone strength. *British Journal of Sports Medicine,* 39, 188–189.

Welch. J. M., & C. M. Weaver. (2005). Calcium and exercise affect the growing skeleton. *Nutrition Reviews,* 63(11), 361–373.

Villemure, I., & I.A.F. Stokes. (2009). Growth plate mechanics and mechanobiology: A survey of present understanding. *Journal of Biomechanics,* 42, 1793–1803.

Wingstrand, H., Wingstrand, A., & Krantz, P. (1990). Intracapsular and atmospheric pressure in the dynamics and stability of the hip: A biomechanical study. *Acta Orthopaedica Scandinavica,* 61(3), 231–235.

Zernicke, R., McKay, C., & Lorincz, C. (2006). Mechanisms of bone remodeling during weight-bearing exercise. *Applied Physiology of Nutrition and Metabolism,* 31, 655–660.

LABORATORY EXPERIENCES

1. By studying a skeleton and observing a living subject, classify the following joints without referring to the textbook: hip, elbow, knee, ankle, wrist, radioulnar, metacarpophalangeal joint of finger, shoulder joint. (Do not confuse the motion at the elbow or wrist joints with that of the radioulnar joints.)
2. Take turns with a partner performing simple movements of the head, trunk, upper extremity, and lower extremity, and identify the planes and axes concerned.
3. Construct a simple device to illustrate the planes and axes in relation to the human body.
4. Study the soccer throw-in (Exercise 5.4 in Appendix G). The action between (a) and (b) represents the "force phase," and between (b) and (c) the "follow-through phase." Following the example given for the right metatarsophalangeal

Name of Joint	Type of Joint	Starting Position	Observed Joint Action	Plane of Motion	Axis of Motion
R. metatarso-phalangeal	Ellipsoid	Sl. hyper-extension	Hyperextension	Sagittal	Bilateral
R. ankle					
R. knee					
R. hip					
Lumbar spine					
R. shoulder					
R. elbow					
R. wrist					
R. fingers					

joint, complete the table above for the force phase. Repeat for the follow-through.

5. Measure the joint ranges of motion of 10 to 15 subjects for the movements indicated, using either a goniometer or a flexometer. Compare the results obtained with the averages given in Table 2.3. Explain why you think the differences among individuals exist. (The figure numbers refer to Appendix B.)
   a. Elbow flexion and hyperextension (Figure B.1)
   b. Shoulder flexion and hyperextension (Figure B.4b)
   c. Shoulder rotation (Figure B.5)
   d. Lateral flexion of trunk (Figure B.11b)
   e. Hip flexion (Figure B.7)
   f. Medial and lateral hip rotation (Figure B.8b)
   g. Plantar flexion and dorsiflexion (Figure B.10)
6. Select one or two joint actions (e.g., shoulder flexion and hip flexion). Perform a comparison study of the range of motion for the actions selected using two groups of people, such as the following.
   a. Males versus females
   b. Varsity athletes from different sports (swimming vs. basketball or wrestling vs. gymnastics)
   c. Different age groups (20–30 vs. 50–60)
   d. Joggers versus sedentary people

   Subjects in each group should be matched on the basis of age and gender. Are any "group" differences apparent? Explain your results.
7. Measure the range of motion in one ankle. Tape the ankle and repeat the measurements immediately and then following 10 to 15 minutes of exercise during which the ankle is used (e.g., jogging, basketball, handball). Record your results and compare the differences. What effect, if any, did the tape have on range of motion for plantar and dorsiflexion? Inversion and eversion? Using the results of your measurements as the basis, discuss the value of taping as a means of preventing ankle injuries.
8. Measure the ranges of motion at the hip and knee joints during the back somersault depicted in Exercise 5.6 in Appendix G.
   a. On each tracing, mark the location of the right hip, knee, and ankle joints with a dot. Also place a dot at the midpoint of the waist. Connect the dots with straight lines so as to make a stick figure of the leg.
   b. Using a protractor, measure and record the angles between the trunk and thigh, and the thigh and lower leg, on each tracing.
   c. Determine the range of motion for each joint action from start to end of takeoff [(a) to (c)] and from peak to touchdown [(b) to (e)].
   d. What effect does range of motion in these joints have on skillful performance of this technique? As a coach or teacher, what specific training techniques would you include in the program of the performer to improve the range of motion where needed?

CHAPTER 3

The Musculoskeletal System

The Musculature

OUTLINE

- ***Skeletal Muscle Structure***
  - Properties of Muscular Tissue
  - The Muscle Fiber
  - Slow- and Fast-Twitch Fibers
  - Muscular Attachment
  - Structural Classification of Muscles on the Basis of Fiber Arrangement
  - Effect of Muscle Structure on Force and Range of Motion
- ***Skeletal Muscle Function***
  - Line of Pull
  - Types of Contraction
  - Influence of Gravity
  - Length-Tension Relationship
  - Force-Velocity Relationship
  - Stretch-Shortening Cycle
- ***Coordination of the Muscular System***
  - Roles of Muscles
  - Cocontraction
  - Action of Biarticular Muscles
  - Types of Bodily Movements
- ***Methods of Studying the Actions of Muscles***
  - Conjecture and Reasoning
  - Dissection
  - Inspection and Palpation
  - Models
  - Muscle Stimulation
  - Electromyography (EMG)
  - Imaging
- ***Muscular Analysis***
- ***Laboratory Experiences***

OBJECTIVES

At the conclusion of this chapter, the student should be able to:

1. Describe the structure and properties of the whole muscle, fast- and slow-twitch muscle fiber, and the myofibril.
2. Explain how the relationship of the muscle's line of pull to the joint axis affects the movement produced by the muscle.
3. Describe the relationship between the skeletal muscle's fiber arrangement and its function.
4. Define the roles a muscle may play (agonist, antagonist, and synergist), and explain the cooperative action of muscles in controlling joint actions by naming and explaining the muscle roles in a specified movement.
5. Define the types of muscular contraction (concentric, eccentric, and static), and name and demonstrate each type of action.
6. Demonstrate an understanding of the influence of gravity and other external forces on muscular action by correctly analyzing several movement patterns in which these forces influence the muscular action.
7. Describe the various methods of studying muscle action, citing the advantages and disadvantages of each method.
8. State the force-velocity and length-tension relationships of muscular contraction, and explain the significance of these relationships in static and dynamic movements.
9. Identify the muscle groups active in a variety of motor skills.

Body parts are moved by external or internal forces. The internal force responsible for the movement and positioning of the bony segments of the body is the action of skeletal muscles. These muscles are able to serve this function because they can contract, they are attached to the bones, and they cross a joint. In addition, they are constructed of bundles of striated muscle fibers, which differ in both structure and function from the highly specialized cardiac muscle and from the smooth muscle of blood vessels, digestive organs, and urogenital organs.

SKELETAL MUSCLE STRUCTURE

Properties of Muscular Tissue

The properties of striated muscle tissue are extensibility, elasticity, and contractility. The first two enable a muscle to be stretched like an elastic band and, when the stretching force is discontinued, to return again to its normal resting length. Tendons, which are simply continuations of the muscle's connective tissue, also possess these properties. Contractility, the ability to shorten and produce tension at its ends, is a unique property possessed by muscle tissue only. The average muscle fiber can shorten to approximately one-half its resting length. It can also be stretched until it is approximately one-half again as long as its resting length. The range between the maximal and minimal lengths of a muscle fiber is known as the amplitude of its action. The elongation varies proportionately with the length of the fiber and inversely with its cross section.

The Muscle Fiber

A single muscle cell is a threadlike fiber about 1 to 20 inches in length and containing the cell nucleus, mitochondria (important in cell metabolism), myoglobin (similar to hemoglobin), and glycogen (form of sugar). In addition, microscopic examination has revealed that the fiber consists

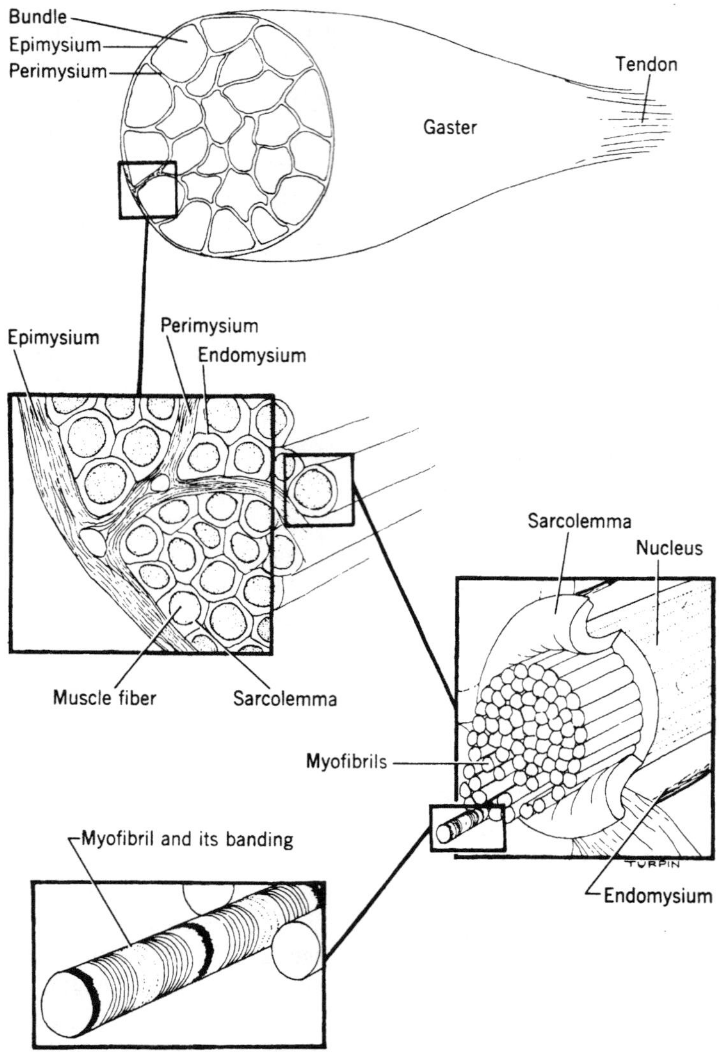

Figure 3.1 Architecture of a skeletal muscle and its fibers. *Source:* From *Morphogenesis of the Vertebrates,* by T. W. Torrey. Copyright © 1962, John Wiley & Sons, New York.

of many hundreds of myofibrils embedded in sarcoplasm, held together by a delicate membrane known as sarcolemma, which has the ability to propagate nerve impulses (Figure 3.1). Each fiber is enclosed within a thin connective tissue sheath called endomysium. The microscopic *myofibrils,* which are the contractile elements, are arranged in parallel formation within the fiber and are made of alternating dark and light bands that give the muscle fibers their striated appearance.

The electron microscope has revealed the striations to be a repeating pattern of bands and lines caused by an interdigitating arrangement of two sets of filaments. These myofilaments of contractile proteins, mainly actin (thin ones) and myosin (thick ones), when stimulated, slide past each other. This is due to the coupling and uncoupling of the cross-bridges, which appear as projections (heads) of the myosin filament attaching to the actin filaments. The myofibril is divided into a series of several sarcomeres, with each sarcomere consisting of the portion of the myofibril between two Z lines (Figure 3.2). The sarcomere is considered the functional contractile unit of skeletal muscle. A concentric contraction (shortening) occurs when the actin filament slides over the myosin filament, pulling the Z lines toward one another; an eccentric contraction is the reverse, with the actin filament sliding outward, resulting in the return of the sarcomere to its original length or longer. An isometric contraction involving no length change results from the continual breaking and rebuilding of the cross-bridges. This is a condensed and highly simplified explanation of contraction, a function that is the unique property of muscle tissue.

The muscle fibers are bound into bundles within bundles (see Figure 3.1). Each individual bundle of muscle fibers, called a *fasciculus,* is enclosed in a fibrous tissue sheath called *perimysium;* the group of bundles that constitutes a complete muscle is in turn encased within a tougher connective tissue sheath called *epimysium.* In long muscles whose fibers run parallel to the long axis of the muscle, the bundles form "chains," which function as though the individual fibers ran the entire length of the muscle. Each enclosing sheath (the endomysium, perimysium, and epimysium) is made of connective tissue, which contains elastic fibers arranged both in series (end to end) and parallel (in the same direction) to the contractile elements. The elements that are in series are those which are

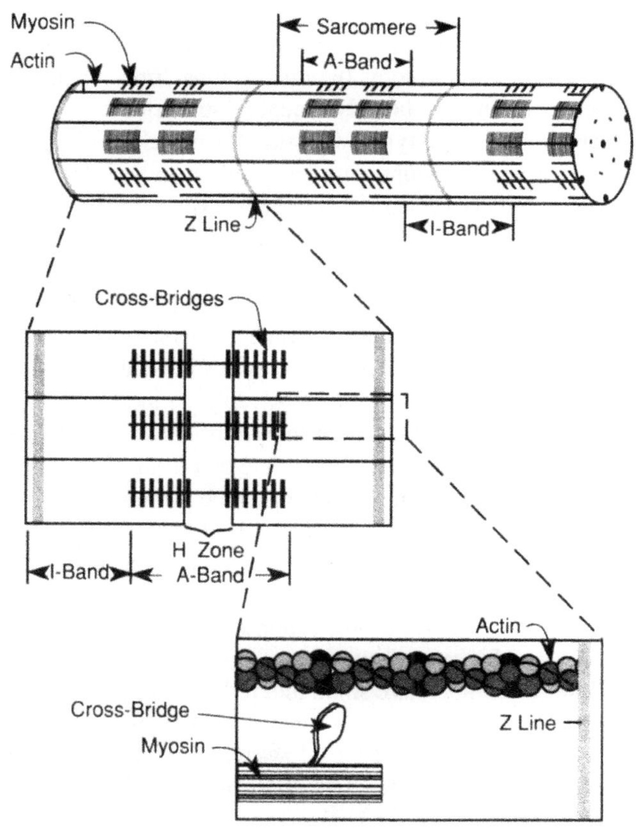

a. Magnification of single muscle fiber showing smaller fibers–myofibrils–in its sarcoplasm.

b. Myofibril magnified further to show thick and thin filaments composing it and producing its cross-striated appearance; dark A (anisotropic) bands alternate with light I (isotropic) bands; H zones, less dense midsections of A-bands; Z lines, more dense midlines of I-bands.

c. Scheme to show how myosin interacts with actin to shorten muscle fibers. The cross-bridges bond to the actin filaments and slide them toward the center of the sarcomere.

Figure 3.2 The single muscle fiber and its myofibrils. *Source:* From *Sports Physiology* (3rd ed.), by Richard W. Bowers & Edward L. Fox.

important in controlling how the tension is applied to the bony levers in moving a load. Those in parallel remain slack in contraction and have a negligible effect during stretching of the muscle fiber.

Muscles are attached to bone by means of their connective tissue, which continues beyond the muscle belly in the form of a tendon or an aponeurosis (a fibrous sheet). The muscle–tendon complex formed by the two tissue types provides the primary series elastic component of muscle. The stiffness of the tendon is largely responsible for the transmission of force from the contracting muscle to the affected bone.

Slow- and Fast-Twitch Fibers

Although four different fiber types (one slow- and three fast-twitch fibers) have been identified in human skeletal muscle, only the two major categories of slow- and fast-twitch fibers are pertinent for the study of kinesiology. In humans, most limb muscles contain a relatively equal distribution of each muscle fiber type, whereas the muscles of the back (i.e., posture muscles) contain more slow-twitch fibers. Where differences exist, the usual variation may be on the order of 2% to 10%. However, rare instances of significant variation between fiber types may be found among muscles and individuals, although not between genders.

The two primary types of fast-twitch muscle fiber are types IIa (fast oxidative glycolytic) and IIb (fast glycolytic). Fast-twitch muscle fibers are large and pale and have a less elaborate blood supply than slow-twitch muscle fibers. Once stimulated, fast-twitch fibers respond rapidly but fatigue easily. This characteristic makes them suitable for activities requiring intense responses over a short period of time, such as those responses found in sprints or weight-training exercises.

Slow-twitch fibers are small and red and have a rich blood supply. They also contain more myoglobin than fast-twitch fibers. Slow-twitch fibers take relatively longer to reach peak isometric tension (80–100 milliseconds [ms] vs. approximately 40–60 ms for fast-twitch fibers), are highly efficient, and do not fatigue easily. Slow-twitch fibers are suitable for activities of long duration, including posture and endurance events.

Research has shown that training does not produce an increase in the number of muscle fibers or major shifts in muscle fiber types. There is evidence that some shift from fast-twitch to slow-twitch fibers, or the reverse, can occur with training (MacIntosh et al., 2006). Training does result in muscle fiber hypertrophy and may change some fast-twitch fiber types, but these changes, such as increased endurance and a greater number of capillaries, are reversible when use is discontinued. With aging, muscle fibers tend to atrophy, although this loss is not as great as once thought. As some fibers are lost, others may hypertrophy to compensate. Most serious sarcopenia (muscle loss) occurs with inactivity. It has been found that even with sarcopenia, muscle-fiber type distribution does not change (Frontera et al., 2008). This is one reason that activity that places demands on the muscle fibers should be done on a lifelong basis.

Muscular Attachment

Historically, anatomy texts designated attachments of the two ends of a muscle as "origin" and "insertion." The origin is usually characterized by stability and closeness of the muscle fibers to the bone. It is usually the more proximal of the two attachments. The insertion, on the other hand, is usually the distal attachment; it frequently involves a relatively long tendon, and the bone into which the muscle's tendon inserts is ordinarily the one that moves. It should be understood, however, that the muscle does not pull in one direction or the other. When it contracts, it exerts equal force on the two attachments and attempts to pull them toward each other. Which bone is to remain stationary and which one is to move depends on the purpose of the movement. A muscle spanning the inside of a hinge joint, for instance, tends to draw the two bones toward one another. However, most precision movements require that the proximal bone be stabilized, whereas the distal bone performs the movement. The stabilization of the proximal bone is achieved by the action of other muscles. Sometimes the greater weight or the more limited mobility of the proximal structure is sufficient to stabilize it against the pull of the contracting muscles.

Reverse Muscle Action

Students often receive the impression that there is some physiological reason for a muscle to pull in a single direction. They fail to grasp the concept of a muscle merely contracting, and do not realize that it cannot pull in a predetermined direction. This misconception makes it difficult for students to understand seeming exceptions. Actually, in many movements the insertion or distal attachment of the muscle is stationary and the origin or proximal attachment is the one that moves. Such is the case in the familiar act of performing pull-ups. The movement of the elbow joint is flexion, but it is the upper arm that moves toward the forearm, just the reverse of what happens when one lifts a book from the table. The grasp of the hands on the bar serves to immobilize the forearm, and thus it provides a stable base for the contracting muscles. To avoid the erroneous idea of a muscle always pulling from its insertion toward its origin, the following terminology for muscular attachments is used in this text.

Terminology for Muscular Attachments

Attachments of muscles of the extremities:
- Proximal attachment
- Distal attachment

Attachments of muscles of the head, neck, and trunk:

Upper attachment Lower attachment	muscles whose line of pull is more or less vertical—that is, parallel with the long axis of the body
Medial attachment Lateral attachment	for muscles whose line of pull is more or less horizontal

Attachments of the diaphragm:
- Peripheral attachment
- Central attachment

Structural Classification of Muscles on the Basis of Fiber Arrangement

The arrangement of the fibers and the method of attachment vary considerably among different muscles. These structural variations form the basis for a classification of the skeletal muscles.

Longitudinal

This is a long, straplike muscle whose fibers lie parallel to its long axis. Two examples are the sartorius, which slants across the front of the thigh, and the rectus abdominis on the front of the abdomen (see Figures 7.15 and 9.17).

Quadrate or Quadrilateral (*Figures 3.3e and f*)

Muscles of this type are four sided and usually flat. They consist of parallel fibers. Examples include the pronator quadratus on the front of the wrist and the rhomboid muscle between the spine and the scapula.

Triangular (*Figure 3.3d*)

This is a relatively flat type of muscle whose fibers radiate from a narrow attachment at one end to a broad attachment at the other. The pectoralis

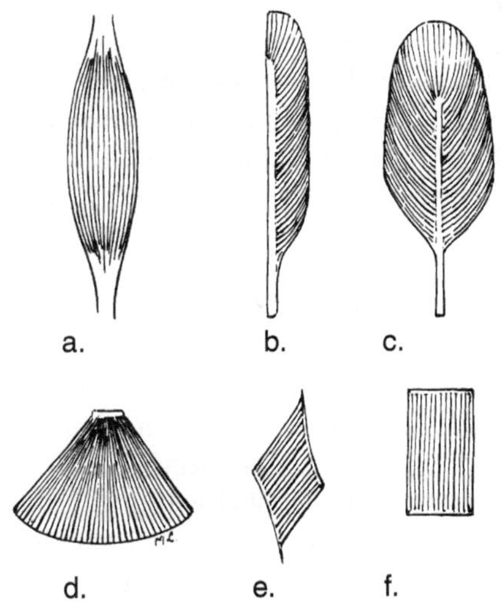

Figure 3.3 Examples of muscles of different shapes and internal structure: (a) fusiform or spindle; (b) pennate; (c) bipennate; (d) triangular or fan shaped; (e) rhomboidal (quadrate); (f) rectangular (quadrate).

major on the front of the chest is an excellent example.

Fusiform or Spindle Shaped (Figure 3.3a)

This is usually a rounded muscle that tapers at either end. It may be long or short, large or small. Good examples are the brachialis and the brachioradialis muscles of the upper extremity.

Pennate (Figure 3.3b)

In this type of muscle, a series of short, parallel, featherlike fibers extends diagonally from the side of a long tendon, giving the muscle as a whole the appearance of a wing feather. Examples include the extensor digitorum longus and tibialis posterior muscles of the leg.

Bipennate (Figure 3.3c)

This double pennate muscle is characterized by a long central tendon with the fibers extending diagonally in pairs from either side of the tendon. It resembles a symmetrical tail feather. Examples include the flexor hallucis longus and rectus femoris of the leg and thigh, respectively.

Multipennate

In this type of muscle several tendons are present, with the muscle fibers running diagonally between them. The middle portion of the deltoid muscle of the shoulder and upper arm is a prime example of a multipennate muscle (see Figures 5.11 and 5.14).

Effect of Muscle Structure on Force and Range of Motion

The force a muscle can exert is proportional to its physiological cross section, a measure that accounts for the diameter of every fiber and whose size depends on the number and thickness of the fibers. A broad, thick, longitudinal muscle exerts more force than a thin one, but a pennate muscle of the same thickness as a longitudinal muscle can exert greater force. The oblique arrangement of the fibers in the various classifications of pennate muscle allows for a larger number of fibers than in comparable sizes of the other classifications. Pennate muscles are the most common type of skeletal muscle and predominate when forceful movements are needed.

The range through which a muscle shortens depends on the length of its fibers, with the average muscle fiber capable of shortening to half its resting length. Those long muscles with fibers longitudinally arranged along the long axis of the muscle, such as the sartorius, can exert force over a longer distance than muscles with shorter fibers. Muscles of the pennate type, with their oblique fiber arrangement and short fiber length, can exert their superior force through only a short range.

SKELETAL MUSCLE FUNCTION

The basis for all muscle function is the ability of muscular tissue to contract. This should be kept in mind as various aspects of muscular function are considered.

Line of Pull

The movement that the contracting muscle produces—flexion, extension, abduction, adduction, or rotation—is determined by two factors: the type of joint that it spans and the relation of the muscle's line of pull to the joint. For instance, the contraction of a muscle whose line of pull is directly anterior to the knee joint may cause the joint to extend, whereas a muscle whose line of pull is anterior to the elbow joint may cause this joint to flex. The possible axes of motion are, of course, determined by the structure of the joint itself. It will be recalled that, from the anatomical standing position, hinge joints have only a bilateral axis, and condyloid (ovoid) joints have both a bilateral and an anteroposterior axis. Ball-and-socket joints have three axes, bilateral and anteroposterior and vertical (longitudinal), whereas pivot joints have a vertical axis only.

A muscle whose line of pull is lateral to the hip joint is a potential abductor of the thigh, but muscles whose lines of pull are lateral to the elbow joint cannot cause abduction of the forearm because the construction of the elbow joint is such that no provision is made for abduction or adduction. Because it is a hinge joint, its only axis of motion is a bilateral one, and the only movements possible are flexion and extension.

The importance of the relation of a muscle's action line to the joint's axis of motion is especially seen in some of the muscles that act on triaxial joints. Occasionally it happens that a muscle's line of pull for one of its secondary movements shifts from one side of the joint's center of motion to the other during the course of the movement. For instance, the clavicular portion of the pectoralis major is primarily a flexor, but it also adducts the humerus. When the arm is elevated sideward (abducted) to a position slightly above shoulder level, however, the line of pull of some of the fibers of the clavicular portion shifts from below to above the anteroposterior axis of the shoulder joint (Figure 3.4). Contraction of these fibers in this position contributes to abduction of the humerus, rather than to adduction. Similarly, several muscles or parts of muscles of the hip joint appear to reverse their customary function. Steindler (1970) pointed out that as the adductor longus adducts the hip joint, it also flexes it until the flexion exceeds 70 degrees. Beyond this point the adductor longus helps extend the hip.

It is not uncommon to classify and name muscles according to the relation of their line of pull to the joint structure. In other words, muscles whose line of pull is such that they produce flexion are called flexors, and those in a position to cause extension are extensors. Similarly there would also be abductors, adductors, and rotators. The difficulty with this type of classification is that it may mislead the student into believing that the muscle is responsible for the related joint action under all circumstances, when in reality this is not the case. The biceps brachii muscle, for instance, is usually listed as a flexor and supinator of the forearm, when in fact the results of electromyographic studies have established that the biceps plays little if any part in flexion of the prone forearm or supination of the extended forearm unless the movements are resisted (Basmajian & DeLuca, 1985). This example is not unusual. Many situations occur in which the presence or absence of resistance governs a muscle's participation in a joint action. Other factors, such as the starting position for the joint action, the direction of the movement, and the speed of the movement may also alter a muscle's involvement in the joint action.

Knowing the general location of a muscle with respect to the joint axis—anterior, superior, lateral, or medial—and knowing the line of pull of the muscle is important information for deducing possible muscle participation during a body movement, but confirmation of those muscle actions must rely on the evidence of electromyography.

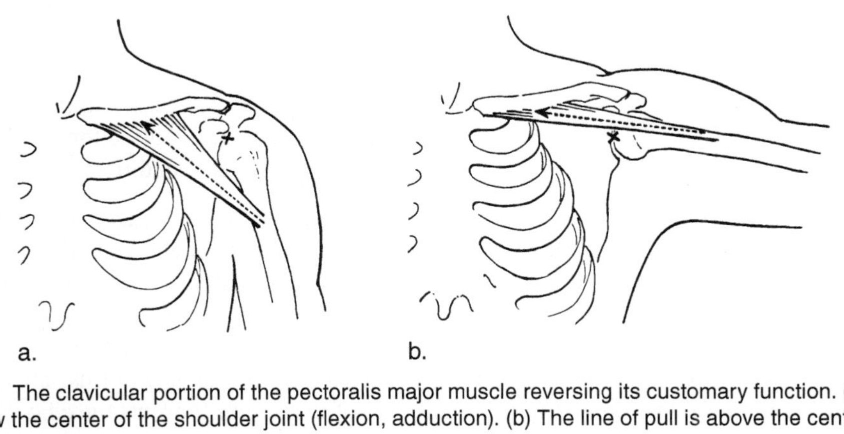

Figure 3.4 The clavicular portion of the pectoralis major muscle reversing its customary function. (a) The line of pull is below the center of the shoulder joint (flexion, adduction). (b) The line of pull is above the center of the shoulder joint (abduction).

Angle of Attachment

The efficiency of a muscle in producing movement at a joint is also affected by the angle of attachment of a muscle to the stationary bone. If the angle of attachment is very shallow (the muscle lies along the line of the bone), most of the tension developed in the muscle will produce a force pulling along the bone. In other words, this muscle will have a very large stabilizing component. Force produced by this muscle will tend to stabilize the joint rather than produce motion. Conversely, a muscle whose angle of attachment is fairly large will have a much larger rotary component of force. The development of tension in this muscle will produce a force that will cause action at the joint. In many muscles the angle between muscle and bone changes as movement occurs. A good example of this is the biceps, whose tendon can be easily palpated where it attaches to the radius. Starting from the neutral position, one can feel that the biceps tendon lies almost parallel to the humerus. As the forearm is slowly moved through elbow flexion, it is possible to feel the change in the angle between the biceps tendon and the radius. When the elbow is at a 90-degree angle, notice that the biceps tendon forms approximately a 90-degree angle with the radius. In this position, all of the force generated by the biceps can act to produce joint motion. As elbow flexion continues beyond 90 degrees, notice that the angle between the biceps tendon and the radius again begins to decrease as the line of pull shifts closer to the bone. As this change occurs, the biceps is becoming less efficient at producing joint motion.

Types of Contraction

Because the word *contract* literally means to "draw together" or to shorten, the nature of muscular contraction may cause some initial confusion. A muscle contraction occurs whenever the muscle fibers generate tension in themselves, a situation that may exist when the muscle is actually *shortening, remaining the same length, or lengthening.*

Concentric or Shortening Contraction

Concentric (toward the middle) *contraction* occurs when the tension generated by the muscle is sufficient to overcome a resistance and to move the body segment of one attachment toward the segment of its other attachment. As the arm is raised sideward, the abductor shoulder muscles shorten to overcome the resistance of the arm. The muscle actually shortens and, when one end is stabilized, the other pulls the bone to which it is attached and turns it about the joint axis (Figure 3.5c).

Eccentric or Lengthening Contraction

When a muscle slowly lengthens as it gives in to an external force (such as gravity) that is greater than the contractile force it is exerting, it is in *eccentric* (away from the middle) *contraction.* The term *lengthening* is misleading because in most instances the muscle does not actually lengthen. It merely returns from its shortened condition to its normal resting length (Figure 3.5a). The abductor shoulder muscles are in eccentric contraction when the arm is slowly lowered from an abducted position. In most instances in which muscles contract eccentrically, the muscles are acting as a "brake," or resistive force, against the moving force of gravity or other external forces. When the muscles contract in this manner, they are said to perform negative work.

Isometric or Static Contraction

Isometric means "equal length." Tension of the muscle in partial or complete contraction without any appreciable change in length is *isometric contraction.* Isometric contraction is likely to occur under two different conditions.

1. Muscles that are antagonistic to each other contract with equal strength, thus balancing or counteracting each other. The part affected is held tensely in place without moving. Tensing the biceps to show off its bulge is an example of this. The contraction of the triceps prevents the elbow from further flexing.

2. A muscle is held in either partial or maximal contraction against another force, such as the pull of gravity or an external mechanical or muscular force. Examples of this are holding a book with outstretched arm, a tug-of-war between two equally matched opponents, and attempting to move an object that is too heavy to move.

Isotonic Contraction

Isotonic means "equal tension." *Isotonic contraction* is a contraction in which the tension remains constant as the muscle shortens or lengthens. It is commonly, although erroneously, used as a synonym for either *eccentric* or *concentric contraction.* The latter terms, however, do not indicate the degree of tension; they merely indicate an increase or decrease in length.

Isokinetic Contraction

Literally, *isokinetic* means "equal or same motion" (*iso* + *kinetic*). Through the use of special equipment, it is possible to have maximum muscle effort at the same speed throughout the entire range of motion of the related lever. The response of the muscles in maximum contraction to the "accommodating resistance" of the machinery is called *isokinetic contraction.*

Influence of Gravity

Movements of the body or its segments may be in the direction of gravitational forces (downward), opposing gravity (upward), or perpendicular to gravity (horizontal). It is essential to consider the direction and speed of the movement when identifying the nature of the muscular involvement of any movement. The muscles may be contracting, either to provide the force for a movement or the force to resist and control the movement, or they may be completely relaxed (Figure 3.5). It may surprise the student to learn that the muscles used when placing a book on a low table or a suitcase on the floor are the same as those used for lifting it. They are used in a different way, however. When the book or suitcase is lifted, the muscles provide the force, and the weight of the object (gravity) is the resistance. In this case the muscles shorten in concentric contraction. When the object is slowly lowered, however, the muscles lengthen in eccentric contraction as they resist, but gradually give in to, the force of gravity. Without the muscular resistance,

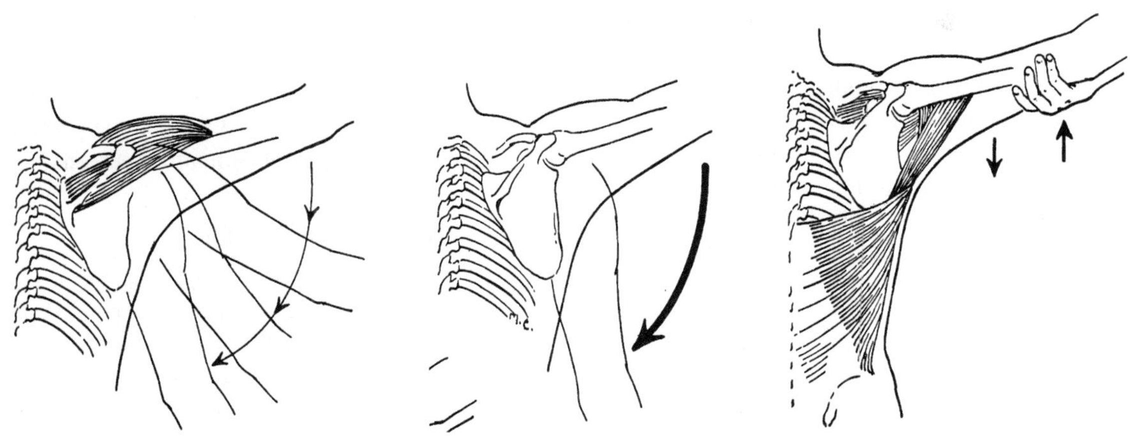

Figure 3.5 Influence of gravitational force on muscular action in sideward depression of the arm (adduction of the humerus): (a) eccentric contraction of the abductors in slow lowering of the arm; (b) absence of muscular action when the arm is dropped to the side; (c) concentric contraction of the adductors when the movement is performed against resistance.

the force of gravity would lower the object at a far more rapid rate! Another example of the influence of gravity on muscular action is the action of the lower extremity muscles when one lowers the body weight by bending the knees to assume a squat or semi-squat position and then returns to the erect position. As the body is lowered, the extensor muscles of the hips and knees are undergoing eccentric contraction. They are indeed lengthening in this instance, yet their tension is increasing as they assume the burden of the body weight and gradually allow it to be lower in a controlled manner. When the joint action is reversed and the body weight is lifted, the extensor muscles are contracting concentrically until the hips and knees are straight and the body is erect.

As has been demonstrated, any slow, controlled movement in the downward direction of gravity's force uses the same muscles in eccentric contraction that would be used in concentric contraction to perform the opposite upward movement (against gravity). Slow lowering of the forearm from a flexed position to one of extension is controlled by eccentric contraction of the elbow flexors, the same muscles that, by contracting concentrically, cause flexion. A forceful movement downward does not follow this pattern, however. When done forcefully, as in the downswing of a golf swing, the same movement of elbow extension uses the elbow extensors in concentric contraction, because gravitational pull is now being exceeded (Figure 3.6).

Muscular involvement in movements performed horizontally is not affected by gravity in the manner just described. Regardless of the force or speed of the movement, the muscle force for extension of the forearm at the elbow in the transverse plane is provided by the elbow extensors. The only exception to this is seen when one is opposing an external force other than gravity, and it proves to be too strong. In a tug-of-war, for instance, the weaker opponents will find their elbows being pulled out straight in spite of themselves. The elbow flexor muscles are in eccentric contraction as they attempt to resist the force causing the extension at the elbow.

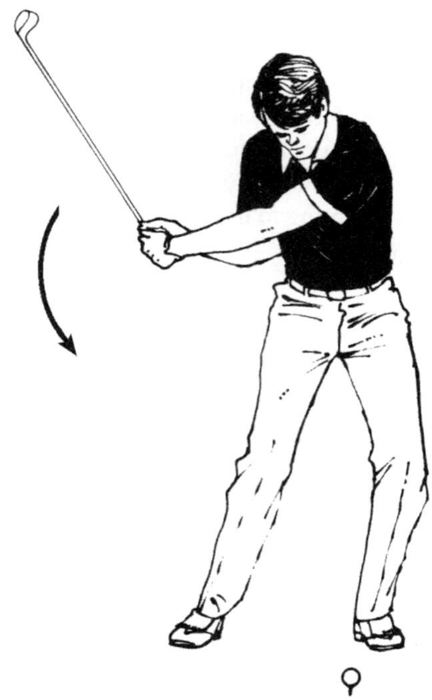

Figure 3.6 Example of a rapid downward action utilizing a concentric muscle contraction.

Finally, at times the movement of the body or its segments occurs without muscular action. In these instances the external force causing the movement is not resisted by eccentric muscle action. Examples are allowing the force of gravity to cause the arm to drop to the side from a flexed or abducted position (Figure 3.5b) and the passive moving of a body segment by another person.

Length-Tension Relationship

There is an optimum length at which a muscle, when stimulated, can exert maximum tension. This length varies somewhat according to both the muscle's structure and its function but, as a general rule, it is slightly greater than the resting length of the muscle. Lengths that are either greater or less produce less tension. This relationship applies for all three types of contraction: isometric, concentric, or eccentric. A typical length-tension curve is depicted in Figure 3.7. The maximum resting length occurs

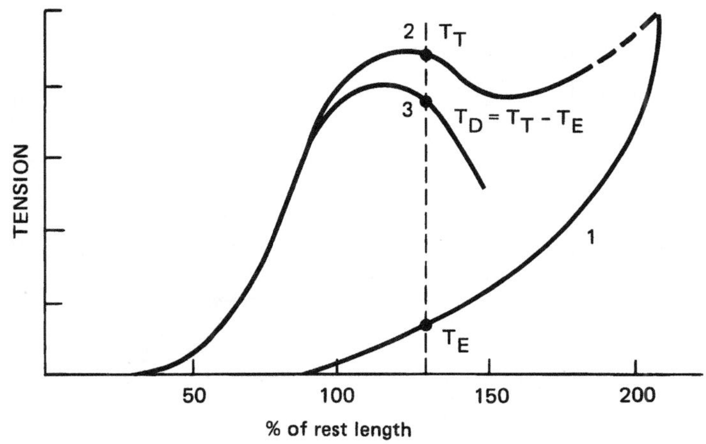

Figure 3.7 Length-tension curves for isolated muscle. Curve 1, passive elastic tension (T_E) in a muscle passively stretched to increasing lengths. Curve 2, total tension (T_T) exerted by muscle contracting actively from increasingly greater initial lengths. Curve 3, developed tension calculated by subtracting elastic tension values on Curve 1 from total tension values at equivalent lengths on Curve 2; i.e., $T_D = T_T - T_E$. *Source:* From *Scientific Bases of Human Movement* (3rd ed.), by B. Gowitzke & M. Milner. Copyright © 1988, Williams & Wilkins, Baltimore, MD. Reprinted by permission.

at 100%. Curve 1 represents the tension generated when the muscle is passively stretched, and curve 2 represents the total tension generated in the muscle. The active tension of the muscle would thus be the difference between the passive and the total tension, curve 2 minus curve 1. This relationship suggests that when maximum force is desired, the muscle should be longer than the resting length. It should also be noted that a longer tendon can generate a higher level of stored elasticity than a shorter tendon. The Achilles tendon, for instance, is able to generate greater velocity than the shorter quadriceps tendon.

Other factors such as the muscle's angle of pull also must be considered. It is rare for the angle of pull for optimum force application to occur when the muscle is in the resting position.

Force-Velocity Relationship

As the speed of a muscular contraction increases, the force it is able to exert decreases. The velocity of contraction is maximal when the load is zero, and the load is maximal when the velocity is zero (Figure 3.8). For any given load there is an optimum velocity that is somewhere between the slowest and fastest rates. As the load increases, the optimum rate decreases. So does the need for more cross-bridges. Because it takes time for the cross-bridge sites to form or break down, the inverse relationship between load and rate is readily understood. Thus, if an activity requires the development of large forces, only a small amount of muscle shortening should be expected. If, on the other hand, high limb or implement velocities are needed, then little force should be expected from the contracting muscles.

Stretch-Shortening Cycle

The synergistic response of a muscle and associated tendinous structures gives rise to the phenomenon known as the stretch-shortening cycle. Both muscle and tendon possess elastic properties. That is, when they are stretched, they store energy and will release this energy when they return to their original length. When a concentric muscle contraction is preceded by an active stretch, the elastic energy stored in the stretch phase is available for use in the contractile phase. The work done by the concentric contraction of muscle immediately following a prestretch is greater than that done by muscles contracting from their resting length. In addition, the work done increases with the speed of the stretch.

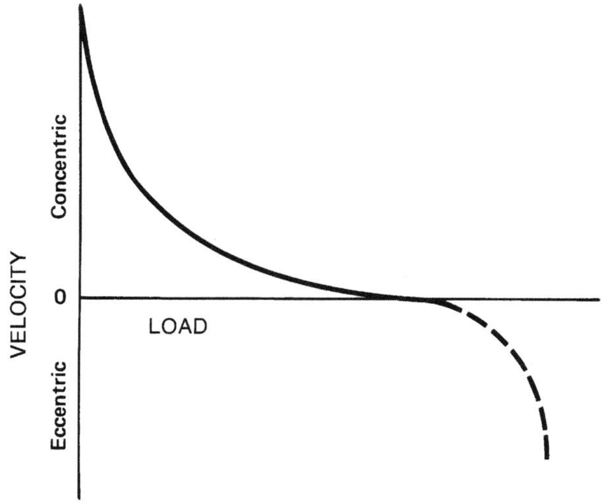

Figure 3.8 Force-velocity relationship. As the velocity of concentric contraction increases, the force that can be exerted decreases. When the velocity drops to zero, the contraction is isometric. In eccentric contraction, tension increases with the increased speed of lengthening.

In the muscle–tendon complex, the tendons are most responsive to speed of stretch and provide the largest percentage of elastic energy release. Tendons, therefore, are the prime providers of the series elastic component. A parallel elastic component of muscle is also active when a prestretch is applied. This parallel component is considered to be the result of cross-bridge and fascicle elasticity (the contractile elements) and possibly the stretch reflex (see Chapter 4).

Many common movement patterns make use of the stretch-shortening cycle to enhance the effects of muscle action. The countermovement action common in the preparatory phase of many sport motions is an example of this. A fast squat before a jump, a rapid backswing before a tennis serve, or a kick are all examples of the utilization of the stretch-shortening cycle and the series elastic component of the muscle–tendon complex. Training using activities that make use of the stretch-shortening cycle have been found to produce gain in muscle fiber force and contraction velocity. Using training methods such as plyometrics and jump training may increase power production through training the elastic as well as the contractile elements of muscle.

COORDINATION OF THE MUSCULAR SYSTEM

An effective, purposeful movement of the body or any of its parts involves considerable muscular activity in addition to that of the muscles that are directly responsible for the movement itself. To begin with, the muscles causing the movement must have a stable base. This means that the bone (or bones) not engaged in the movement but providing attachment for one end of such muscles must be stabilized by other muscles. In some movements, such as those in which the hands are used at a high level, the upper arms may need to be maintained in an elevated position. This necessitates contraction of the shoulder muscles to support the weight of the arms. Many muscles, especially those of biaxial and triaxial joints, can cause movements involving more than one axis, yet it may be that only one of their actions is needed for the movement in question. A similar situation exists in regard to the muscles of the scapula. A muscle cannot voluntarily choose to effect one of its movements and not another; it must depend on other muscles to contract and prevent the unwanted movement. Even a simple movement such as threading a needle or hammering a nail may require the cooperative action of a relatively large number of muscles, each performing its own particular task in producing a single, well-coordinated movement.

Roles of Muscles

Muscles have various roles. Their particular roles in a given movement depend on the requirements of that movement. These roles are designated prime movers (or agonists), antagonists, and synergists. Furthermore, if one concedes that the negative function of remaining relaxed can be viewed as a role, then the muscles that are antagonistic to the movers may also be included as participants in the total cooperative effort. The definitions of these roles are as follows.

Movers, or Agonists

A mover is a muscle that is directly responsible for producing a movement. In the majority of movements there are several movers, some of them of greater importance than others. These are the principal, or prime, movers. The muscles that help perform the movement but seem to be of less importance, or contract only under certain circumstances, are the assistant movers. Muscles that help only when an extra amount of force is needed, as when a movement is performed against resistance, are sometimes called emergency muscles. This distinction between the various muscles that contribute to a movement is an arbitrary one. There may well be some difference of opinion as to whether a muscle is a prime or an assistant mover in a given movement.

Synergists

The term *synergy* is often used to describe muscles in various ways, from mutual neutralizer to stabilizer. In this text, synergistic muscle action will be used to indicate cooperative muscle functioning in various roles. Muscles acting as synergists may fill one of several roles. The way in which a muscle aids in the production of the desired motion determines its synergistic role.

Stabilizing, Fixator, and Supporting Muscles
This group includes the muscles that contract statically to steady or support some part of the body against the pull of the contracting muscles, against the pull of gravity, or against the effect of momentum and recoil in certain vigorous movements. One of the most common functions of stabilizers is steadying or fixating the bone to which a contracting muscle is attached. It is only by the stabilizing of one of its attachments that the muscle is able to cause an effective movement of the bone at which it has its other attachment (Figure 3.9). The term *supporting* may be used when a limb or the trunk must be supported against the pull of gravity

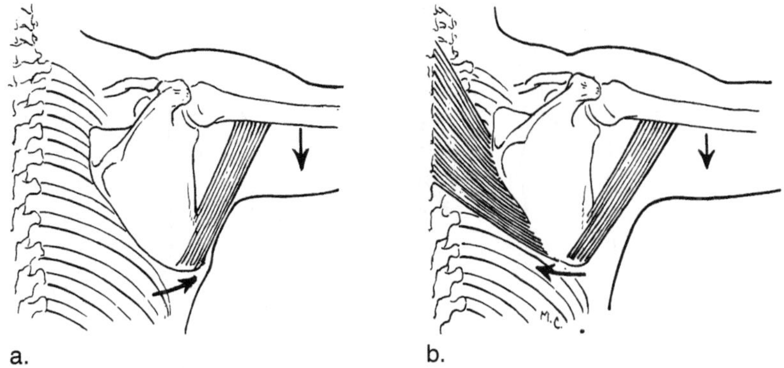

Figure 3.9 If the scapula were not stabilized, the teres major would increase the upward rotation of the scapula as it adducted the humerus. This dual action on the humerus and scapula is shown in (a). In (b) the scapula is stabilized by the scapular adductors and downward rotators. This permits the teres major to concentrate its force on the adduction of the humerus.

while a distal segment such as the hand, foot, or head is engaging in the essential movement.

Neutralizers A neutralizer is a muscle that acts to prevent an undesired action of one of the movers. Thus, if a muscle both flexes and abducts, but only flexion is desired in the movement, an adductor contracts to prevent the abduction action of the mover.

Occasionally two of the movers have one action in common but can also perform second actions that are antagonistic to each other. For instance, one muscle may upward rotate and adduct while the other may downward rotate and adduct. When they contract together to cause adduction, their rotary functions counteract each other (Figure 3.10). Muscles that behave this way in a movement are mutual synergists as well as movers.

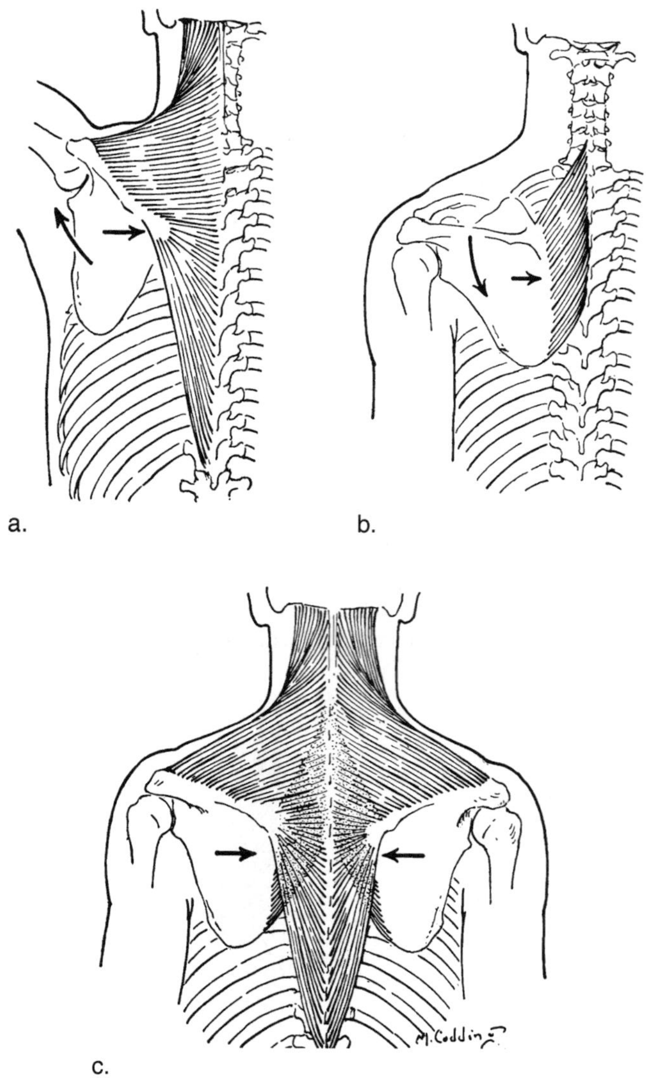

Figure 3.10 The trapezius and rhomboids as mutual movers and neutralizers. (a) The trapezius alone adducts the scapula and rotates it upward. (b) The rhomboids alone adduct the scapula and rotate it downward. (c) Together the trapezius and rhomboids adduct the scapula without rotating it either upward or downward.

Antagonists

Muscles that have an effect opposite to that of movers, or agonists, are labeled antagonists. Because they are located on the opposite side of the joint from the movers, they are also called contralateral muscles. The elbow flexors, located on the anterior arm, are antagonistic to the elbow extensors located on the posterior arm. When the forearm is extended at the elbow, as in doing a push-up, the extensors are the movers and contract concentrically to provide the force for the movement. The flexors are the antagonists and are relaxed. In the return movement, the letdown, the joint action at the elbow is flexion but the flexors do not contract—they remain relaxed. The contracting muscles, once again, are the extensors, but now they are contracting eccentrically to resist gravity and control the speed of the elbow flexion. When a body segment is moved by muscular effort, the contracting muscles are the movers in concentric contraction. When movement of a segment is effected by the force of gravity and resisted by muscle force, the contracting muscles are the antagonists in eccentric contraction.

Now that the general rule has been stated, it is necessary to describe what may at first appear to be a contradiction. If a movement performed with great force and rapidity is not checked, it will subject the ligamentous reinforcements of the joint to sudden strain. The tissues would probably be severely damaged. This is particularly true of quick movements of the arm or leg because of the tremendous momentum that can be developed in a long lever. This is often referred to as a ballistic movement, which by definition is a movement carried on by its own momentum. To prevent injury from the momentum of the limbs, the muscles that are antagonistic to the movers contract momentarily to check the movement. As they contract, the movers relax, if indeed they have not already relaxed, allowing momentum to complete the movement. The situation is a little like taking the foot off the accelerator to put it on the brake. At the moment when the movement is being checked, the so-called antagonistic muscles are not truly antagonistic. In a vigorous movement, the antagonistic muscles may be said to perform two functions. Their first function is to relax in order to permit the movement to be made without hindrance; their second function is to act as a brake at the completion of the movement and, by doing so, to protect the joint.

Summary of Muscle Classification Based on Role in Total Movement

Mover or agonist: A muscle that is directly responsible for effecting a movement.

Synergist:

- *Fixator, stabilizer, supporting muscle:* Muscles that contract statically to steady or to support some part of the body against the pull of contracting muscles, the pull of gravity, or any other force that interferes with the desired movement.
- *Neutralizer:* A muscle that acts to prevent an undesired action of one of the movers.

Antagonist: A muscle that causes the opposite movement from that of the movers.

Example of the Different Roles of Muscles in a Total Movement

Let us consider the movement of the right upper arm when playing shuffleboard (pushing a disk with a cue). The movement of the humerus at the shoulder joint is flexion, and this is accompanied by slight upward rotation and abduction of the scapula. The *movers of the humerus* are the anterior deltoid, the clavicular portion of the pectoralis major, and the coracobrachialis. (Look up these terms if you are not yet familiar with them.) The two former muscles are also inward rotators of the humerus, but because this movement is not desired, it must be prevented. The infraspinatus and the teres minor take care of this. Therefore, they are serving as *neutralizers* in this pushing action. Meanwhile, the scapula is rotating upward through the action of the serratus anterior and trapezium II and IV, which are serving as *shoulder girdle movers.* Trapezius II, which is an elevator as well as an upward rotator of the scapula, and trapezium IV, which is a depressor as well as an upward rotator, mutually neutralize each other with respect to elevation and depression while they are cooperating in rotating the scapula upward. Hence they are both *movers* and *mutual neutralizers.*

Consider the movers of the humerus once again, keeping in mind that muscles tend to pull both their distal and proximal ends toward each other. Note that the proximal attachments of both the anterior deltoid and the pectoralis major are side by side on the anterior border of the clavicle. As they contract, they not only raise the humerus forward but also tend to pull the clavicle laterally, a movement that would put a strain on the sternoclavicular joint. They are prevented from doing this by the action of the subclavius muscle, which pulls the clavicle medially and thus serves as a stabilizer. So in this simple pushing movement we see that we have muscles acting as movers, neutralizers, and stabilizers, which, by their cooperative action, ensure an efficient movement.

Cocontraction

The patterns of muscle activation that can occur in the production of human movement are vast in number. Recent research in muscle activation has shown that the relationships between muscle actions is, by nature, task dependent. That is, the relationships will depend on the nature of the motion to be produced. Simultaneous cocontraction or coactivation of agonist and antagonist muscles across one or more joints does occur. Cocontraction is most often associated with stabilization, either during postural loading or in dynamic, unstable situations. The cocontraction of the abdominal muscles, for instance, helps stabilize the trunk during lifting tasks. In a similar fashion, cocontraction of the muscles of the arm stabilizes the arm when learning an accuracy task (Granata & Marras, 2000; Gribble et al., 2003).

Cocontraction of biarticular muscles is common. The muscles that act as an agonist–antagonist pair for the motion of one joint often reverse roles for the second joint. In this situation, both muscles are active, but for different reasons. A more detailed description of the actions of biarticular muscles follows.

Action of Biarticular Muscles

Another type of coordination of the muscular system may be seen in the action of the biarticular muscles—that is, the muscles that pass over and act on two joints. Examples of these are the hamstrings (the semitendinosus, the semimembranosus, and the biceps femoris), which flex the leg at the knee and extend the thigh at the hip; the rectus femoris, which flexes the thigh and extends the leg; the sartorius, which flexes both the thigh and the leg; the gastrocnemius, which helps flex the leg in addition to its primary function of extending the foot; and the long flexors and extensors of the fingers. The latter are actually multijoint muscles because they cross the wrist and at least two of the joints of the fingers. A characteristic of all these muscles, whether they act on joints that flex in the same direction, as in the case of the wrist and fingers, or in the opposite direction, as in the case of the knee and hip, is that they are not long enough to permit complete movement in both joints at the same time. This results in the tension of one muscle being transmitted to the other, in much the same manner that a downward pull on a rope that passes through an overhead pulley is transmitted in the form of a pull in the reverse direction to the rope on the other side of the pulley. Thus, if the hamstrings contract to help extend the hip, tension in the form of a stretch is placed on the rectus femoris, causing it to extend the knee. Or if the rectus femoris contracts to help flex the hip, tension in the form of a stretch is placed on the hamstrings, causing them to flex the knee. This is a simplified version of what in actuality is a rather complex coordination.

When monoarticular (one-joint) muscles contract, their shortening is accompanied by a corresponding loss of tension. In quick movements of the limbs, monoarticular muscles rapidly lose their tension. The advantage of biarticular muscles is that they can continue to exert tension without shortening. The biarticular muscles have two different patterns of action, described as *concurrent* and *countercurrent* movements.

Concurrent Movements

An example of concurrent movement is seen in the simultaneous extension of the hip and knee and also in the simultaneous flexion of these joints. As the muscles contract, they act on each other in such a way that they do not lose length; thus their tension is retained. It is as though the pull traveled up one muscle and down the other in a continuous circuit. In simultaneous extension of the hip and knee, for instance, the rectus femoris's loss of tension at the distal or knee end is balanced by a gain in tension at the proximal or hip end. Similarly, the hamstrings, which are losing tension at their proximal end, are gaining it at their distal end.

Countercurrent Movements

The countercurrent pattern presents a different picture. In this type of movement, while one of the biarticular muscles shortens rapidly at both joints, its antagonist lengthens correspondingly and thereby gains tension at both ends. An example of this action is seen in the rapid loss of tension in the rectus femoris and corresponding gain of tension in the hamstrings when the hip is flexed and the knee is extended simultaneously. A vigorous kick is a dramatic illustration of this kind of muscle action. The backward swing of the lower extremity preparatory to kicking is a less spectacular but equally valid example. The forward swing in walking is another. In both patterns of movement the monoarticular and biarticular muscles appear to supplement each other and thus, by their cooperative action, produce smooth, coordinated, efficient movements (Figure 3.11).

When a biarticular muscle contracts, it acts on both joints it crosses. If action is desired in only one joint, the other joint must be stabilized by another muscle or by some external force. In such circumstances, Basmajian (Basmajian & DeLuca, 1985) found that the rectus femoris shows maximum activity in either pure hip flexion or pure knee extension, and the medial hamstrings,

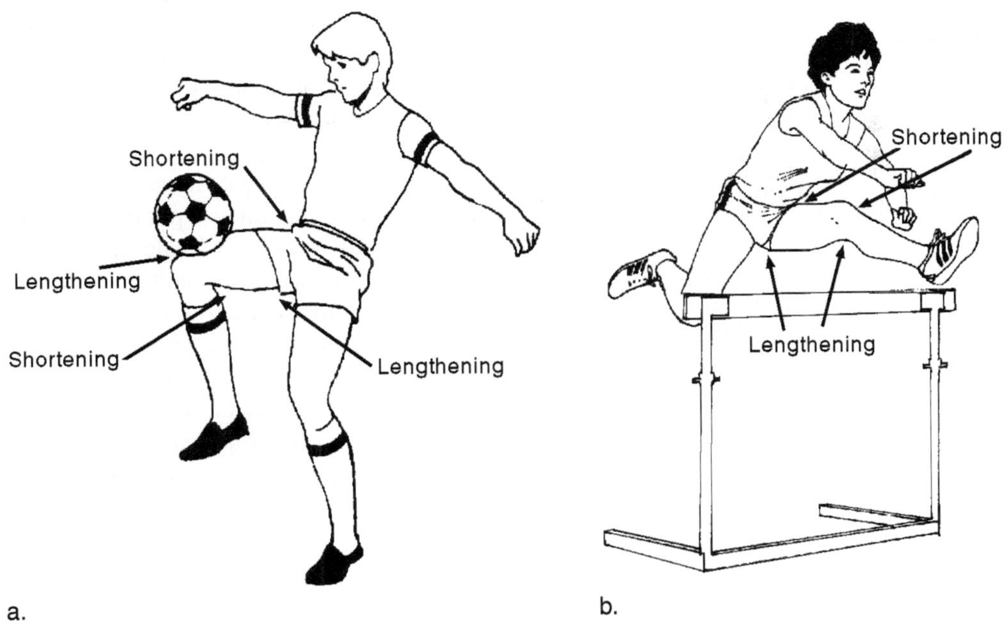

Figure 3.11 (a) A concurrent muscle action of the rectus femoris on top of the thigh and the hamstrings on the underside of the thigh occurs when each of the antagonist muscles lengthens at one joint and shortens at the other. (b) A countercurrent muscle action occurs as the rectus femoris shortens concentrically at both joints while the hamstrings are stretched at both joints.

similarly, are most active in either hip extension or knee flexion. In the biarticular countercurrent movements of hip flexion and knee extension, the rectus femoris exhibited strong activity. The medial hamstrings exhibited similar strong activity during hip extension and knee flexion. When the movement was concurrent hip and knee flexion, however, the rectus femoris showed no activity, but the hamstring did. Similarly, during knee and hip extension, the hamstrings were inhibited and the rectus femoris was active. The activity of the rectus femoris and hamstrings was thus inhibited when they were antagonists.

Types of Bodily Movements

Movements may be passive or active, and if active, they may be slow or rapid. They may involve the constant application of force, or after the initial impetus has been given, they may continue without further muscular effort.

A *passive* movement requires no effort on the part of the person involved. It is performed by another person such as a therapist giving a treatment or an instructor or partner stretching tight ligaments, fascia, and muscles in an attempt to increase the range of motion of a particular joint. In some cases, it is a movement that has been started by the subject's own effort but is continued by momentum. It might also be caused by the force of gravity if the subject remained relaxed and used no muscular effort to aid, restrain, or guide the moving part. To avoid injury, care must be taken that the subject does not resist the movement and that the person applying the force to cause the movement is not too aggressive.

An *active* movement is produced by the subject's own muscular activity. It is usually performed volitionally, but it may be a reflex reaction to an external or internal stimulus. It may be rapid or slow. In slow movements, muscular tension is maintained throughout the range of motion. Pushing a heavy piece of furniture across the room is an example of this type of movement. In rapid movements, tension could also be maintained throughout the range of motion, but this would be an inefficient way of performing. For efficiency, rapid movements should be performed ballistically. The concept of *ballistic* movement was introduced a number of years ago by experimental psychologists. They used the term for movements that were initiated by vigorous muscular contraction and completed by momentum. This type of movement is characteristic of throwing, striking, and kicking. It is also seen in the finger movements used for typing and piano playing. When such movements are performed nonballistically—that is, with constant muscular contraction—they are uneconomical and hence not skillful. In fact, they are characteristic of the way in which beginners tend to attempt new coordinations, especially if they are concentrating on accuracy of aim rather than on a ballistic type of motion. They need to be encouraged in the early stages of learning a skill to concentrate on form rather than accuracy if they are to master the skill of moving ballistically.

Ballistic movements may be terminated by one of three methods: (1) by contracting antagonistic muscles, as in the forehand drive in tennis; (2) by allowing the moving part to reach the limit of motion, in which case it will be stopped by the passive resistance of ligaments, other tissues, or the braking action of antagonistic muscles, as in the case of the forceful overarm throw; or (3) by the interference of an obstacle, as when chopping wood.

In many movements found in both sports and activities of living, three types of muscular action cooperate to produce a single act. This kind of cooperation is seen especially in striking activities that require the use of an implement, such as a tennis racket, golf club, or ax. Movements such as these involve (1) fixation to support the moving part and to maintain the necessary position, (2) ballistic movement of the active limb, and (3) fixation in the fingers as they grasp the implement.

Methods of Studying the Actions of Muscles

In addition to the obvious method of studying the actions of muscles in a textbook, a number of procedures may be more meaningful to the student.

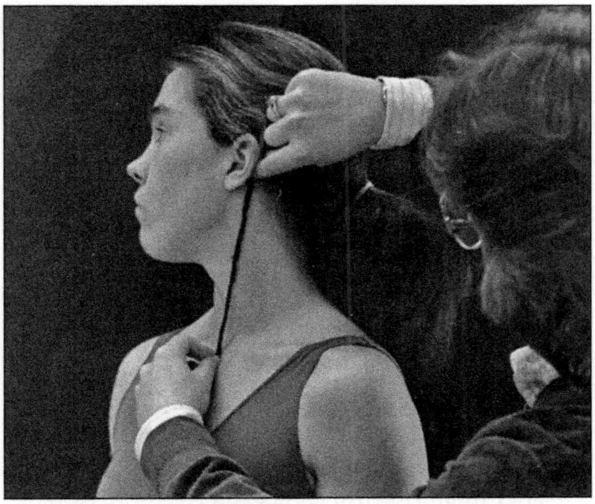

Figure 3.12 Locating a muscle's line of pull by placing ends of a string or elastic at the location of the muscle's attachment. The line of pull of the sternocleidomastoid is located using this procedure.

Conjecture and Reasoning

Using knowledge of the location and attachments of a muscle and the nature of the joint or joints it spans, one can deduce a great deal about a muscle's actions. Conjecture and reasoning is a valuable method to use in conjunction with other methods. Although the use of this method does not identify which muscles are actually contracting in a given action, a careful study of the muscles' attachments and line of pull (Figure 3.12) will enable one to see what movements a muscle is *capable* of causing.

Dissection

An excellent way of studying the location and attachments of a muscle and its relation to the joint it spans is dissection. This method provides a more meaningful basis for visualizing the muscle's potential movements, but it sometimes leads to misinterpretations and erroneous conclusions.

Inspection and Palpation

Even though its use is limited to superficial muscles, inspection and palpation of normal living subjects is a valuable method, as far as it goes. Much of the information in early anatomy textbooks was based on the combination of dissection of the cadaver and inspection and palpation of living subjects. Before the days of electromyography, these were the chief methods of determining the actions of the muscles. There is a possibility of misinterpretation, however, against which students should be warned. When the force of a muscle contraction is weak, it is sometimes difficult to feel its contraction. If the subject repeats the action against greater resistance, the contraction may be stronger and more easily felt. The conclusion may be drawn erroneously that the muscle is a major mover for the action involved, when in fact it comes into action only as an assistant under conditions of heavy resistance.

Models

Numerous devices, both commercial and homemade, can be used for demonstrating and studying the actions of muscles. Probably the most commonly used device is the simplest of all—a long rubber band (or chain of short ones) held against the bones of a skeleton in such a way as to represent a single muscle. The movement is demonstrated by holding the elastic on a stretch with one end representing the proximal attachment and the other the distal attachment. The tendency of both bones to move toward each other can easily be demonstrated, as well as the necessity for stabilizing one bone so that the muscle can be effective in moving the other bone.

Muscle Stimulation

To most kinesiologists, the term *muscle stimulation* means G. B. Duchenne, the pioneer in the use of electrical stimulation as a means of studying the actions of the muscles and the author of *Physiologie des Mouvements.* This classic work was translated into English and published in 1949. It made a tremendous contribution to the science of kinesiology, yet its limitations must be recognized. It demonstrates the contraction of individual muscles when they are stimulated electrically. Unfortunately, it cannot analyze the sequence of muscular actions that occur in an everyday act such as walking, lifting a package, or working with a common tool.

Neither can it reveal the complex combinations of muscular actions in ordinary sport techniques.

In spite of its limitations, muscle stimulation is being used in many modern kinesiology laboratories as a device for studying the responses of individual muscles to electrical stimulation and to rehabilitate muscles. One of the more promising areas of research in the rehabilitation field has been that of functional electrical stimulation (FES). FES combines electrical stimulation with computer control systems to offer some movement in muscles that have no functional nerves. The development of FES technology is aimed at providing mobility to disabled individuals. At this writing, much work remains to be done. FES systems have been used with some success in a number of settings, but the complexity of human movement, even the simple act of walking, has made the task of programming computers to stimulate the appropriate muscles in the appropriate sequence a daunting one. It is possible, however, that in this century, disabled individuals may be able to walk with the aid of electrical stimulation and computer control.

Electromyography (EMG)

Although few undergraduate students may have the opportunity of personal experience with electromyography, all may benefit by reading the reports of EMG investigations. A wealth of information concerning muscular action is available in such reports. Electromyography is based on the fact that contracting muscles generate electrical impulses. It is a technique of recording such impulses or action potentials, as they are also called (Figure 3.13). It provides specific information about muscular actions that we have only been able to guess at in the past, information that has proved much of our guessing to be inaccurate. The unique advantages of EMG are that it reveals both the intensity and duration of a muscle's action and, in fact, discloses the precise time sequences of muscular activity in a movement. Furthermore, it reveals the actions not only of the agonists and antagonists but also of the muscles serving as stabilizers and neutralizers. Perhaps its greatest contribution to our knowledge of muscular action is its ability to record the impulses of deep as well as superficial muscles. Basmajian, the apostle of electromyography, says that it surpasses all the older methods of studying muscular action in that it reveals what the individual muscles are actually doing, not just what they *can do* or *probably do* (Basmajian & DeLuca, 1985).

Imaging

The introduction of magnetic resonance imaging (MRI) has provided a method for actually "seeing" a muscle or muscle group. MRI images are based on the water and compounds that make up tissue. An MRI image clearly shows the structure of muscle and can be used to determine such factors as cross-sectional area, fiber orientation, fiber length, and tendon structure. From the changes that occur with muscle activation, it is possible to determine which muscles are active during movement. This is done in several ways. One might examine the change in muscle-fiber length on the image, or the relative change in the pennations of a muscle. MRI findings have been found to agree well with EMG and are much more accurate than palpation (Yuen & Orendurff, 2006). Currently, MRI imaging is expensive and available primarily to hospitals and large research institutions.

Muscular Analysis

The approach to the analysis of the muscle participation in a given motion is exactly the same as that used for joint action. Using the same anatomical analysis model (see Table 1.1), the analyst adds a description of muscular involvement to the previously completed analysis of joint and segment involvement. The muscular action is identified for each joint movement and recorded next to the joint actions on the chart (see Table 1.2). This implies identifying not only the muscle groups (flexors, extensors, abductors, adductors, etc.) that are contracting but also their function in the movement and the kind of contraction they are undergoing (concentric, eccentric, or static). Identification of the force causing the motion facilitates the subsequent

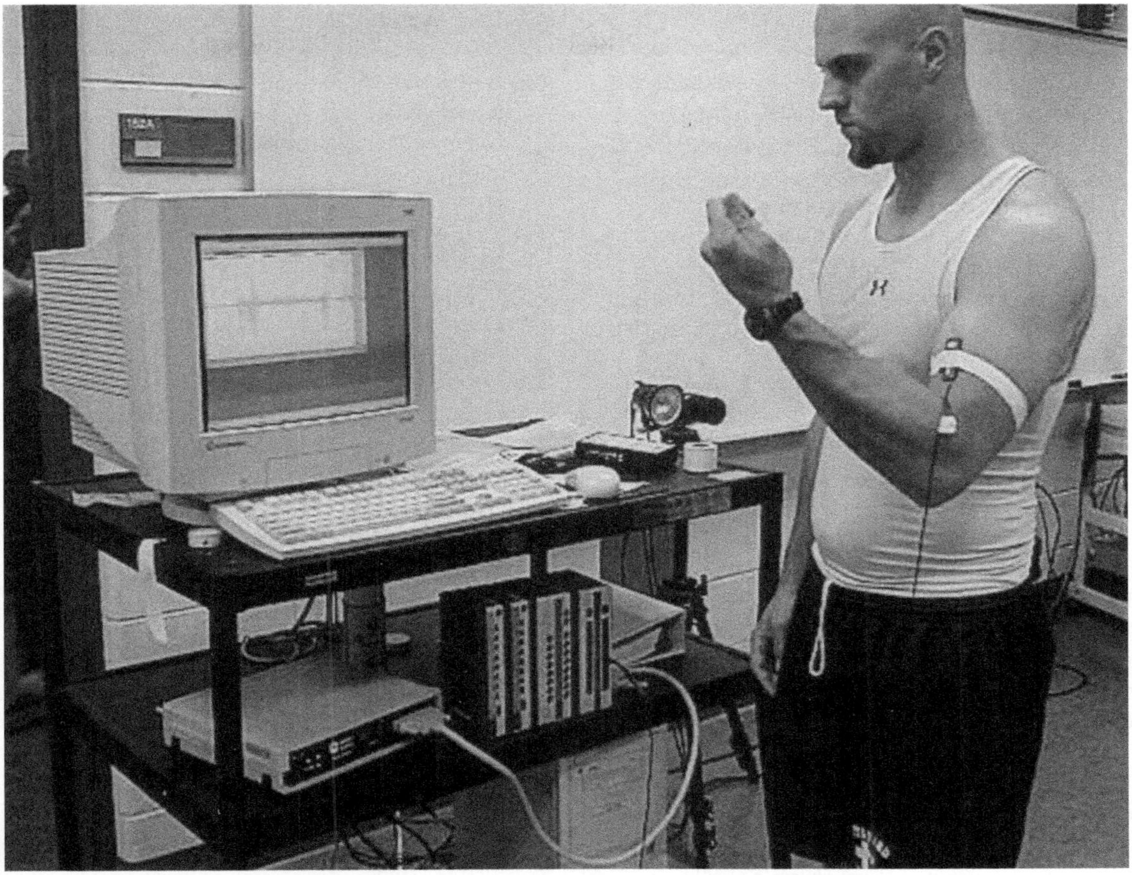

Figure 3.13 Electromyography is a valuable tool for studying muscle activity.

identification of the muscle and type of contraction involved. In those instances where the force causing the motion is gravity, the muscle contraction type is most likely to be eccentric. If muscle is the force causing the motion, the contraction is concentric. It is critical to remember the influence of gravity during this portion of the analysis. When gravity is the force producing motion, the muscle group that is active will be that which is antagonistic to the *observed* motion. In other words, extension produced by the pull of gravity is controlled by eccentric contraction of the *flexor* muscles.

Any of the methods described for studying muscle actions may be used to determine which muscle groups are active during a performance. Once the general muscle groups have been identified, the analyst may wish to identify specific prime movers (agonists) and synergists. Chapters 5 through 9 provide the knowledge required concerning individual muscles and their actions.

A condition of efficient movement is to use only those muscles that are appropriate to the motion. Tension in muscles that are not active in the skill produces fatigue and often a performance that is both inefficient and ineffective. Failure to use all requisite muscle groups can also seriously impair movement. A common fault in unskilled jumpers, for example, is tension in the anterior muscles of the lower leg (the ankle dorsiflexors). This tension can restrict the forceful plantarflexion muscle action and related ankle motion necessary for an efficient and effective jump.

REFERENCES AND SELECTED READINGS

Basmajian, J. V., & Deluca, C. J. (1985). *Muscles alive* (5th ed.). Baltimore: Williams & Wilkins.

Bojsen-Møller, J. S., Magnusson, P., Rasmussenn, M. K., & Aagaard, P. (2005). Muscle performance during maximal isometric and dynamic contractions is influenced by the stiffness of the tendinous structures. *Journal of Applied Physiology,* 99, 986–994.

Ford, K. R., van den Bogert, J., Myer, G. D., Shapiro, R., & Hewett, T. E. (2008). The effects of age and skill level on knee musculature co-contraction during functional activities: A systematic review. *British Journal of Sports Medicine,* 42(7), 561–566.

Frontera, W. R., Reid, K. F., Phillips, E. M., Krivickas, L. S., Hughes, V. A., Roubenoff, R., et al. (2008). Muscle fiber size and function in elderly humans: a longitudinal study. *Journal of Applied Physiology,* 105, 637–642.

Fukashiro, S., Hay, D. C., & Nagano, A. (2006). Biomechanical behavior of the muscle-tendon complex during dynamic human movements. *Journal of Applied Biomechanics,* 22, 131–147.

Granata, K. P., & Marras, W. S. (2000). Cost-benefit of muscle cocontraction in protecting against spinal instability. *Spine,* 25, 1398–1404.

Gribble, P. L., Mullin, L. I., Cothros, N., & Mattar, A. (2003). Role of cocontraction in arm movement accuracy. *Journal of Neurophysiology,* 89, 2396–2405.

Griffin, T. M., & Guilak, F. (2005). The role of mechanical loading in the onset and progression of osteoarthritis. *Exercise and Sport Science Review,* 33(4), 195–200.

Harris, A. J., Duxson, M. J., Butler, J. E., Hodges, P. W., Taylor, J. L., & Gandevia, S. C. (2005). Muscle fiber and motor unit behavior in the longest human skeletal muscle. *Journal of Neuroscience,* 25(37), 8528–8533.

Kawakami, Y., & Fukunaga, T. (2006). New insights into in vivo human skeletal muscle function. *Exercise and Sport Science Review,* 34(1), 16–21.

Krosshaug, T., Andersen, T. E., Olsen, O. E., Myklebust, G., & Bahr, R. (2005). Research approaches to describe the mechanisms of injuries in sport: Limitations and possibilities. *British Journal of Sports Medicine,* 39(6), 330–339.

MacIntosh, B. R., Gardiner, P., & McComas, A. J. (2006). *Skeletal muscle—form and function* (2nd ed.). Champaign, IL: Human Kinetics.

MacWilliams, B. A., Wilson, D. R., DesJardins, J. D., Romero, J., & Chao, E. Y. (1999). Hamstrings cocontraction reduces internal rotation, anterior translation, and anterior cruciate ligament load. *Journal of Orthopedic Research,* 17(6), 817–822.

Malisoux, L., Francaux, M., Nielens, H., & Theisen, D. (2006). Stretch-shortening cycle exercises: An effective training paradigm to enhance power output of human single muscle fibers. *Journal of Applied Physiology,* 100(3), 771–779.

Mayer, J. M., Graves, J. E., Clark, B. C., Formikell, M., & Ploutz-Snyder, L. L. (2004). The use of magnetic resonance imaging to evaluate lumbar muscle activity during trunk extension exercise at varying intensities. *Spine,* 30(22), 2556–2563.

Milner, T. E. (2002). Adaptation to destabilizing dynamics by means of muscle cocontraction. *Experimental Brain Research,* 143(4), 406–416.

Perez, M. A., & Nussbaum, M. A. (2002). Lower torso muscle activation patterns for high-magnitude static exertions: Gender differences and the effects of twisting. *Spine,* 27(12), 1326–1335.

Reeves, N. D., & Narici, M. V. (2003). Behavior of human muscle fascicles during shortening and lengthening contractions in vivo. *Journal of Applied Physiology,* 95, 1090–1096.

Steindler, A. (1970). *Kinesiology of the human body.* Springfield, IL: Charles C. Thomas.

Takeda, Y., Kashiwaguchi, S., Matsuura, T., Higashida, T., & Minato, A. (2006). Hamstring muscle function after tendon harvest for anterior cruciate ligament reconstruction: Evaluation with T2 relaxation time of magnetic resonance imaging. *American Journal of Sports Medicine,* 34(2), 281–288.

Thompson, L. V. (2002). Skeletal muscle adaptations with age, inactivity, and therapeutic exercise. *Journal of Orthopedic & Sports Physical Therapy,* 32(2), 44–57.

Van Dieén, J. H., Kingma, I., & van der Bug, J. C. E. (2003). Evidence for a role of antagonist cocontraction in controlling trunk stiffness during lifting. *Journal of Biomechanics,* 36, 1829–1836.

Yuen, T. J., & Orendurff, M. S. (2006). A comparison of gastrocnemius muscle-tendon unit length during gait using anatomic, cadaveric and MRI models. *Gait and Posture,* 23(1), 112–117.

LABORATORY EXPERIENCES

1. Take two sticks that are joined at one end by a hinge. Attach a single piece of elastic or a long rubber band to the opposite ends of the two sticks.
   a. Separate the ends of the sticks as far as the elastic will permit and then demonstrate the way the elastic will pull both sticks together.
   b. Demonstrate the way in which the elastic will move only one of the sticks if the other one is stabilized.
   c. Repeat both a and b, using the arm of the skeleton instead of the sticks.
2. Get a subject to hold a heavy dumbbell in the right hand and slowly raise the arm sideward/upward without bending the elbow. Keep your fingers on the clavicular portion of the pectoralis major. Does it contract? If so, at what position of the arm does it begin?
3. Flex the fingers hard. Keep them flexed and flex the hand at the wrist as far as possible. What happens to the fingers? Explain.
4. Extend the fingers, and then hyperextend the hand at the wrist as far as possible. What happens to the fingers? Explain.
5. Get a subject to lie on the left side with the hip and knee in a partly flexed position and the right leg fully extended. The right thigh should now be flexed passively by an operator. The subject should attempt to keep the knee straight but not to the point of interfering with the hip flexion. What happens? Where does the subject feel discomfort? Explain.
6. Have the subject, in the same starting position as in Experience 5, flex both the right thigh and right leg completely. The right thigh should now be passively extended by an operator, with the subject attempting to keep the leg flexed at the knee. As the thigh becomes fully extended, what happens to the knee? Where does the subject feel discomfort? Explain.

(*Caution:* Do not use an acrobat or acrobatic dancer as a subject for Experience 5 or 6, or the experiments may not work. Why?)

7. Have a subject lie supine on a table with the knees at the edge and the lower legs hanging down. Ask the subject to extend one leg at the knee while you attempt to stop the motion by applying strong resistance at the front of the ankle. Note the amount of resistance you have to apply. Now ask the subject to flex the leg at the knee while you attempt to stop the movement by resisting at the rear of the ankle. Which action requires more resistance on your part?

   Now ask the subject to sit up and flex the trunk well forward from the hips. Repeat the same two actions of knee flexion and extension against resistance. Which action requires more effort on your part this time? How does this compare with the first result? Explain.

   It may help you to know that the rectus femoris crosses the front of the hip joint and the front of the knee joint. Hence, it is a flexor of the hip and an extensor of the knee. The biceps femoris is located on the back of the thigh and therefore is an extensor of the hip and flexor of the knee.
8. Following the analysis model presented in Table 1.2, do an analysis of the muscle groups (i.e., flexors, extensors, etc.) active in the performance of a motor skill that involves a number of joints.

   Note: Laboratory exercises on the action of muscles as movers, stabilizers, and neutralizers are not included here because, in order to do them, it is necessary to know the individual muscles. They will be found in the laboratory sections of Chapters 5 through 9.

CHAPTER 4

The Neuromuscular Basis of Human Motion

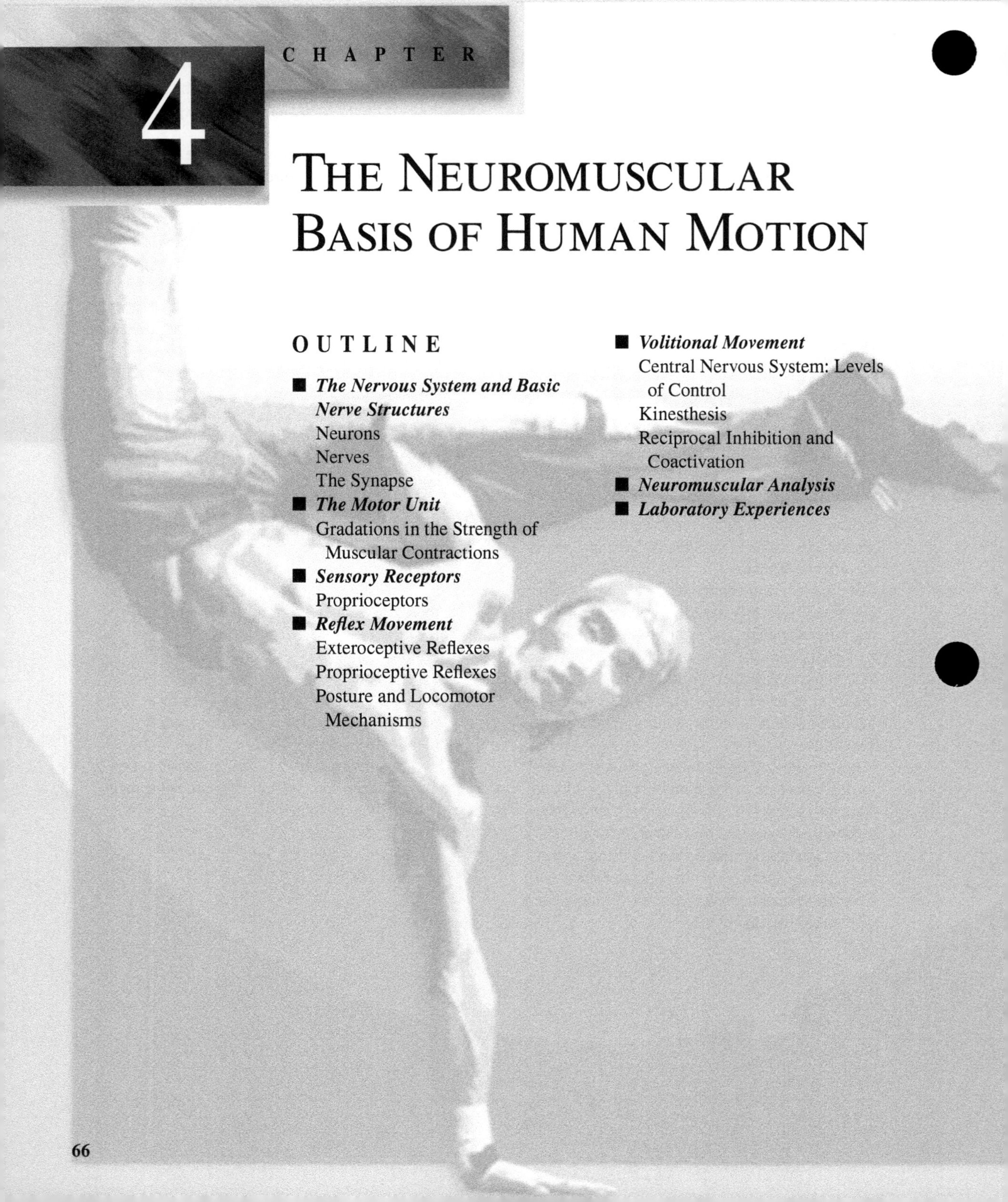

OUTLINE

- ***The Nervous System and Basic Nerve Structures***
  - Neurons
  - Nerves
  - The Synapse
- ***The Motor Unit***
  - Gradations in the Strength of Muscular Contractions
- ***Sensory Receptors***
  - Proprioceptors
- ***Reflex Movement***
  - Exteroceptive Reflexes
  - Proprioceptive Reflexes
  - Posture and Locomotor Mechanisms
- ***Volitional Movement***
  - Central Nervous System: Levels of Control
  - Kinesthesis
  - Reciprocal Inhibition and Coactivation
- ***Neuromuscular Analysis***
- ***Laboratory Experiences***

OBJECTIVES

At the conclusion of this chapter, the student should be able to:

1. Name and describe the functions of the basic structures of the nervous system.
2. Explain how gradations in strength of muscle contraction and precision of movements occur.
3. Name and define the receptors important in musculoskeletal movement.
4. Explain how the various receptors function, and describe the effect each has on musculoskeletal movement.
5. Describe reflex action, and enumerate and differentiate among the reflexes that affect musculoskeletal action.
6. Demonstrate a basic understanding of volitional movement by describing the nature of the participation of the anatomical structures and mechanisms involved.
7. Perform an analysis of the neuromuscular factors influencing the performance of a variety of motor skills.

The role of the bones, joints, and muscles in human movement were presented in the previous two chapters. The appropriate function of these systems requires an intact nervous system. Therefore, this chapter takes up the role of the nervous system in initiating, modifying, and coordinating muscular action.

Loofbourrow (1973) presented this topic so succinctly and vividly that his classic and still applicable introductory paragraph is quoted here in full as an introduction to this chapter:

> The forces which move the supporting framework of the body are unleashed within skeletal muscles on receipt of signals by way of their motor nerves. In the absence of such signals, the muscles normally are relaxed. Movement is almost always the result of the combined action of a group of muscles which pull in somewhat different directions, so the control of movement involves a distribution of signals within the central nervous system (CNS) to appropriate motor nerves with precise timing and in appropriate number. In order for movements to be useful in making adjustments to external situations, it is necessary for the central nervous system to be appraised of these situations, which are continually changing. A means of providing this information promptly exists in a variety of receptors sensitive to changes in temperature, light, pressure, etc. These receptors are signal generators which dispatch signals (nerve impulses) to the CNS over afferent nerve fibers. The CNS receives these signals together with identical ones from within the muscles, joints, tendons, and other body structures and is led thereby to generate and distribute in fantastically orderly array myriads of signals to various muscles. This, despite the enormous complexity of the machinery involved, enables the individual to do one main thing at a time. This is integration. It is what Sir Charles Sherrington meant by "the integrative action of the nervous system."

The following discussion does not presume to be an exhaustive treatise on neuromuscular mechanisms. It attempts rather to present as simply as possible those mechanisms that are pertinent to the study of kinesiology. Because of techniques made possible by electronic sensing and imaging devices, great strides have been made in acquiring more accurate information concerning the intricacies of neuromuscular function.

THE NERVOUS SYSTEM AND BASIC NERVE STRUCTURES

It is assumed that the kinesiology student is already familiar with the general plan of the nervous system; hence, it will not be described in full here. Only a brief outline of the major divisions will be presented to give the reader a framework for the topics selected for discussion:

I. Central nervous system
   A. Brain
   B. Spinal cord
II. Peripheral nervous system
   A. Cranial nerves (12 pairs)
   B. Spinal nerves (31 pairs)
III. Autonomic nervous system (sympathetic and parasympathetic)

The autonomic nervous system is not a distinct system based on structure and geographic location, as are the central and peripheral systems, but is rather a functional division that overlaps with those in specific areas. It includes those portions of the brain, spinal cord, and peripheral nervous system that supply cardiac muscle, smooth muscle, and gland cells.

Neurons

A neuron, the structural unit of the nervous system, is a single nerve cell consisting of a cell body and one or more projections. Three kinds of neurons propagate impulses. Two kinds of neurons whose long fibers constitute the peripheral nervous system are the sensory (or afferent) and motor (or efferent) neurons (Figure 4.1). The primary motor neurons are also referred to as alpha motor neurons. There are also numerous connector neurons located only within the central nervous system.

The cell bodies of the majority of efferent, or motor, neurons are situated within the anterior horns of the spinal cord. (Some also exist in the brainstem and sympathetic ganglia.) Many short, threadlike extensions of the cell body, known as dendrites, synapse with the axons of other cells, the latter being either sensory or connector neurons.

Each motor and connector neuron has a specialized process termed an axon. The axon of the motor neuron emerges from the spinal cord in a ventral root. It then travels by way of a peripheral nerve to the muscle that it helps activate. There it divides and subdivides into smaller and smaller branches, the most distal being known as the terminal branches. Each terminal branch ends within a single muscle fiber in the structure called the motor endplate or neuromuscular junction.

The cell body of a spinal afferent, or sensory, neuron, unlike that of a motor neuron, is situated in a dorsal root ganglion just outside the spinal

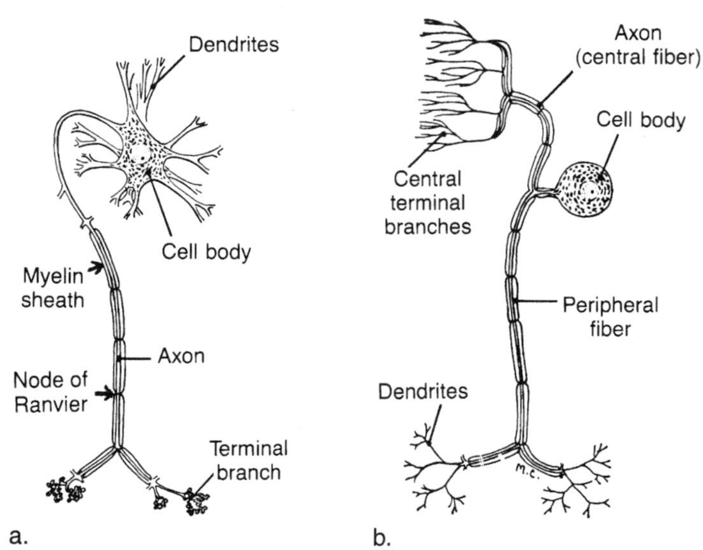

Figure 4.1 Neurons: (a) motor neuron; (b) sensory neuron.

cord. (The cell bodies of cranial sensory neurons are in cranial nerve ganglia.) The neuron has a single short process that projects from the cell body and then bifurcates into two branches that go in opposite directions. One, the so-called central fiber, travels in the dorsal root of the nerve to the posterior horn of the spinal cord, where it divides into numerous branches. It may terminate in the cord, or it may ascend in the cord to the brain and terminate there. The other branch of the afferent neuron is the long peripheral fiber, which comes from a receptor. It travels in a nerve trunk (peripheral nerve) to the vicinity of the appropriate dorsal root ganglion, where it unites with the cell body via the short stemlike process mentioned earlier (Figure 4.1b).

An axon is the fiber over which impulses are conducted *away from* the cell body, as opposed to dendrites, which convey impulses toward the cell body. When referring to a sensory neuron, the term *dendrite* is applied not to the long fiber that conveys impulses from peripheral regions to the cell body, but rather to its branches. The long sensory fiber itself is known simply as the peripheral fiber.

It was noted earlier that the dendrites of efferent (motor) neurons make contact within the spinal cord, either with the terminal branches of afferent (sensory) neurons or with connector neurons. Connector neurons, also known as interneurons, are a third type of nerve cell. They exist completely within the central nervous system and serve as connecting links. They may vary from a single small neuron, connecting a sensory neuron with a motor neuron, to an intricate system of neurons whereby a sensory impulse may be relayed to many motor cell bodies. We know from common experience that a complex motor act may result from a single sensory impulse. For instance, a sudden loud noise may cause us to jump, turn around, and tense nearly every muscle in our body. The connector neurons are responsible for this widespread response to the single sensory impulse. Thus only one connector neuron may be participating in a movement, or there may be an intricate network making possible an almost limitless number of connections with other neurons.

Nerves

Just as an electric cable is an insulated bundle of wires for the transmission of electric currents, so a nerve is a bundle of fibers, enclosed within a connective tissue sheath, for the transmission of impulses from one part of the body to another. A nerve, or nerve trunk as it is frequently called, may consist entirely of efferent fibers from the central nervous system to the muscles and other tissues, or it may consist only of afferent fibers from the sensory organs to the central nervous system. The typical spinal (peripheral) nerve, however, is mixed; that is, it contains both efferent and afferent fibers. Each spinal nerve is attached to the spinal cord by an anterior (motor) root and a posterior (sensory) root (Figure 4.2). The posterior root bears a ganglion (a collection of cell bodies), and it is just beyond the ganglion that the two roots unite to form the spinal nerve. Once outside the vertebral canal, each spinal nerve divides into an anterior and a posterior branch, each of which contains both motor and sensory fibers. The anterior branches supply the trunk and limbs, the posterior branches the back. Motor nerves that activate skeletal muscle fibers are referred to as the alpha motor system.

The 31 pairs of mixed peripheral nerves exit from both sides of the vertebral column between every two vertebrae, with the first spinal nerve exiting from between the skull and the first cervical vertebra. Therefore, there are 8 cervical,

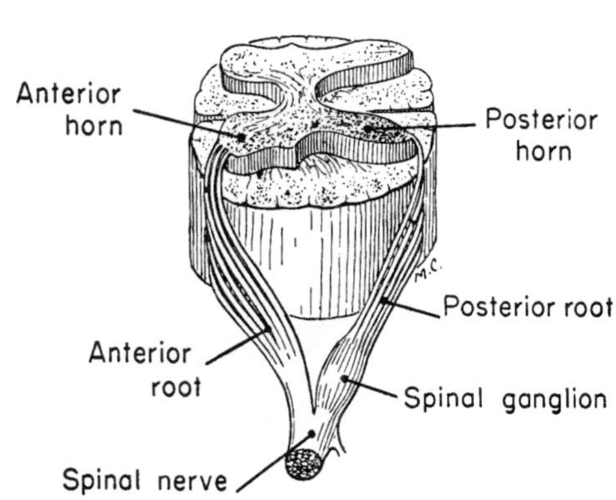

Figure 4.2 Section of the spinal cord showing the anterior and posterior roots of a spinal nerve.

12 thoracic, 5 lumbar, 5 sacral, and 1 coccyx spinal nerves. Specific areas of the body are activated by fibers from specific peripheral nerves. Table 4.1 outlines the spinal nerve innervation patterns.

The Synapse

Synapses are connections between and among neurons and occur only within the central nervous system (Figure 4.3). A synapse, and there may be thousands between any two neurons, is a proximity of the membrane of an axon and the membrane of a dendrite or a cell body. No physical union occurs between or among neurons. Conduction of impulses takes place in one direction only, from the axon of one neuron to the dendrites, cell body, or, rarely, to the axon of another. Synapses are influenced by use and disuse. The more often one is crossed, the easier it becomes for signals to pass through it. Conduction velocity is very rapid along

TABLE 4.1 Peripheral Nerve Innervation Pattern

Vertebrae	Peripheral Nerves	Plexus	General Innervation
Cervical (7)	8 pairs (between skull and C1)	Cervical (C1–C4)	Head and neck
		Brachial (C5–T1)	Upper extremities
Thoracic (12)	12 pairs		Trunk, including abdomen
Lumbar	5 pairs	Lumbar (L1–4)	Lower extremities
			Pelvis
		Lumbosacral (L4–S3)	Lower extremities
Sacral (5 fused)	5 pairs	Sacral (S1–5)	Pelvis and lower extremities
Coccyx	1 pair	Coccygeal (S4–C)	Coccyx

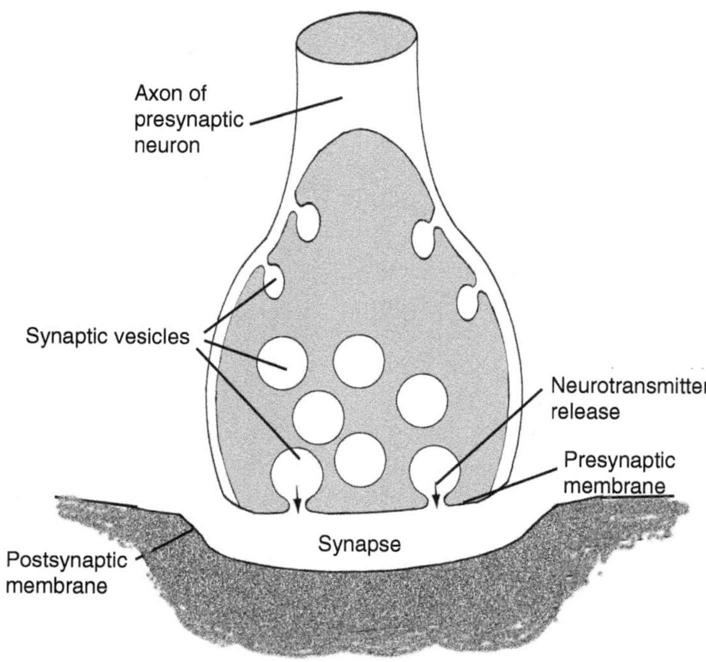

Figure 4.3 Nerve ending and synapse.

the nerve fiber. Whenever there is a delay, it occurs at the synapses. The greater the number of synapses from receptor to effector, the longer the time from stimulus to response.

The transmission of an impulse across a synapse depends on the release of a chemical transmitter substance by the axon. This substance diffuses throughout the membranes, and an action potential is created in the postsynaptic neuron. The action potential may be excitatory or inhibitory. Threshold level is the minimum level of stimulus (chemical transmitter) necessary to result in the initiation or propagation of a signal. Too little transmitter results in no impulse being carried to the next neuron, but an increase in this transmitter beyond the threshold level produces a response equal to but not greater than that needed for the threshold level. It must be remembered that it is at the synapse where facilitation (making it easier) or inhibition (making it more difficult) occurs. If the threshold level is altered so that only a small amount of additional neurotransmitter needs to be released for the threshold level to be achieved, facilitation will occur. Conversely, if a larger quantity of the chemical is needed before threshold level is reached, inhibition will occur. The student is reminded that more than one motor neuron may attach to a single muscle fiber, and therefore neurotransmitters released from several neurons simultaneously may have an additive or inhibitory effect.

THE MOTOR UNIT

The structural units of the nervous and motor systems are, respectively, the neuron and the muscle fiber. Functionally, the two systems combine to form the neuromuscular system. The functional unit of the neuromuscular system is the *motor unit,* and it consists of a single motor neuron (see Figure 4.1a), together with all of the muscle fibers that its axon supplies (Figure 4.4). All muscle fibers activated by the same motor neuron are of the same muscle fiber type.

Motor units vary widely in the number of muscle fibers supplied by one motor neuron. Some motor units may have as many as 2,000 or more muscle fibers (gastrocnemius); others may have fewer than 10 (eye muscles). A muscle that has a small ratio of muscle fibers to alpha motor neurons is capable of more precise movements than is the muscle with a small number of motor neurons for the same number of muscle fibers. Hence, the ratio of muscle fibers to motor neurons has a direct bearing on the precision of the movements executed by the muscle. For example, the small muscles of the thumb and index finger are capable of movements of great precision because their motor units have such a low ratio of muscle fibers to motor neurons or, to state it differently, such a large number of motor neurons per muscle. By way of contrast, the gluteus maximus has a relatively small number of motor neurons for its size, hence a large number of muscle fibers per neuron. It does not need to be pointed out that the movements for which the gluteus maximus is responsible can scarcely be described as precise.

Gradations in the Strength of Muscular Contractions

Common experience indicates that the same muscles contract with various gradations of strength according to the requirements of the task. The elbow flexors, for example, are able to contract just enough to enable the hand to lift a piece of paper from the desk; they can also contract forcefully enough to lift a 15-pound briefcase. How do they adjust to such extremes? Two major factors influence the gradation of contraction. These are (1) the number of motor units that participate in the act and (2) the frequency of stimulation. If the stimulus is of threshold value, all the muscle fibers in the motor unit will contract maximally. If the stimulus is subliminal—in other words, below threshold value—none of the muscle fibers in the unit will contract at all. This characteristic is known as the *all-or-none principle of muscular contraction.* It must be emphasized that the principle applies only to individual motor units, not to entire muscles. To reiterate, if the stimulus is of threshold value, each muscle fiber in the participating unit whose threshold level has been reached will contract. Hence, it follows that, other things

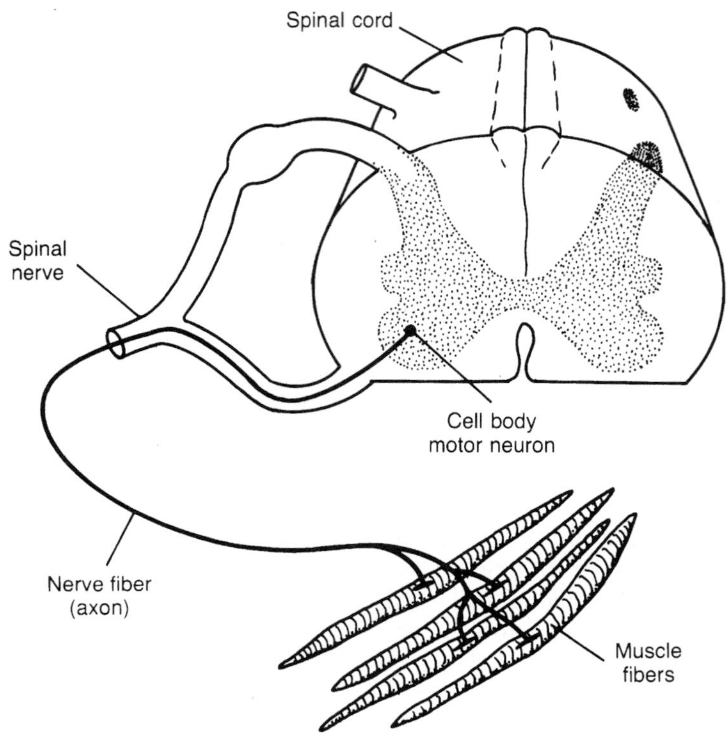

Figure 4.4 The organization of a motor unit. *Source:* Adapted from *Muscles Alive* (5th ed.), by J. V. Basmajian & C. Deluca. Copyright © 1985, Williams & Wilkins, Baltimore, MD. Reprinted with permission.

being equal, the more motor units that contract, the greater will be the total strength developed.

There is an orderly sequence to the recruitment of motor units. Innervation begins with the recruitment of the smaller slow-twitch fiber motor units, which have lower thresholds. They are followed by the larger fast-twitch motor units, which have high threshold levels. The recruitment patterns of the various fiber types are also determined by the mechanical requirements of the task. This is especially true for cyclic actions such as walking and running. The sequence of recruitment is reversed with the release of tension—that is, "last on" is "first off."

If stimuli are discharged at low frequency, the muscle fibers will partially relax between impulses, but if the stimuli are discharged at high frequency, the fibers will have insufficient time to relax and the result is summation or maximal contraction. If these two factors are combined—that is, if the maximum number of fibers are stimulated with the impulses being discharged at high frequency—the resulting contraction is of maximal strength. It has been noted that during prolonged contractions, motor units will cycle through on/off stages to rest, with the contraction shifting from motor unit to motor unit periodically (Bawa et al., 2006).

It should be noted that motor unit areas overlap, with a single muscle fiber often belonging to more than one motor unit. It takes a number of motor units firing to result in joint angle changes. The ability of a single muscle fiber to respond to more than one motor unit also becomes important with aging; there is evidence to suggest that with age, the number of active motor units decreases (Deschenes, 2004).

SENSORY RECEPTORS

Most activities of the nervous system begin with stimuli that activate sensory nerve terminals. Whereas motor nerves end on muscle fibers, forming motor units, sensory nerves are attached to specialized endings referred to as receptors. These receptors are specialized cells or organs that are selective in their response to different types of stimuli, although they often respond to more than one type of stimulus. There are two major classifications: exteroceptors and interoceptors.

Exteroceptors are located at or near a body surface and receive and transmit stimuli that come from outside the body, including the receptors of the familiar five senses: sight, hearing, smell, taste, and touch.

Interoceptors include the receptors for other cutaneous sensations, such as heat, cold, pain, and pressure (Figure 4.5). The interoceptors may be subdivided into receptors that receive impulses from the viscera and those that receive impulses from the tissues directly concerned with musculoskeletal movements and positions. The former are known as visceroceptors, and the latter are called proprioceptors.

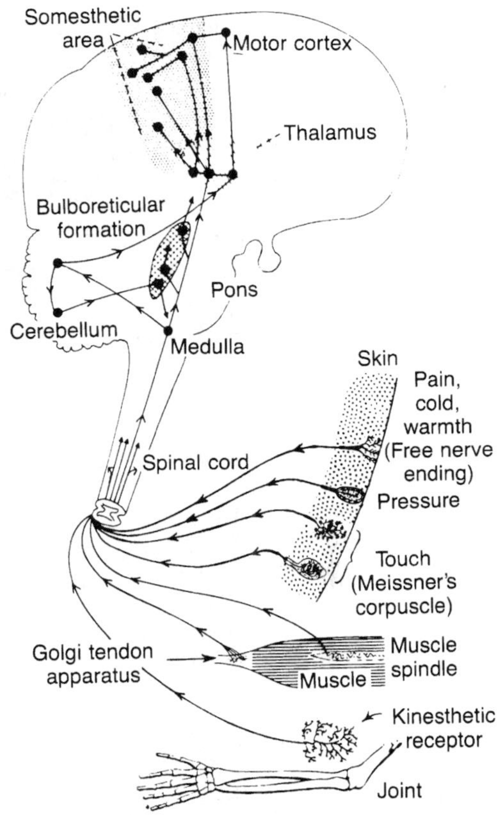

Figure 4.5 Transmission of proprioceptive sensations to the brain, showing the sensory receptors and the nerve pathways for transmitting these sensations into the brain. From A. C. Guyton, *Textbook of Medical Physiology,* 5th ed. Copyright © 1976 W. B. Saunders, Orlando, FL. Reprinted by permission.

Proprioceptors

Students of motor activity and posture find the proprioceptors of special interest, for these are the receptors that receive impulses that occur because of body movements or positions. They are located in the muscles, tendons, and joints, including the surrounding and protective tissues such as capsules, ligaments, and other fibrous membranes, and in the labyrinth of the inner ear. The proprioceptors are stimulated by motions of the body and in turn are responsible for transmitting a constant flow of information from these structures to the central nervous system. This information involves the appropriateness of the response in regard to the degree, direction, and rate of change of body movements. Without these sensory reports, effective coordination in motor patterns would not occur. Information from the receptors is directed both to the conscious and unconscious levels and, in addition to giving us a sense of awareness of body and limb positions, provides us with automatic reflexes. Proprioceptors are classified as muscle proprioceptors (muscle spindles and Golgi tendon organs), joint and skin proprioceptors (Ruffini endings and pacinian corpuscles), and labyrinthine and neck proprioceptors (Figures 4.5 and 4.6).

Muscle Proprioceptors

An abundance of two types of receptors are located within muscles and tendons. Both are responsive to stretch tension. The *muscle spindle*

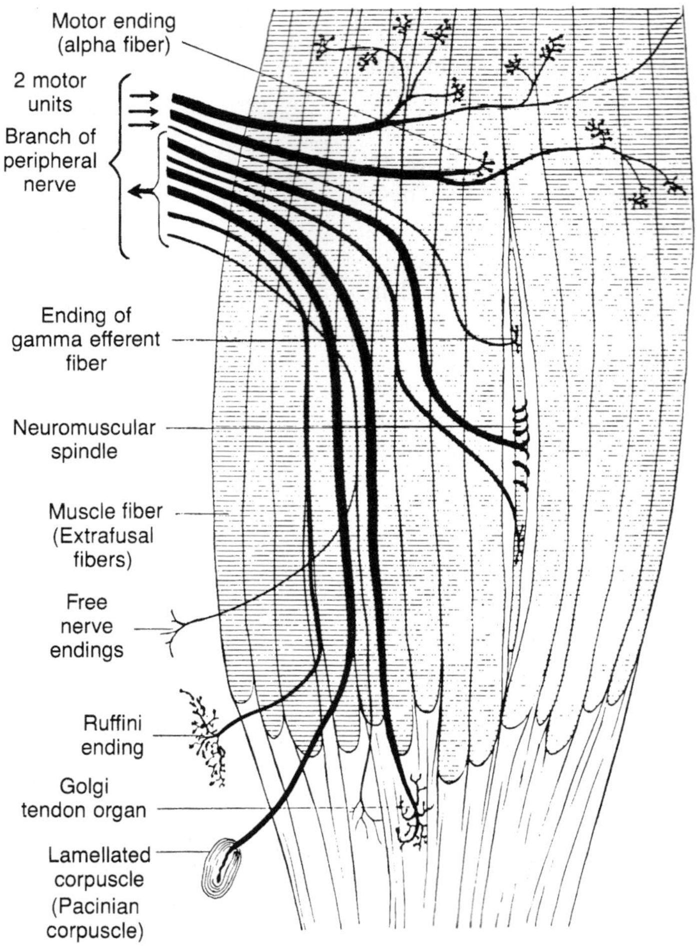

Figure 4.6 Schematic representation of a muscle and its nerve supply. *Source:* From *Fundamentals of Neurology* (6th ed.), by E. Gardner. Copyright © 1975, W. B. Saunders, Orlando, FL. Reprinted by permission.

detects relative muscle length and the *Golgi tendon organ (GTO)* detects muscle tension and active contraction through tension in the tendon.

Muscle spindles The muscle spindles are scattered throughout the muscle but predominate in the belly of the muscle, lying between the muscle fibers and parallel with them. More spindles are located in muscles controlling precise movements than are located in postural muscles. When the spindle is stretched, a sensory nerve located in its center sends impulses to the CNS, which in turn activates the motor neurons innervating the muscle, thus causing it to contract. The muscle spindle is responsive to both length (tonic response) and rate of change in length (phasic response). A single spindle is a tiny capsule (about 1 millimeter [mm] long), filled with fluid and containing some specialized muscle fibers known as intrafusal (fusimotor) fibers, to distinguish them from the extrafusal (skeletomotor) or "regular" muscle fibers (Figure 4.7). There are two kinds of intrafusal fibers, nuclear bag fibers and nuclear chain fibers. They are similar in that they both have

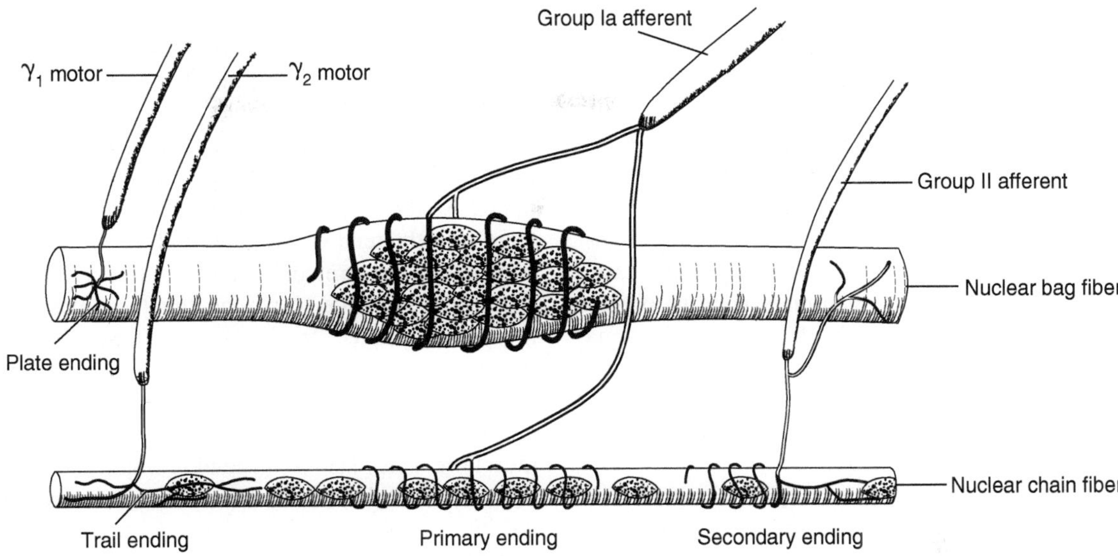

Figure 4.7 A muscle spindle containing a nuclear bag fiber and a nuclear chain fiber. *Source:* From *Skeletal Muscle: Form and Function* (2nd ed.), by B. R. MacIntosh, P. Gardiner, & A. J. McComas. 2006, Champaign, IL: Human Kinetics Publishers.

central noncontractile areas in which the nuclei are situated, and both have polar ends that are contractile. They differ in size and in the arrangement of the nuclei. The nuclear bag fiber is the larger of the two, and the nuclei appear crowded into the baglike central area, which gives the fiber its name. The small nuclear chain fiber is named for the single-line, chainlike arrangement of the nuclei in its slim, noncontractile central portion. There are differences also in the intricate system of innervation.

Each spindle is supplied with a type Ia afferent neuron that has a characteristic ending known as the *primary,* or *annulospiral,* ending. This ending is divided into as many branches as there are intrafusal fibers, and each branch is coiled around the noncontractile midsection of the intrafusal fiber. The annulospiral (AS) ending is highly sensitive to the velocity of changes in fiber length (phasic response), but only while the change is occurring. It also reacts to static (tonic) or length responses but with a sharp decline in frequency of impulse.

Most muscle spindles also have from one to five sensory endings that, because of their appearance, are given the picturesque name of *flower-spray (FS)* endings. Each FS ending has its own sensory (type II) fiber. The FS endings (also called secondary endings) are found at either end of the noncontractile midsection of the intrafusal fibers. They are believed to register static muscular length only (tonic response). The impulses transmitted by the FS endings increase almost directly in proportion to the amount of stretch and continue for a prolonged period of time. The FS endings are less sensitive to muscle stretch than the AS endings and therefore require a greater stimulus before responding. Because both the AS and FS endings activate the nuclear chain fibers, it is assumed that these fibers are responsible for the static response of both AS and FS endings. In contrast, only the AS endings activate the nuclear bag fibers. These fibers, then, must be responsible for the strong phasic response of the AS endings (Gowitzke & Milner, 1988; Park et al., 1999).

Muscle spindles are also supplied with their own small efferent fibers. To differentiate these fibers from the motor neurons of the "regular" muscle fibers, they are termed *gamma fibers,* in contrast to the "regular" motor neurons whose axons are termed *alpha fibers* (see Figure 4.6).

As a group, the gamma fibers form a *gamma fiber system.* Approximately one-third of the fibers in the peripheral nerve are gamma fibers. Impulses conveyed by gamma fibers (also called gamma efferents) cause the intrafusal muscle fibers to contract. This shortening of the spindle muscle fibers stretches their central noncontractile region where the AS endings are situated, and this stimulates them, causing their rate of firing to increase. Hence the effect of the gamma system is to control the sensitivity of the spindle afferents (gamma bias). The AS endings can be caused to fire, not only by passive stretch of the muscle as a whole, but also in the absence of such stretch by the function of the gamma system.

An exaggerated but familiar example of a simple adjustment of this nature is seen when picking up an object that is thought to be heavy. When the opposite proves to be the case, the correction in muscular effort is almost instantaneous. Less spectacular examples of this kind of coordination occur in all movements all the time. The gamma system provides a means of maintaining a position regardless of the tension put on it and enables smooth rather than jerky muscle response.

In summary, a muscle spindle can be stimulated in two different ways: (1) by stretching the whole muscle, causing the spindle to stretch; and (2) by contracting the ends of the intrafusal fibers via the gamma efferent system, thus stretching the center receptor portion of the spindle. The muscle spindle response is *tonic* in reacting to a static length and *phasic* in reacting to the rate at which length changes. Primary (AS) endings are sensitive to both tonic and phasic stretches, but secondary (FS) endings respond only to tonic stretch. Muscle spindles are very complex organs that are responsible for controlling the coordination of our muscular behavior. The feedback, which they supply continually, ensures a constant adjustment of muscular contraction.

Golgi tendon organ In contrast to the muscle spindle, the *Golgi tendon organ,* when stretched, sends signals to the central nervous system and causes the muscle to relax rather than contract. It consists of a mass of nerve endings, which are enclosed within a connective tissue capsule and embedded in a muscle tendon (Figure 4.8). It is situated close to the junction of the tendon with the fleshy part of the muscle in such a way that it has an end-to-end relationship with the muscle fibers. It is said to be "in series" with the muscle fibers. As the muscle shortens in contraction, the tension in the tendon increases and the Golgi tendon organs are stretched and activated. They are much less sensitive to stretch than spindles and require a stronger stretch to be activated. When the stress is greater than the Golgi tendon organ stretch threshold, the reflex contraction that is due to spindle stimulation is overridden and the muscle relaxes. The Golgi tendon organ provides instantaneous information about the degree of tension on each small segment of muscle. It is, therefore, a protective mechanism, and when the tension is extreme, its inhibitory effect can be great enough to effect a whole muscle relaxation.

Joint and Skin Proprioceptors

Two important receptors located in the joints or skin are the *Pacinian corpuscles* and the *Ruffini endings.* Pacinian corpuscles are found beneath the skin, concentrated in regions around the joint capsules, ligaments, and tendon sheaths. They are large end organs consisting of a tip of nerve fiber surrounded by many concentric layers of capsule. They are activated by rapid joint angle changes and by pressure that compresses and distorts the capsule, but only for a very brief period of time. Consequently, they are important for detecting rapid changes in pressure but useless for constant pressure awareness. In running, the information provided by the Pacinian corpuscles allows the nervous system to predict where the feet will be at any time so that appropriate adjustments in limb position can be anticipated and effected as needed. Ruffini endings are also activated by mechanical deformation and, in contrast to the Pacinian corpuscles, are important for signaling continuous states of pressure. They adapt slowly at first but then transmit a steady signal thereafter. Ruffini endings are located in the deep layers of the skin and are scattered throughout the collagenous fibers of the joint capsules. They are

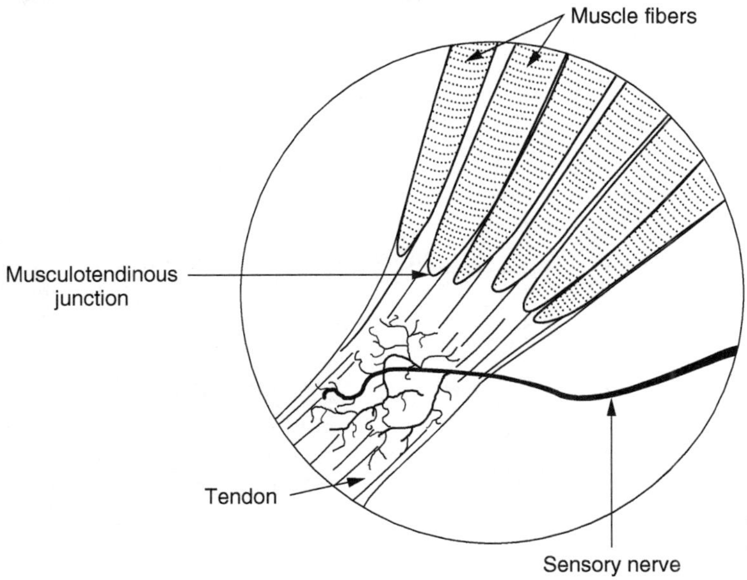

Figure 4.8 Golgi tendon organ located in series at the musculotendinous junction. *Source:* From *The Physiological Basis of Physical Education and Athletics* (4th ed.), by E. L. Fox, R. W. Bowers, & M. L. Foss. Copyright © 1988, W. B. Saunders Company. Reprinted by permission of Times Mirror Higher Education Group, Inc., Dubuque, IA. All rights reserved.

stimulated strongly by sudden joint movements and are thus important in sensing joint position and changes in joint angle of as little as 2 degrees. Each joint receptor monitors a specific section of the total range of motion of the joint. By knowing which receptor is stimulated, the brain can tell how far the joint is bent. The sensing of the complete movement by the central nervous system is the result of the integration of the stimuli received from the individual receptors.

Although *cutaneous* receptors are fundamentally exteroceptors, the ones that receive stimuli from touch (Meissner's corpuscles), pressure (Pacinian corpuscles), and pain (free nerve endings) serve as proprioceptors when they show sensitivity to texture, hardness, softness, and shape and when they participate in the extensor thrust reflex, pain, or flexion withdrawal reflex.

Labyrinthine and Neck Proprioceptors

These proprioceptors detect sensations concerned with determination of body position and changes in position as they relate to equilibrium. The labyrinths detect orientation and movements only in the head, whereas the neck proprioceptors inform the nervous system of the orientation of the head in relation to the body.

The labyrinths of the inner ear consist of the cochlea, the three semicircular canals, and the utricle and saccule (Figure 4.9). The cochlea is concerned with hearing, but the rest of the labyrinth is concerned with the sense of balance, or equilibrium. Each of the canals contains a membranous tube, and the bony spaces for the macule of the utricle and the saccule contain membranous sacs correspondingly named. The entire membranous labyrinth is filled with fluid called endolymph and is lined with hair cells that are sensitive to the movement of the fluid as the head moves. These hair cells are intimately related to branches of the eighth cranial nerve. Thus, movement of the head is translated into nerve impulses that reach the brain.

In addition to hair cells located throughout the labyrinth, there is a gelatinous substance in which otoliths (small carbonate of lime crystals) are embedded. The otoliths accentuate the effects of gravity on the hair cells and thus are able to

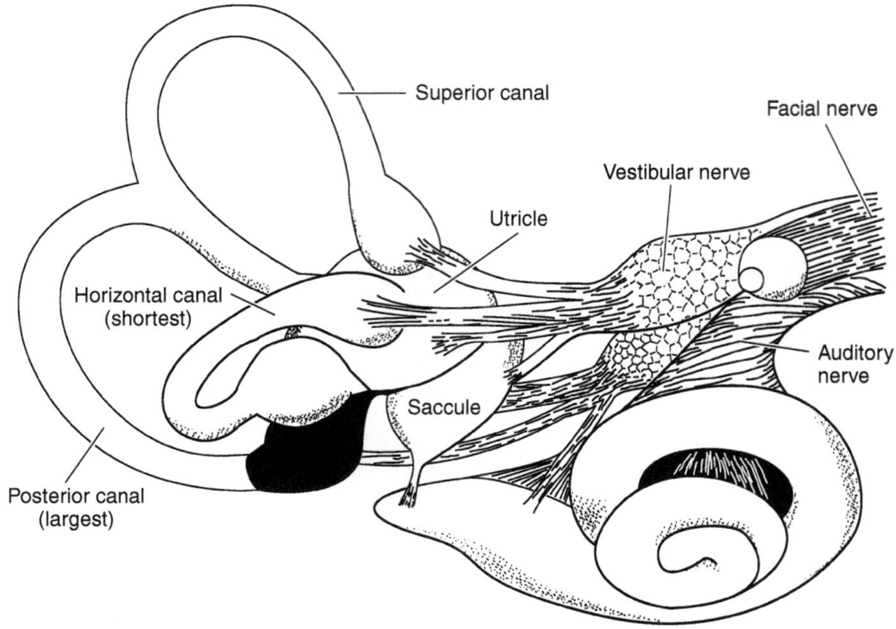

Figure 4.9 The labyrinthine system of the inner ear. *Source:* From *Scientific Bases of Human Movement* (3rd ed.), by B. A. Gowitzke & M. Milner (p. 290). Copyright © 1988, Williams & Wilkins, Baltimore, MD. Reprinted by permission.

detect changes in position that upset static equilibrium. They are also sensitive to linear acceleration by the head.

The semicircular canals are each in a different plane at right angles to each other. When the head turns, the canals move with it, but at first the fluid in them tends to remain stationary owing to inertia. When the head stops, the canals do also, but again, because of inertia, the fluid does not stop moving immediately. Relative motion in the endolymph produces motion in the hair cells, triggering impulses to the cranial nerve. This process enables the canals to detect any changes in angular velocity of the head. The anatomical arrangement of the entire labyrinth is such that some part of it is especially sensitive to any position or direction of movement of the head with respect to gravity.

The most important proprioceptive information needed for the maintenance of equilibrium is that provided by the joint (ligament) receptors of the neck (C1–C3) because they are sensitive to the angle between the body and the head. When the head is bent in one direction, the impulses from the neck prevent the labyrinthine proprioceptors from producing a feeling of imbalance. They do this by sending signals exactly opposite to those transmitted by the labyrinth. If the entire body's orientation with respect to gravity is altered, however, the neck receptors do not counteract the labyrinthine receptors, and change in equilibrium is sensed.

Reflex Movement

Reflexes are integrated at various levels of the nervous system. A reflex movement is a specific pattern of response that occurs without volition and without the need of direction from the cerebrum. The anatomical basis for a reflex act is the reflex arc (Figure 4.10). This consists of an afferent neuron that comes from a receptor organ,

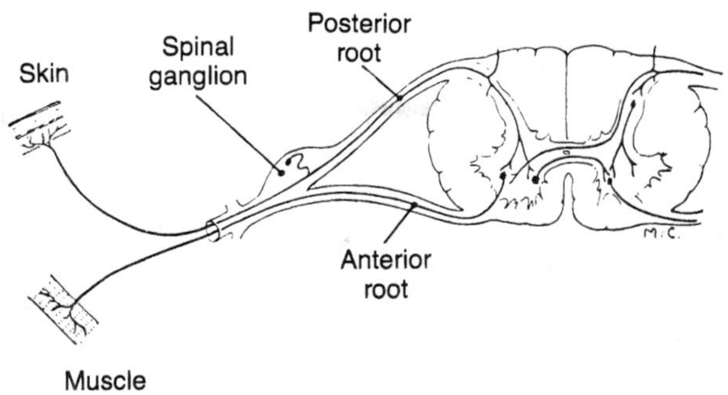

Figure 4.10 Reflex arc mechanism.

enters the spinal cord, and there makes a synaptic connection either directly with the dendrites and the cell body of an efferent neuron or indirectly through one or more connector neurons. The axon of the efferent neuron extends from the cord to the muscle, where its distal branches terminate in muscle fibers. The point of contact between an axon and a muscle fiber is known as a myoneural junction, or motor endplate. The number of reflex arcs and the number of motor units involved depend both on the nature of the reflex and on the extent of muscular activity needed. Automatic reflex motions accompany all normal voluntary motion. Indeed, very few muscles in most movement patterns are under conscious control.

Reflex action, by its very nature, is complex and highly integrated with other control mechanisms. The complicated relationship between propioceptive afferents, exteroceptive afferents, and subconscious levels of control is even now not well understood. What is presented here is a highly simplified discussion of reflex activity, intended as a basic introduction to the concepts of reflex activity. A simplistic but useful list of the reflexes covered is presented in Table 4.2.

Exteroceptive Reflexes

Although some overlap occurs, as could be inferred from the discussion of receptors, two main classes of reflexes are related to skeletal movements—namely, exteroceptive and proprioceptive. Many of the exteroceptor reflexes exhibited by animals and human beings are familiar to us. A horse will twitch its skin when flies alight on it; a dog will scratch when its skin is irritated by a flea, or perhaps tickled by a person. A human jumps upon hearing a sudden loud noise. A person also blinks when a foreign body strikes the eyeball, or even threatens to strike it. Three exteroceptive reflexes that may be of special interest are the extensor thrust, flexor, and crossed extensor reflexes.

Extensor Thrust Reflex

Pressure against the sole of the foot stimulates the Pacinian corpuscles in the subcutaneous tissue and elicits the reflex contraction of the extensor muscles of the lower extremity. When the weight is supported by the feet, the pressure of the floor is sufficient to bring about this reaction. As the weight is shifted to the balls of the foot in preparation for a jump, or to the palms of the hand in preparation for a handspring, the pressure results in the extensor thrust reflex facilitating contractions of the extensor muscles of the legs or arms, respectively, thus assisting the push-off from the floor (Figure 4.11). Similarly in archery, the Pacinian corpuscles in the bow hand are stimulated, and facilitation of the extensor muscles of the bow arm occurs. However, in this instance, the archer must counteract this reflex action and prevent full extension at the elbow or suffer a painful lesson of being whipped by the released strings. The extensor thrust reflex is often included as a proprioceptive reflex in some classifications.

TABLE 4.2 Simplified Reflexes

Reflex	Stimulus	Receptor	Response
Extensor thrust reflex	Deep pressure in subcutaneous tissue	Pacinian corpuscles	Contraction of extensor muscles
Flexor reflex	Pain or noxious stimuli	Free nerve endings	Contraction of flexor muscles
Crossed extensor reflex	Flexor reflex, or unweighting (release of pressure)		Contraction of extensor muscles in opposite limb
Stretch reflex	Stretch	Muscle spindle	
Phasic	High-velocity stretch, short duration	Annulospiral endings	Reflex contraction of same muscle proportional to stimulus; uses alpha efferent motor neuron
Tonic	Slow, sustained stretch	Flower-spray endings	Reset tension in muscle spindle, low-level contraction of same muscles; uses gamma efferent motor neuron
Tendon organ reflex	Tendon stretch	Golgi tendon organ	Relaxation of stretched muscle
Tonic neck reflex	Change in head/neck position	Joint receptors in neck	
Symmetrical	Head/neck flexion or hyperextension		Head/neck flexion, upper extremity flexion; head/neck hyperextension, upper extremity extension
Asymmetrical	Head/neck rotation		Chin side, upper extremity abduction and extension; back of head side, upper extremity flexion and adduction
Labyrinthine reflex	Change in head/neck position	Joint receptors in neck	
Symmetrical	Head/neck flexion or hyperextension		Head/neck flexion, lower extremity flexion; head/neck hyperextension, lower extremity extension
Asymmetrical	Head/neck rotation		Chin side, lower extremity adduction and flexion; back of head side, lower extremity extension and abduction
Righting reflex	Change in head position with respect to gravity	Utricle	Bring head upright with respect to gravity; integrated with the tonic neck and labyrinthine reflexes to produce movements of the extremities to restore balance

Flexor (Nociceptive) Reflex

The flexor reflex most frequently operates in response to pain and is a device for self-protection. Because of the flexor reflex, we quickly withdraw a part of the body the instant it is hurt. If a finger is pricked by a pin or if it inadvertently touches a hot pan, we do not have to decide to remove our hand from the source of pain; we jerk it back even before we realize what happened to it. Furthermore, all the necessary muscles for withdrawing it are activated promptly, not just those in the immediate vicinity of the injury. Although we are

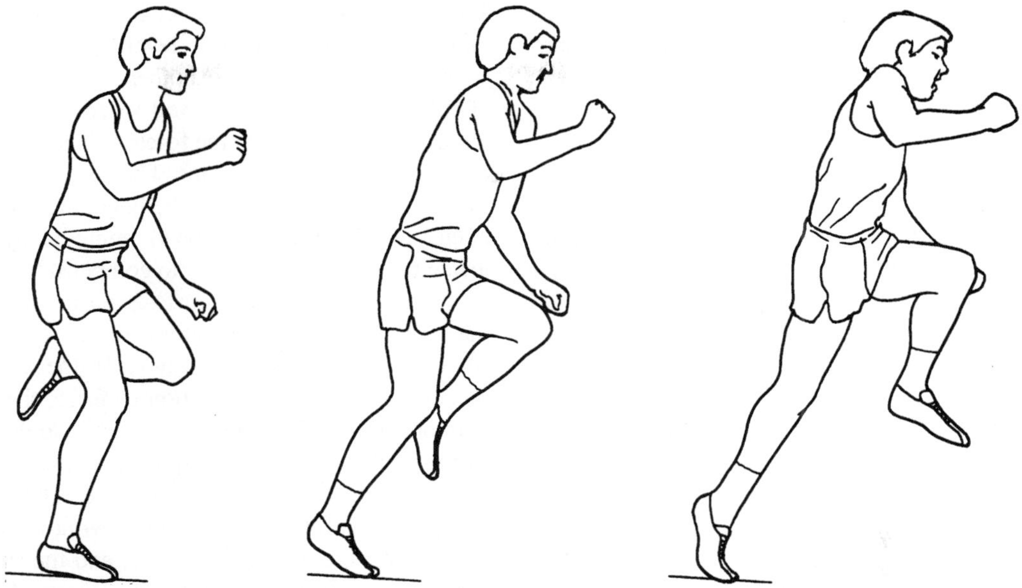

Figure 4.11 Extensor thrust reflex. As the weight is transferred to the ball of the foot in preparation for the hurdle, the concentrated pressure on the ball of the foot may enable the extensor thrust reflex to facilitate the push-off from the ground.

all too aware of the pain, this awareness occurs after the withdrawal and plays no part in the reflex action. The value of the awareness is rather in teaching us to avoid repeating the act that caused the pain. This reflex is also called the nociceptive withdrawal reflex.

Crossed Extensor Reflex

This reflex functions cooperatively with the flexor reflex in response to pain in a weight-bearing limb. For instance, when an animal injures its paw, the flexor reflex causes it to withdraw the paw. Simultaneously, owing to the crossed extensor reflex, the extensor muscles of the opposite limb contract to support the additional weight thrust upon it. Similarly, if a person who is barefoot happens to step on a tack with the right foot, the body weight quickly shifts to the left foot and the right foot is withdrawn from the floor. As the flexors of the right limb contract to enable the lifting of the right foot, the extensors of the left limb contract more strongly to support the weight of the entire body.

Applications of the crossed extensor reflex have also been made to a non-weight-bearing limb. When a pain stimulus is applied to one hand, at the same moment that the hand is withdrawn, the opposite arm will extend as though to push the body away. Some individuals have also suggested that walking may reflect an application of the crossed extensor reflex. Release of pressure from the sole of the back foot results in facilitation of the extensor muscles of the front leg to accommodate the shift in weight over that foot.

Proprioceptive Reflexes

Earlier in this chapter, receptors were classified as exteroceptors and interoceptors, the latter being subdivided into visceral receptors and proprioceptors. Proprioceptive reflexes are generally described as those reflexes that occur in response to stimulation of receptors located in the skeletal muscles, tendons, joints, and labyrinths of the inner ear. According to this interpretation, the proprioceptive reflexes are those interoceptors related to motions and positions of the body. The stretch, or myotatic, reflex is always included among these. Some classifications also include the extensor thrust, the labyrinth and neck, and the tendon organ reflex.

Stretch Reflex

The stretch reflex is so named because stretch on the muscle stimulates the muscle spindle, resulting in the reflex contraction of the stretched muscle and its synergists and relaxation of its antagonists. The muscle spindle picks up the stretch stimulus and transmits it by way of the afferent neuron to the spinal cord. There the central terminal branches of the sensory neuron synapse directly with the dendrites of the motor neuron, which activates the same muscle fibers that were stretched. These fibers then contract. This two-neuron reflex arc is the simplest type of reflex arc, consisting of a single sensory neuron and single motor neuron, which may involve one or more synapses. The important characteristic of this type of reflex arc is that it does not make use of connector neurons in the spinal cord.

There are two responses to the stretch reflex—phasic (short latency) or tonic (long latency)—depending on the velocity at which the stretch occurs. The frequency of discharge from the primary endings of the muscle spindle is directly related to the velocity at which the muscle fibers are being stretched. The greater the frequency of these impulses, the greater will be the resulting muscle fiber contraction.

Phasic response The phasic type includes familiar clinical tests, such as the knee jerk. Reflexes of this type are extremely rapid and the contraction is of brief duration. The word *jerk* gives an accurate picture. Although it is true that the cause of the stimulus in this instance is exteroceptive in nature (a rubber-headed hammer or the edge of the hand), it is nevertheless classed as a proprioceptive reflex. If the stretch is sudden and sufficiently strong, the stretched muscle contracts quickly and forcefully due to the response of the primary endings of the muscle spindles.

Tonic response A slow stretch, such as is elicited in postural sway, will result in a tonic response (Figure 4.12). Another demonstration of this reflex may be observed when a weight is placed in the hand, with the forearm in 90 degrees of flexion at the elbow joint. The result is likely to be a subtle depression of the hand and forearm (slight extension at the elbow) immediately followed by a return movement to compensate.

Movements that put muscles on a stretch in the backswing or preparatory phase can take advantage of the stretch reflex. If the desired outcome is a strong application of force, the preparatory movement should be rapid, to benefit from the phasic increase in spindle discharge, and long, to increase the tonic response. The backswing in forceful striking and throwing patterns, the crouch before a vertical jump, and the stretch before a tuck dive are all examples (Figure 4.13a). If, however, the desired outcome is accuracy, as in a badminton low serve or a golf putt, the backswing should be short and slow, with a pause before the force application (Figure 4.13b). This approach allows the phasic frequencies of the primary endings to slow down to tonic level.

In the static type of stretch reflex, the muscle is stretched slowly. This causes primary and secondary endings of several spindles to be stimulated and results in a more sustained muscular contraction. The importance of the static stretch is that it causes muscle contraction as long as a muscle is put on excessive stretch. When such a reflex is elicited by the stretch caused by the tendency of weight-bearing joints to flex, the response of the extensor muscles is commonly referred to as the *antigravity reflex*. Some also use this term to include the response of lower extremity and trunk muscles to the involuntary forward-backward swaying that usually occurs when a person stands in one position for a long time.

The gamma efferent system functions to adjust the muscle spindle length by causing the intrafusal fibers to contract (see p. 75). This mechanism receives signals whenever the alpha motor system stimulates the extrafusal (skeletal muscle) fibers. Thus, a balance between the length of the skeletal and spindle fibers is maintained.

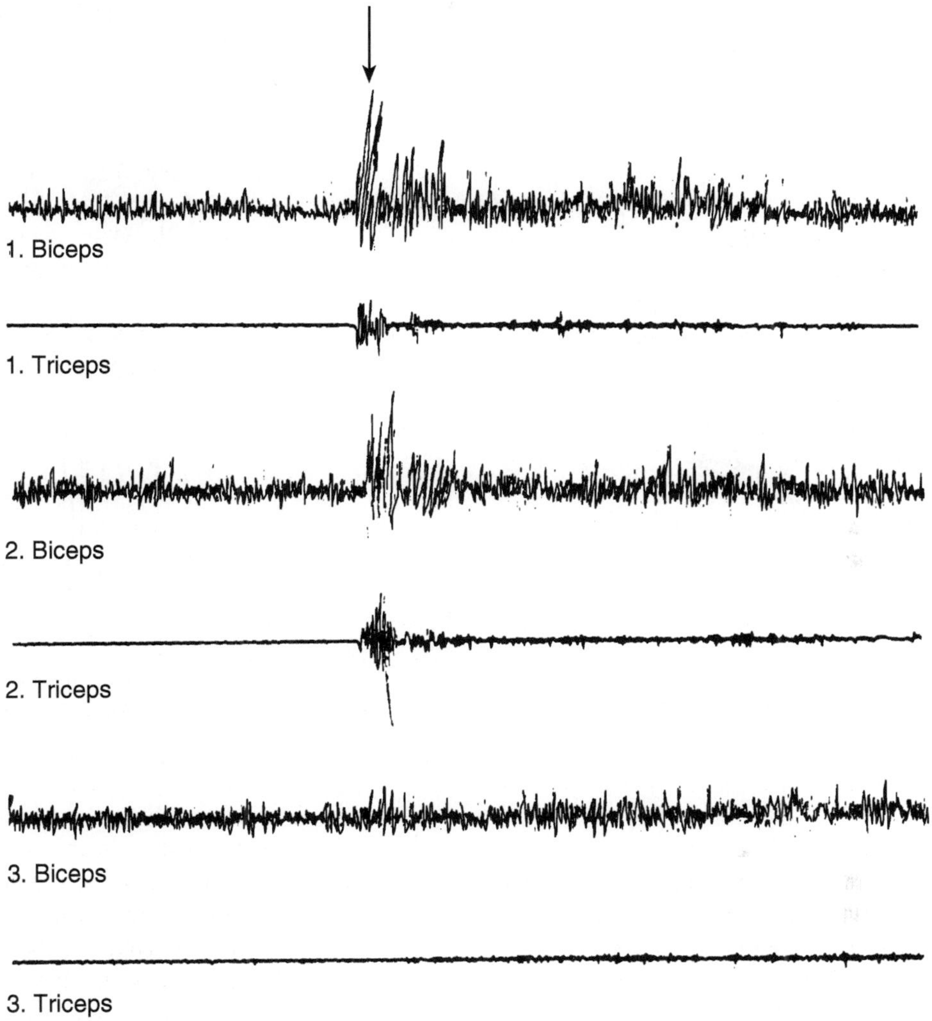

Figure 4.12 Electromyograms: Stretch reflex. Subject is maintaining the elbow joint at 90 degrees of flexion while holding a bucket. Arrow (↓) indicates loading the bucket. Tracings 1 and 2 show the biceps and triceps muscle activity when the load is dropped from decreasing heights (phasic response). Tracing 3 shows muscle activity when the load is placed into the bucket (tonic response).

In addition, the gamma efferent system is under voluntary control (gamma bias). For example, this mechanism is at work when a subject anticipates receiving a weight. Impulses are sent along the gamma system, adjusting the threshold level of the muscle spindle so that as soon as any change occurs, a reflex contraction results. Remember what happens when lifting an empty box after thinking it would be weighted.

The flower-spray endings, or secondary afferents, are less sensitive to stretch and only result in the tonic response. Therefore, a greater or prolonged stretch is necessary to stimulate the secondary endings. Whereas the primary endings always facilitate the contraction of the muscle in which they are located, the influence of the secondary afferents depends on the type of muscle in which it is located. Secondary afferents

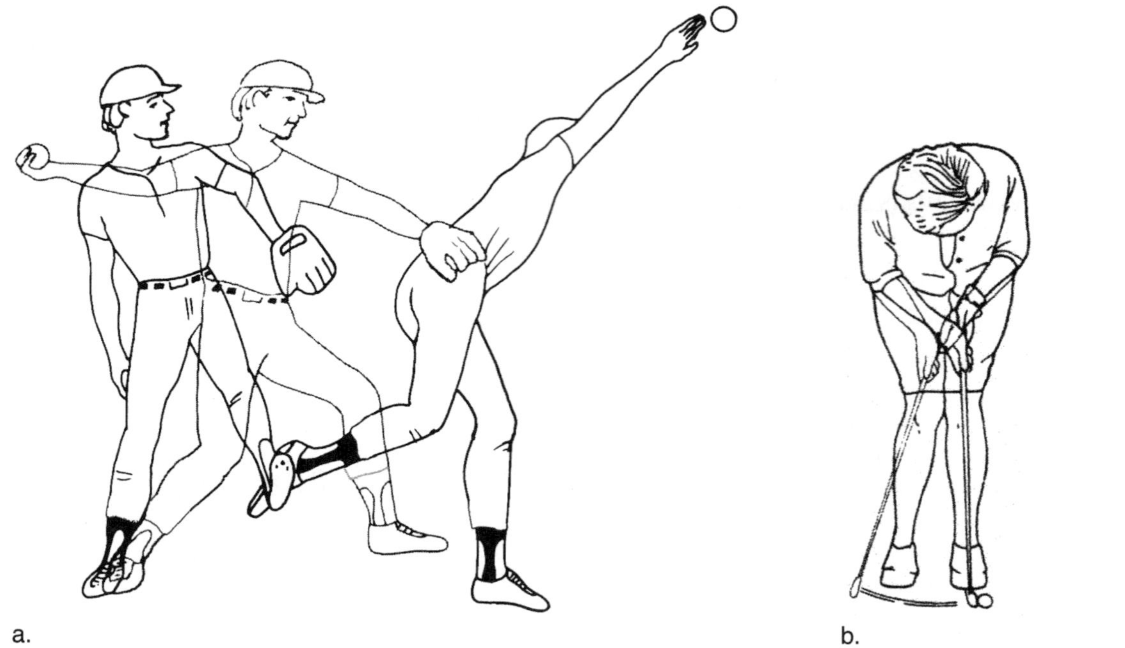

Figure 4.13 (a) The phasic type of stretch reflex will facilitate force development if the backswing is long and rapid with little pause between the backswing and force phase, as demonstrated in a forceful overarm throw. (b) To take advantage of the tonic type of stretch reflex when accuracy is desired, the backswing should be short and slow, with a pause before the force phase. An example is the golf putt.

facilitate flexor muscles and inhibit extensor muscle contraction. Therefore, the secondary afferent response would reinforce the primary afferent response if the stimulated spindle was located in a flexor muscle but would result in a cocontraction if the stimulated spindle were in an extensor muscle. This would be due to the reflex contraction facilitated by the primary endings in the extensor muscle and the facilitation of the flexor muscle by the secondary ending. Two-joint muscles respond to secondary afferent stimulation as though they are flexor muscles.

Spindles may also be stimulated by pressure and vibration. This fact is important whenever pressure must be placed on another individual. In gymnastics, if pressure is placed on flexor muscles, the gymnast may fall rather than be helped to hold a position. Similarly, pressure on the extensor muscles when working in rehabilitation may inhibit elbow flexion. Use of this technique may provide additional variations to the rehabilitation setting.

In some instances it would be desirable to minimize the effect of the stretch reflex, as in flexibility exercises. This can be done if the stretch is done slowly and is held, as in static stretching. A quick stretch or bounce will evoke a stronger, phasic, reflex contraction.

Tendon Reflex

The second muscle proprioceptor, the *Golgi tendon organ (GTO)*, is located in series at the musculotendinous junction. It too is stimulated by tension, but because of its location, the stretch may be induced on the tendon when the muscle contracts as well as when the muscle is stretched. The threshold of the GTO muscle stretch is higher than that of the muscle spindle. That is, if the stimulus is strong enough to stimulate the GTO, the muscle spindle response is overridden. On the other hand, the GTO is very sensitive to tension when it is produced by tendon stretch resulting from muscle contraction. In either case, the reflex effect is to inhibit impulses from the motor nerve to the muscle and its synergists, thus causing the muscle to relax. Simultaneously, the antagonist contracts from being facilitated.

When tension on the muscle is extreme, the Golgi tendon organs' inhibiting action results in sudden relaxation of the muscle. This effect is called the *lengthening reaction* and undoubtedly serves as protection for muscles or tendons that could be torn or ruptured by the strong contractile force. Guyton (2000) has suggested that the tendon reflex serves as a feedback mechanism to control the tension in the muscle. If the tension in the muscle became too great, the inhibiting action of the receptors would cause relaxation. If the muscle tension became too little, the receptors would stop firing, and the muscle tension would be able to increase.

The behavior of the tendon reflex in the performance of some skills by beginners is also a matter of interest. It may be that the reason beginners do not follow through has to do with the fact that the tendon reflex causes relaxation of vigorously contracting muscle. It is suggested that until an increase in the Golgi tendon organ threshold develops with learning, beginners may need voluntary effort to counteract the inhibitory effect of the tendon reflex.

Labyrinth and Neck Reflexes

Tonic labyrinth reflex Newborn infants start out with very simple reflexes, which in the process of normal motor development are suppressed or modified. This phenomenon is especially evident in the labyrinth and neck reflexes. The tonic labyrinth reflexes emanate from utricle and semicircular canal receptors, which are sensitive to changes in position of the head with respect to gravity. Because of the primitive tonic labyrinth reflex present in the newborn child, a supine position of the head facilitates extension of the extremities, whereas a prone position inhibits extension and facilitates flexion. At a few months of age or more, this primitive reflex is suppressed, and the labyrinth righting reflex is evident. In cooperation with other righting reflexes of the neck and eyes, it evokes muscular responses to restore the body to a normal upright position.

Righting reflex Righting reflexes can be demonstrated in adults. They respond to any body-tilting action by attempting to restore balance through facilitating limb actions, such as an arm or leg being thrust out. In spinning, the limbs facilitate restoration of the normal head position by actions that inhibit the rotation. The arm on the same side as the direction of the spin is thrust out during the spin, and the opposite arm is thrust out at the termination of the spin. This latter action is probably a response to the imbalance caused by the dizziness experienced at the conclusion of the spin because of the continuation of movement (inertia) of the fluid and resulting stimulation of the hair cells.

Tonic neck reflex Tonic neck reflexes are evident when the joint receptors in the neck are stimulated by any movement in the neck. They are also present at birth, and even though they are masked by further development, they remain in adults. Like the tonic labyrinth reflex, they can also be demonstrated in adults. Actions due to tonic neck reflexes in the primitive infant form are predictable. If the head is flexed, flexion will occur in the upper extremities and extension in the lower ones. With head extension, the opposite occurs—extension in the upper extremities and flexion in the lower ones. Rotation of the head to the right is accompanied by extension and abduction of the limbs on the chin side, and flexion and adduction on the opposite side.

Tonic neck and tonic labyrinth reflexes become most apparent in adults in stressful situations. They are hard to distinguish from each other because movements of the head and neck occur together, and labyrinth and neck receptors are stimulated simultaneously. In some instances they reinforce each other in their effect on joint actions of the extremities, and in some instances they oppose each other. There are times when we should take advantage of them to facilitate actions and other times when it would be beneficial to suppress them.

The neck reflexes are more effective in modifying upper extremity actions, and the labyrinthine in modifying those of the lower extremities, and these results are still accepted. There is no question that head position influences the actions of the arms. When a strong pulling action is required, flexion of the head will facilitate it to some extent. On the other hand, the neck reflex facilitation suggests that the head should be extended for strong pushing actions. For facilitating a one-armed pull, the head should be turned away in addition to being flexed and, in a one-armed push, the head should be turned toward the pushing arm. Other examples of reflex facilitation include extension of the head in a handstand to reinforce extension in the arms, flexion of the head to reinforce trunk, arms, and leg flexion in forward or backward rolls, and head rotation in archery to facilitate bow arm pushing on the chin side and bowstring arm pulling by the opposite side (Deutsch et al., 1987; Gowitzke & Milner, 1988; Le Pellec & Maton, 1993).

Undoubtedly one of the difficulties in learning new motor skills is the failure to suppress reflex responses. In falling backward, our natural reaction is to extend the arms and throw the head forward. If a beginner did this in attempting a back dive, the entry into the water would be uncomfortable, to say the least. The labyrinth righting reflex must be suppressed consciously so that the head may be extended back and the body follow. Belly flops in front dives can also be attributed to the labyrinth righting reflex.

Posture and Locomotor Mechanisms

Whether because of reflex action or some other mechanism, it seems apparent that the human body has certain provisions for remaining more or less erect and for engaging in locomotion and that these follow the general pattern of reflex behavior. The coordinated efforts of the body to resist the downward pull of gravity include the extensor thrust reflex, the static type of stretch reflex in response to gravitational pull, the muscular action evoked by forward-backward swaying, and the various mechanisms for preserving equilibrium, including visual orientation and labyrinthine reflexes.

In regard to locomotion, the action of the legs of a four-footed animal has been attributed to reflex action. Some classify this reflex as a division of the crossed extensor reflex. Because research in this area has been done primarily on dogs and cats, it has been suggested that this reflex exists only in quadrupeds. Nevertheless, it is logical to assume that it exists also in humans inasmuch as the early forms of locomotion—creeping and crawling—resemble the locomotion of quadrupeds. Even after the erect position is assumed, the swing of the arms in opposition to the lower extremities reflects the earlier four-footed gait.

Volitional Movement

This topic involves such an extensive and complex body of knowledge that only the bare essentials and a few concepts can be touched on here. The chief anatomical structures concerned with volitional movement, in addition to those mentioned earlier (skeletal muscle, basic nerve structures, motor units, and sensory receptors), are the cerebral cortex, the cerebellum, the brainstem, spinal cord, and the numerous motor pathways, both pyramidal (corticospinal tracts) and extrapyramidal tracts.

Volitional movement is goal directed where the higher centers of the brain have the most general control, with each succeeding level having more specific control. The central nervous system is often divided into five levels in hierarchical order.

Central Nervous System: Levels of Control

The *cerebral cortex* (Figure 4.14) is the first and highest level of control. It is the level at which consciousness occurs and the level responsible

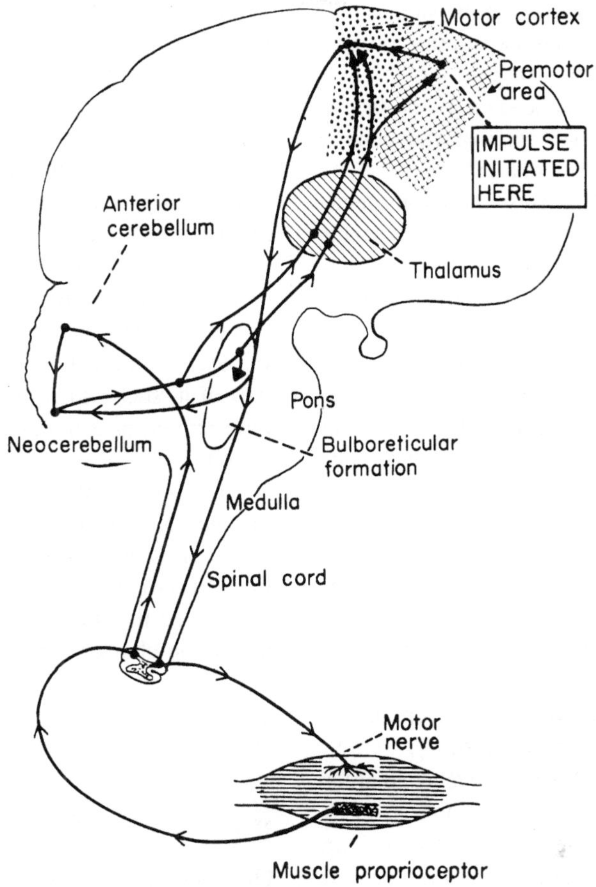

Figure 4.14 Feedback circuits of the cerebellum for damping motor movements. *Source:* From *Function of the Human Body* (4th ed.), by A. C. Guyton. Copyright © 1974, W. B. Saunders, Orlando, FL. Reprinted by permission.

for the initiation of voluntary movement. The cerebral cortex contains a motor area situated in front of the transverse central fissure known as the precentral gyrus. Within this area, all body parts are represented by an area whose size correlates with the complexity or precision of the body part. Therefore, the area representing the thumb and fingers requires a larger area than that representing the foot. Movements, not muscles, are represented here. The premotor area located in front of the motor cortex is responsible for learning complex acts.

The basal ganglia area is the second level of control. This area is located at the thalamus level and is often identified as containing the subcortical nuclei. The basal ganglia area is responsible for homeostasis; that is, for maintaining a level of constancy within prescribed ranges before adjustments are made. It is responsible for the coordination and control of some learned acts involving posture and equilibrium, including the sensory integration for the righting reflexes.

Level three is in the cerebellum (Figure 4.14). The cerebellum is often referred to as the "little brain." It plays a key role in sensory integration, receiving diverse inputs and acting as a feedback center comparing what should have been with the motion that occurred. The cerebellum is a vital center for regulating the timing and intensity of muscle activity to produce smooth, precise movement.

The pons–medulla area, known as the *brainstem* (Figure 4.14), is level four of the central nervous system. This area contains the reticular formation, which encompasses numerous neurons and nuclei and houses important centers for arousal and monitoring of physiological parameters from the cardiorespiratory mechanisms. The brainstem also contains key facilitory and inhibitory centers, thereby having a direct effect on muscle sensitivity.

The lowest level of control of the central nervous system, level five, is the *spinal cord* (Figure 4.14), containing cell bodies of the lower motor neurons that control the skeletal muscles. It has the most specific control and is the common pathway between the central and peripheral nervous systems. Because signal integration occurs at synapses, and all synaptic connections between and among neurons occur within the central nervous system, the spinal cord is the final point for nerve impulse integration and control.

Although reported as discrete levels and areas with specific functions, functions of the five levels and areas of the central nervous system overlap depending on the classification scheme used. It is true, however, that higher centers may override lower centers, but the reverse is not true. For accurate volitional movement to occur, sensory information is imperative, and continuous sensory stimulation is necessary for accurate volitional action. Moreover, the response of the central nervous system depends on the initial position of the segment or limb (joint angle) for the intensity of muscle contraction.

Kinesthesis

The conscious awareness of position of body parts and the amount and rate of joint movement is known as kinesthesis. Kinesthetic sensations originate primarily in the sensory receptors of the joint capsules and ligaments and include the Ruffini endings, Pacinian corpuscles, and Golgi tendon organs. Signals from these receptors are transmitted rapidly to the cord and brain in beta type A nerve fibers so that the central nervous system is instantaneously aware (at the cerebral cortex level of conscious awareness) of the exact position of the body parts. Without this rapid transmission and processing of information, accurately controlled movements could not proceed. Kinesthetic perception and memory are the basis of voluntary movement and motor learning. This perception and memory enable the performer to initiate a whole movement pattern or modify a part of it, such as the elimination or addition of a joint action, or a change in timing or speed of an action.

Current thinking in kinesthesia is that the muscle spindles and motor afferents play a large role in position sense. For this to be true, some CNS processing has to be occurring. It has been speculated that the "sense of effort" in producing a position change contributes greatly to this. The most logical explanation at this time is that multiple sources of information are centrally processed (Walsh et al., 2009; Proske, 2006).

Reciprocal Inhibition and Coactivation

One of the mechanisms that provides for economical and coordinated movement is known as reciprocal inhibition. According to this concept, when motor neurons are transmitting impulses to muscles, causing them to contract, the motor neurons that supply their antagonists are simultaneously and reciprocally inhibited. The antagonistic muscles, therefore, remain relaxed and the movers, or agonists, contract without opposition. The relaxation occurs to the degree to which the agonists are activated. Reciprocal inhibition operates automatically in movements elicited by the stretch reflex and also in familiar volitional movements. In more complicated and in less familiar coordinations, its operation depends on the degree of skill developed by the performer.

Coactivation, or reciprocal activation, most frequently appears in movement when there is uncertainty about the movement task. As practice or training increases familiarity with the movement, coactivation decreases in favor of reciprocal inhibition. In this way efficiency of movement also increases. Further evidence suggests that coactivation also occurs in order to maintain joint stiffness, especially when faced with an unstable or perturbed posture.

NEUROMUSCULAR ANALYSIS

The muscle-response patterns of well-learned motor skills involve the integrated action of many reflexes and the inhibition of others. After repeated viewing of the performance "live" or on film, the student should name and discuss the reflexes that could be acting at various points in each phase. The reflexes that should be considered are spindle reflexes (stretch reflex), the Golgi tendon organ reflex, joint reflexes, cutaneous responses, labyrinthine reflexes, neck reflexes, and visual righting reflexes. For each reflex, the receptors involved should be identified, the expected action facilitated by the reflex described, and the actual results explained. To return to the standing long jump in Figure 1.3, the following reflex actions are plausible examples of reflex action:

1. Reflex: Labyrinthine head-righting reflex is present.
   Receptor: Labyrinthine system—inner ear.
   Time: Preparation for takeoff.
   Evidence: As the trunk leans farther forward, the head and neck become more hyperextended.
2. Reflex: Stretch reflexes in extensors of hip, knee, and ankle are present.
   Receptor: Muscle spindle.
   Time: Early preparation for takeoff (crouch).
   Evidence: The stretch reflexes are activated in the extensors as flexion occurs in the hips, knees, and ankles. The result is facilitation of contraction of the extensor muscles.
3. Reflex: Extensor thrust reflexes.
   Receptor: Pacinian corpuscles (soles of the feet).
   Time: As force is applied to the floor for takeoff.
   Evidence: Pressure facilitates extensor muscle contraction of the lower extremities.

REFERENCES AND SELECTED READINGS

Asseman, F., & Gahery, Y. (2005). Effect of head position and visual condition on balance control in inverted stance. *Neuroscience Letters,* 375(2), 134–137.

Basta, D., Todt, I., Scherer, H., Clarke, A., & Ernst, A. (2005). Postural control in otolith disorders. *Human Movement Science,* 24(2), 268–279.

Bawa, P., Pang, M.Y., Oleson, K.A., & Calancie, B. (2006). Rotation of motoneurons during prolonged isometric contractions in humans. *Journal of Neurophysiology,* 96(3), 1135–1140.

Bent, L. R., Potvin, J. R., Brooke, J. D., & McIlroy, W. E. (2001). Mediolateral balance adjustments preceding reflexive limb withdrawal are modified by postural demands. *Brain Research,* 914(1–2), 100–105.

Chalmers, G. (2002). Do Golgi tendon organs really inhibit muscle activity at high force levels to save muscles from injury, and adapt with strength training? *Sports Biomechanics,* 1(2), 239–249.

Deschenes, M. R. (2004). Effects of aging on muscle fibre type and size. *Sports Medicine,* 34(12), 809–824.

Deutsch, H., Kilani, H., Moustafa, E., & Hamilton, N. (1987). Effect of head-neck position on elbow flexor muscle torque production. *Physical Therapy,* 67, 517–521.

Gowitzke, B. A., & Milner, M. (1988). *Understanding the scientific basis of human movement* (3rd ed.). Baltimore: Williams & Wilkins.

Guyton, A. C. (2000). *Textbook of medical physiology* (10th ed.). Philadelphia: Saunders.

Highstein, S. M., Rabbitt, R. D., Holstein, G. R., & Boyle, R. D. (2005). Determinants of spatial and temporal coding by semicircular canal afferents. *Journal of Neurophysiology,* 93(5), 2359–2370.

Hughes, B. W., Kusner, L. L., & Kaminski, H. J. (2005). Molecular architecture of the neuromuscular junction. *Muscle and Nerve,* 33(4), 445–461.

Ito, Y., Corna, S., von Brevern, M., Bronstein, A., & Gresty, M. (1997). The functional effectiveness of neck muscle reflexes for head-righting in response to sudden fall. *Experimental Brain Research,* 117(2), 266–272.

Lackner, J. R., & DiZio, P. (2005). Vestibular, proprioceptive, and haptic contributions to spatial orientation. *Annual Review of Psychology,* 56, 115–147.

Le Pellec, A., & Maton, B. (1993). The influence of tonic neck reflexes on voluntary fatiguing elbow movements in humans. *European Journal of Applied Physiology,* 67, 237–238.

Loofbourrow, G. N. (1973). Neuromuscular integration. In *Science and medicine of exercise and sports* (2nd ed.), edited by W. R. Johnson & E. Buskirk. New York: Harper & Row.

MacIntosh, B. R., Gardiner, P., & McComas, A. J. (2006). *Skeletal muscle: Form and function* (2nd ed.). Champaign, IL: Human Kinetics.

Nakazawa, K., Kawashima, N., Akai, M., & Yano, H. (2004). On the reflex coactivation of ankle flexor and extensor muscles induced by a sudden drop of support surface during walking in humans. *Journal of Applied Physiology,* 96(2), 604–611.

Ogiso, K., McBride, J. M., Finni, T., & Komi, P. V. (2005). Effects of effort and EMG levels on short-latency stretch reflex modulation after varying background muscle contractions. *Journal of Electromyography and Kinesiology,* 15(4), 333–340.

Park, S., Toole, T., & Lee, S. (1999). Functional roles of the proprioceptive system in the control of goal directed movement. *Perceptual and Motor Skills,* 88, 631–647.

Proske, U. (2006). Kinesthesia: The role of muscle receptors. *Muscle Nerve,* 34, 545–558.

Wakeling, J. M., Uehli, K., & Rozitis, A. I. (2006). Muscle fibre recruitment can respond to the mechanics of the muscle contraction. *Journal of the Royal Society Interface,* 3, 533–544.

Walsh, L. D., Smith, J. L., Gandevia, S. C., & Taylor, J. L. (2009). The combined effect of muscle contraction history and motor commands on human position sense. *Experimental Brain Research,* 195, 603–610.

Yakovenko, S., Gritsenko, V., & Prochazka, A. (2004). Contribution of stretch reflexes to locomotor control: A modeling study. *Biological Cybernetics,* 90(2), 146–155.

Zehr, E. P., & Stein, R. (1999). What functions do reflexes serve during human locomotion? *Progress in Neurobiology,* 58, 185–205.

LABORATORY EXPERIENCES

1. Engage a partner in arm wrestling until one of you loses. Explain the sudden cessation of muscle tension in the loser that resulted in the end of the contest.
2. Record and explain what happens neurologically when an individual is upset from a blow in front of the knees as opposed to behind them.
3. Explain what happens neurologically when an individual pushes a door at the same time a person on the other side pulls it open.
4. Ask your partner to stand facing you with eyes closed. By moving body segments, place your partner in some novel pose. Ask your partner, with eyes still closed, to describe the position exactly. After once again assuming the original standing position, ask your partner to reproduce the novel position. Explain the neuromuscular mechanisms that enable your partner to sense and reproduce the movement.
5. Record the distance of your best of three standing broad jumps. Repeat the jumps, but this time flex the head and neck vigorously as the legs are extended. After a few practice trials record the distance of the three jumps, which incorporate the reflex pattern. Compare your results with those of others in the class. What effect did the reflex pattern have? Explain.

6. Stand in a doorway with your arms at your side. Now press the backs of your hands strongly against the door jambs. Hold this position for at least 30 seconds. Step clear of the doorway and turn your head to the right. What happens to your arms? Explain.
7. Look at the sequence of film tracings for the volleyball serve depicted in Exercise 5.3 in Appendix G. Which proprioceptive reflexes could be present in the position represented in frames b and c? For each reflex named, state the evidence that would suggest the presence of the reflex, the expected effect the reflex could have on the movement, and the verification of the effect as shown by the action in the next frames. Were there any expected reflex actions that apparently did not occur? Explain.

CHAPTER 5

The Upper Extremity

The Shoulder Region

OUTLINE

OBJECTIVES

At the conclusion of this chapter, the student should be able to:

1. Name, locate, and describe the structure and ligamentous reinforcements of the articulations of the shoulder region.
2. Name and demonstrate the movements possible in the joints of the shoulder region regardless of starting position.
3. Name and locate the muscles and muscle groups of the shoulder region, and name their primary actions as agonists, stabilizers, neutralizers, or antagonists.
4. Analyze the fundamental movements of the arm and trunk with respect to joint and muscle actions.
5. Describe the common injuries of the shoulder region.
6. Perform an anatomical analysis of the shoulder region in a motor skill.

SCAPULOHUMERAL RHYTHM

Anatomical cooperation is beautifully illustrated in the movements of the arms on the trunk. The arm travels through a wide range of movements, and in each of these the scapula cooperates by placing the glenoid fossa in the most favorable position for the head of the humerus. This is known as *scapulohumeral rhythm*. When the arm is elevated sideward (abducted), for instance, the scapula rotates upward; when it is elevated forward (flexed), the scapula not only rotates upward but it tends to slide partially around the rib cage (abducted). Although occasionally movement of the scapula is deliberately repressed (as in some stylized dance movements, and in some exercises), in all natural movements, the scapula shares with the humerus in the movements of the arm on the trunk. In abduction of the arm, for instance, the movements of the scapula and humerus are continuous throughout the movement, with the humeral movement accounting for approximately two-thirds of the total movement and the scapular movement for one-third. It is important to remember, however, that this cooperative scapulohumeral rhythm is not a linear relationship. It varies with individuals and with the phase of the movement. Scapulohumeral rhythm may vary across age groups and with certain types of activity, including throwing. Load and speed of movement may also produce variations. In the normal adult, however, this cooperation is fairly predictable.

The upper extremity is suspended from the axial skeleton (head and trunk) by means of the shoulder girdle. The latter consists of the sternum and two clavicles in front, and two scapulae in back. The sternoclavicular joints connect the sternum and each clavicle, and the acromioclavicular joints connect the acromion process of each scapula with the corresponding clavicle. Because there is no union between the two scapulae in back, this is an incomplete girdle. The upper extremity's connection with the shoulder girdle is made through the glenohumeral joint, the joint between the head of the humerus and the glenoid fossa of the scapula, better known as the shoulder joint.

The sternoclavicular joint is an exceedingly small one, about the size of the joint between the great toe and the first metatarsal bone, yet it is the sole skeletal connection between the upper extremity and the trunk. This anatomical arrangement accounts for the extensive freedom of motion enjoyed by the upper extremity and is a vital factor in the superb cooperation that exists between the shoulder joint and the shoulder girdle. The upper arm has a remarkably wide range of motion owing largely to its ball and shallow socket construction. Its movements are further amplified by the cooperative actions of the shoulder girdle, as just described.

To understand and appreciate the great variety of movements of the arm on the trunk, it is essential that one be thoroughly familiar with the structure and function of each joint involved and be able to distinguish between the contributions of each in any given movement.

The Shoulder Girdle (Acromioclavicular and Sternoclavicular Articulations)

Structure of Acromioclavicular Articulation

The articulation between the acromion process of the scapula and the outer end of the clavicle (Figure 5.1) belongs to the diarthrodial classification. Within this group it is further classified as an irregular (arthrodial) joint. A small wedge-shaped disc may be found between the upper part of the joint surfaces, but this is frequently absent. The articular capsule is strengthened above by the acromioclavicular ligament, which passes from the upper part of the outer end of the clavicle to the upper surface of the acromion process. The joint is strengthened behind by the aponeurosis of the trapezius and deltoid muscles. The clavicle is further stabilized by means of the coracoclavicular ligament (actually two ligaments, the conoid and the trapezoid), which, as the name suggests, binds the clavicle to the coracoid process.

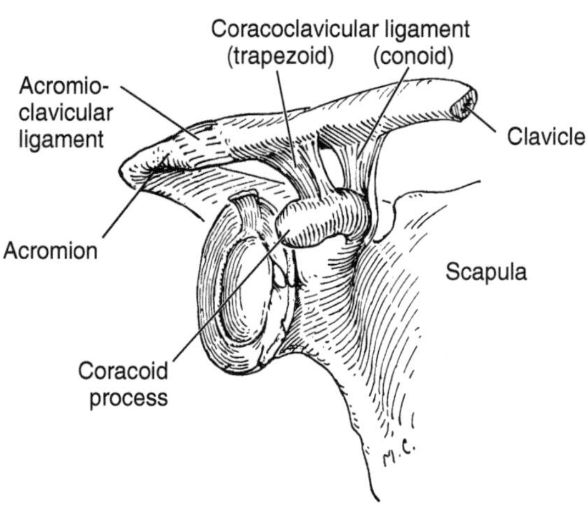

Figure 5.1 Anterior view of acromioclavicular articulation.

The conoid ligament passes from the base of the coracoid process to the conoid tubercle on the underside of the clavicle. The trapezoid ligament extends from the top of the coracoid process to the trapezoid ridge on the underside of the clavicle.

Structure of Sternoclavicular Articulation

The sternal end of the clavicle articulates with both the sternum and the cartilage of the first rib (Figure 5.2). It is classified as a double arthrodial joint because there are two joint cavities, one on either side of the articular disc. This round, flat disc of white fibrocartilage is attached above to the upper, posterior border of the articular surface of the clavicle and below to the cartilage of the first rib near its junction with the sternum. The articular capsule is thin above and below but is thickened in front and behind by bands of fibers called the anterior and posterior sternoclavicular ligaments.

The sternoclavicular articulation is of great importance in the movements of the shoulder girdle and of the arm as a whole because it is the only bony connection between the humerus and axial skeleton. It permits limited motion of the clavicle in all three planes and, because of the bone's attachment to the scapula at its distal end, is partially responsible for the latter's movements. It is reinforced by four ligaments: the anterior sternoclavicular, a band of fibers blending with the anterior fibers of the articular capsule limiting anterior clavicular motion; the posterior sternoclavicular, which blends with the posterior fibers of the articular capsule limiting posterior clavicular motion; the interclavicular, consisting of a flat band that passes across the upper margin of the sternum and attaches to the sternal end of each clavicle and limits downward clavicular motion; and the costoclavicular, a short, strong band of fibers that connects the upper border of the first costal cartilage with the costal tuberosity on the underside of the clavicle and restricts clavicular elevation, protraction, and retraction.

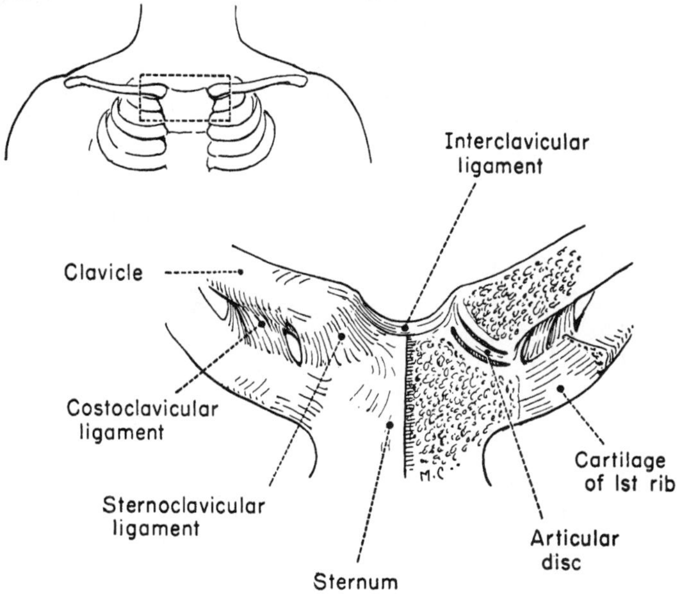

Figure 5.2 Anterior view of sternoclavicular articulation.

The movements of the clavicle at the sternoclavicular joint are as follows: elevation and depression, which occur approximately in the frontal plane about an anteroposterior axis; horizontal forward-backward (protraction and retraction) movements, which occur in the horizontal plane about a vertical axis; and a limited degree of forward and backward rotation, which occurs approximately in the sagittal plane about the bone's own longitudinal axis. (In forward rotation, the top of the clavicle revolves forward-downward.)

Movements

It is customary to define the movements of the shoulder girdle (Figure 5.3) in terms of the movements of the scapulae. In doing this, there is some danger that the reader will visualize the movement as taking place solely in the joint between the scapula and the clavicle. It is well to emphasize that every movement of the scapula involves motion in both joints, the acromioclavicular and the sternoclavicular. The movements of the shoulder girdle expressed in terms of the composite movements of the scapula are as follows.

Elevation

An upward movement of the scapula (Figure 5.3a), with the vertebral border remaining approximately parallel to the spinal column. The elevation of the scapula is the direct result of elevation of the outer end of the clavicle, a movement that takes place at the sternoclavicular joint. This movement occurs to a slight extent during elevation of the humerus and to a greater extent in lifting the shoulders in a hunching gesture. The farther the clavicles depart from the horizontal position, the closer the scapulae move toward each other. The latter movement might well be called passive adduction, because it is caused by the movement of the clavicles rather than by the adductor muscles of the scapulae.

Depression

The return from the position of elevation. There is no depression below the normal resting position.

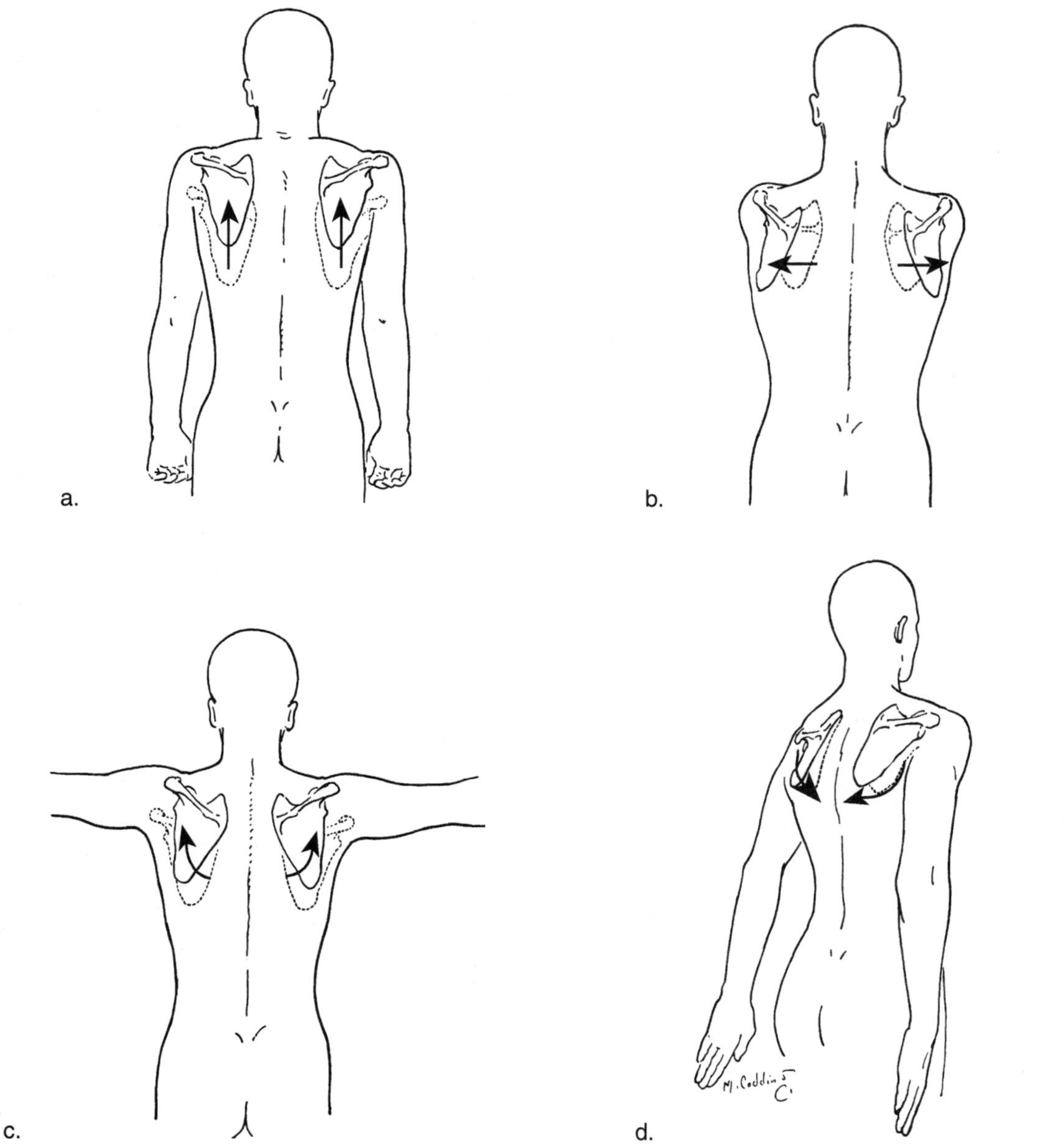

Figure 5.3 Movements of the shoulder girdle: (a) elevation; (b) abduction (combined with lateral tilt and upward rotation); (c) upward rotation; (d) anterior tilt.

Abduction, or Protraction

A lateral movement of the scapula away from the spinal column with the vertebral border remaining approximately parallel to it (Figure 5.3b). Pure abduction of the scapula is a hypothetical movement. Actually, because of two factors, the rounded contour of the thorax and the forward movement of the clavicle about a vertical axis at the sternoclavicular joint, a pure lateral movement of the scapula in the frontal plane is impossible. As the scapula abducts, it turns slightly about its vertical axis in a movement known as a lateral tilt.

This turning is characterized by a slight backward movement of the vertebral border and a corresponding forward movement of the axillary border. This movement causes the glenoid fossa to face slightly forward and the arms, if relaxed, to hang in a more forward position and in slight inward (medial) rotation.

Adduction, or Retraction

A medial movement of the scapula toward the spinal column combined with a reduction of lateral tilt.

Upward Rotation

A rotation of the scapula in the frontal plane so that the glenoid fossa faces somewhat upward (Figure 5.3c). The movement occurs largely at the acromioclavicular joint but is accompanied by elevation of the outer end of the clavicle. Upward rotation is always associated with elevation of the humerus, either sideward or forward. This scapular motion puts the glenoid fossa in a favorable position for upper extremity movement, positioning the small glenoid fossa beneath the larger head of the humerus and contributing significantly to the stability of the shoulder joint as well as maintaining the position of the deltoid muscle for effective action.

Upward rotation produces the greatest range of motion in the scapula. Studies have found this range to be 50 to 60 degrees. Upward rotation will usually also include some amount of posterior tilt and some medial tilt, although this will not be considered in this text. Those students proceeding to clinical practice will become more familiar with this phenomenon.

Downward Rotation

The return from the position of upward rotation. There may be slight downward rotation beyond the normal resting position so that the glenoid fossa faces slightly downward.

Anterior Tilt

A turning of the scapula on its mediolateral axis so that the posterior surface faces slightly upward and the inferior angle protrudes from the back (Figure 5.3d). This action is accompanied by a rotation of the clavicle about its mechanical axis so that the superior border turns slightly forward-downward, and the inferior border turns backward-upward. It occurs only in conjunction with hyperextension of the humerus.

Posterior Tilt

A tipping of the posterior surface slightly downward and forward. This most often accompanies elevation of the arm and upward rotation of the scapula.

MUSCLES OF THE SHOULDER GIRDLE

Location

The muscles of the shoulder girdle are classified as anterior or posterior muscles according to their location on the trunk.

Anterior	**Posterior**
Pectoralis minor	Levator scapulae
Serratus anterior	Rhomboids
Subclavius	Trapezius (4 parts)

Characteristics and Functions of Shoulder Girdle Muscles

Pectoralis Minor

This muscle (Figure 5.4) participates in several movements of the *scapula—downward rotation, anterior tilt, depression,* and the combined movements of *abduction* and *lateral tilt.* In addition to its action on the scapula, an important function of the pectoralis minor is its lifting effect on the ribs, both in forced inspiration and in maintaining good chest posture. When the scapulae are stabilized by the adductors, contraction of the pectoralis minor *elevates* the third, fourth, and fifth ribs. Even without contracting, it exerts a slight upward and outward pull on these ribs if the muscle is well developed. The pectoralis minor can therefore contribute either to good or to poor posture, depending on whether its more effective pull is on the ribs or on the scapula. The key to its function as a muscle influencing good posture is stabilization of

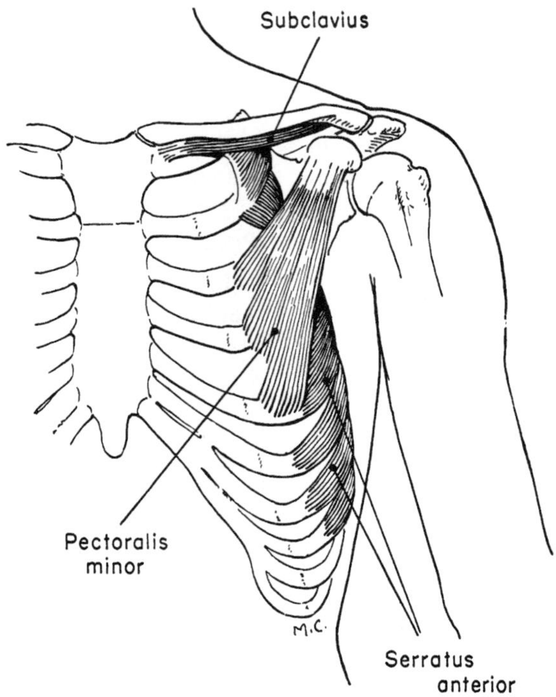

Figure 5.4 Anterior muscles of shoulder girdle.

the scapulae by the adductors—that is, the rhomboids and the middle trapezius. The pectoralis minor may be palpated midway between the clavicle and the nipple when the arm is elevated backward against resistance, provided the pectoralis major is relaxed, and also when the subject sits with the forearm resting on a table and pushes both downward and laterally simultaneously.

Serratus Anterior

The upper portion causes *abduction* and *lateral tilt* (protraction) of the scapula close to the ribs (see Figures 5.4 and 5.16). The upper and lower portions of the serratus anterior and trapezius combine to form a force couple for upward rotation of the scapula. Activity of these muscles is especially evident during elevation of the arm, with the lower trapezius the more active of the two during abduction and the serratus anterior the more active during flexion. This muscle is important in reaching and pushing. A paralyzed serratus anterior prevents elevation of the arm above 100 degrees.

The muscle may be palpated on the anterior-lateral surface of the upper thorax, especially on a thin, muscular subject.

Subclavius

The pull of this muscle (see Figure 5.4), which is slightly downward and strongly toward the sternum, suggests that its chief function is to protect and stabilize the sternoclavicular articulation. It is also in a position to depress the scapula. It is not possible to palpate this muscle.

Levator Scapulae

This muscle is also listed with the muscles of the neck. As a muscle of the shoulder girdle, the levator scapula (Figure 5.5) causes elevation and downward rotation of the scapula when the trunk is in the erect position. The weight of the arm at

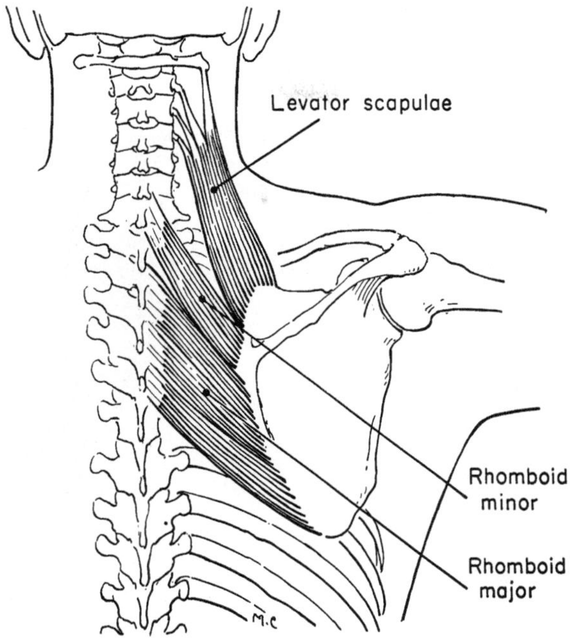

Figure 5.5 Posterior muscles of shoulder girdle, deep layer.

the acromial end of the scapula pulls that end down at the same time that the levator is lifting the medial angle. These two forces act as a force couple to rotate the scapula.

Rhomboids, Major and Minor

Functionally, the rhomboids may be regarded as one muscle (Figure 5.5). They cause downward rotation, adduction, and elevation of the scapula. Their cooperative action with trapezius III (see next section) is an important factor in the maintenance of good shoulder posture. When the tonus of these two muscles is deficient, the unbalanced pull of the pectoralis minor and the serratus anterior results in habitually abducted and tilted scapulae (round shoulders). This, in turn, results in the failure of the pectoralis minor and serratus anterior to hold the chest in good posture. Thus, one weak link in the chain of postural relationships leads to another. The rhomboids are also most active with the middle trapezius in stabilizing the scapula during abduction of the arm. Little activity occurs in these muscles during arm flexion until 150 degrees of flexion is reached, when activity increases markedly (Basmajian & DeLuca, 1985).

Trapezius

The trapezius (Figure 5.6) is a fascinating muscle to study. Because it is located directly under the skin, it is easy to palpate. Although some anatomists treat the muscle in three parts, it is more accurate to consider the four parts shown in Figure 5.6 separately. Parts I and II compose the upper trapezius, part III the middle, and part IV the lower. Its actions include the following:

- Part I. Elevation.
- Part II. Elevation; upward rotation; adduction.
- Part III. Adduction.
- Part IV. Upward rotation; depression; adduction.

The trapezius shows definite activity during both elevation and adduction (retraction) of the scapula.

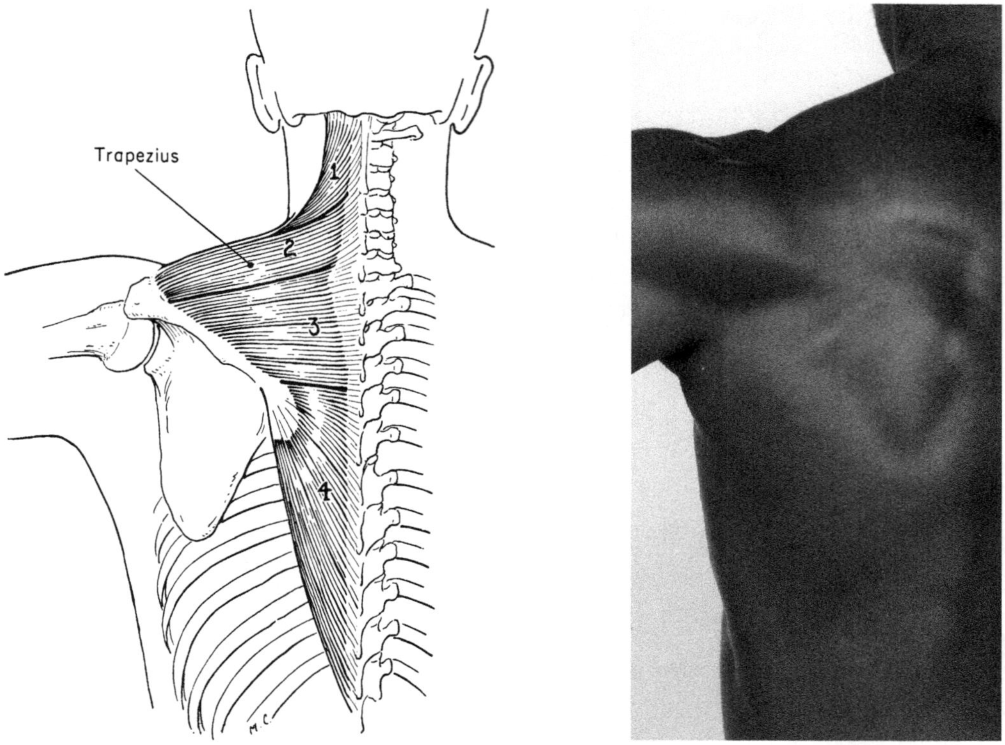

Figure 5.6 Trapezius.

In elevation the upper portion shows the greatest activity, and in retraction the middle and lower portions are most active. During abduction of the humerus and the accompanying upward rotation of the scapula, the lower two-thirds of the trapezius is most active, and during flexion of the humerus the lower third is most active. The greatest activity of the muscle as a whole is seen in the upward rotation of the scapula accompanying abduction of the humerus (Basmajian & DeLuca, 1985; Ludewig et al., 1996).

The relation of the trapezius to the rhomboids and serratus anterior is interesting. The rhomboids and part III of the trapezius both adduct the scapulae and have similar activity patterns during elevation of the arm. In these actions they are partners. Parts II and IV, however, rotate the scapulae upward; the rhomboids rotate them downward. In this respect, then, they are antagonists.

Trapezius III and the upper serratus anterior are antagonistic, the former adducting and the latter abducting the scapulae. But trapezius II and IV are partners with the lower serratus because they act on the scapula as a force couple to rotate the scapula upward, with part II pulling up on the acromial end of the scapular spine and part IV and the serratus anterior pulling down on the medial end or root. (See the discussion of a force couple on pp. 334–335 and Figure 13.7.) This action facilitates elevation of the arm. The lower and middle parts of the trapezius are quite active during the entire range of abduction. They are less active during the early stages of flexion when the scapula is being abducted. It is here that the serratus anterior, a scapular abductor as well as rotator, dominates.

Trapezius I and II have one important function that may be overlooked because little, if any, actual movement is involved. This is support for the distal end of the clavicle and the acromion process of the scapula when a heavy weight is held by the hand with the arm down at the side. Anyone who has carried a heavy suitcase for a long distance has doubtless experienced tension and subsequent soreness in these parts of the muscle. When no weight is carried, however, the capsule of the sternoclavicular articulation provides all the support necessary for the fully depressed clavicle.

These various combinations of function are an excellent illustration of the cooperative action of the muscles and of the astonishing versatility of the musculoskeletal mechanism.

THE SHOULDER JOINT (GLENOHUMERAL ARTICULATION)

Structure

The shoulder joint is formed by the articulation of the spherical head of the humerus with the small, shallow, somewhat pear-shaped glenoid fossa of the scapula (Figure 5.7). It is a ball-and-socket joint. The structure of the joint and the looseness of the capsule (permitting between 10 and 20 mm of separation between the two bones) account for the remarkable mobility of the shoulder joint. Both the humeral head and the glenoid fossa are covered with hyaline cartilage. The cartilage on the head of the humerus is thicker at the center, whereas that which lines the cavity is thicker around the circumference. The glenoid fossa is further protected by a flat rim of white fibrocartilage, also thicker around the circumference. Called the glenoid labrum, this cartilage serves both to deepen the fossa by about 50% and to cushion it against the impact of the humeral head in forceful movements (Figure 5.8).

The joint is completely enveloped in a loose, sleevelike articular capsule that is attached proximally to the circumference of the glenoid cavity and distally to the anatomical neck of the humerus. The capsule is lined with synovial membrane that folds back over the glenoid labrum, covers all but the upper portion of the anatomical neck of the humerus, and extends through the intertubular or bicipital groove in the form of a sheath for the tendon of the long head of the biceps. There are several bursae in the region of the shoulder joint. Among the larger are the one between the deltoid muscle and the capsule and the one on top of the acromion process. All of these

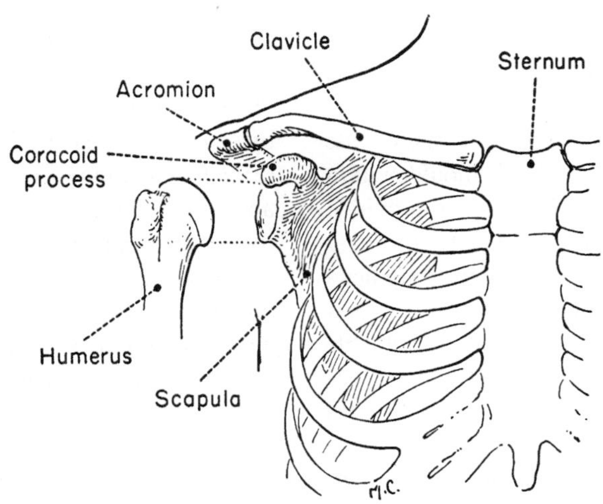

Figure 5.7 Anterior view of shoulder joint and shoulder girdle.

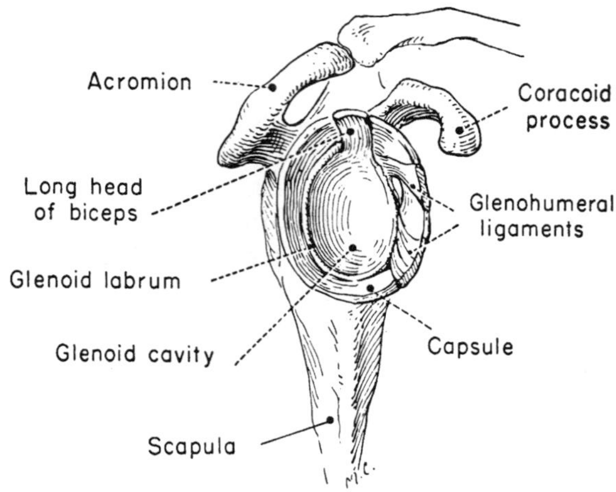

Figure 5.8 Lateral view of right scapula showing glenoid cavity.

soft tissue structures are sealed, producing a negative pressure in the joint capsule, which may contribute in a small way to joint stability.

Ligamentous and Muscular Reinforcements

The shoulder joint is protected and stabilized by both ligaments and muscles. Inspection of the illustrations on these pages (supplemented by study of the table of muscular attachments in Appen-dix C) will help the reader understand the relationships of the ligaments and muscles to the joints they reinforce.

The coracohumeral ligament, the three bands of the glenohumeral ligament, and the bridge-like coracoacromial ligament constitute the *ligamentous reinforcements* of the shoulder joint (Figure 5.9). Muscular reinforcement is provided above by the supraspinatus muscle and the long head of the biceps brachii, below by the long head of the triceps brachii, in front by the subscapularis muscle and the fibrous prolongations of both the pectoralis major and teres major muscles, and behind by the infraspinatus and teres minor muscles (see Figures 5.11 through 5.15).

Apparently these reinforcements alone do not prevent downward dislocation, however. In 1959 Basmajian and Bazant investigated the muscles whose fibers cross the shoulder joint vertically, as compared with those whose fibers cross it horizontally. To their surprise, they discovered that it was the horizontal fibers and not the vertical that were active in preventing downward dislocation of the humerus. After doing a dissection of the shoulder joint, they agreed that the slope of the glenoid fossa was an important factor. Because of this slope, the head of the humerus was forced laterally as it was pulled downward, and it took the horizontally directed muscle fibers to check this lateral movement which, in turn, stopped the downward movement. A number of investigators have studied the mechanisms of stability in downward motion. They concluded that downward dislocation of the humerus is prevented primarily by four factors: (1) the slope of the glenoid fossa; (2) the tightening of the upper part of the capsule and of the coracohumeral ligament; (3) the activity of the supraspinatus muscle and the middle and posterior fibers of the deltoid; and (4) the combined actions of the infraspinatus, teres minor, and subscapularis, which compress the head of the humerus into the glenoid fossa, adding to vertical stability. Veeger and van der Helm (2007) have concluded that stability in the glenohumeral joint relies heavily on active muscle control in these muscles.

The shoulder joint is relatively stable when in extension but very vulnerable when flexed. That is

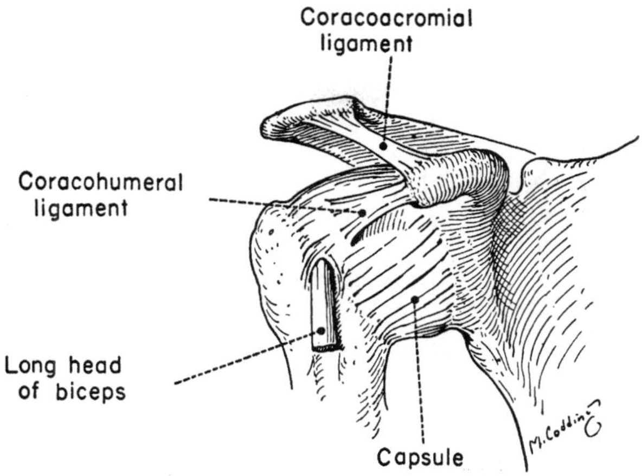

Figure 5.9 Anterior view of shoulder joint showing ligaments.

why it is dangerous in sports to have force applied when the arm is raised overhead, such as when the quarterback is throwing a pass.

Movements

The movements of the humerus, all of which take place at the glenohumeral articulation, are illustrated in Figure 5.10. The expected average ranges of these movements are summarized in Table 2.3. They are defined as follows.

Flexion and Hyperflexion

A forward-upward movement in a plane at right angles to the plane of the scapula (sagittal plane). If the movement exceeds 180 degrees, it is hyperflexion.

Extension

Return movement from flexion (sagittal plane).

Hyperextension

A backward movement in a plane at right angles to the plane of the scapula (sagittal plane).

Abduction

A sideward-upward movement in a plane parallel with the plane of the scapula (frontal plane).

Adduction

Return movement from abduction (frontal plane).

Outward (External) Rotation

A rotation of the humerus around its mechanical axis so that when the arm is in its normal resting position, the anterior aspect turns laterally (horizontal plane).

Inward (Internal) Rotation

A rotation of the humerus around its mechanical axis so that when the arm is in its normal resting position, the anterior aspect turns medially (horizontal plane). The full range of inward and outward rotation is best observed when the forearm is held in 90 degrees of flexion and the humerus is held in 90 degrees of abduction.

Horizontal Adduction

A forward movement of the abducted humerus in a horizontal plane (i.e., from a plane parallel to the plane of the scapula to a plane at right angles to it). Sometimes identified as *horizontal flexion* in other textbooks.

Horizontal Abduction

A backward movement of the flexed humerus in a horizontal plane (i.e., from a plane at right angles to the plane of the scapula to a plane parallel to it).

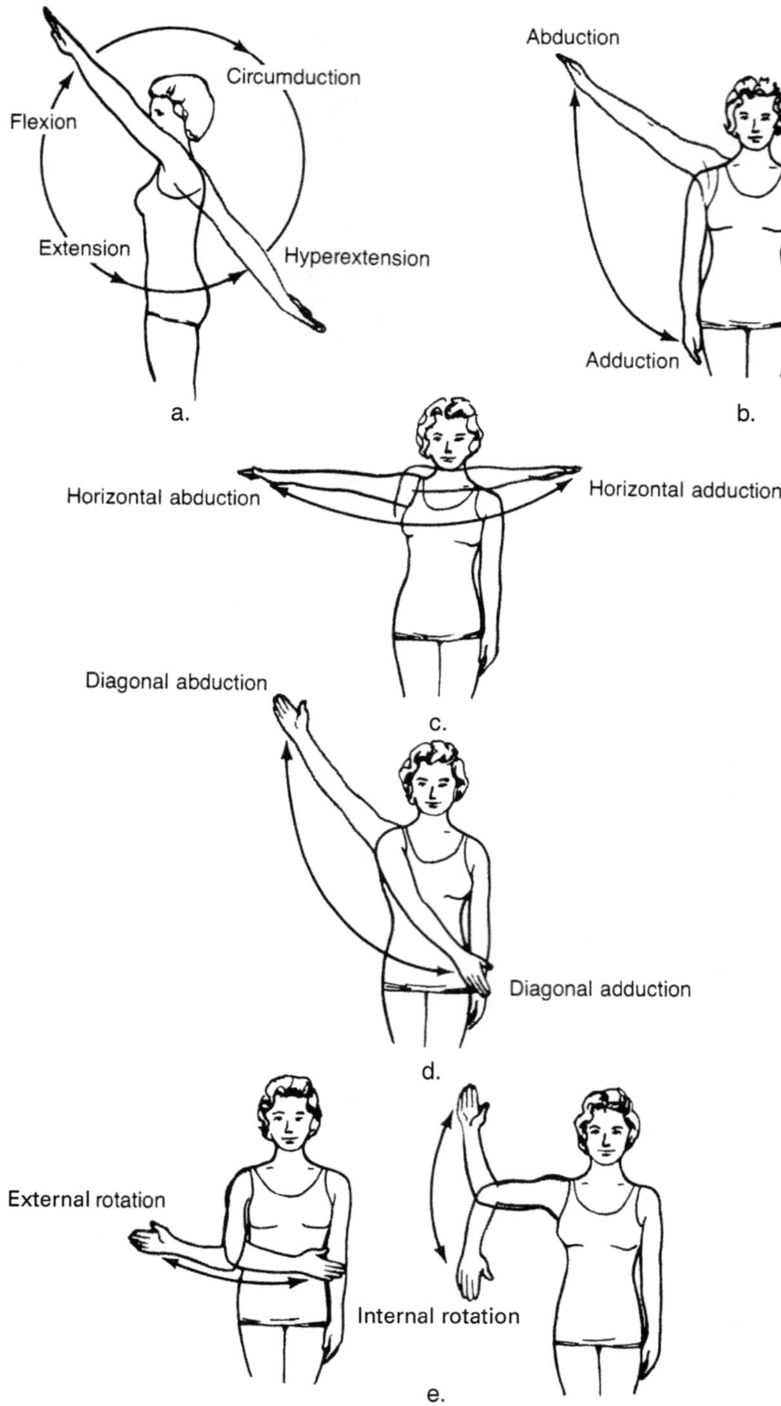

Figure 5.10 Movements of the humerus: (a) flexion, extension, hyperextension, circumduction; (b) abduction and adduction; (c) horizontal adduction and abduction; (d) diagnonal adduction and abduction; (e) internal and external rotation.

Sometimes called *horizontal extension* in other texts.

Circumduction

A combination of flexion, abduction, extension, hyperextension, and adduction performed sequentially in either direction so that the extended arm describes a cone and the fingertips a circle.

MUSCLES OF THE SHOULDER JOINT

Location

The muscles of the shoulder joint are listed according to their position in relation to the joint. This position is not always apparent, as a look at the illustrations will show. All muscles in this classification pass either from the trunk or the scapula to the arm.

Anterior
Pectoralis major
Coracobrachialis
Subscapularis
Biceps brachii

Posterior
Infraspinatus
Teres minor

Superior
Deltoid
Supraspinatus

Inferior
Latissimus dorsi
Teres major
Triceps brachii, long head

Characteristics and Functions

Pectoralis Major

This large fan-shaped muscle of the chest (Figure 5.11) converges to a flat tendon, which twists on itself so that the lowest fibers become the uppermost at its point of attachment. The muscle is divided functionally into two parts, clavicular and sternal (or sternocostal). The clavicular portion lies close to the anterior deltoid muscle and acts with it in flexion, horizontal adduction, and inward rotation of the humerus.

Ordinarily the line of pull of the clavicular portion of the pectoralis major lies below the axis of the shoulder joint. However, when the arm is raised sideward well above the horizontal, the line of pull of the upper clavicular fibers shifts above the center of the shoulder joint, and these fibers then cease to adduct and become abductors of the humerus (see Figure 3.4). The clavicular fibers of the pectoralis major are significantly active in abduction at the level of 110 degrees. The sternocostal portion is generally antagonistic to the clavicular portion in its actions in the sagittal plane. It acts in downward and forward movements of the arm and in inward rotation when accompanied by adduction. The pectoralis major as a whole is most powerful for actions in the sagittal plane and is particularly important in all pushing, throwing, and punching activities. The clavicular portion may be palpated just below the medial two-thirds of the clavicle, the sternal portion just lateral to the sternum and below the clavicular part, and the muscle as a whole at the anterior border of the axilla.

Coracobrachialis

The muscle's line of pull passes in front of the shoulder joint (Figure 5.12), which suggests that it participates in *forward movements of the humerus*. Because the proximal attachment and line of pull of the coracobrachialis and the long head of the biceps are so similar, it has been difficult to determine the specific actions of the coracobrachialis. However, Stevens et al. (1976) were successful in isolating and recording activity in the coracobrachialis, confirming that it serves as a main force in horizontal adduction movements. Their research also verified the belief that this muscle, the middle deltoid, and the long head of the triceps, acting like guy wires on a mast, serve to stabilize the shoulder joint. It may be palpated on the front of the upper arm between the anterior deltoid and the pectoralis major, but it is a difficult muscle to identify.

Biceps Brachii

Although essentially a muscle of the elbow joint, the biceps (see Figure 5.12) crosses the shoulder joint and is active in some of the movements of the humerus. Both heads are always active in flexion and in abduction with resistance when the elbow is

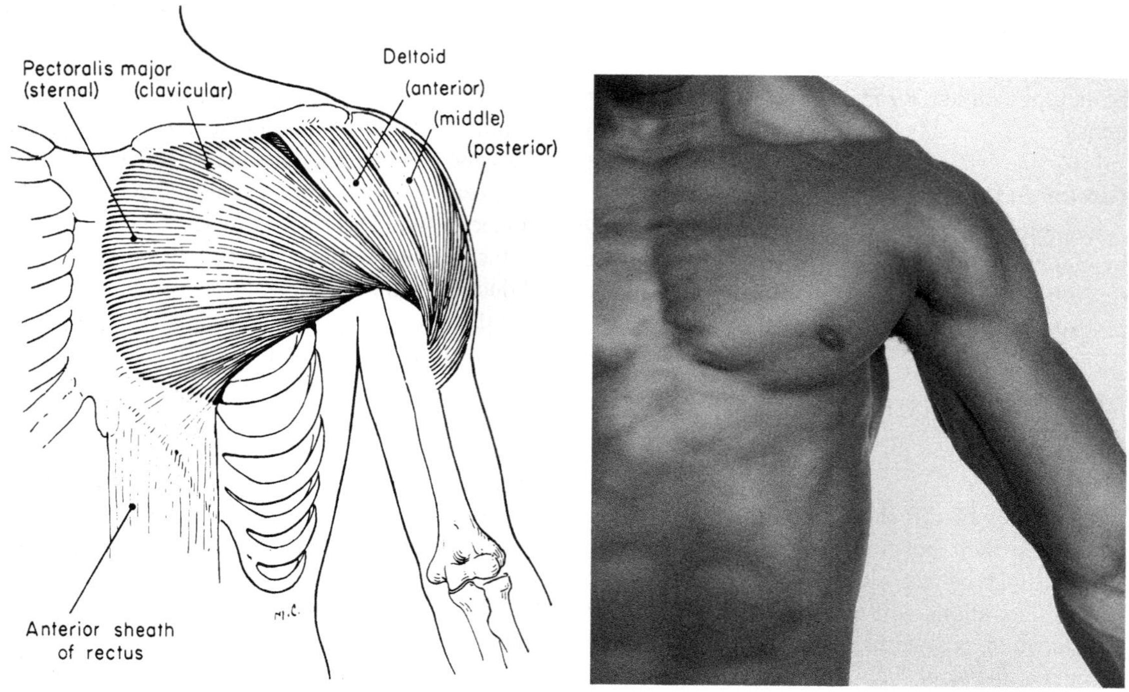

Figure 5.11 Anterior view of muscles of shoulder joint, superficial layer.

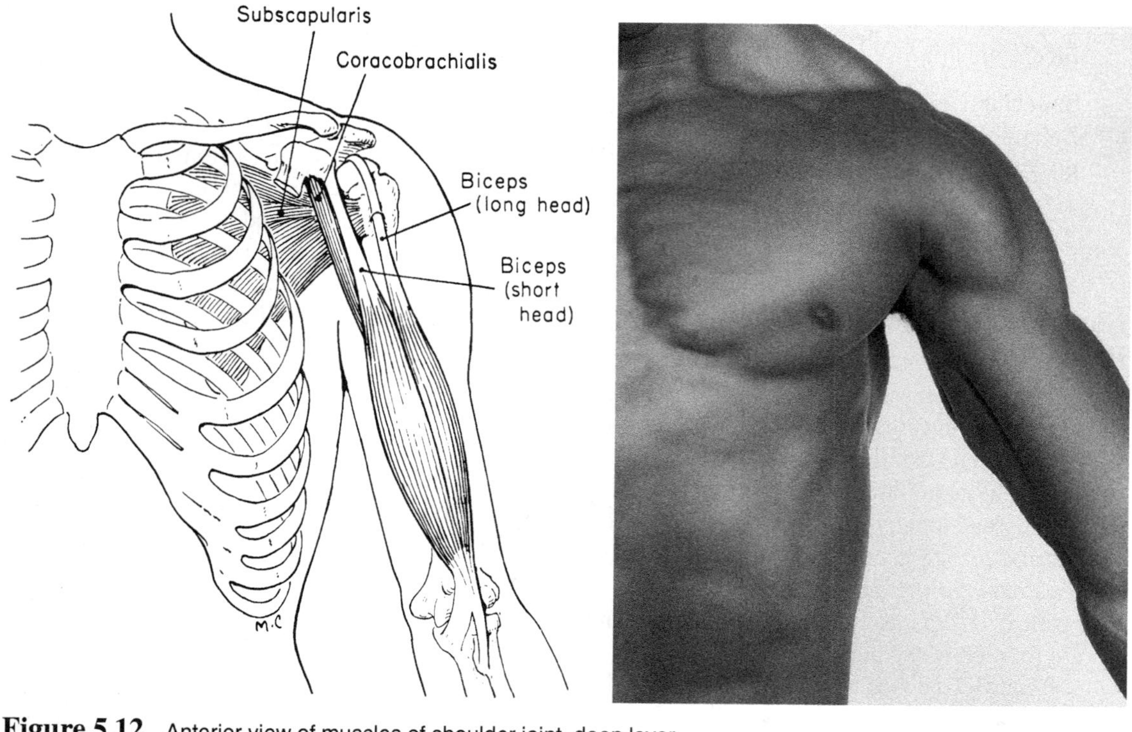

Figure 5.12 Anterior view of muscles of shoulder joint, deep layer.

straight. The muscle is also active in horizontal adduction, and the short head sometimes participates in adduction against resistance and in medial rotation. The biceps also stabilizes the shoulder joint.

Deltoid

The complex structure of the deltoid (Figures 5.11 and 5.14), with the multipenniform arrangement of the bundles making up the middle portion, gives it a potential for great strength without undue bulk. The middle portion of the muscle is a *powerful abductor of the humerus,* its greatest activity occurring when the humerus is raised between 90 and 120 degrees. It is capable of supporting the weight of the upper extremity for long periods while the hand is working at a height. The multipenniform arrangement of fibers compensates for the middle deltoid's rather poor angle of pull. The angle of pull, however, serves the useful purpose of providing the muscle with a strong stabilizing component force. This is fortunate because, in the raised position, the shoulder joint depends more on its muscles than on its ligaments for holding the head of the humerus on the glenoid fossa. The middle portion has also been found to be active in horizontal abduction.

The anterior portion of the deltoid aids in all *forward movements* of the arm and in *inward rotation* of the humerus. It is also active in abduction. There is disagreement in the literature concerning the movements effected by the posterior deltoid, but there seems to be sufficient evidence to conclude that, in addition to extension and lateral rotation, the lowest fibers, being situated below the axis of motion, assist in forceful adduction of the humerus from an overhead position. On the other hand, some of the upper fibers (those closest to the middle deltoid) probably act with the latter in contributing to abduction.

Rotator Cuff

The muscles of the rotator cuff (subscapularis, supraspinatus, infraspinatus, and teres minor) serve dual roles as stabilizers and primary movers. During overhead throwing activities, the rotator cuff has been found to be very active in providing shoulder stability during arm deceleration (Escamilla & Andrews, 2009). Although the rotator cuff is frequently treated as a single entity in research studies, each of the muscles of the rotator cuff will be dealt with separately in this text.

Subscapularis

As one of the *rotator cuff* muscles, the subscapularis (Figures 5.12 and 5.13a) contributes significantly to stabilization of the glenohumeral joint, especially in the prevention of dislocation during forced lateral rotation of the abducted arm. It is also one of the depressors of the humeral head during abduction and flexion of the arm. Its chief action as a mover is inward rotation, which it performs most effectively when the arm is at the side or is elevated posteriorly. It has also shown significantly more electrical activity in horizontal abduction than in horizontal adduction.

Supraspinatus

This muscle (Figures 5.13 and 5.15) acts together with the deltoid in abduction of the arm throughout the entire range. It also acts in flexion and horizontal extension. Action potentials reach their maximum when the arm is at 100 degrees of flexion. As part of the rotator cuff, it plays a significant part in the stability of the shoulder joint and is important in preventing downward dislocation. It may be palpated above the spine of the scapula, provided that the scapula is supported, as when the armpit rests over the back of a chair.

Infraspinatus and Teres Minor

In addition to their outward rotary action, these two muscles (see Figures 5.13b, 5.14, and 5.15), which seem to act as one, have two additional noteworthy functions. Together with the subscapularis, they depress the head of the humerus and thus prevent it from jamming against the acromion process during flexion and abduction of the arm. They are also part of the rotator cuff muscles (infraspinatus, teres minor, subscapularis, and supraspinatus), whose important function it is to aid materially in holding the head of the humerus in the glenoid fossa. Their

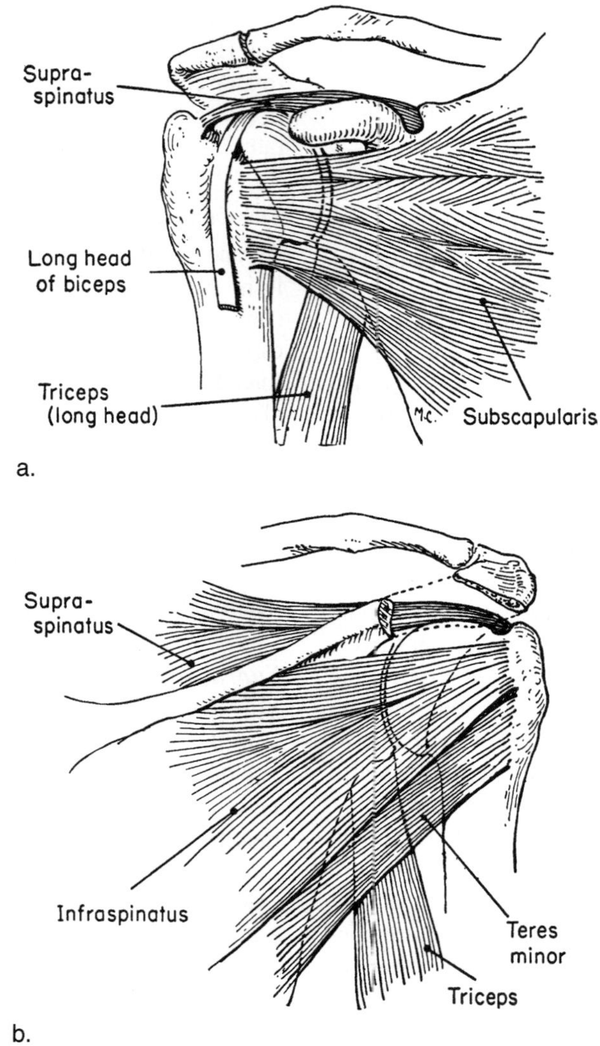

Figure 5.13 Muscular reinforcement of shoulder joint: (a) anterior view; (b) posterior view.

important function in this capacity is to prevent dislocation of the shoulder joint, especially when the humerus is in the abducted position. They may be palpated on the posterior surface of the scapula, medial to and below the posterior deltoid muscle.

Latissimus Dorsi

This is a broad sheet of muscle (see Figure 5.14) that covers the lower and middle portions of the back. Coming mainly from the lower half of the thoracic spine and the entire lumbar spine, the fibers gradually converge as they pass upward and laterally toward the axilla. Here the fibers twist on themselves in such a way that the lowest fibers become the uppermost. They end in the narrow, flat tendon of the distal attachment. The muscle has a favorable angle of pull for extension and adduction of the arm, particularly when the latter is raised between 30 and 90 degrees. EMG has confirmed the action of the latissimus dorsi in extension and

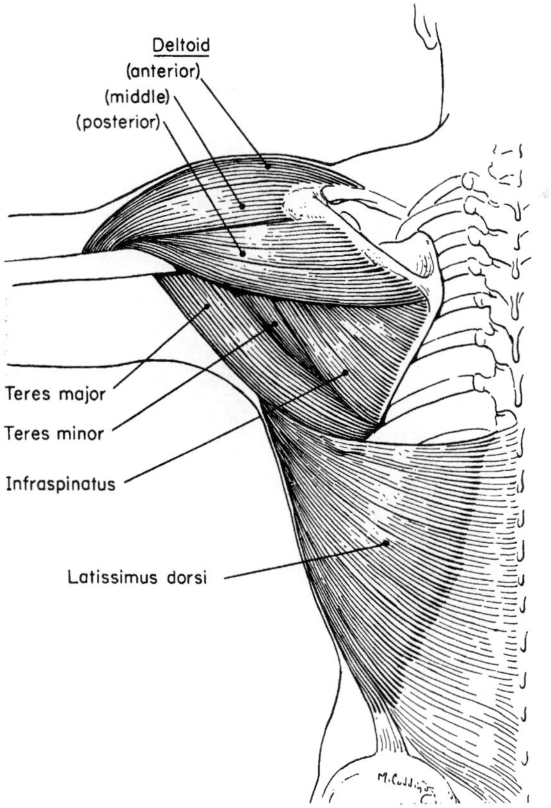

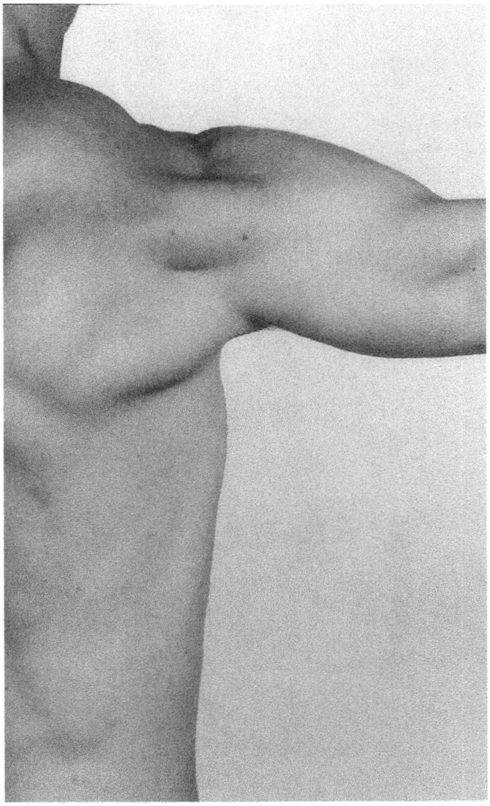

Figure 5.14 Posterior view of muscles of shoulder joint, superficial layer.

adduction during static and dynamic, resisted and unresisted movements. Electromyographic evidence confirms that the latissimus dorsi muscle is also very active during inward rotation of the humerus (Basmajian & DeLuca, 1985; Suenaga et al., 2003). The latissimus dorsi is also an active spinal extensor and rotator muscle. Action of the muscle on the vertebral column is covered in Chapter 9. The muscle may be palpated on the posterior border of the axilla just below the teres major.

Teres Major

Structurally, this muscle (see Figures 5.14 and 5.15) appears to be in a favorable position to work with the latissimus dorsi in *downward and backward movements* of the humerus and also in *inward rotation,* but Basmajian & DeLuca (1985) detected no sign of activity in this muscle during these movements unless external resistance was applied. Against active resistance, activity was evident during internal rotation, adduction, and extension. No added resistance is needed, however, for the teres major to be active during hyperextension and adduction when the arm is behind the back.

Triceps Brachii

Although primarily a muscle of the elbow joint, the triceps (see Figures 5.13 and 5.15) is active in movements of the humerus because its long head crosses the shoulder joint. It assists in adduction, extension, and hyperextension of the humerus and acts to stabilize the shoulder.

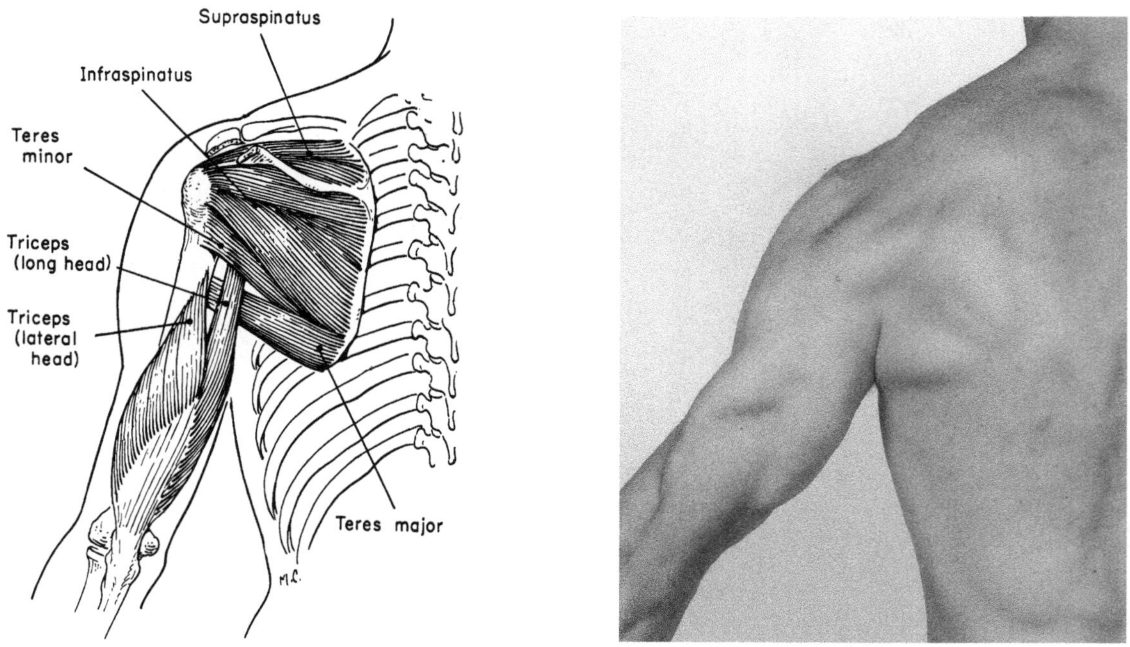

Figure 5.15 Posterior view of muscles of shoulder joint, deep layer.

Joint and Muscular Analysis of the Fundamental Movements of the Arm on the Trunk

As stated earlier, the movements of the arm on the trunk involve the cooperative action of the shoulder girdle and the shoulder joint, the former including both the acromioclavicular and the sternoclavicular joints. To correctly analyze the great variety of movements of the upper extremity, it is essential to understand this cooperative action of the three joints and their muscles. The fundamental movements of the arm on the trunk, together with the anatomical analysis of each, are presented next.

Movements in the Frontal Plane

Abduction

This movement may occur from any distance up to the vertical (Figure 5.16).

Shoulder joint *Abduction* of the humerus by the deltoid and supraspinatus accompanied by slight depression of the humeral head because of the action of the subscapularis, infraspinatus, and teres minor. This is the least forceful of shoulder joint actions. True humeral abduction is the sideward elevation of the humerus in a plane parallel with the scapula.

Outward or *external rotation* by the infraspinatus and teres minor when palms are turned either out or up. Possible abduction by the biceps when the arm is in complete external rotation.

Shoulder girdle *Upward rotation* of the scapula by the serratus anterior and trapezius II and IV.

Adduction

This movement may occur from any degree of sideward elevation, either against resistance or in any position that rules out the help of gravitational force (Figure 5.17).

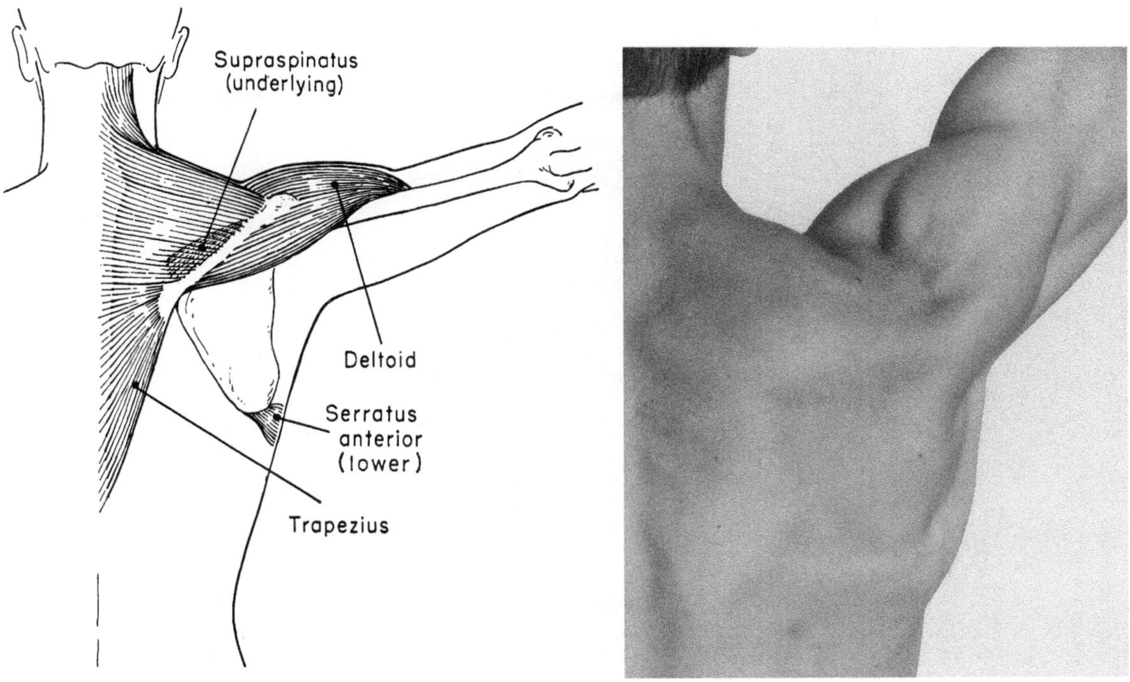

Figure 5.16 Muscles that contract to produce abduction of the upper extremity.

Shoulder joint *Adduction* of the humerus by the latissimus dorsi, the teres major (against resistance), sternal portion of the pectoralis major, and probably the lowest fibers of the posterior deltoid. *Reduction of outward rotation* mainly by the subscapularis and the teres major. The teres major is also active in adduction when the arm moves behind the back.

Shoulder girdle *Reduction of upward rotation* by the rhomboids and pectoralis minor, with help from the levator scapulae.

Movements in the Sagittal Plane

Flexion

This movement may occur up to the horizontal (Figure 5.18).

Shoulder joint *Flexion* of the humerus by the anterior deltoid and clavicular portion of the pectoralis major, probably with some participation of the coracobrachialis (against resistance) and biceps brachii.

Slight external rotation by the infraspinatus and teres minor.

Shoulder girdle *Upward rotation* of the scapula by the serratus anterior and trapezius II and IV (slight).

Abduction and lateral tilt of the scapula by the serratus anterior and pectoralis minor, unless intentionally inhibited.

Continued Flexion

This movement may occur from the horizontal to the vertical and beyond.

Shoulder joint *Flexion* of the humerus by the same muscles as above; hyperflexion if the humerus moves beyond the vertical.

Continued *external rotation* by the infraspinatus and teres minor if the palms turn to face each other when the arms reach the vertical.

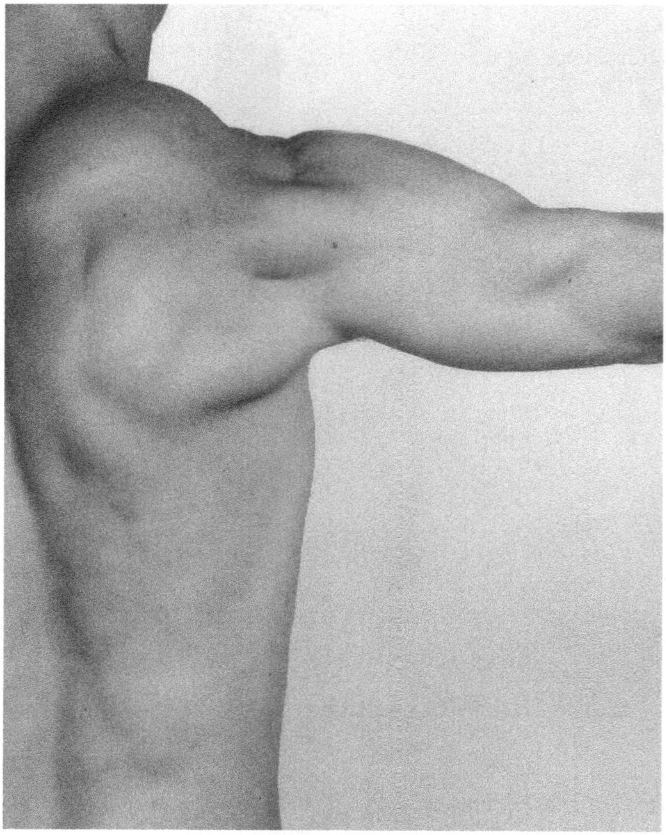

Figure 5.17 Adduction of the upper extremity against resistance. The latissimus dorsi, teres major, and rhomboids are in strong contraction.

Shoulder girdle *Upward rotation* of the scapula by the serratus anterior and trapezius II and IV (increased).

Slight to moderate *elevation* of the scapula by the levator scapulae, trapezius I and II, and rhomboids, unless effort is made to inhibit elevation. This action would be evident in reaching activities such as the high jump, long jump, or the pushing phase of the pole vault.

Reduction of abduction and lateral tilt mainly by virtue of the overhead position.

Extension

This movement may occur from the overhead vertical to the starting position, either against resistance or in a position that rules out the help of gravitational force (Figure 5.19).

Shoulder joint *Extension* of the humerus by the sternal portion of the pectoralis major (diminishing as the movement progresses), teres major (against resistance), latissimus dorsi (especially during the lower 60 degrees of motion), and possibly the posterior deltoid and the long head of the triceps brachii. Extension is the most powerful of shoulder movements.

Reduction of external rotation, probably by relaxation of outward rotator muscles but possibly aided by the subscapularis, teres major, latissimus dorsi, and pectoralis major.

Shoulder girdle *Reduction of elevation and upward rotation* by relaxation of muscles. If the movement is performed against resistance, the pectoralis minor, trapezius IV, subclavius, and

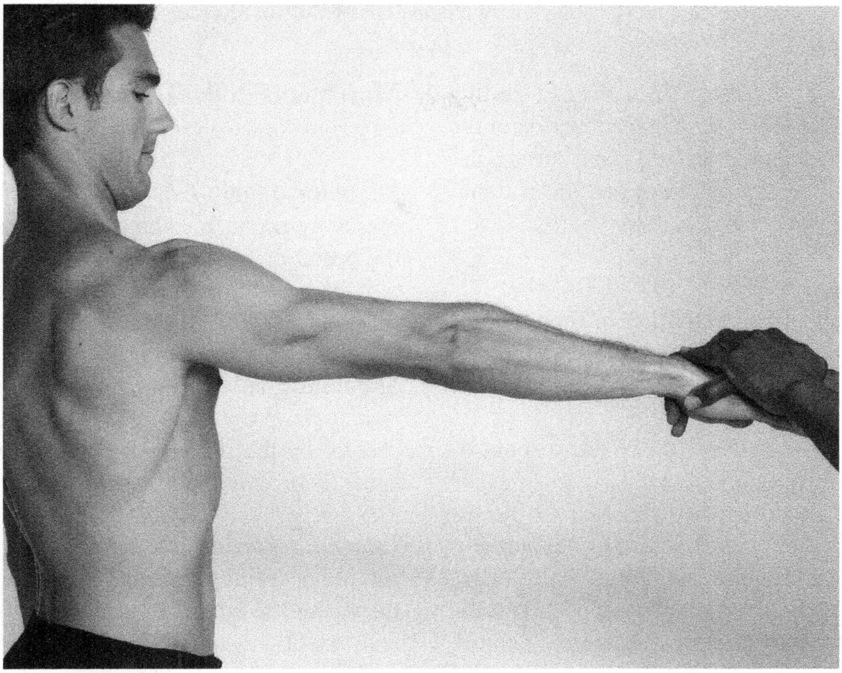

Figure 5.18 Flexion of the upper extremity against resistance. The anterior and middle deltoid, upper trapezius, and serratus anterior are in strong contraction.

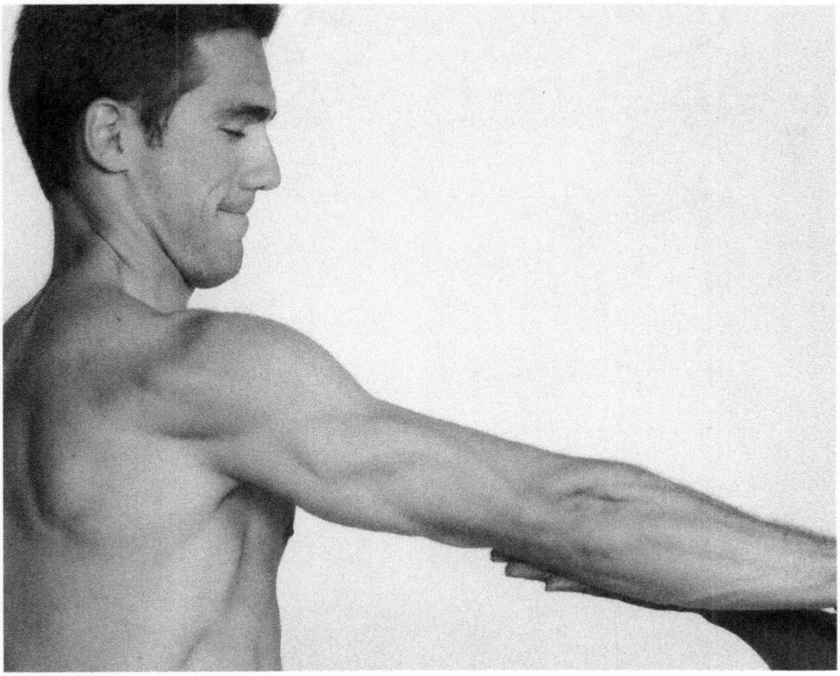

Figure 5.19 Extension of the upper extremity against resistance. The latissimus dorsi and teres major are in strong contraction.

rhomboids would doubtless be active. In pulling movements like a chin-up, strong adduction of the middle trapezius and rhomboids and strong depression by the pectoralis minor and lower trapezius would also be evident.

Hyperextension *(Figure 5.20)*
Shoulder joint *Hyperextension* of the humerus by the posterior deltoid, latissimus dorsi, and teres major.

Shoulder girdle *Anterior tilt* of the scapula by the pectoralis minor.

Elevation if movement is carried to the extreme. Possibly the hyperextension of the humerus pushes the scapula into a position of slight elevation. If any scapular muscles are acting, they would probably be the levator scapulae, trapezius I and II, and rhomboids, with possibly the clavicular portion of the sternocleidomastoid (a neck muscle) helping.

Movements in the Horizontal Plane

External Rotation (Figures 5.21 and 5.22)

Shoulder joint *External rotation* of the humerus by the infraspinatus and teres minor with the posterior deltoid acting only if the humerus is also being adducted and extended, as in a calisthenic or postural exercise.

Shoulder girdle *Adduction* of the scapulae and *reduction of any lateral tilt,* which may have been present by the rhomboids and trapezius III, with some involvement of trapezius II and IV.

Internal Rotation
Shoulder joint *Internal rotation* of the humerus by the subscapularis, teres major (against resistance), latissimus dorsi, anterior deltoid, and pectoralis major. If the upper extremity is in a position of outward rotation to start with, the

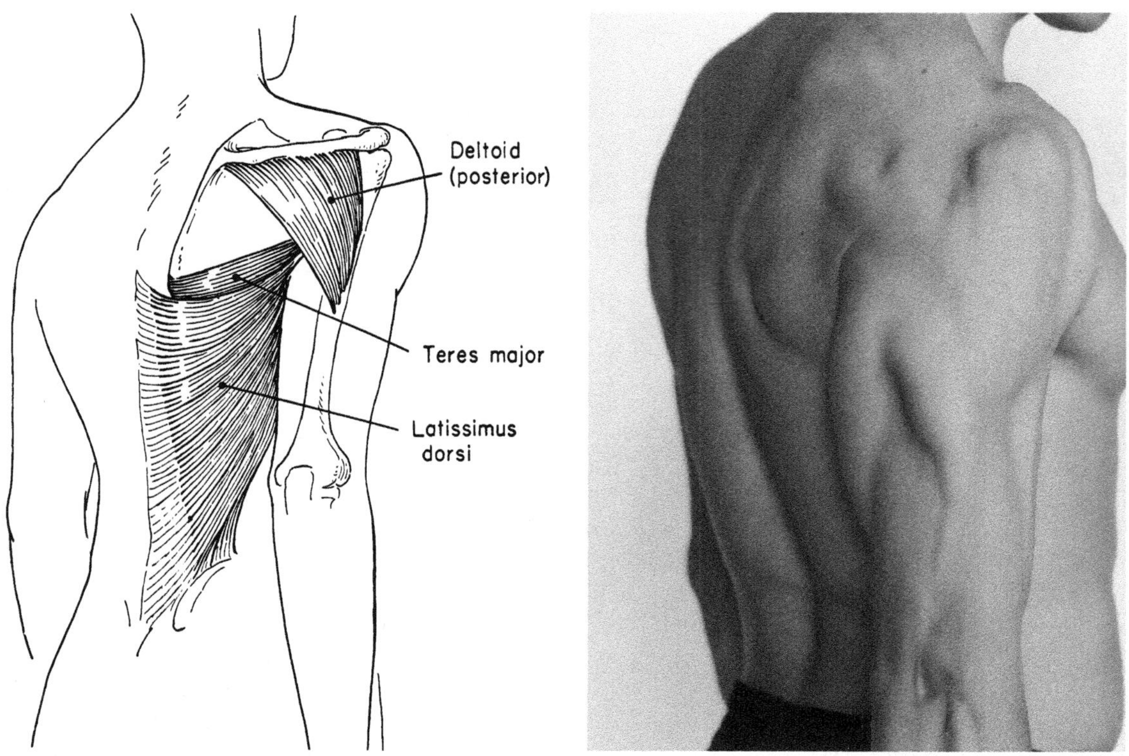

Figure 5.20 Muscles that contract to produce hyperextension of the upper extremity.

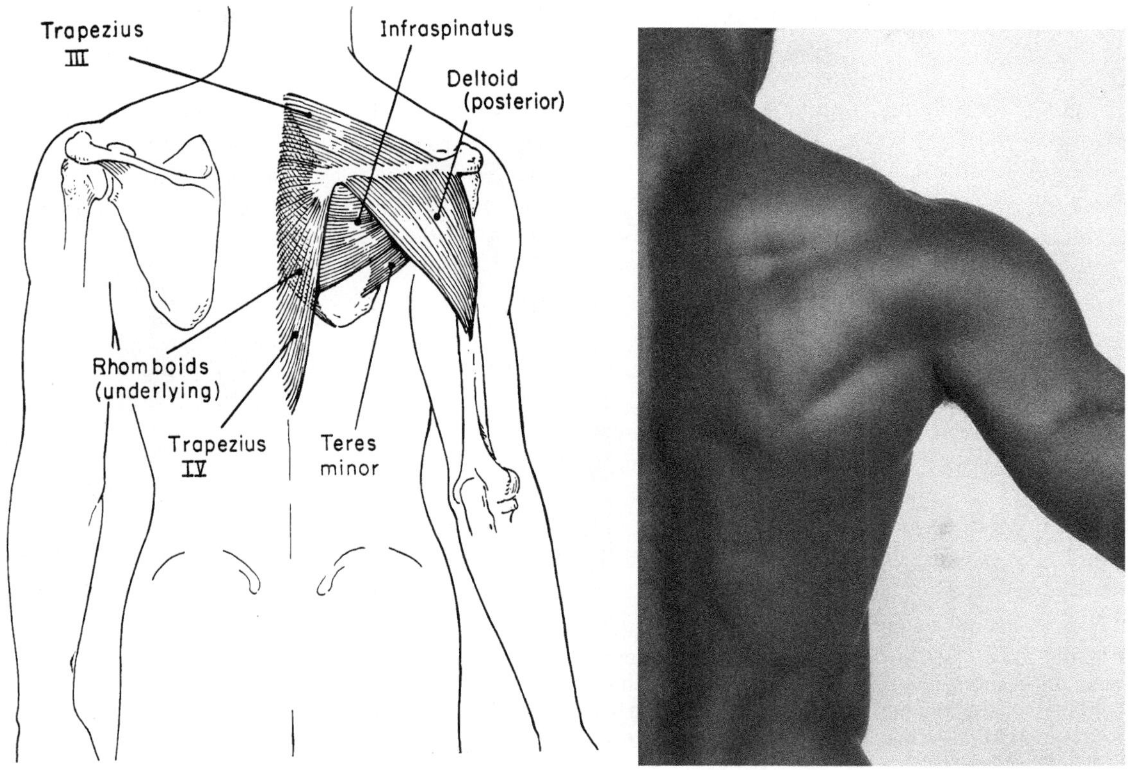

Figure 5.21 Muscles that contract to produce outward rotation of the arm and accompanying adduction of the scapula.

coracobrachialis and short head of the biceps would be active in the first part of the movement.

Shoulder girdle *Abduction and lateral tilt* by the serratus anterior and pectoralis minor, with a tendency toward elevation by the levator scapulae, trapezius I and II, and rhomboids.

Horizontal Adduction

Shoulder joint *Horizontal adduction* of humerus by the pectoralis major, anterior deltoid, and coracobrachialis, with the short head of the biceps helping if the forearm is extended.

Shoulder girdle *Abduction and lateral tilt* of scapula, unless deliberately inhibited. The movement is produced by the serratus anterior and pectoralis minor.

Horizontal Abduction

Shoulder joint *Horizontal abduction* of the humerus by the posterior deltoid, posterior portion of middle deltoid, infraspinatus, teres minor, and long head of the triceps.

Shoulder girdle *Adduction and reduction of lateral tilt* of scapula by the rhomboids and trapezius III in particular, with II and IV also participating.

Diagonal Movements

Unless performing calisthenic or gymnastic exercises, one rarely performs pure fundamental movements of the arm on the trunk. Most athletic and everyday movements are "in-between" or combination movements. To analyze these in terms of their

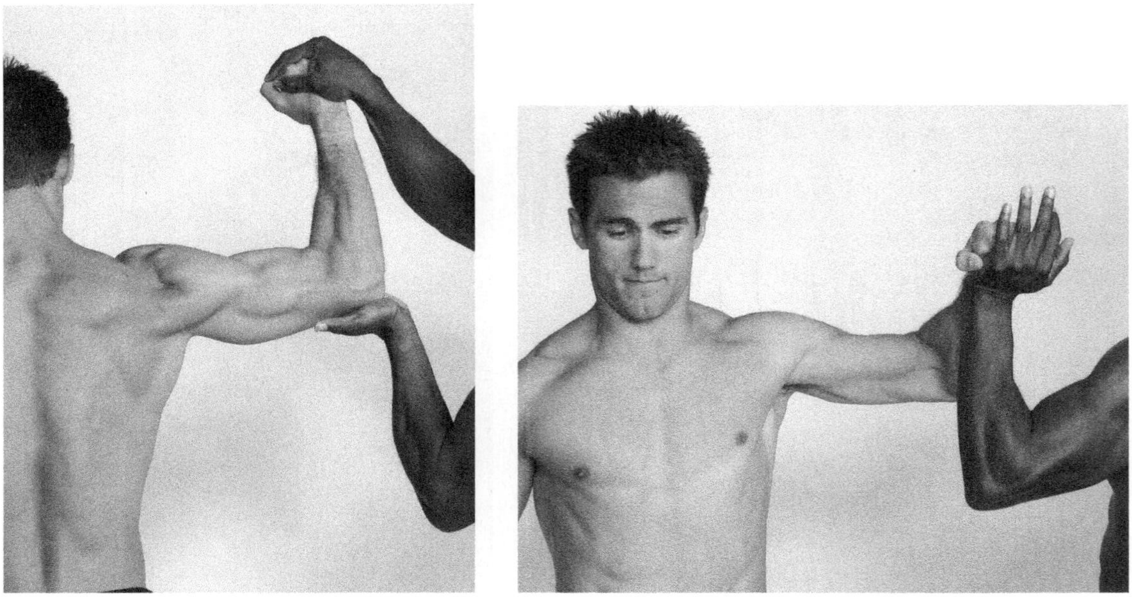

a. b.

Figure 5.22 (a) Outward rotation of the arm against resistance. The posterior deltoid, infraspinatus, and teres minor are in strong contraction. (The hyperextension and lateral flexion of the trunk are caused by the extreme effort. The latissimus is contracting because he is pushing his elbow down.) (b) Inward rotation. The pectoralis major, anterior deltoid, teres major, and latissimus dorsi are in strong contraction.

muscular action, it is necessary to estimate the approximate proportions of the fundamental joint motions. For instance, the follow-through on a tennis serve might involve extension of the arm, or it might consist of extension combined with a slight amount of "horizontal" adduction swing. In other words, this could be described as a diagonal forward-downward and slightly inward movement of the arm, consisting mainly of extension of the humerus combined with a slight degree of adduction. An appropriate term proposed is *diagonal adduction* (Figures 5.10 and 5.23). After the server's racket is moved forward-upward to ball contact by internal rotation of the humerus at the shoulder and extension at the elbow, the arm movement is diagonally down and across the body in a combination of extension and adduction—that is, diagonal adduction.

An underhand volleyball serve or the motion of a snow shovel, which are likely to have an upward as well as a forward component, would consist of a horizontal forward swing from the side horizontal position of the arm combined with a slight amount of forward-upward elevation. This would involve slight shoulder joint flexion accompanied by a combination of abduction, lateral tilt, and upward rotation of the shoulder girdle.

Shoulder Girdle Movements Not Involving the Arm

In addition to these coordinated movements of the arm on the trunk, there are three movements of the shoulder girdle in which movements of the arm are passive because they are produced by the changes in position of the shoulder girdle from which they are suspended. These are (1) a lifting or hunching of the shoulders, (2) protraction of the shoulders, and (3) retraction of the shoulders.

Shoulder Lifting or Hunching

Shoulder girdle *Elevation* by the levator scapulae, trapezius I and II, and rhomboids, with assistance by the sternocleidomastoid if the movement

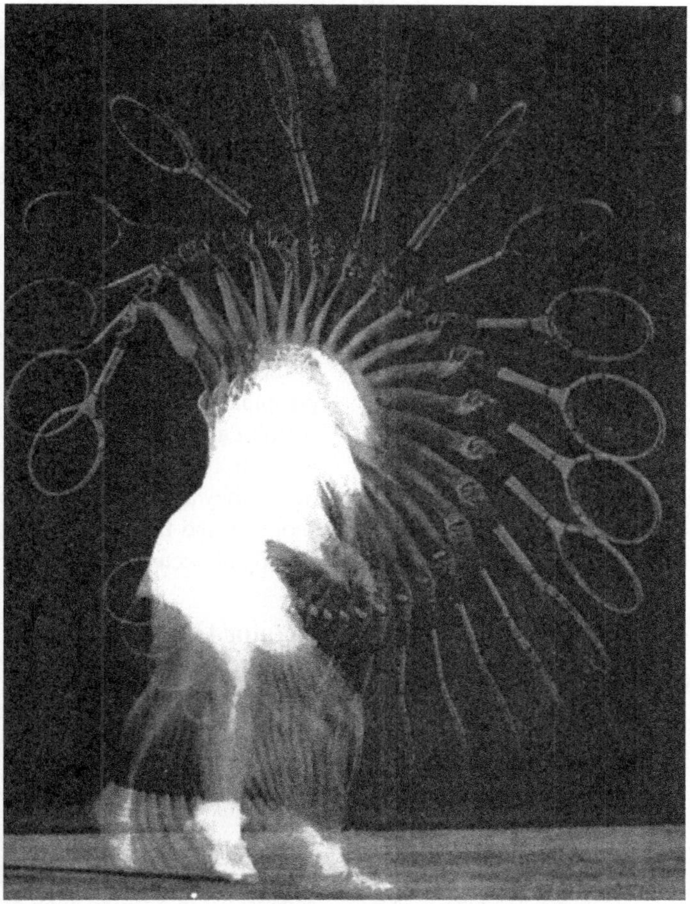

Figure 5.23 A tennis serve showing diagonal adduction of arm at shoulder joint during follow-through. Courtesy of H. E. Edgerton.

is performed against resistance. Reduction of the elevation is achieved by relaxing the muscles and letting the force of gravity have its way.

Shoulder Protraction

Shoulder girdle *Forceful abduction and lateral tilt* of scapula by the serratus anterior and pectoralis minor.

Shoulder joint Slight *passive internal rotation.* Reduction of the movement is achieved by relaxation of the muscles but may be followed by slight retraction.

Shoulder Retraction

Shoulder girdle *Adduction and reduction of lateral tilt* by the rhomboids, trapezius III, and possibly II and IV.

Common Injuries of the Shoulder Region

Acromioclavicular Sprain

This injury occurs if the acromioclavicular joint is forced beyond its normal range of motion, such as from a downward blow against the outer end of the shoulder, causing the acromion to be driven downward away from the clavicle. It is also caused by a fall in which the person lands on an outstretched hand or flexed elbow when the arm is in a vertical position and at an angle of 45 to 90 degrees of flexion or abduction from the trunk. The damage consists of the tearing or severe stretching of the acromioclavicular ligaments.

Fracture of the Clavicle

A fracture of the clavicle in its middle third may result from the same type of injury that causes acromioclavicular sprains—namely, either a direct downward blow to the acromion process, or, more commonly, landing on the hand from a fall with the arm rigidly outstretched. Such a fracture may be recognized or at least suspected if the injured person tends to support the injured arm with the good arm and carries the head tilted toward the injured side with the face turned to the opposite side. Teenagers and preteenagers are more likely to have a greenstick fracture from such injuries (Arnheim & Prentice, 1998).

Dislocation of the Shoulder

There are three types of these dislocations: forward or subcoracoid (Figure 5.24a); downward or subglenoid (Figure 5.24b); and posterior (Figure 5.24c). The most common type among young athletes is the forward (subcoracoid) type, which is most likely to occur when the humerus is abducted and laterally rotated or when the pectoralis major is forcefully contracting. In this circumstance, the head of the humerus, having slipped forward out of the glenoid fossa, comes to rest beneath the coracoid process (Figure 5.24a). The injured arm is usually held out from the side in a position of slight abduction and lateral rotation. The shoulder is well protected from downward dislocations because of the upward tilt of the glenoid fossa and the effectiveness of the supraspinatus, posterior deltoid, and the superior part of the capsule in tightening to hold the humeral head in the socket. When these dislocations do occur, they are caused by a blow from the top of the shoulder and happen more easily when the arm is slightly abducted.

Rotator Cuff Tears

The supraspinatous muscle is the rotator cuff muscle most often injured, although the nature of the muscle injury is dependent on the kinematics of the shoulder joint action. In some situations, all muscles of the cuff might be involved. The complex motions that occur at the shoulder place strains on all of these muscles, especially in actions such as throwing (Whiting

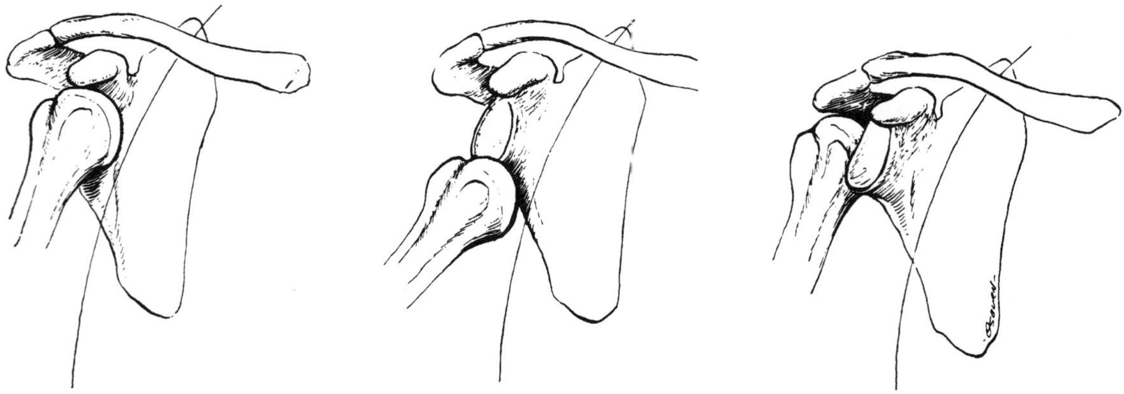

a. b. c.

Figure 5.24 Dislocations of the shoulder: (a) typical subcoracoid dislocation; (b) subglenoid dislocation; (c) posterior dislocation. *Source:* From *Treatment of Injuries to Athletes* (3rd ed.), by D. H. O'Donoghue. Copyright © 1976, W. B. Saunders, Orlando, FL. Reprinted by permission.

and Zernicke 1998). Tears in the rotator cuff may be caused by overuse, falls, or violent, fast arm motions.

Shoulder Impingement

Impingement syndrome occurs when the soft tissue structure superior to the head of the humerus is pressed against the acromion process. This painful condition may be the result of overuse, a trapped or inflamed bursa, a sports-related injury, or degeneration due to age. In the young these injuries are often ascribed to abduction pressure, whereas in the elderly bone spurs and joint degeneration are contributing factors (Whiting & Zernicke, 1998).

REFERENCES AND SELECTED READINGS

Arnheim, D. D., & Prentice, W. W. (1998). *Essentials of athletic training* (4th ed.). St. Louis, MO: McGraw-Hill.

Basmajian, J. V., & Deluca, C. J. (1985). *Muscles alive* (5th ed.). Baltimore: Williams & Wilkins.

Dayanidhi, S., Orlin, M., Kozin, S., Duff, S., & Karduna, A. (2005). Scapular kinematics during humeral elevation in adults and children. *Clinical Biomechanics,* 20, 600–606.

Escamilla, R. F., & Andrews, J. R. (2009). Shoulder muscle recruitment patterns and related biomechanics during upper extremity sports. *Sports Medicine,* 39(7), 569–590.

Kumar, S., Narayan, Y., & Garand, D. (2002). Electromyography of trunk muscles in isometric graded axial rotation. *Journal of Electromyographic Kinesiology,* 12(4), 317–328.

Ludewig, P. M., Cook, T. M., & Nawoczenski, D. A. (1996). Three-dimensional scapular orientation and muscle activity at selected positions of humeral elevation. *Journal of Orthopedic and Sports Physical Therapy,* 24(2), 57–65.

Lugo, R., Kung, P., and Ma, C. B. (2008). Shoulder biomechanics. *European Journal of Radiology,* 68, 16–24.

McClure, P. W., Michener, L. A., Sennett, B. J., & Karduna, A. R. (2001). Direct 3-dimensional measurement of scapular kinematics during dynamic movements in vivo. *Journal of Shoulder and Elbow Surgery,* 10(3), 269–270.

McGill, S. M. (1991). Electromyographic activity of the abdominal and low back musculature during the generation of isometric and dynamic axial trunk torque: Implications for lumbar mechanics. *Journal of Orthopedic Research,* 9, 91–103.

Myers, J. B., Laudner, K. G., Pasquale, M. R., & Lephart, S. M. (2005). Scapular position and orientation in throwing athletes. *American Journal of Sports Medicine,* 33(2), 263–271.

Pascoal, A. G., van der Helm, F., Correia, P. P., & Carita, I. (2000). Effect of different arm external loads on the scapulo-humeral rhythm. *Clinical Biomechanics,* 15(S1), S21–S24.

Reinold, M. M., Wilk, K. E., Fleisig, G. S., Zheng, N., Barrentine, S. W., Chmielewski, T., et al. (2004). Electromyographic analysis of the rotator cuff and deltoid musculature during common shoulder external rotation exercises. *Journal of Orthopedic Sports Physical Therapy,* 34(7), 385–394.

Stevens, A. J., Rosselle, N. E., & Michels, A. A. (1976). Possibility of a selective activity in the coracobrachialis. In *Biomechanics,* edited by V.-A. Komi (pp. 267–271). Baltimore: University Park Press.

Suenaga, N., Minami, A., & Fujisawa, H. (2003). Electromyographic analysis of internal rotational motion of the shoulder in various arm positions. *Journal of Shoulder and Elbow Surgery,* 12, 501–505.

Veeger, H. E. J., & van der Helm. F. C. T. (2007). Shoulder function: The perfect compromise between mobility and stability. *Journal of Biomechanics,* 40, 2119–2129.

Whiting, W. C., & Zernicke, R. F. (1998). *Biomechanics of musculoskeletal injury.* Champaign, IL: Human Kinetics.

Laboratory Experiences

Joint Structure and Function

1. Facing your partner's back, hold your thumb against the inferior angle of one scapula and your index or middle finger against the root of the spine at the scapula. Try to follow the movements of the scapula as your partner performs all the fundamental movements of the arm on the body.
2. Study the movements of the glenohumeral, acromioclavicular, and sternoclavicular articulations. Classify each joint according to structure (see pp. 27–29). For each joint, name and describe briefly the articulating processes and surfaces, ligaments, and cartilages. Explain how the joint structure influences the ranges of identified motions and prevents motions not observed.
3. In five different subjects, measure the amount of abduction that occurs in the shoulder girdle (i.e., the separation of the scapulae) when the arms are flexed 90 degrees at the shoulder joint. How much can this vary in one individual? In measuring the distance between the scapulae, measure the horizontal distance between the midpoints of the vertebral borders.
4. Using a protractor or goniometer, measure the amount of upward rotation of the scapula that occurs when the arm is abducted to the overhead position. To make this measurement, center the instrument over the medial angle of the scapula and adjust one of its arms in line with the normal resting position of the inferior angle and the other in line with the inferior angle after maximum upward rotation of the scapula has taken place.

Muscular Action

Directions: Work in groups of three, with one person serving as the subject, the second as an assistant helping to support or steady the stationary part of the body and giving resistance to the moving part, and the third palpating the muscles and recording the results according to the format used in Table 1.2.

5. **Abduction of the Arm.** Shoulder joint: abduction and possibly external rotation; shoulder girdle: upward rotation.
   Subject: In erect position, abduct the arm to shoulder level, keeping the forearm extended.
   Assistant: Resist movement by exerting pressure downward on subject's elbow. See to it that subject does not elevate shoulder.
   Observer: Palpate the three portions of the deltoid and tell which portions contract. Palpate the four parts of the trapezius. Which parts contract? Does the pectoralis major contract during any part of the movement?
6. **Adduction of the Arm** (see Figure 5.17). Shoulder joint: adduction and possibly reduction of external rotation; shoulder girdle: downward rotation.
   Subject: In erect position with arm abducted to shoulder level, lower arm until 45 degrees from side.
   Assistant: Place hand under subject's elbow and resist movement. (If no resistance is given, the muscle action will be the same as in abduction, except that the contraction will be eccentric instead of concentric.)
   Observer: Palpate the latissimus dorsi, teres major, pectoralis major, and posterior deltoid. Do they each contract and, if so, during which part of the movement?
7. **Flexion of the Arm** (see Figure 5.18). Shoulder joint: flexion; shoulder girdle: upward rotation and probably abduction.
   Subject: In erect position, flex arm to shoulder level, keeping elbow extended.
   Assistant: Resist movement by exerting pressure downward on the subject's elbow. See that subject does not elevate shoulder.
   Observer: Palpate the anterior deltoid and the pectoralis major. Do both the sternal and clavicular portions of the latter muscle contract?
8. **Extension of the Arm** (see Figure 5.19). Shoulder joint: extension; shoulder girdle: downward rotation and probably adduction.
   Subject: In erect position with arm flexed to shoulder level, lower it until 45 degrees from side.
   Assistant: Resist movement at underside of elbow.

Observer: Palpate the latissimus dorsi and the pectoralis major. Do they contract with equal force throughout the movement?

9. **Hyperextension of the Arm** (see Figure 5.20). Shoulder joint: hyperextension; shoulder girdle: upward tilt.
   Subject: Either in erect position or lying facedown: hyperextend upper extremity, keeping elbow extended.
   Assistant: Place hand over subject's elbow and resist movement.
   Observer: Palpate the posterior deltoid, latissimus dorsi, and teres major.
10. **Horizontal Abduction of the Arm** (from horizontal adduction). Shoulder joint: horizontal abduction and slight external rotation; shoulder girdle: adduction and reduction of lateral tilt.
    a. *Subject:* In erect position with arms flexed to shoulder level, palm down, horizontally abduct the arms as far as possible.
    Assistant: Stand facing subject between the arms and resist movement by grasping the outstretched elbows.
    Observer: Palpate the posterior deltoid and latissimus dorsi. What other muscles can be palpated?
    b. *Subject:* Lying facedown on narrow plinth or on table close to edge with arm hanging straight down (flexed), horizontally abduct the arms as far above the horizontal as possible.
    Assistant: Resistance may be given at elbow but is not necessary, because gravity furnishes sufficient resistance.
    Observer: Same as in a.
11. **Horizontal Adduction of the Arm** (from abducted position). Shoulder joint: horizontal adduction and slight internal rotation; shoulder girdle: abduction and lateral tilt.
    a. *Subject:* In erect position with arm abducted to shoulder level, palm down, horizontally adduct the arms.
    Assistant: Stand behind subject's arm and resist movement by holding elbow.
    Observer: Palpate pectoralis major and anterior deltoid.
    b. *Subject:* Lie on back on table with arm horizontally extended, palm up. Horizontally adduct the upper extremity to a vertical position, keeping elbow extended.
    Assistant: Resistance may be given at elbow but is not necessary, because gravity furnishes sufficient resistance.
    Observer: Same as in a.
12. **Outward Rotation of Arm.** Shoulder joint: external rotation; shoulder girdle: possibly adduction and reduction of lateral tilt.
    a. *Subject:* Lying facedown on a table with upper arm at shoulder level, resting on table and forearm hanging down off edge of table. Keeping forearm at right angles to upper arm, outward rotate arm at the shoulder joint to limit of motion without allowing upper arm to leave table.
    Assistant: Steady upper arm and resist movement of forearm by holding wrist.
    Observer: Palpate infraspinatus and teres minor.
    b. *Subject:* Sitting erect with upper arm abducted and elbow flexed at right angles with forearm at forward horizontal position. Without moving upper arm, externally rotate at the shoulder joint so that the forearm is in a vertical position (see Figure 5.22).
    Assistant: Support upper arm at elbow and give resistance to forearm at wrist.
    Observer: Same as in a.
13. **Inward Rotation of Arm.** Shoulder joint: internal rotation; shoulder girdle: abduction and lateral tilt, and tendency toward elevation.
    a. *Subject:* Same position as in 12a. Internally rotate arm at the shoulder joint.
    Assistant: Steady upper arm and resist movement of forearm by holding wrist.
    Observer: Palpate teres major and latissimus dorsi.
    b. *Subject:* Lie on back on table with upper arm abducted resting on table and forearm raised to vertical position. Internally rotate arm at shoulder joint to the limit of motion.
    Assistant: Steady upper arm and resist forearm motion by holding wrist.
    Observer: Palpate anterior deltoid and clavicular portion of pectoralis major.
14. **Elevation of Shoulder.**
    Subject: In erect position, elevate shoulder girdle, keeping arm muscles relaxed.

Assistant: Resist movement by pressing down on shoulder.
Observer: Palpate trapezius I and II.

15. **Depression of Shoulder.**
    a. *Subject:* In erect position with shoulder girdle elevated and elbow flexed, push down with elbow and depress shoulder girdle to normal position.
    Assistant: Resist movement by holding hand under elbow.
    Observer: Palpate trapezius IV.
    b. *Subject:* Take a cross-rest position between two chairs or parallel bars.
    Observer: Palpate trapezius IV.
16. **Adduction of Shoulder Girdle** (retraction).
    Subject: In erect position with arms abducted, elbows flexed, and fingers resting on shoulders, push elbows backward (horizontally extend at the shoulder joint), keeping the elbows at shoulder level.
    Assistant: Stand facing subject and resist movement by pulling elbows forward (horizontally flex at the shoulder joints).
    Observer: Palpate middle and lower trapezius (parts III and IV). (This movement is somewhat similar to the one in Experience 10, but here the emphasis is on the shoulder girdle rather than on the arm.)
17. **Abduction of Shoulder Girdle** (protraction).
    Subject: In erect position with arm abducted, elbows flexed, and fingers resting on shoulders, horizontally flex at the shoulder joints, attempting to touch the elbows in front of chest.
    Assistant: Stand behind subject and resist movement by pulling elbows back (horizontally extend at the shoulder joint).
    Observer: Palpate serratus anterior.

Action of the Muscles Other Than the Movers

18. **Stabilization of the Scapula During Forceful Extension of the Arm.**
    Subject: In erect position with arm flexed above shoulder level, lower arm against strong resistance.
    Assistant: Resist the arm movement by placing hand under the arm just above the subject's elbow.
    Observer: Palpate trapezius IV. Explain.
19. **Stabilization of Scapula During External Rotation of Humerus.**
    Subject: Rotate the arm externally as it hangs at the side.
    Observer: Palpate the scapular adductors. Explain.
20. **Rotation of Arm in Abducted Position.**
    Subject: With one arm abducted to shoulder level, rotate it first outward, then inward.
    Observer: Palpate middle deltoid. Explain its action.

Applications

21. Work in groups of three with the members designated respectively as A, B, and C. Equipment for each group: a volleyball and an empty 12-ounce frozen juice can or another can of approximately the same size.
    A stands at one end of playing area with left side toward the opposite end.
    B stands facing A about two arm lengths away and holds can vertically in right hand with arm flexed and with volleyball balanced on open end of can.
    A adjusts distance and swings extended right arm horizontally backward with thumb side up and palm flat. A then swings arm vigorously forward and strikes ball forcefully with palm, attempting to project ball as far as possible.
    C observes A's action and writes answers to the following questions without saying them aloud.
    a. What is the movement of A's humerus at the shoulder joint in the preparatory movement?
    b. Same for the striking movement?
    c. What is the position of A's humerus at the moment of impact?
    Repeat until each person has taken a turn at being A, B, and C. Report answers to the rest of the group, and discuss if not in agreement.
22. Work in partners with one observing while the other performs.
    Starting position: Hang from horizontal bar with palms facing body and with feet hanging clear or, if necessary, with toes just touching floor or bench.

Movement: Chin self with steady pull and hold end position.

Observer: Write joint analysis of (a) starting position of humerus at shoulder joint, and of scapulae; and (b) movement of each. Discuss with partner.

23. Choose a simple motor skill from Appendix G. Do a complete anatomical analysis of the shoulder region, following the analysis outline in Table 1.2.

CHAPTER

6

THE UPPER EXTREMITY

The Elbow, Forearm, Wrist, and Hand

OUTLINE

OUTLINE

OBJECTIVES

At the conclusion of this chapter, the student should be able to:

1. Name, locate, and describe the structure and ligamentous reinforcements of the articulations of the elbow, forearm, wrist, and hand.
2. Name and demonstrate the movements possible in the joints of the elbow, forearm, wrist, and hand regardless of the starting position.
3. Name and locate the muscles and muscle groups of the elbow, forearm, wrist, and hand, and name their primary actions as agonists, stabilizers, neutralizers, or antagonists.
4. Analyze the fundamental movements of the forearm, hand, and fingers with respect to joint and muscle actions.
5. Describe the common athletic injuries of the forearm, elbow, wrist, and fingers.
6. Perform an anatomical analysis of the elbow, forearm, wrist, and hand in a motor skill.

In much the same way that the shoulder girdle's cooperation with the shoulder joint contributes to the wide range of motion available to the hand, the cooperative movements of the elbow, radioulnar, and wrist joints contribute to the versatility and precision of its movements. Although the hand is intrinsically skillful, its usefulness is greatly impaired when anything interferes with the motions of the forearm or wrist. Injury to any one of the joints involved makes this painfully obvious to the sufferer.

THE ELBOW JOINT

Structure

The elbow is far more complex than the simple hinge joint that it appears to be. The two bones of the forearm attach to the humerus in totally different ways. The humeroulnar joint is indeed a true hinge joint, but the humeroradial joint is far from it. It has been classified as an arthrodial or gliding type of joint, but it is more accurately described as a restricted ball-and-socket joint. Inspection of the articulating surfaces as depicted in Figure 6.1 or of the skeleton itself will help make this clear. The distal end of the humerus presents a spool-like process (trochlea) on the medial side and a spherical knob (capitulum) on the lateral side. The ulna articulates with the humerus by means of a semicircular structure that is cupped around the back and underside of the trochlea. The inner surface of this is known as the semilunar notch. It terminates below and in front in the small coronoid process, and above and in back in the broad olecranon process.

The radius articulates with the humerus by means of a slightly concave, saucerlike disc, which is directly beneath the capitulum when the arm is hanging straight down. In spite of the joint's

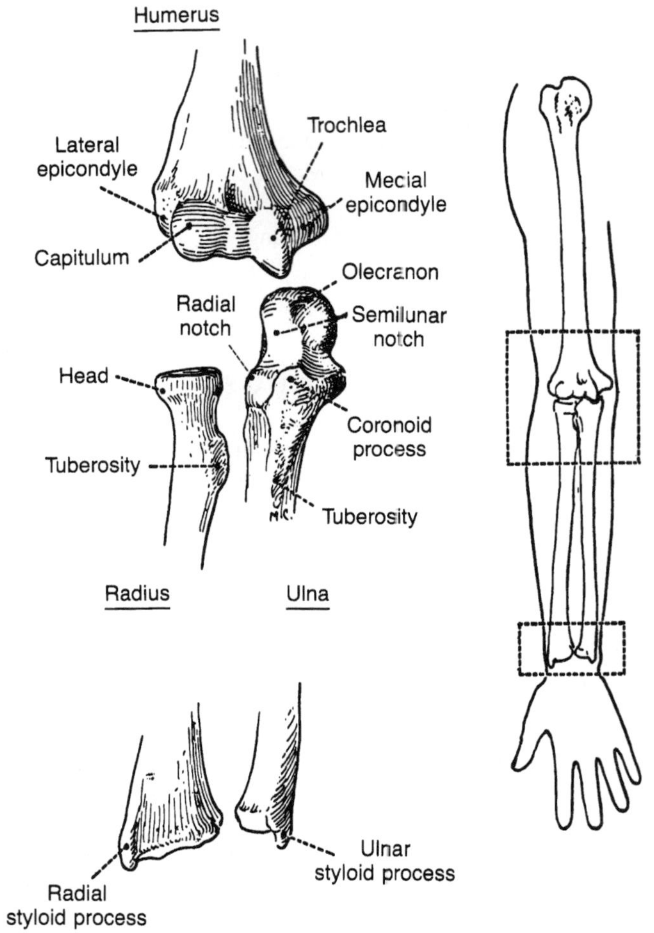

Figure 6.1 The bony structures of the elbow and radioulnar joints, anterior view.

ball-and-socket structure, the radius is unable to abduct or adduct because of the annular ligament that encircles the radial head and binds it to the radial notch of the ulna. Furthermore, because of this and other ligamentous connections with the ulna, the radius is unable to rotate independently (Figures 6.2 and 6.3). Hence, the only movements it is free to engage in at the elbow are flexion and extension. For this reason, one is justified in classifying the elbow joint as a hinge joint.

Joint Stability

The two articulations of the elbow joint, as well as the proximal radioulnar articulation, are completely enveloped in a single, extensive capsule.

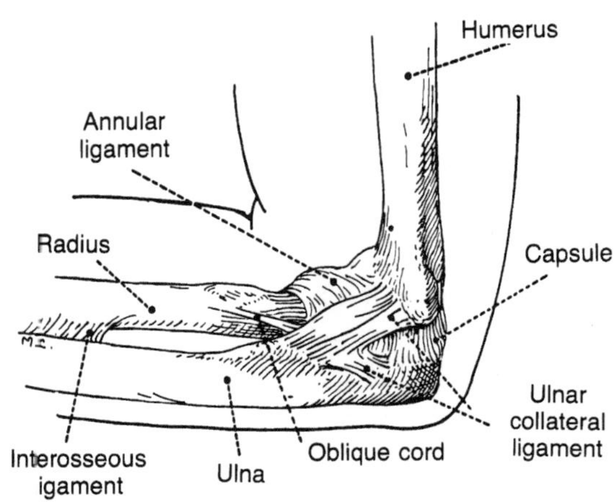

Figure 6.2 Medial aspect of elbow joint showing ligaments.

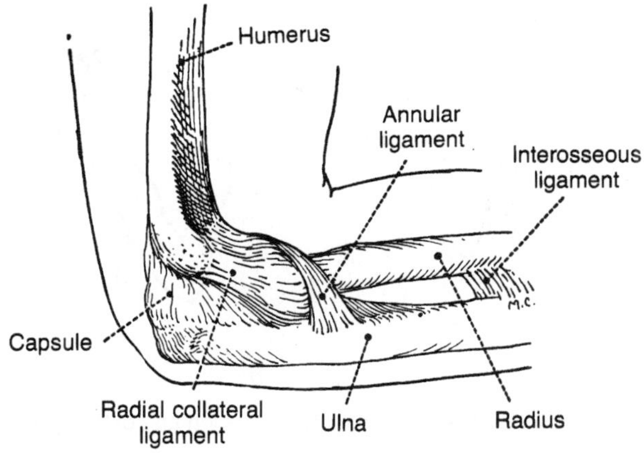

Figure 6.3 Lateral aspect of elbow joint showing ligaments.

This is lined by the synovial membrane, which extends into the proximal radioulnar articulation, covers the olecranon, coronoid, and radial fossae, and lines the annular ligament. The capsule is strengthened by five ligaments: the *anterior, posterior, lateral collateral, lateral ulnar collateral* (not pictured), and *ulnar collateral.* The last named is the strongest. It is a thick triangular band attached above by its apex to the medial epicondyle of the humerus and below by its base to the medial margins of the coronoid and olecranon processes of the ulna and the intervening ridge.

The stabilizing components of muscle pull also add to the stability of the elbow joint. In weight bearing (such as falling onto the hands), the compression on the elbow can be very high. The muscle surrounding the joint will contract to provide joint stability against forces that may exceed the capabilities of the ligamentous structures. The same holds true for many throwing activities.

Carrying Angle

In the anatomical position, the forearm is abducted in relation to the humerus, an alignment caused by the angle of articulation of the humerus and ulna at the elbow joint. Normally this angle, called the carrying angle, is larger in women than in men. If the forearm were to hang straight down in women as it does in men, it would not clear the female pelvis. Not only is the female's pelvis broader than the male's, her shoulders also are narrower. This exaggerated carrying angle, referred to as cubitus valgus, disappears during elbow flexion or forearm pronation.

Movements

Flexion

From the anatomical position this is a forward-upward movement of the forearm in the sagittal plane (Figure 6.4a).

Extension

Return movement from flexion. A few individuals are able to hyperextend the elbow joint. This is probably because of a short olecranon process rather than loose ligaments (Figure 6.4a).

THE RADIOULNAR JOINTS

Structure of Proximal Radioulnar Joint

The disc-shaped head of the radius fits against the radial notch of the ulna and is encircled by the annular ligament (see Figures 6.1, 6.2, and 6.3). The notch and annular ligament between them form a complete ring within which the radial head rotates. Inasmuch as the superior surface of the radial head articulates with the capitulum of the humerus, rotation must occur here, too, although strictly speaking, this is not part of the radioulnar joint. The three joints in this region, the humeroulnar, humeroradial, and proximal radioulnar, all share a common capsule.

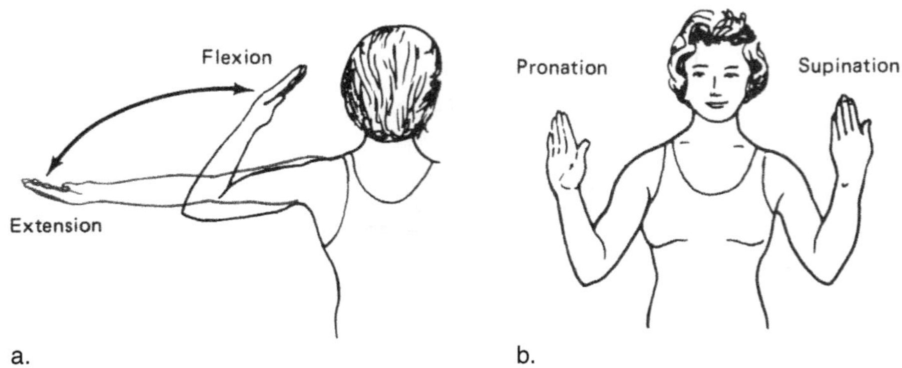

Figure 6.4 Movements of the elbow and radioulnar joints: (a) flexion and extension; (b) right radioulnar joints pronated; left radioulnar joints supinated.

Structure of Distal Radioulnar Joint

At the distal end of the forearm the radius articulates with the head of the ulna by means of a small notch (see Figure 6.1). A triangular fibrocartilaginous disc lies between the head of the ulna and the proximal row of wrist bones (see Figure 6.12) and serves to reinforce the joint, as well as to separate it from the wrist. The joint is also strengthened by the *volar radioulnar* and *dorsal radioulnar* ligaments. Both the proximal and distal radioulnar joints are classified as pivot joints.

Movements

Pronation

This is a rotation of the forearm around its longitudinal axis in such a way that the palm turns medially. It corresponds to medial or inward rotation of the humerus.

Supination

This is a rotation of the forearm around its longitudinal axis in such a way that the palm turns laterally. It corresponds to lateral or outward rotation of the humerus. During pronation and supination, the distal end of the radius moves about the ulna, whereas the proximal end of the radius rotates or pivots about its long axis.

Note: When the elbow is in an extended position, pronation of the forearm tends to accompany inward rotation of the upper arm, and supination tends to accompany outward rotation. In the anatomical position of the arm, the humerus is rotated outward and the forearm is supinated. The full range of forearm pronation and supination is best seen when the elbow is maintained at a 90-degree angle (see Figure 6.4). When the upper arms are at the sides of the body and the forearms are extended forward in the horizontal position, the mid or neutral position relative to pronation, and supination is with the thumbs up and the palms facing each other. An excellent way to study what happens to the two forearm bones in these movements is suggested in Laboratory Experience 4.

Muscles of the Elbow and Radioulnar Joints

Location

The muscles of the elbow and radioulnar joints are listed here according to their positions relative to the joints involved:

Anterior (Elbow Region)
Biceps brachii
Brachialis
Brachioradialis
Pronator teres

Anterior (Wrist Region)
Pronator quadratus

Posterior
Triceps brachii
Anconeus
Supinator

Characteristics and Functions of Individual Muscles

Biceps Brachii

This is primarily a muscle of the elbow and radioulnar joints (Figure 6.5), but, as noted in the last chapter, it also acts at the shoulder joint. Unless prevented from doing so (by the action of neutralizers or by fixation of the hand when the subject is hanging from a bar), it simultaneously *flexes* and *supinates* the forearm. Studies by Basmajian and others (Basmajian & DeLuca, 1985) have shown that the biceps is active during flexion of the supine forearm under all conditions of static and dynamic contraction. In most instances in which the forearm is pronated, however, the biceps shows little activity unless external resistance is applied (Figure 6.6). This is because its tendon wraps around the radius and therefore has a poor line of pull. External resistance is also necessary for the biceps to be active in supination of the extended arm. It may be palpated on the anterior surface of the upper arm when the forearm is flexed, especially in the supinated position.

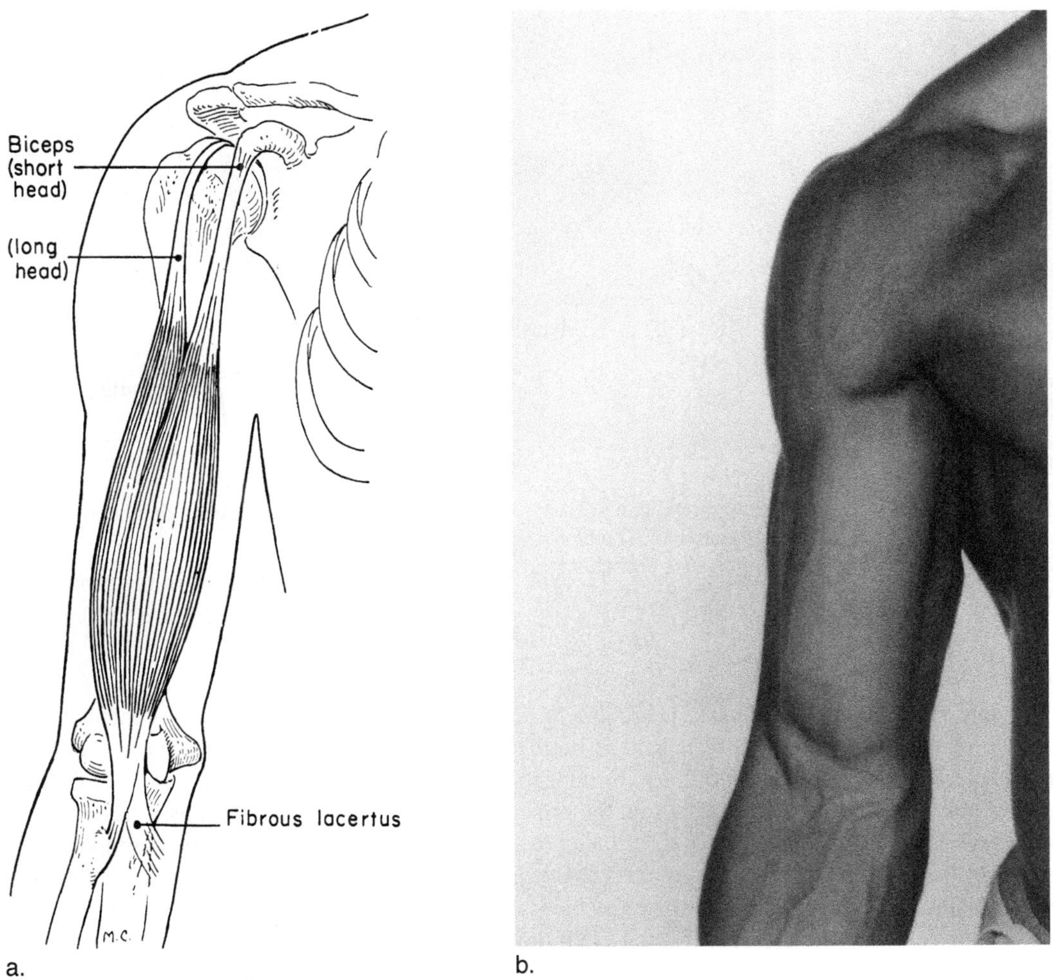

Figure 6.5 Biceps muscle of the arm.

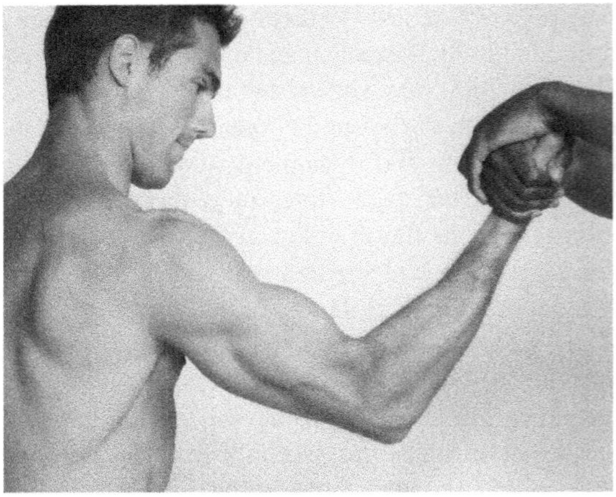

a.

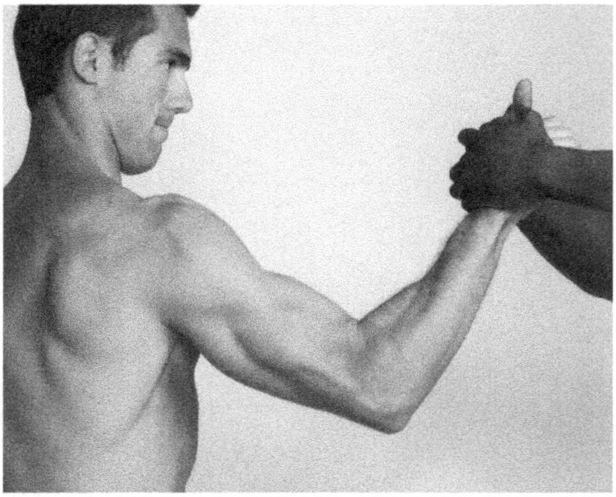

b.

Figure 6.6 Flexion of the forearm: (a) in a position of supination; (b) in a position of pronation. The biceps brachii is less active when the forearm is pronated than when it is supinated.

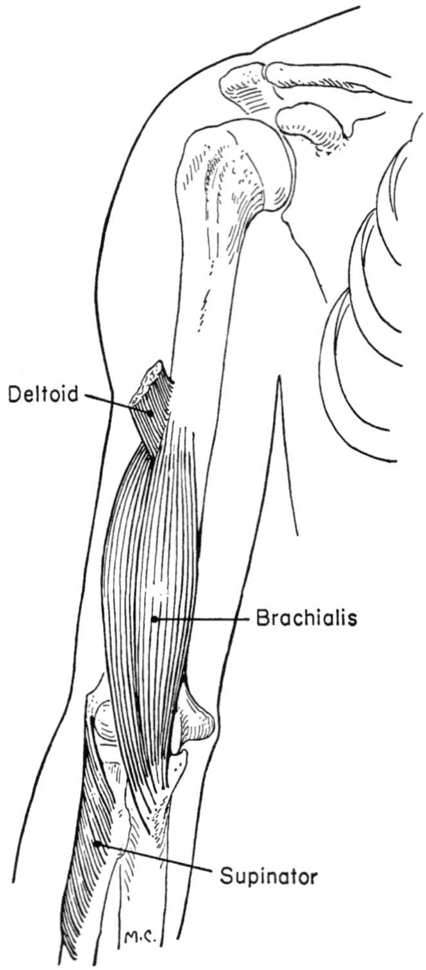

Figure 6.7 Deep muscles on front of right arm.

Brachialis

The sole function of this muscle (Figure 6.7) is *flexion* of the elbow joint, and it is said to be the unexcelled flexor under all conditions (Basmajian & DeLuca, 1985). Because it attaches on the proximal end of the ulna, its line of pull remains the same regardless of whether the forearm is pronated or supinated. It is partially covered by the biceps but can be palpated just lateral to this muscle if the contraction is sufficiently strong, and especially if the forearm is maintained in the pronated position as it is being flexed (see Figure 6.6b).

Brachioradialis

In addition to its role as a contributor to elbow *flexion* when the movement is resisted, it has been suggested that this muscle (Figure 6.8) may tend to "derotate" the forearm as it flexes. This has not been confirmed by electromyographic research. It has been found, however, that the brachioradialis neither supinates nor pronates the fully extended forearm unless the movement is strongly resisted. It has also been noted that this muscle is most

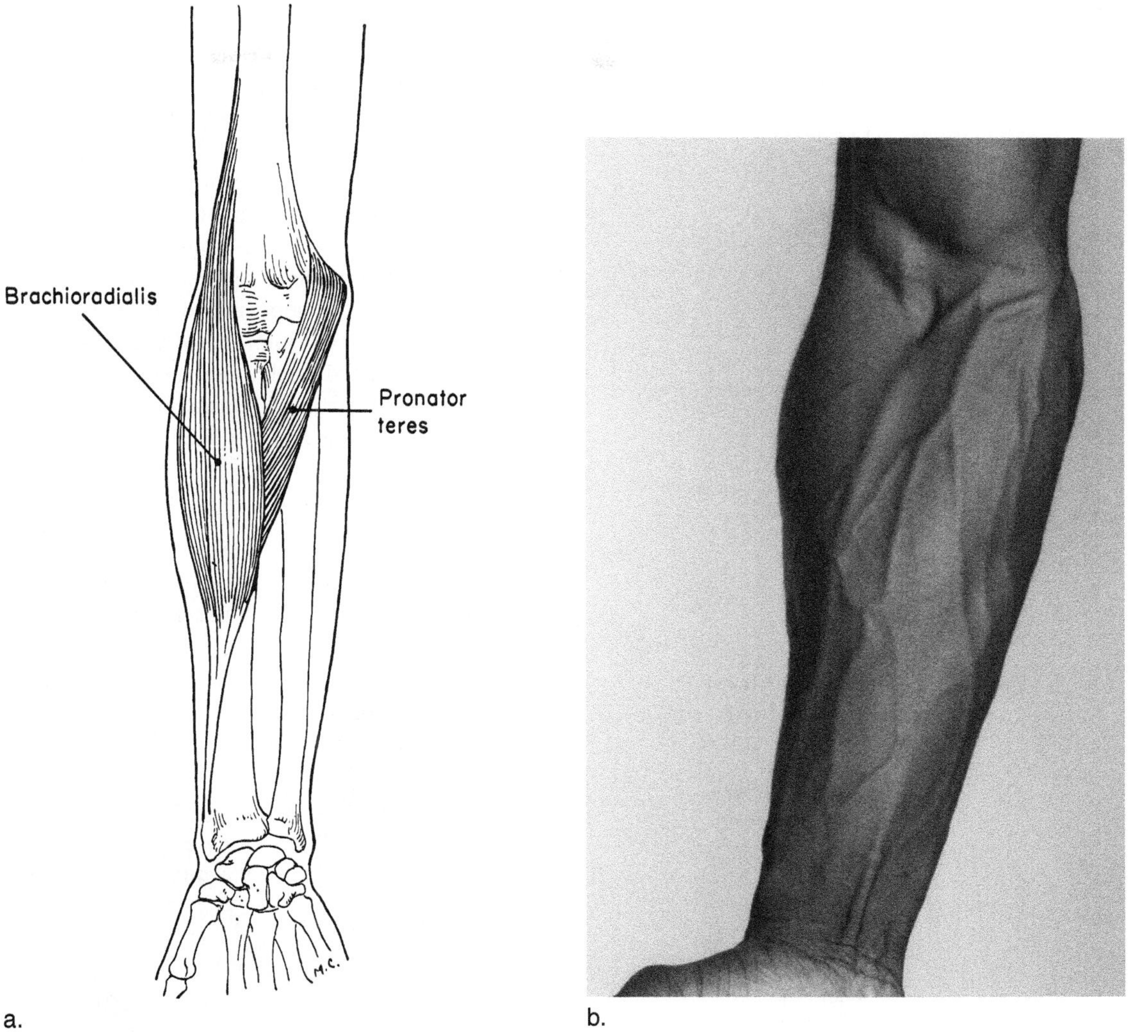

Figure 6.8 Superficial muscles on front of right forearm.

active in quick movements. It is more active in a semipronated than a supinated forearm position (Basmajian & DeLuca, 1985). It may be palpated on the anteroradial aspect of the upper half of the forearm.

Pronator Teres

This is primarily a *pronator* of the forearm (Figure 6.8), but it assists in elbow flexion against resistance. The angle of the elbow joint does not influence the pronation activity of this muscle (Basmajian & DeLuca, 1985). It is difficult to palpate.

Pronator Quadratus

This muscle's (Figure 6.9) sole action is *pronation* of the forearm. EMG experiments have shown that the electrical activity of the pronator quadratus is definitely greater than that of the pronator teres, irrespective of the speed of the movement or the degree of elbow flexion. It is too deep to palpate successfully.

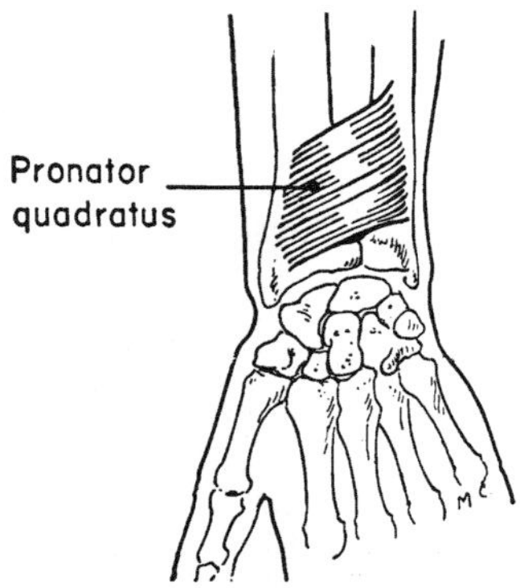

Figure 6.9 Anterior view of distal end of forearm showing pronator quadratus.

Triceps Brachii

Virtually three muscles in one (Figures 6.10 and 6.11), the triceps covers the entire posterior surface of the upper arm. Its long head is the only one of the three to cross the shoulder joint. It is a powerful *extensor of the elbow joint* and has two factors in its favor: the number and size of its fibers (p. 48), and a favorable angle of pull (p. 50). In a comparison of the three heads, it was noted that the medial head appeared to be the principal extensor of the elbow joint, usually accompanied by the lateral head. All three heads participate when there is resistance (Basmajian & DeLuca, 1985). The muscle is an easy one to see as well as to palpate.

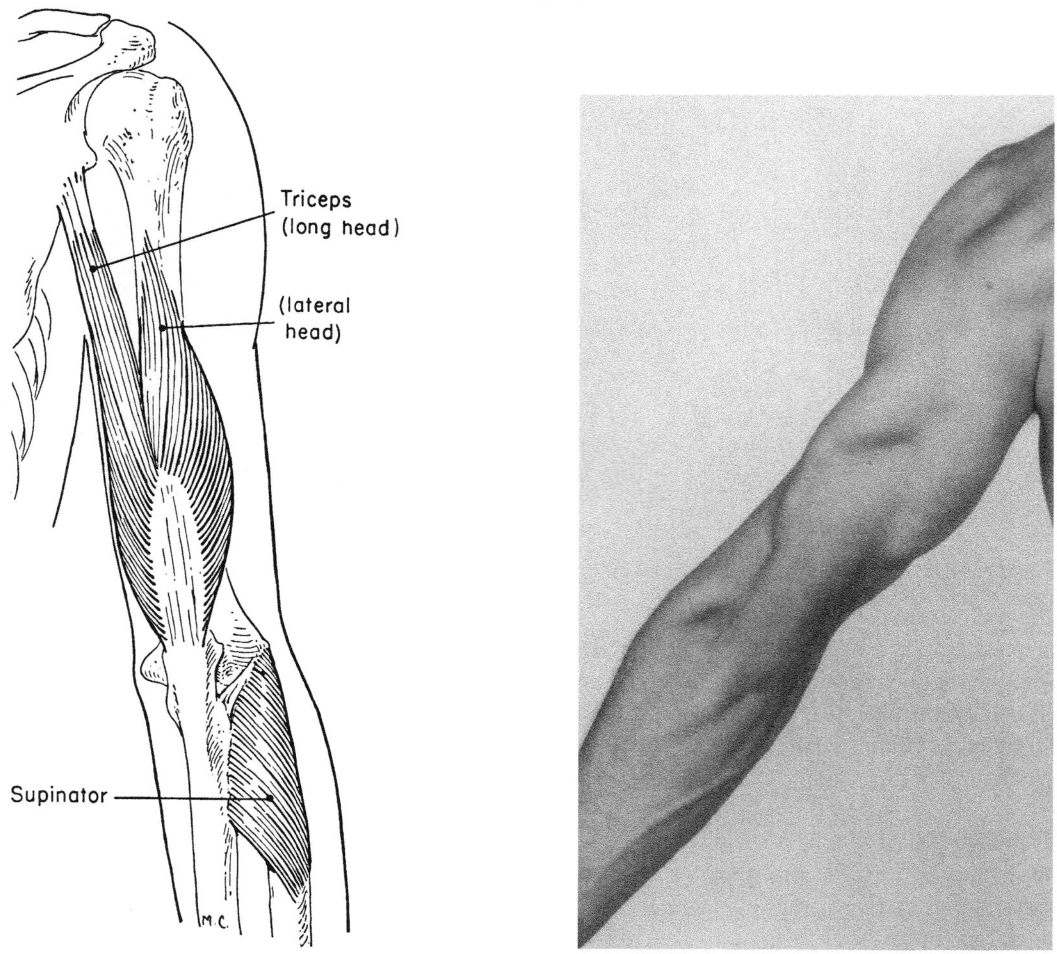

a. b.

Figure 6.10 Triceps and supinator.

Anconeus

This muscle, working with the triceps, *extends* the forearm (Figure 6.11). This muscle is moderately active during pronation and supination of the forearm, and therefore it is suggested that the anconeus acts as a stabilizer of the elbow joint (Basmajian & DeLuca, 1985). The muscle may be palpated on the back of the elbow at the lateral margin of the olecranon process.

Supinator

Although assisted by others, this muscle (see Figures 6.7 and 6.10) is the primary one for *supination* under all conditions. Palpation with any degree of success is extremely difficult.

MUSCULAR ANALYSIS OF THE FUNDAMENTAL MOVEMENTS OF THE FOREARM

Flexion

There are three important flexors of the forearm: the brachialis, the brachioradialis, and the biceps—the three Bs. Their relative participation in and contribution to flexion of the forearm have been the subjects of much study. Because elbow flexion may be performed with the forearm pronated, semipronated, or supinated, with or without resistance, slowly or rapidly, with or against gravity, there have been many variables to study.

Investigators agree that the brachialis serves as a flexor under all conditions, and there is general agreement that the biceps is more active in flexion when the arm is supinated than when it is pronated.

It is now generally accepted that during maximal isometric contractions, (1) the biceps is most active when the forearm is supinated and least active when it is pronated; (2) the brachioradialis is most active when the forearm is either in the midposition or in supination and least active when the forearm is in extreme pronation or supination; (3) the pronator teres, as a moderate flexor, is most active in a position of pronation; and (4) the isometric force exerted by the elbow flexors during maximal voluntary contractions is greatest when

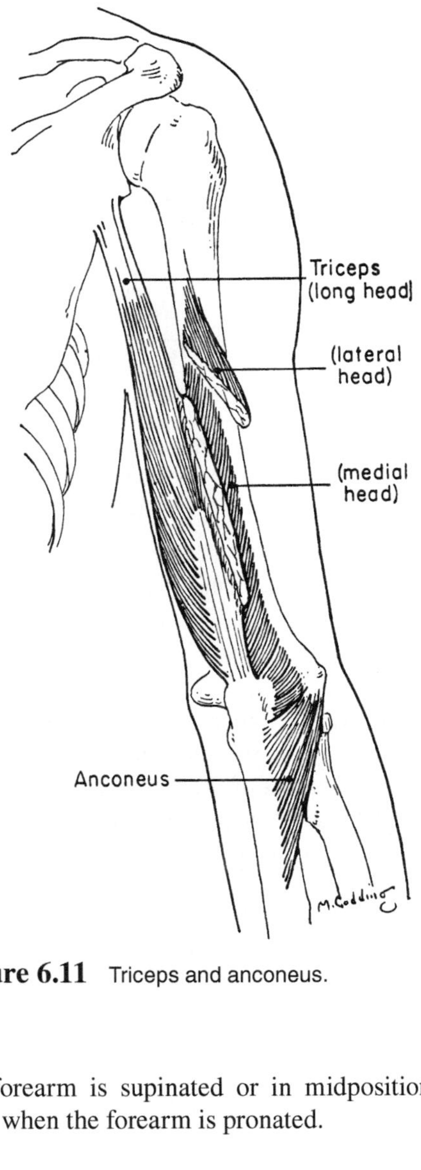

Figure 6.11 Triceps and anconeus.

the forearm is supinated or in midposition and least when the forearm is pronated.

Extension

When not produced by the force of gravity, the forearm is extended at the elbow joint by the triceps and anconeus.

Pronation

Movement of the forearm at the two radioulnar joints. Produced by the combined action of the pronator teres and pronator quadratus.

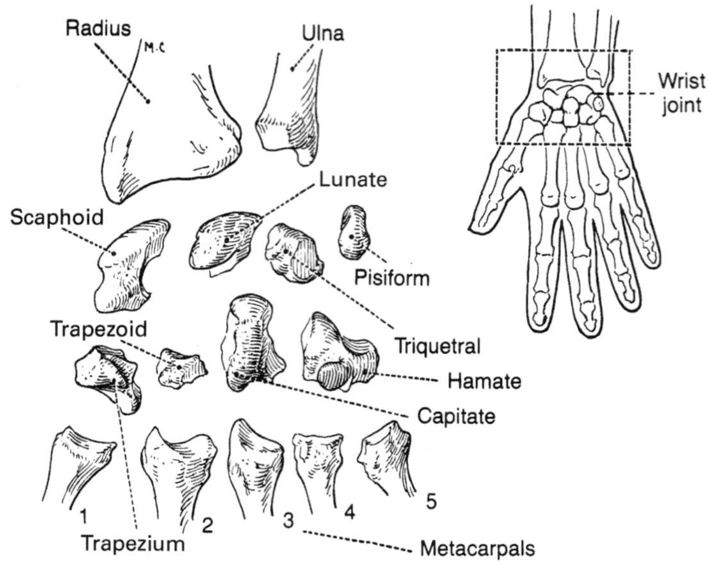

Figure 6.12 Bones of the wrist, anterior view.

Supination

Movement of the forearm at the two radioulnar joints. Produced by the supinator and biceps brachii. The two heads of the biceps are not equally active in all supination motions. Functional capacity in each of the heads is related to initial muscle length. The long head of the biceps was found to be more active with a greater muscle length (elbow extension), whereas the short head was more active with a shortened initial muscle length (elbow flexion) (Murray et al., 2000).

THE WRIST AND HAND

The hand and wrist owe their mobility to their generous supply of joints (Figure 6.12). The most proximal of these is the radiocarpal, or wrist, joint. Just beyond this are the two rows of carpal bones, each row consisting of four bones. The carpal joints include the articulations within each of these rows, as well as the articulations between the two rows. The carpometacarpal joints (Figure 6.13a) are located at the base of the hand. Closely associated with them are the intermetacarpal joints, those points of contact between the

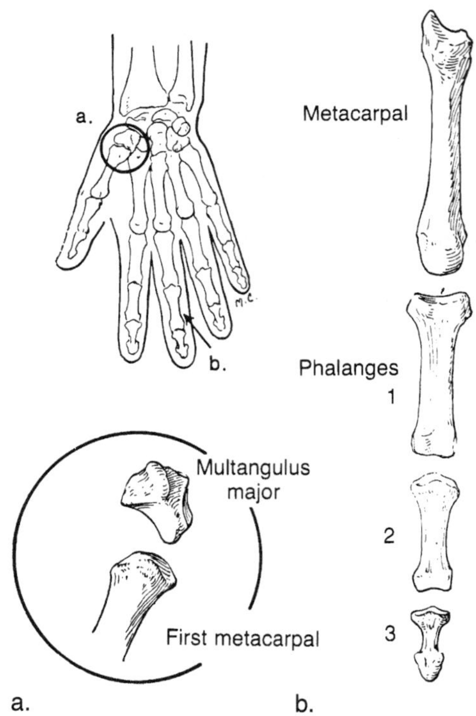

Figure 6.13 Bones of the hand showing selected joint surfaces: (a) carpometacarpal joint of thumb (a saddle joint); (b) metacarpal bone and phalanges of middle finger, anterior view.

bases of the metacarpal bones of the four fingers. The fingers unite with the hand at the metacarpophalangeal joints. Within the fingers themselves are two sets of interphalangeal joints, the first between the proximal and middle rows of phalanges and the second between the middle and distal rows. The thumb differs from the four fingers in having a more freely movable metacarpal bone and in having only two phalanges instead of three. The metacarpal bone of the thumb is so similar to a phalanx that it might well be described as a cross between a phalanx and a metacarpal (Figure 6.13b).

Structure of the Wrist (Radiocarpal) Joint

The wrist joint is a condyloid (ovoid) joint formed by the union of the slightly concave, oval-shaped surface of the proximal row of carpal bones (i.e., the scaphoid, lunate, and triquetral bones, but not the pisiform). The distal radioulnar joint is in close proximity to the wrist joint and shares with it the articular disc that lies between the head of the ulna and the triquetral bone of the wrist. However, it is not a part of the wrist joint because each joint has its own capsule. The capsule of the wrist consists of four ligaments that merge to form a continuous cover for the joint. These are the volar radiocarpal, dorsal radiocarpal, ulnar collateral, and radial collateral (Figures 6.14 and 6.15).

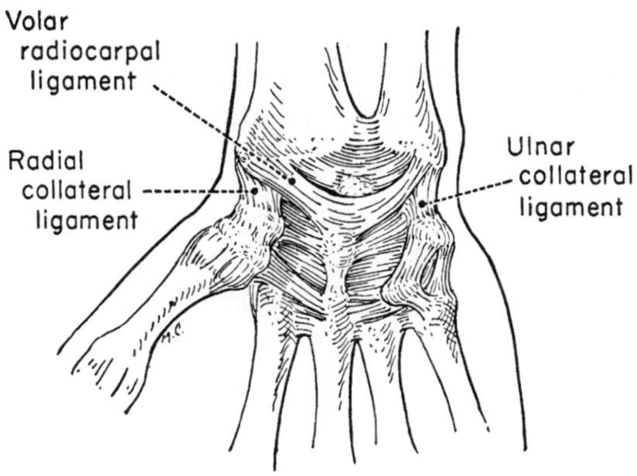

Figure 6.14 Anterior view of right wrist joint showing ligaments.

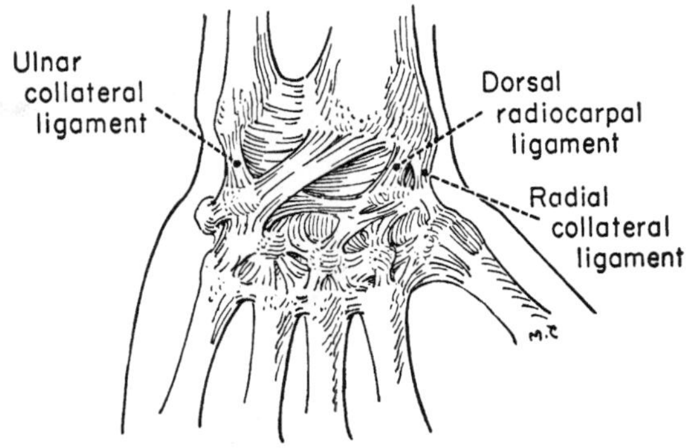

Figure 6.15 Posterior view of right wrist joint showing ligaments.

Movements of the Hand at the Wrist Joint

Flexion

From the anatomical position (Figure 6.16a), this is a forward-upward movement in the sagittal plane, whereby the palmar surface of the hand approaches the anterior surface of the forearm.

Extension

Return movement from flexion.

Hyperextension

A movement in which the dorsal surface of the hand approaches the posterior surface of the forearm—the exact opposite of flexion.

Radial Flexion (Abduction)

From the anatomical position this is a sideward movement in the frontal plane, whereby the hand moves away from the body with the thumb side leading (Figure 6.16b). The movement corresponds to abduction of the humerus. This motion is also referred to as radial deviation.

Ulnar Flexion (Adduction)

From the anatomical position this is a sideward movement in the frontal plane, whereby the hand moves toward the body with the little finger side leading. The movement corresponds to adduction of the humerus. This motion is also referred to as ulnar deviation.

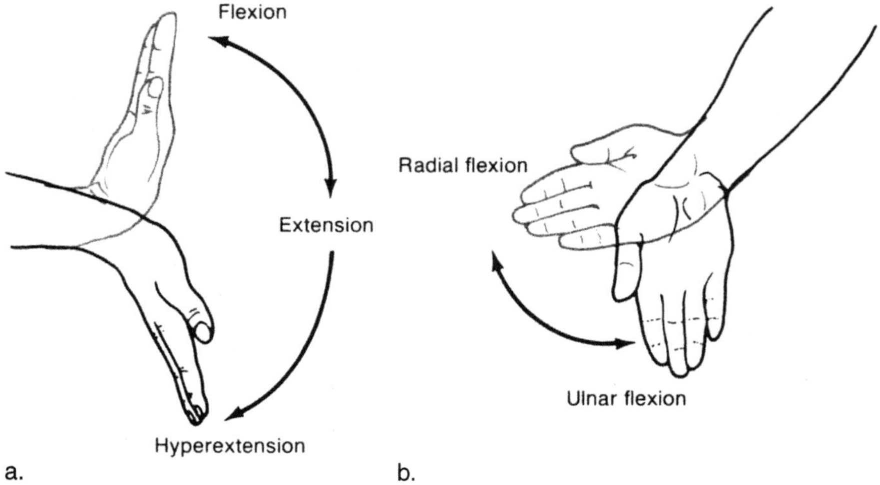

Figure 6.16 Movements of the hand at the wrist joint: (a) flexion, extension, and hyperextension; (b) ulnar and radial flexion.

Circumduction

A movement of the hand at the wrist whereby the fingertips describe a circle, and the hand as a whole describes a cone. It consists of flexion, radial flexion, hyperextension, and ulnar flexion occurring in sequence in either this order or the reverse. If there appears to be rotation when one performs this movement, it is taking place in the radioulnar joints, not the wrist joint.

Structure and Movements of the Midcarpal and Intercarpal Joints

These are the joints within the wrist itself. The articulation between the four carpal bones in the proximal row with the four in the distal row is known as the midcarpal articulation. The joints between the adjacent bones within either row are known as the intercarpal joints of the proximal and distal rows, respectively. These joints are all diarthrodial in structure. Within this classification they belong to the nonaxial group and thus permit only a slight gliding motion between the bones. These slight movements, however, add up to a modified hinge type of movement for the midcarpal joint as a whole.

A further characteristic of the carpal region is that the bones are shaped and arranged in such a way that the anterior surface is slightly concave from side to side. This provides a protected passageway for the tendons, nerves, and blood vessels supplying the hand. Referred to as the carpal tunnel, this is the site of many pathologies of the hand and wrist. Among the many carpal ligaments, the volar radiocarpal ligament is the strongest. Its fibers radiate from the capitate to the scaphoid, lunate, and triquetral bones on the anterior surface of the wrist.

Structure of the Carpometacarpal and Intermetacarpal Joints

(Figures 6.13, 6.17, and 6.18)

The carpometacarpal joint of the thumb is a prime example of a saddle joint (see Figure 6.13a). It is enclosed in an articular capsule that is stronger in back than in front. The capsule is thick but loose and serves to restrict motion rather than to prevent it. There are no additional ligaments.

The carpometacarpal joints of the four fingers not only are encased in capsules but also are protected by the dorsal, volar, and interosseous

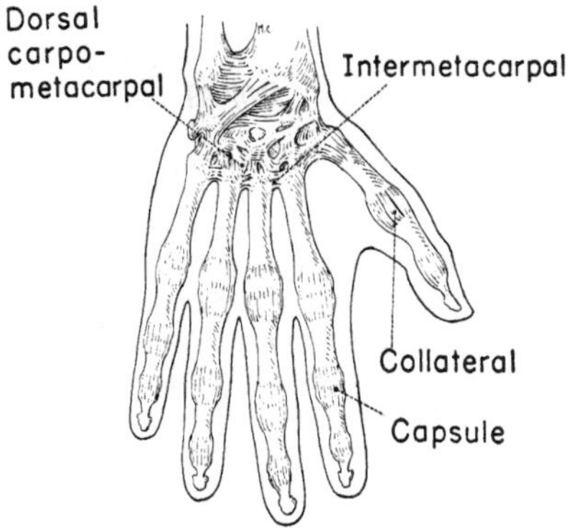

Figure 6.17 Posterior view of ligaments of right hand.

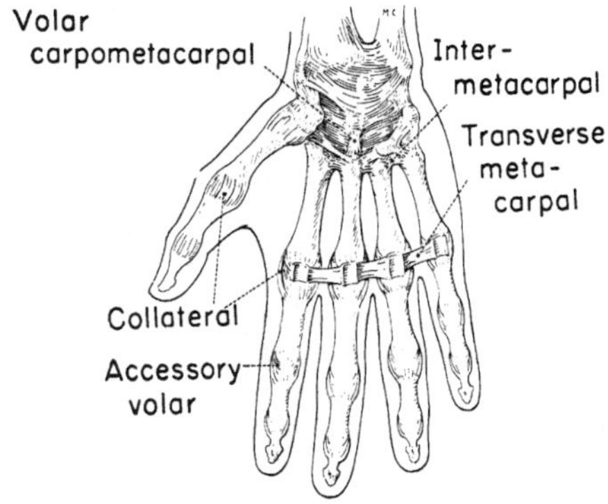

Figure 6.18 Anterior view of ligaments of right hand.

carpometacarpal ligaments (Figures 6.17 and 6.18). Closely associated with these joints are the intermetacarpal articulations, the joints between the bases of the metacarpal bones of the four fingers. These are irregular joints. They share the capsules of the carpometacarpal joints and are further reinforced by the dorsal, volar, and interosseous basal ligaments and also by the transverse metacarpal ligament, a narrow fibrous band that connects the heads of the four outer metacarpal bones.

Movements of the Carpometacarpal Joint of the Thumb

The names of the movements of the thumb may seem illogical until they are viewed in the context of the resting thumb position; that is, turned on its axis so that it faces in a plane perpendicular to the other fingers.

Abduction *(Figure 6.19a)*

A forward movement of the thumb at right angles to the palm.

Adduction

Return movement from abduction.

Hyperadduction *(Figure 6.19b)*

A backward movement of the thumb at right angles to the hand.

Extension *(Figure 6.19c)*

A lateral movement of the thumb away from the index finger, on a level with the palm.

Flexion *(Figure 6.19d)*

Return movement from extension.

Hyperflexion *(Figure 6.19e)*

A medially directed movement of the thumb from a position of slight abduction. The thumb slides across the front of the palm.

Circumduction

A movement in which the thumb as a whole describes a cone and the tip of the thumb describes a circle. It consists of all the movements just described, performed in sequence in either direction.

Opposition *(Figure 6.19f)*

This movement, which makes it possible to touch the tip of the thumb to the tip of any of the four fingers, is essentially a combination of abduction and hyperflexion and, according to some investigators, slight inward rotation. Others, including the authors, claim that what appears to be inward rotation of the metacarpal is actually a slight medial movement of the trapezium with which the metacarpal articulates. The movements of the metacarpal are accompanied by flexion of the two

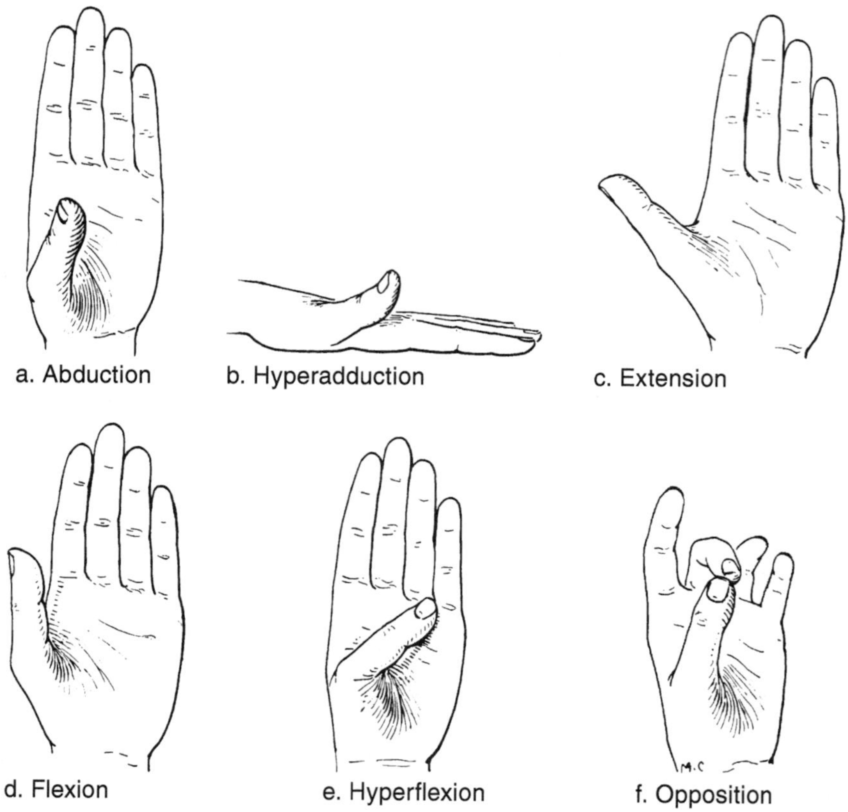

Figure 6.19 Movements of the thumb at the carpometacarpal joint.

phalanges, especially the distal. The apparent rotary movement is explained in part by the oblique axis of motion about which abduction and adduction of the thumb occur, and in part by the movement of the trapezium that accompanies flexion of the thumb. The total movement of the thumb in opposition might well be described as a movement of partial circumduction.

Movements of the Carpometacarpal and Intermetacarpal Joints of the Fingers

Largely because of the short ligaments in this region, especially in the case of the second, third, and fourth digits, the motion in both the carpometacarpal and intermetacarpal joints is almost nonexistent, being limited to slight gliding. The fifth carpometacarpal joint is slightly more mobile and permits a limited motion of the fifth metacarpal bone, resembling in small degree the motion of the thumb.

Structure of the Metacarpophalangeal Joints (Figures 6.13, 6.17, and 6.18)

The joint at the base of the four fingers, uniting the proximal phalanx with the corresponding metacarpal bone, is a condyloid (ovoid) joint. The oval, convex head of the metacarpal fits into the shallow oval fossa at the base of the phalanx. The fossa is deepened slightly by the fibrocartilaginous volar accessory ligament. The joint is encased in a capsule and is protected on each side by strong collateral ligaments.

The metacarpophalangeal joint of the thumb has flatter joint surfaces than do the corresponding joints of the four fingers and has more of the characteristics of a hinge joint. In addition to the articular capsule, it is protected by a collateral ligament on each side and by a dorsal ligament.

Movements of the Metacarpophalangeal Joints of the Four Fingers (Figure 6.20)

Flexion

The anterior surface of the finger approaches the palmar surface of the hand.

Extension

Return movement from flexion. Most individuals are able to achieve slight hyperextension in these joints.

Abduction

For the fourth, fifth, and index fingers this is a lateral movement away from the middle finger. This movement is limited and cannot be performed when the fingers are fully flexed.

Adduction

Return movement from abduction.

Note: In abduction and adduction of the fingers, a different point of reference is used than in abduction and adduction of the hand as a whole. The centerline of the hand—that is, the line passing through the middle finger when the latter is in its normal, extended position—is the reference line for the second, fourth, and fifth digits. Comparable movements of the middle finger are called radial and ulnar flexion.

These lateral finger movements are actually movements of the proximal phalanx, with the action occurring at the metacarpophalangeal joint, but the entire finger moves as a unit because no lateral action is possible at the interphalangeal joints.

Circumduction

The combination of flexion, abduction, extension, and adduction performed in sequence in either direction.

Movements of the Metacarpophalangeal Joints of the Thumb

Flexion

The volar surface of the thumb approaches that of the thenar eminence (base of thumb).

Extension

Return movement from flexion. Individuals vary greatly in their ability to hyperextend the thumb at this joint.

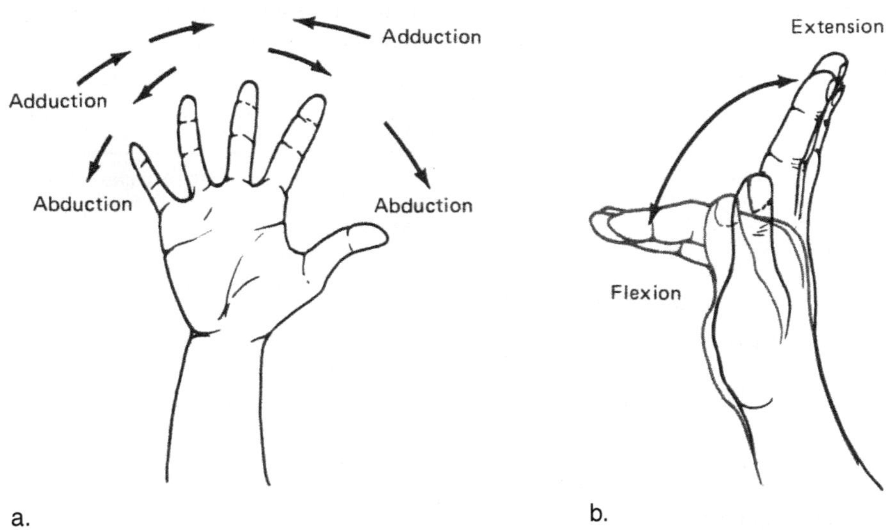

Figure 6.20 Movements of the metacarpophalangeal joints: (a) abduction and adduction; (b) flexion and extension.

The Interphalangeal Joints

These are the joints between the adjacent phalanges of any of the five digits. They are all hinge joints; hence, their only movements are flexion and extension. These correspond to flexion and extension of the first phalanx at the metacarpophalangeal joints. Hyperextension is slight, if present at all. Each joint is enclosed within an articular capsule, which is strengthened in front by an accessory volar ligament and on each side by a strong collateral ligament.

MUSCLES OF THE WRIST AND HAND

Location

The muscles of the wrist, fingers, and thumb are classified according to their location on the forearm or the hand and within each group are listed alphabetically (Table 6.1). Of the nineteen muscles of the fingers and thumb, ten are located entirely within the hand and are called intrinsic muscles. Those located outside the hand on the forearm but with tendon attachments on the thumb or fingers are extrinsic muscles.

The wrist flexor muscles originate (proximal attachments) on the medial epicondyle of the humerus or ulna; the wrist extensors have their proximal attachments on the lateral epicondyle of the humerus. These attachments allow these muscles to remain effective across the wrist joint regardless of the position of the forearm. They also contribute to stabilization of the elbow joint, which contributes further to enhancing effective action of these muscles at the wrist joint. The major disadvantage, as with most multijoint arrangements, is the limiting of the range of motion when there is simultaneous movement across all joints.

TABLE 6.1 Wrist and Hand Muscles

Muscles of the Wrist	
Anterior	**Posterior**
Flexor carpi radialis	Extensor carpi radialis brevis
Flexor carpi ulnaris	Extensor carpi radialis longus
Palmaris longus	Extensor carpi ulnaris
Muscles of the Fingers and Thumb	
On the Forearm (Extrinsic Muscles) (9)	**In the Hand (Intrinsic Muscles) (10)**
Fingers*	Fingers
Extensor digiti minimi	Abductor digiti minimi
Extensor digitorum	Flexor digiti minimi brevis
Extensor indicis	Interossei dorsales manus
Flexor digitorum profundus	Interossei palmaris
Flexor digitorum superficialis	Lumbricales manus
	Opponens digiti minimi
Thumb	Thumb
Abductor pollicis longus	Abductor pollicis brevis
Extensor pollicis brevis	Adductor pollicis
Extensor pollicis longus	Flexor pollicis brevis
Flexor pollicis longus	Opponens pollicis

*To understand the actions of these muscles, it is important to have an exact knowledge of their distal attachments.

Characteristics and Functions of Muscles

Wrist Muscles (Figures 6.21, 6.22, and 6.23a)

As one would expect from their location, the *flexor carpi radialis* and *flexor carpi ulnaris* are important flexors of the wrist. The palmaris longus, however, is a weak contributor to wrist flexion and is absent in a small part (6–25%) of the population. The flexor carpi radialis is also active in radial flexion (abduction) and the flexor carpi ulnaris in ulnar flexion. The tendons of these muscles may be readily palpated on the anterior surface of the wrist (see Figure 6.21). The palmaris longus tendon, if present, is clearly visible if the hand is flexed against slight resistance (see Figure 6.21). The ulnaris tendon (see Figure 6.21) is best identified by its relation to the pisiform bone. It should not be confused with the tendon lying close on the ulnar side of the palmaris tendon. This is a tendon of the flexor digitorum superficialis, probably the one for the fourth finger (Figure 6.24a).

Both *radial extensor* muscles of the wrist are active in extension and radial flexion (abduction), with the *extensor carpi radialis brevis* more active in extension than the *extensor carpi radialis*

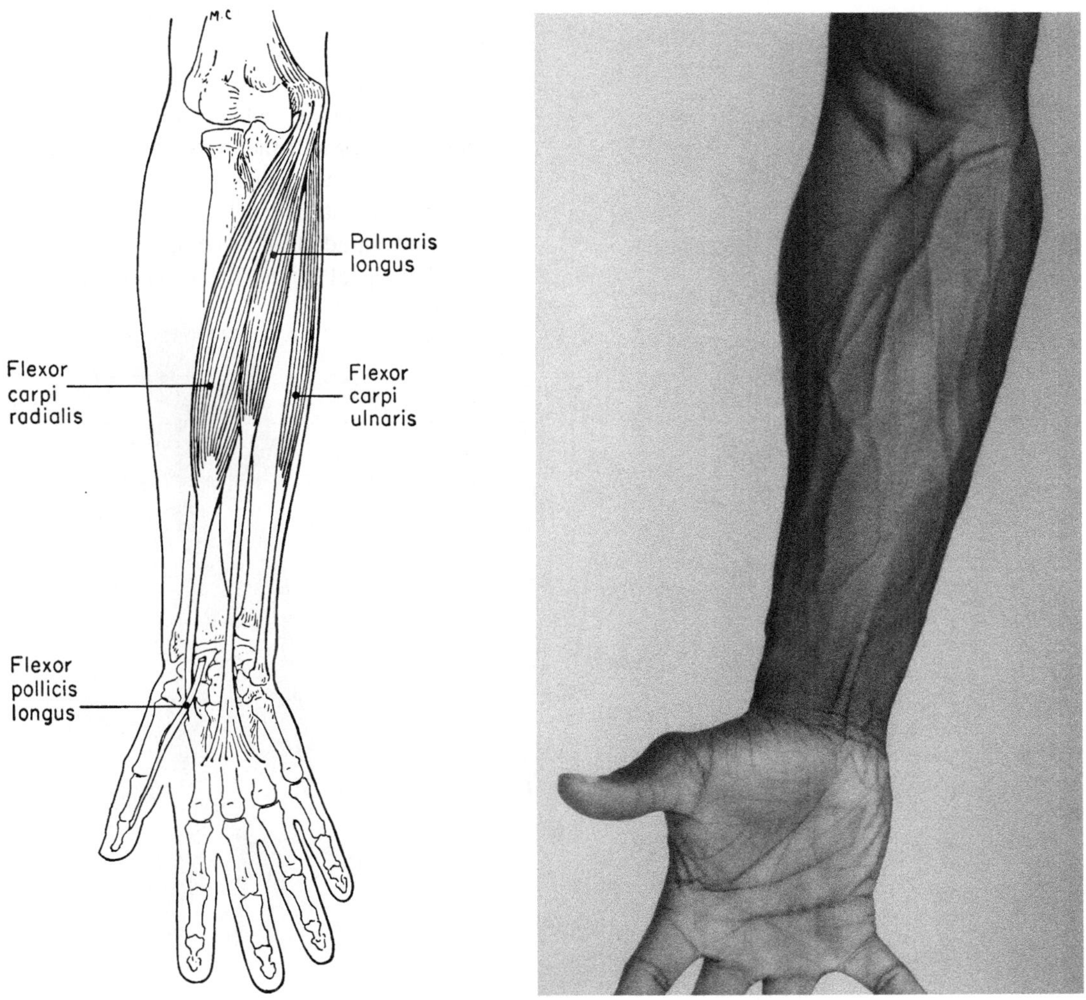

Figure 6.21 Superficial muscles on front of right forearm.

longus. The *extensor carpi ulnaris* works cooperatively with the extensor carpi radialis muscles in wrist extension and participates in ulnar flexion (adduction; see Figure 6.23).

The three *wrist extensor muscles* may be palpated on the dorsal surface of the forearm when the forearm and hand are resting palm down on a table, the *carpi radialis longus* on the radial side at elbow level and slightly below, the *brevis* slightly below the *longus,* and the *carpi ulnaris* on the ulnar margin of the dorsal surface about midway between the elbow and wrist. The tendon of the carpi radialis longus may be palpated on the dorsal surface of the wrist in line with the index finger.

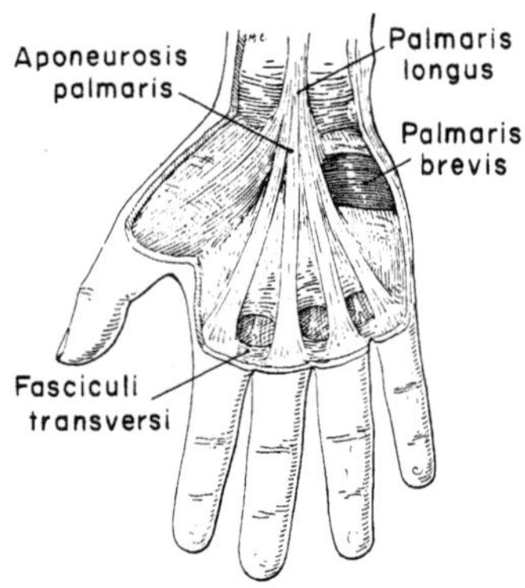

Figure 6.22 Palmar aponeurosis and palmaris muscles of right palm.

The *flexor carpi radialis* and *extensor carpi radialis longus,* together with the *abductor pollicis longus* of the thumb, team up to produce *radial flexion (abduction)* of the wrist. The *extensor* and *flexor carpi ulnaris* muscles team up similarly to produce *ulnar flexion (adduction).*

Muscles of the Fingers and Thumb

(Figures 6.22 through 6.29)

In most instances, the names of the muscles of the fingers and thumb indicate their chief function. These muscles will therefore not be discussed individually. Some of these muscles, however, have important additional roles, and these should be identified. In addition to being an extensor of the interphalangeal joints, the *extensor digitorum* is

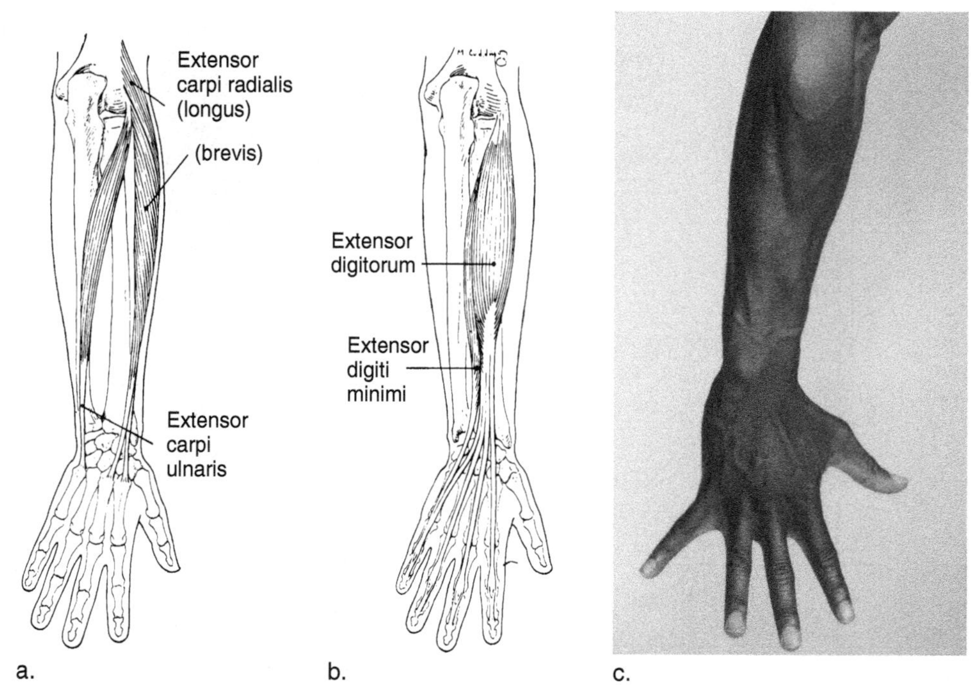

Figure 6.23 Muscles on back of right forearm: (a) extensor carpi radialis longus and brevis and extensor carpi ulnaris; (b) extensor digitorum and extensor digiti minimi.

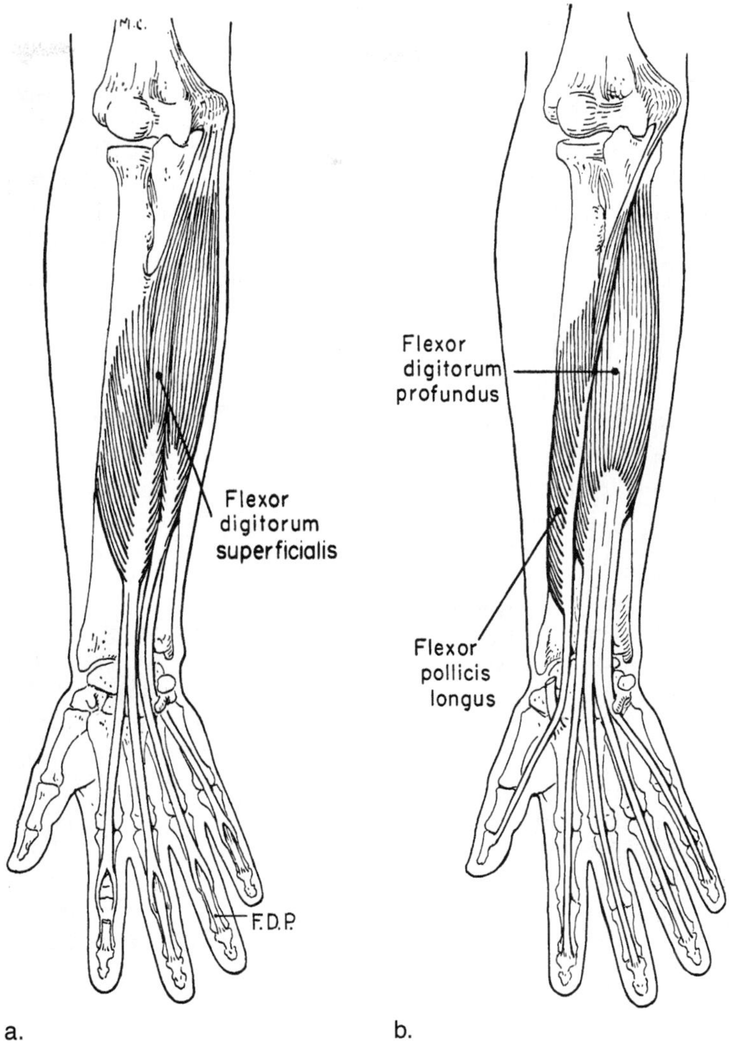

Figure 6.24 Deep muscles on front of right forearm: (a) flexor digitorum superficialis; (b) flexor digitorum profundus and flexor pollicis longus. (F.D.P. = Flexor digitorum profundus.)

an important wrist extensor. Similarly, the *flexor digitorum superficialis* is active in wrist flexion as well as in flexion at the proximal phalangeal joints. The *abductor pollicis longus* both abducts and flexes the metacarpophalangeal joint of the thumb, and the *abductor pollicis brevis,* together with the *opponens pollicis,* is active in extension and abduction of the thumb. Both the *flexor* and *extensor pollicis longus* are active in adduction and opposition of the thumb, and the *adductor pollicis* participates in opposition and flexion.

Muscular Analysis of the Fundamental Movements of the Wrist, Fingers, and Thumb

The Wrist

Fundamental movements of the wrist are movements of the hand as a unit. They occur chiefly at the radiocarpal joint but involve the midcarpal and intercarpal joints when flexion or hyperextension is carried to the limit of motion.

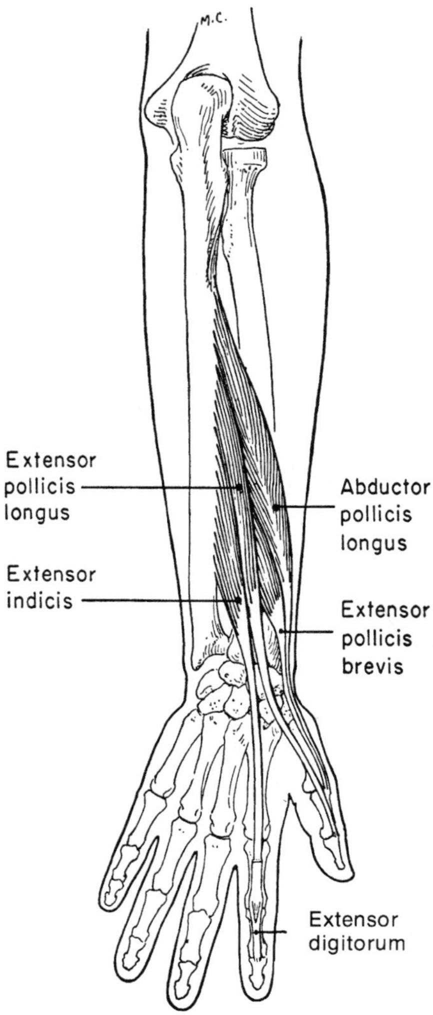

Figure 6.25 Posterior muscles of thumb and index finger.

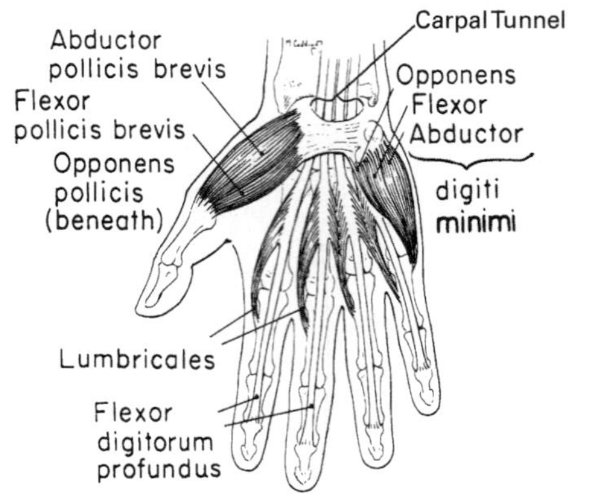

Figure 6.26 Anterior view of muscles of right hand.

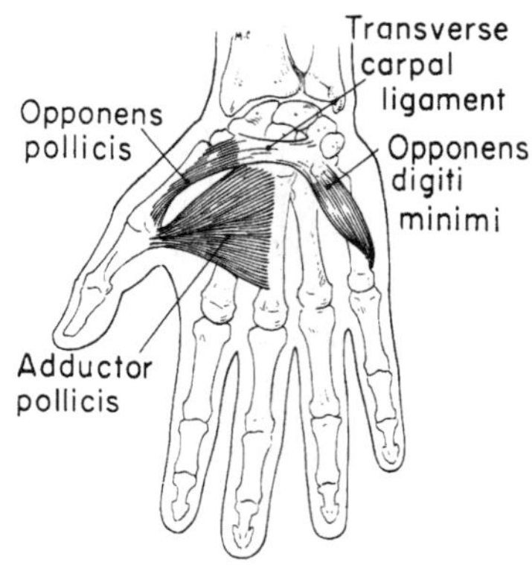

Figure 6.27 Deep muscles of thumb and fifth metacarpal.

Flexion

Performed by the flexors carpi radialis, carpi ulnaris, and digitorum superficialis, with possible help from the palmaris longus, flexor pollicis longus, and flexor digitorum profundus.

Extension and Hyperextension

Performed synchronously by the extensors carpi radialis longus, carpi radialis brevis, carpi ulnaris, and extensor digitorum, with possible help from the pollicis longus and extensors indicis and digiti minimi.

Radial Flexion (Abduction)

Performed by the extensors carpi radialis longus and brevis and flexor carpi radialis, with possible help from the abductor pollicis longus and the extensors pollicis longus and brevis.

Ulnar Flexion (Adduction)

Performed by the extensor carpi ulnaris and the flexor carpi ulnaris.

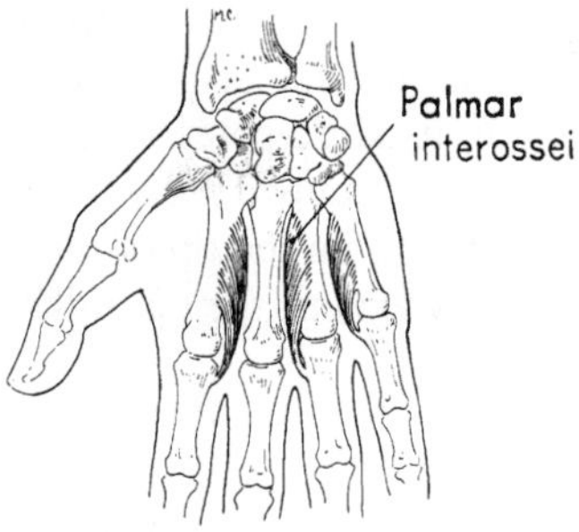

Figure 6.28 Palmar interossei, right hand.

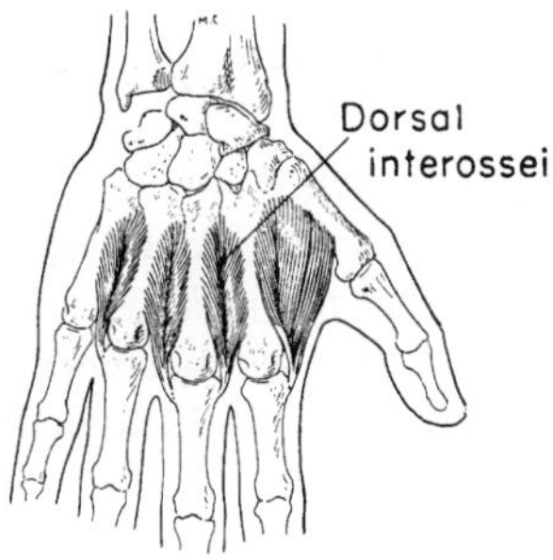

Figure 6.29 Dorsal interossei, right hand.

The Fingers

For a better understanding of all the actions of the finger and thumb muscles, they should be studied both on the skeleton (using elastic bands to represent muscles) and on another person. Particular attention should be paid to the relation of each muscle to every joint it crosses, to the muscle's line of pull, and to the leverage involved.

As an aid to recognizing the secondary actions of the muscles, a record of all the joints crossed by all the finger and thumb muscles is included here.

Forearm Muscles of the Fingers

All five of these muscles cross four sets of joints: wrist, carpometacarpal, metacarpophalangeal, and proximal interphalangeal. The extensor digitorum and extensor digiti minimi also cross both the elbow and the distal interphalangeal joint, making a total of six joints crossed. The flexor digitorum superficialis crosses the elbow but not the distal interphalangeal joint, and both the extensor indicis and flexor digitorum profundus cross the distal interphalangeal joint but not the elbow.

Intrinsic Muscles of the Fingers

Of these six muscles, only the abductor digiti minimi and flexor digiti minimi brevis cross both the carpometacarpal and the metacarpophalangeal joints. The two interossei muscles, dorsales and palmaris, and the lumbricales cross only the metacarpophalangeal joint. The opponens digiti minimi, like the opponens pollicis, crosses only the carpometacarpal joint. The two work together in the cupping action of the palm as well as independently in other opposition movements.

Forearm Muscles of the Thumb

All four of these muscles cross both the wrist and carpometacarpal joints, and all but the abductor pollicis longus also cross the metacarpophalangeal joint. The extensor and flexor pollicis longus muscles cross the interphalangeal joint as well. The thumb, of course, has no second interphalangeal joint.

Intrinsic Muscles of the Thumb

All four of these muscles cross the carpometacarpal joint, and all but the opponens pollicis cross the metacarpophalangeal joint.

The muscular action of the fingers is given in terms of the movement of each phalanx. Movement of the proximal phalanx occurs at the metacarpophalangeal joint, of the middle phalanx at the proximal interphalangeal joint, and of the distal phalanx at the distal interphalangeal joint. For convenience in referring to individual fingers, numbers are assigned as follows: 2 for the index finger, 3 for the middle finger, 4 for the ring finger, and 5 for the little finger.

Flexion

Proximal phalanx Flexed by the lumbricales manus (all fingers), interossei palmaris (palmar interossei; 2,4,5), interossei dorsales manus (2,3,4), flexor digiti minimi brevis (5), and opponens digiti minimi (5), with possible help from the flexors digitorum superficialis and profundus.

Middle phalanx Flexed by the flexor digitorum superficialis, which acts on all four fingers and at the same time contributes to flexion of the metacarpal bones.

Distal phalanx Flexed by the flexor digitorum profundus, which also acts on all four fingers and at the same time contributes to flexion of the proximal and middle phalanges.

Extension

Proximal phalanx Extended by the extensor digitorum (all fingers), extensor indicis (2), and extensor digiti minimi (5). The extensor digitorum is also able to help extend the middle and distal phalanges.

Middle and distal phalanges Extended by the lumbricales manus (all fingers) and interossei dorsales manus (dorsal interossei; 2,3,4). The abductor digiti minimi (5) and the extensor digitorum (all fingers) are also able to help extend the middle and distal phalanges at the same time that they are extending the proximal phalanx.

Note: When all the fingers flex or extend, the antagonists relax in reciprocal innervation. However, if a single finger moves, the antagonists will contract in an attempt to keep the other fingers still.

Abduction and Adduction

Abduction is brought about by the interossei dorsales manus (2,4) and abductor digiti minimi (5), and adduction by the interossei palmaris (2,4,5).

Radial and ulnar flexion of the middle finger is performed by the interossei dorsales manus (3).

Opposition

The fifth digit, or little finger, being at the outer margin of the hand, has greater freedom of movement than do the other fingers. Through the action of the opponens digiti minimi, the metacarpal bone of this finger can engage in a slight degree of opposition at the carpi metacarpal joint. Together with the thumb, it participates in this movement when the hand is "cupped," as when scooping up water, and also when the tip of the little finger is brought forcibly against the tip of the thumb.

The Thumb

The muscular action of the thumb is given in terms of the movements of the metacarpal bone and the two phalanges, proximal and distal.

The Thumb Metacarpal

Flexion

The metacarpal is flexed and hyperflexed after being slightly abducted by the flexor pollicis brevis and the adductor pollicis. The flexor pollicis longus also participates and becomes more dominant when the action is full flexion (Basmajian & DeLuca, 1985).

Extension

Performed chiefly by the abductor pollicis longus, with help from the opponens pollicis, the abductor pollicis brevis, and the extensors pollicis longus and brevis.

Abduction

Four muscles are responsible for this movement, two from the forearm, the abductor pollicis longus and the extensor pollicis brevis, and two from the thenar eminence, the abductor pollicis brevis and the opponens pollicis. Under some conditions these may be helped by the flexor pollicis brevis.

Adduction

This movement is performed mainly by the adductor pollicis, with some help from the flexor pollicis brevis and, in certain positions, from the extensor pollicis longus.

Opposition

This action is performed mainly by the opponens, but with appreciable help from the flexor pollicis brevis. As opposition is not a single, well-defined movement but varies according to the finger that is being opposed and to the exact position of that finger, the muscles controlling the thumb must adapt to the demands of the situation. This includes the action of the phalanges as well as that of the metacarpal.

The Thumb Phalanges

Flexion

The flexor pollicis longus flexes both of the phalanges. Additional flexors of the proximal phalanx include the flexor pollicis brevis and the adductor pollicis, with help from the abductor pollicis brevis when necessary.

Extension

The extensor pollicis longus extends both of the phalanges. This is joined by the brevis in the extension of the proximal phalanx.

The plane in which flexion and extension of the thumb phalanges occurs is determined by the position of the metacarpal bone of the thumb.

Cooperative Actions of the Wrist and Digits

Length of Long Finger Muscles Relative to Range of Motion in Wrist and Fingers

An interesting characteristic of the long finger muscles is that they do not have sufficient length to permit the full range of motion in the joints of the fingers and wrist at the same time. For instance, one cannot achieve complete flexion of the fingers and wrist simultaneously, because the extensor digitorum will not elongate enough to permit it. If maximum *finger* flexion is maintained, the wrist is able to flex only slightly. Similarly, if maximum *wrist* flexion is maintained, it will be impossible to achieve a real grip with the fingers. They flex incompletely and without appreciable force. Or, if one makes a tight fist and then determines to flex the wrist completely, the individual will soon discover that the fingers loosen their grip and tend to open up in spite of efforts to prevent it. This is not caused by contraction of the finger extensors but by their inability to elongate sufficiently, due to the countercurrent nature of the muscle action of the multiarticular muscles, as discussed in Chapter 3.

The same type of reaction occurs if one attempts to achieve maximum extension of the fingers when the wrist is fully hyperextended. This involuntary movement due to the tension of opposing muscles is known as the tendon or pulley action of multijoint muscles. Because of this arrangement of the muscles, the strongest finger flexion can be obtained when the wrist is held rigid in either a straight or slightly hyperextended position, and the strongest finger extension when the wrist is rigid in either a straight or slightly flexed position. The most powerful wrist action—either flexion or hyperextension—can occur only when the fingers are relaxed. In other words, strong finger action requires a rigid wrist; strong wrist action requires relaxed fingers.

Using the Hands for Grasping

Grasping, or prehension, is a fairly complex act that is used more frequently than almost any other human motion. Reaching for a thrown ball, grasping a badminton racquet, moving a computer mouse, or gripping a door key all combine action of the hand, wrist, and forearm, often with involvement of the shoulder as well. To produce a grasping motion, one must first position the hand in space, often through arm motion. The hand must then be shaped for the task by moving the thumb and fingers. The hand and fingers are then moved into position around the object. Finally, the fingers close and grasp the object.

The nature of the grasp (or grip) pattern is determined by both the object to be handled and by the objective of the handling. Grasps are often divided into the major categories of power grip and precision grip. A power grip involves flexion of all the fingers. The thumb may participate in the grip, or it may simply stabilize the hand or the object. There are three basic classifications of the power grip: (1) cylindrical (Figure 6.30d), (2) spherical (Figure 6.30e and g), and (3) hook (Figure 6.30h).

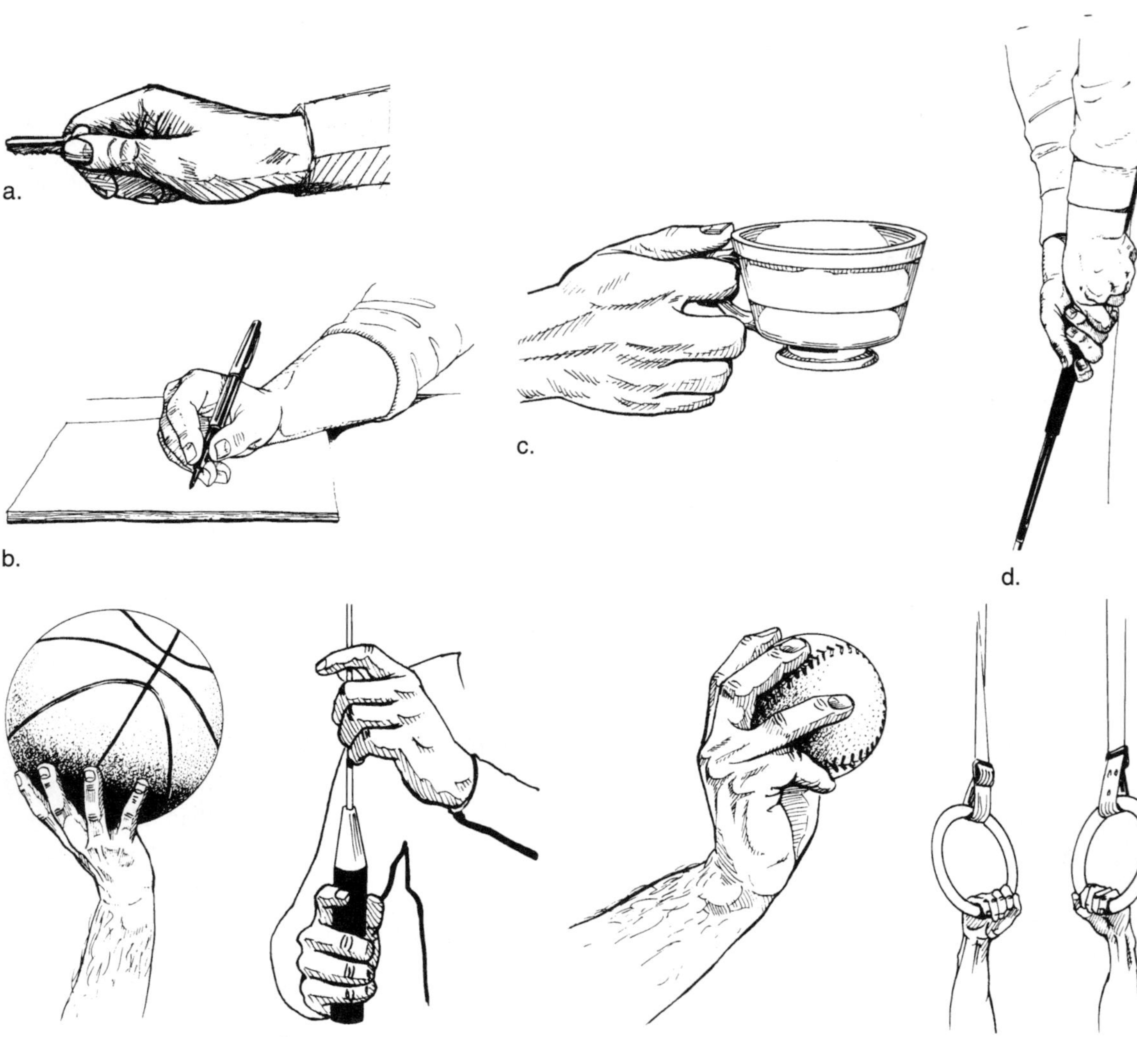

Figure 6.30 Examples of grasps. The muscular involvement depends on the nature of the grasp.

Ulnar deviation of the wrist enhances the force of the cylindrical grip. The spherical grip is similar to the cylindrical grip but with a greater spread of the fingers. The hook grip excludes use of the thumb but sometimes includes use of the palm. Therefore, the hook grip is sometimes categorized as precision handling.

Precision handling involves the use of the thumb and one or two fingers in various positions in order to accommodate a multiplicity of grasping functions. It entails great variability in pressure and fine motor control to manipulate efficiently the various objects (Figure 6.30a–c).

The muscular involvement also depends on the nature of the grasp. A complex interplay occurs between the extrinsic and intrinsic muscular involvement, which varies with the force and spread of the grasp. Generally speaking, the extrinsic rather than the intrinsic muscles appear to be the major force for compression actions, power gripping, and the gross movements associated with precision gripping. The intrinsic muscles are of greater significance in the refinements of precision movements and the adduction actions that are part of these movements. The wrist extensors are also active during grasping motions, because they stabilize the wrist against the flexion tendencies of those finger flexors that cross the front of the wrist joint (Basmajian & DeLuca, 1985).

In sports and gymnastics there is probably less concern with the fine, precise movements of the fingers and thumb than with the grosser movements such as the grasping of balls, striking implements, and suspension apparatus. In general, grasping activities involve flexion of the fingers (usually all three joints), opposition of the thumb metacarpal, and flexion of the phalanges. The degrees of these movements, together with the degree of abduction that may be present in the fingers, depend on the shape and size of the object being grasped, as well as on the purpose of the movement (Figure 6.30).

In sport, whether pitching, throwing for distance, or tossing a ball straight upward, the movements of the forearm and hand are of prime importance. The greater the force desired for moving the ball, the greater the contribution of the upper arm, but because this discussion applies only to the forearm and hand, the upper arm is not considered here. Ignoring the finer movements, the essential action of the forearm in both overhand pitching and in throwing for distance is extension; of the wrist, "flexion" from the hyperextended to the extended position (with an abrupt check of the motion when the wrist is straight); and of the fingers, extension.

In a vertical toss, starting with the forearm forward at a slight downward slant—that is, with the elbow at a slightly obtuse angle—the movements are elbow flexion followed by finger extension and wrist flexion from the hyperextended position. The active muscles are mainly the elbow flexors, the wrist flexors in static contraction, and the finger extensors. The reader may find it of interest to analyze the joint and muscle actions in other kinds of throws.

Common Injuries of the Forearm, Elbow, Wrist, and Fingers

Fractures of the Forearm

These are common among children, teenagers, and the elderly and are usually caused either by a direct blow or by falling on a rigidly outstretched arm. It is more usual for both the radius and ulna to break than for either one to break alone, and in the younger age group the fracture of either or both bones is likely to be of the greenstick type.

It is important to immobilize the elbow joint in the treatment of a fractured radius, even though the fracture is close to the wrist. This is because in pronation and supination, as the radial head rotates against both the capitulum of the humerus and the radial notch of the ulna, the broad distal end swings halfway around the ulna. The need for immobilizing the elbow joint in the event of a radial fracture should be apparent to anyone who is conversant with kinesiology.

Elbow Dislocation and Fracture

The majority of these dislocations consist of the backward displacement of the ulna and radius in relation to the humerus. The most common cause is catching oneself from a fall by taking the weight on the outstretched hand with the elbow in rigid extension or hyperextension. This can be a very serious injury because it is likely to involve blood vessels and nerves.

Elbow dislocations are frequently accompanied by fractures, the most common being a fracture of the medial epicondyle, especially in the middle- to late-adolescent age group in those whose epicondylar epiphyses have not yet closed. These dislocations often occur because of repeated forceful acts such as pitching or serving in tennis.

Sprained or Strained Wrist

This type of wrist injury is very common and, like so many of the other upper extremity injuries, is caused by catching oneself from a fall by thrusting the arm downward and taking the weight on the palm with the hand hyperextended at the wrist and the elbow rigidly extended. Although the injury is usually called a sprain, it is often a strain, because the site of the trouble may be at the tendon attachments rather than at the attachments of the anterior ligaments (Arnheim & Prentice, 1998). It may also involve fracture of a carpal bone.

Carpal Tunnel Syndrome

In the wrist, the carpal arch and transverse carpal ligament form the carpal tunnel through which the finger flexors and median nerve pass (Figure 6.26). Overuse may result in pain caused by nerve compression and numbing of the fingers caused by blood vessel involvement. Carpal tunnel syndrome is a classic example of a repetitive stress injury (RSI). Such injuries are becoming more common as more people spend longer hours working with small hand tools and keyboards. This condition is often treated with rest followed by support and intermittent use. Extreme or very painful conditions may require surgery.

Avulsion Fracture

An avulsion fracture occurs when an external force applied to a tendon pulls off the bit of bone to which it is attached. It occurs at the weakest link in the structure. Avulsion fractures of the forearm and hand are often the result of high stress on the tendon, frequently from very rapid pronation or supination actions in the radioulnar joints or high-energy flexion of the fingers. The probability of occurrence is greatest in youth at the epiphyseal plates, and in the elderly because of osteoporosis.

Epicondylitis

Lateral epicondylitis ("tennis elbow") and medial epicondylitis ("golfer's elbow") are further examples of repetitive stress injuries. Although the term *epicondylitis* implies an inflammatory condition, most such injuries are actually microtraumas or tears in the muscle and soft tissue in the region of the proximal attachment sites of the flexor (medial) or extensor (lateral) muscles of the wrist. The valgus load on the elbow during the overhand throwing motion in pitching puts high-energy stress on the medial side of the elbow and is a leading cause of medial epicondylitis in throwing athletes. In extreme cases medial epicondylitis may be accompanied by an avulsion fracture (Grana, 2001). Rest, ice, anti-inflammatory drugs, and cortizone injections are often prescribed for these conditions. In some cases, pain can be reduced through surgery or counterforce bracing (Field & Savoie, 1998; Whiting & Zernicke, 1998).

REFERENCES AND SELECTED READINGS

Alcid, J. G., Ahmad, C. S., & Lee, T. Q. (2004). Elbow anatomy and structural biomechanics. *Clinics in Sports Medicine,* 23(4), 503–517.

Arnheim, D. D., & Prentice, W. W. (1998). *Essentials of athletic training* (4th ed.). St. Louis, MO: McGraw-Hill.

Basmajian, J. V., & Deluca, C. J. (1985). *Muscles alive* (5th ed.). Baltimore: Williams & Wilkins.

Bryce, C. D., & Armstrong, A. D. (2008). Anatomy and biomechanics of the elbow. *Orthopedic Clinics of North America,* 39(2), 141–154.

Field, L. D., & Savoie, F. H. (1998). Common elbow injuries in sport. *Sports Medicine,* 26(3), 193–205.

Grana, W. (2001). Medial epicondylitis and cubital tunnel syndrome. *Clinics in Sports Medicine,* 20(3), 541–548.

Haugstvedt, J. R., Berger, R. A., & Berglund, L. J. (2001). A mechanical study of the moment-forces of the supinators and pronators of the forearm. *Acta Orthopaedica Scandinavica,* 72(6), 629–634.

Lockard, M. 2008. Clinical biomechanics of the elbow. *Journal of Hand Therapy,* 19(2), 72–80.

Loftice, J., Fleisig, G. S., Zheng, N., & Andrews, J. R. (2004). Biomechanics of the elbow in sports. *Clinics in Sports Medicine,* 23(4), 519–530.

Mair, S. D., Uhl, T. L., Robbe, R. G., & Brindle, K. A. (2004). Physical changes and range-of-motion differences in the dominant shoulders of skeletally immature baseball players. *Journal of Shoulder and Elbow Surgery,* 13(5), 487–491.

Murray, W. M., Buchanan, T. S., & Delp, S. L. (2000). The isometric functional capacity of muscles that cross the elbow. *Journal of Biomechanics,* 33(8), 943–952.

Peters, T., & Baker, C. L. (2001). Lateral epicondylitis. *Clinics in Sports Medicine,* 20(3), 549–564.

Schweizer, A., Frank, O., Ochsner, P. E., & Jacob, H. A. (2003). Friction between human finger flexor tendons and pulleys at high loads. *Journal of Biomechanics,* 36(1), 63–71.

Sebastin, S. J., Puhaindran, M. E., Lim, A. Y., Lim, I. J., & Bee, W. H. (2005). The prevalence or absence of the palmaris longus—a study in a Chinese population and a review of the literature. *Journal of Hand Surgery* [European Volume], 30(5), 525–527.

Terada, N., Yamada, H., & Toyama, Y. (2004). The appearance of the lateral ulnar collateral ligament on magnetic resonance imaging. *Journal of Shoulder and Elbow Surgery,* 13(2), 214–216.

Thompson, N. W., Mockford, B. J., & Cran, G. W. (2001). Absence of the palmaris longus muscle: A population study. *Ulster Medical Journal,* 70(1), 22–24.

Van Roy, P., Baeyens, J. P., Fauvart, D., Lanssiers, R., & Clarijs, J. P. (2005). Arthro-kinematics of the elbow: Study of the carrying angle. *Ergonomics,* 48, 1645–1656.

Whiting, W. C., & Zernicke, R. F. (1998). *Biomechanics of musculoskeletal injury.* Champaign, IL: Human Kinetics.

Yilmaz, E., Karakurt, L., Belhan, O., Bulut, M., Serin, E., & Avci, M. (2005). Variation of carrying angle with age, sex, and special reference to side. *Orthopedics, 28*(11), 1360–1363.

Laboratory Experiences

Elbow and Forearm: Joint Structure and Function

1. Record the essential information regarding the structure, ligaments, and cartilages of the two articulations of the elbow joint and, likewise, the two radioulnar articulations. Study the movements of these joints both on the skeleton and on the living body, and explain how their structure facilitates or inhibits movement.
2. Using a protractor or goniometer, measure the range of motion on five subjects for the following movements: flexion, pronation, and supination of the forearm.
3. Repeat Experience 22 from Chapter 5, this time writing the joint analysis of (a) the starting position of the forearm at the elbow and radioulnar joints, and (b) the movement from the starting position to the final pull-up position. Discuss with partner.
4. Assume a handshaking grasp with a skeleton with the elbow flexed and the forearm approximately horizontal. Slowly pronate your forearm and note the movement of the skeleton's forearm. Observe carefully each end of the radius and ulna and describe what happens. Now supinate your forearm as far as possible and carefully observe the radioulnar movements of the skeleton. Note the way the edge of the radial head rotates against the notch of the ulna and the way the superior surface of the radial head revolves against the capitulum of the humerus. At the distal end, note the way the broad articular process of the radius swings around the head of the ulna and the radial shaft crosses over that of the ulna. Note that the ulna itself does not rotate, although it may appear to do so when the elbow is fixed in extension and pronation of the forearm occurs in conjunction with inward rotation of the humerus.

Elbow and Forearm: Muscular Action

Record the results using a format similar to that found in Table 1.2.

5. **Flexion**

   Subject: Sit with the entire arm resting on a table. Flex the forearm (a) with palm up (forearm supinated), (b) with thumb up (forearm in neutral position), and (c) with palm down (forearm pronated).

   Assistant: Resist the movement by holding the wrist. Steady the upper arm if necessary.

Observer: Palpate as many of the forearm flexors as possible. Do you notice any difference in the muscular action in a, b, and c?

6. **Extension**
   a. *Subject:* Lie facedown on a table with one arm raised to shoulder level with the upper arm resting on the table, the forearm hanging down. Extend the forearm without moving the upper arm.
   Assistant: Steady the upper arm and resist the forearm at the wrist.
   Observer: Palpate the triceps and anconeus.
   b. *Subject:* On hands and knees, flex and extend the arms at the elbows in a push-up exercise.
   Observer: Palpate the triceps and anconeus.
7. **Supination**
   Subject: Assume a handshaking position with the assistant and supinate the forearm.
   Assistant: Assume the same position with the subject and resist the movement.
   Observer: Palpate and identify the muscles that contract.
8. **Pronation**
   Subject: Assume a handshaking position with the assistant and pronate the forearm.
   Assistant: Assume the same position with the subject and resist the movement.
   Observer: Palpate and identify the muscles that contract. What is their function? Can you palpate the principal movers?

Action of Muscles Other Than Movers

9. **Supination Without Flexion**
   Subject: Sit with the arm supported, elbow in a slightly flexed position and relaxed. Supinate the forearm without increasing or decreasing flexion at the elbow.
   Observer: Palpate the triceps. Explain.
10. **Vigorous Flexion of Forearm**
    Subject: Flex forearm vigorously, then check the movement suddenly before completing the full range of motion.
    Observer: Palpate the triceps. Does it contract during any part of the movement? Explain.
11. Perform a movement in which the supinator acts as a neutralizer.

Elbow and Forearm: Applications

12. Working with a partner, execute a knee push-up; that is, a push-up from the front lying position, onto the knees instead of the toes, until the elbows are fully extended. Keep the body straight from the knees to the top of the head. Return to the starting position slowly and in good form.
    a. Analyze the joint and muscular action of the elbows in the push-up.
    b. Do the same for the return movement.
    c. What force is responsible for the movement in a? In b?
    d. What is the chief difference in the type of muscular action used in the push-up and in the letdown (return movement)? (See pp. 50–52.)
13. In reading the section on common injuries it may have been noted that several injuries to the forearm, elbow, and wrist are caused by taking the weight on the outstretched hand with the elbow rigidly extended when catching oneself from a fall. The following exercise is designed to accustom one to the practice of giving at the elbow and other upper extremity joints at the moment the hand strikes the ground. If practiced frequently, this technique should become a habit.
    Kneel on a gymnasium mat with the knees slightly separated, hips in extension, and body erect. Shift your weight to the side until you lose your balance and fall to a side sitting position with your arm outstretched and your hand reaching to catch your weight. At the moment of contact let your elbow give (i.e., flex) and, if the force is sufficient, roll onto your shoulder and back with knees drawn up. Practice this many times, both to right and left. Experiment with variations.

Wrist and Hand: Joint Structure and Function

14. Record the essential information regarding the structure, ligaments, and cartilages of the radiocarpal, carpometacarpal, metacarpophalangeal, and interphalangeal articulations. Study the movements both on the skeleton and on the living body, and explain how the joint structure affects functions. Pay particular attention to the carpometacarpal joint of the thumb.
15. With a protractor or goniometer, measure the amount of hyperextension possible at the wrist (a) with the fingers flexed, (b) with fingers extended. Likewise measure the amount of flexion possible at the wrist (a) with fingers flexed, (b) with fingers extended. Explain.

Wrist and Hand: Muscular Action

(See procedures for anatomical analysis of movements in Chapter 1.) If possible, get someone who plays the piano to serve as a subject.

16. **Flexion at Wrist**
    Subject: Sit with forearm resting on a table with palm up. Flex hand at wrist.
    Assistant: Resist movement by holding palm.
    Observer: Palpate, identify, and explain the action of as many muscles as possible.
17. **Extension and Hyperextension at Wrist**
    Subject: Sit with forearm resting on a table with palm down. Extend hand at wrist.
    Assistant: Resist movement by holding back of hand.
    Observer: Palpate, identify, and explain the action of as many muscles as possible.
18. **Radial Flexion at Wrist**
    Subject: Sit with forearm resting on a table, ulnar side (little finger side of hand) down. Keeping thumb against hand, raise hand from table without moving forearm.
    Assistant: May give slight resistance to hand.
    Observer: Palpate and identify the muscles responsible for radial flexion.
19. **Ulnar Flexion at Wrist**
    Subject: Lie facedown or bend forward in such a way that radial side of hand (thumb side) is on supporting surface, with forearm supported and wrist neither flexed nor hyperextended. Keeping little finger against hand, raise hand without moving forearm.
    Assistant: May give slight resistance to hand.
    Observer: Palpate and identify the muscles responsible for ulnar flexion.
20. **Finger Flexion**
    Subject: Sit with forearm resting on a table with palm up. Flex fingers without flexing wrist.
    Assistant: Resist movement by hooking own fingers over those of subject.
    Observer: Palpate, identify, and explain the action of as many muscles as possible.
21. **Finger Extension**
    Subject: Sit with forearm resting on a table with palm down, fingers curled over edge of table. Extend fingers.
    Assistant: Resist movement by holding hand over subject's fingers.
    Observer: Palpate, identify, and explain the action of as many muscles as possible.
22. **Abduction of Thumb**
    Subject: Place the hand on a table with the palm up and the thumb slightly separated from the index finger. Abduct the thumb at the carpometacarpal joint by raising it vertically upward.
    Assistant: Give slight resistance to the thumb at the proximal phalanx.
    Observer: Palpate the abductor pollicis brevis in the thenar eminence.
23. **Hyperflexion of Thumb in Position of Slight Abduction**
    Subject: Place the hand on a table with the palm up and the thumb slightly raised from the table. Hyperflex the thumb at the carpometacarpal joint.
    Assistant: Give slight resistance to the proximal phalanx of the thumb.
    Observer: Palpate the flexor pollicis brevis in the thenar eminence.
24. **Extension of Thumb**
    Subject: Rest the fully extended hand on its ulnar border with the thumb uppermost. Extend the thumb as far as possible.
    Observer: Identify the tendons of the abductor pollicis longus, extensor pollicis longus, and extensor pollicis brevis.
25. **Opposition of Thumb**
    Subject: Press the thumb hard against the tip of the middle finger.
    Observer: Palpate and identify the opponens pollicis and adductor pollicis.

Action of Muscles Other Than Movers

26. Perform a movement in which the extensor carpi ulnaris and extensor carpi radialis longus and brevis act as neutralizers to prevent flexion at the wrist.
27. Perform a movement in which the extensor carpi ulnaris and flexor carpi ulnaris act as mutual neutralizers.

Hands: Application

28. Inspect the various styles of grasping sport objects in Figure 6.30 and analyze a few of these. First identify the joint position of the wrist, fingers, and thumb, and then determine the chief muscular involvement.

Kinesiological Analysis

29. Choose a simple motor skill from Appendix G. Do a complete anatomical analysis of the elbow, forearm, wrist, and hand, following the analysis outline in Tables 1.1 and 1.2.

CHAPTER

7

THE LOWER EXTREMITY

The Hip Region

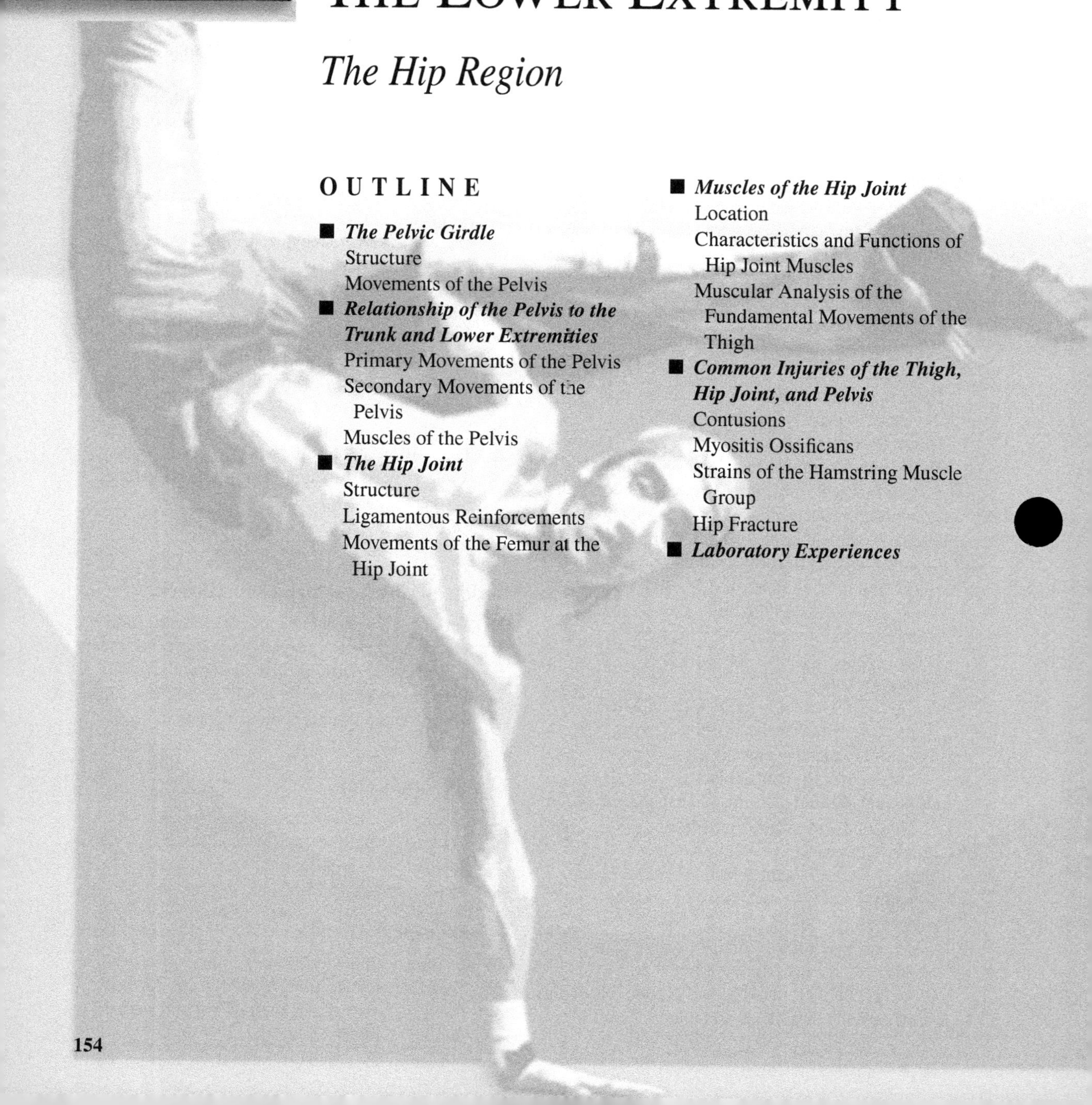

OUTLINE

- ***The Pelvic Girdle***
  - Structure
  - Movements of the Pelvis
- ***Relationship of the Pelvis to the Trunk and Lower Extremities***
  - Primary Movements of the Pelvis
  - Secondary Movements of the Pelvis
  - Muscles of the Pelvis
- ***The Hip Joint***
  - Structure
  - Ligamentous Reinforcements
  - Movements of the Femur at the Hip Joint
- ***Muscles of the Hip Joint***
  - Location
  - Characteristics and Functions of Hip Joint Muscles
  - Muscular Analysis of the Fundamental Movements of the Thigh
- ***Common Injuries of the Thigh, Hip Joint, and Pelvis***
  - Contusions
  - Myositis Ossificans
  - Strains of the Hamstring Muscle Group
  - Hip Fracture
- ***Laboratory Experiences***

OBJECTIVES

At the conclusion of this chapter, the student should be able to:

1. Name, locate, and describe the structure and ligamentous reinforcements of the articulations of the pelvic girdle and hip joint.
2. Name and demonstrate the movements possible in the pelvic girdle and hip joint, regardless of starting position.
3. Name and locate the muscles and muscle groups of the pelvis and hip, and name their primary actions as agonists, stabilizers, neutralizers, or antagonists.
4. Analyze the fundamental movements of the pelvis and thigh with respect to joint and muscle actions.
4. Describe the common athletic injuries of the pelvis, hip, and thigh.
5. Perform an anatomical analysis of the hip region in a motor skill.

The relationship between the pelvic girdle and hip is somewhat similar to that between the shoulder girdle and shoulder joint. Just as the scapula tilts or rotates to put the glenoid fossa in a favorable position for the movements of the humerus, so does the pelvic girdle tilt and rotate to put the acetabulum in a favorable position for the movements of the femur. There are these differences, however. Whereas the left and right sides of the shoulder girdle can move independently, the pelvic girdle can move only as a unit. The difference in depth of socket also limits the movement at the hip joint but is vital to accommodate the weight-bearing function of this joint. Furthermore, whereas the movements of the shoulder girdle take place in its own joints (sternoclavicular and acromioclavicular), the pelvic girdle is dependent on the lumbosacral and other lumbar joints, and the hip joints, for its movements. Hence, an analysis of the movements of the pelvic girdle must always be stated in terms of both spinal and hip action.

THE PELVIC GIRDLE

Structure

The pelvis (Figure 7.1) is a rigid, bony basin that serves as a massive connecting link between the trunk and the lower extremities. Each pelvic bone (os innominatum) is made up of three bones: the ilium, ischium, and pubis. These bones become fused into a single bone by about the time of puberty. The two pelvic bones together form the pelvic girdle. This bony girdle or basin is firmly attached to the sacrum at the sacroiliac articulation, an articulation that is difficult to classify. It presents some of the characteristics of a diarthrodial joint, an articular cavity being present for part of the articulation. It is unlike other diarthrodial joints in one important respect, however. No movement can be voluntarily effected at the sacroiliac joint. Any movement that does occur is involuntary. Just how much motion can occur at the sacroiliac joint is debatable. Some anatomists say that a slight "giving" may occur there as a shock absorption device; others claim that no motion occurs at the joint normally, except in women during pregnancy and parturition, when the ligaments relax to permit a slight spreading of the bones.

The sacrum is firmly bound to the two iliac bones by means of the anterior, posterior, and interosseous sacroiliac ligaments (Figures 7.2 and 7.3). It is further reinforced by the iliolumbar, sacrotuberous, and sacrospinous ligaments and by the lower portion of the erector spinae muscle. Because of this firm attachment, the sacrum might well be considered a part of the pelvic girdle. From the point of view of function, it is more truly a part of the pelvis than of the spine.

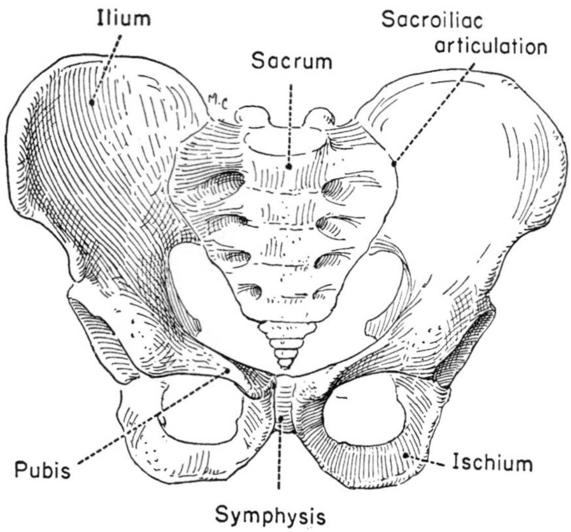

Figure 7.1 Anterior view of pelvis.

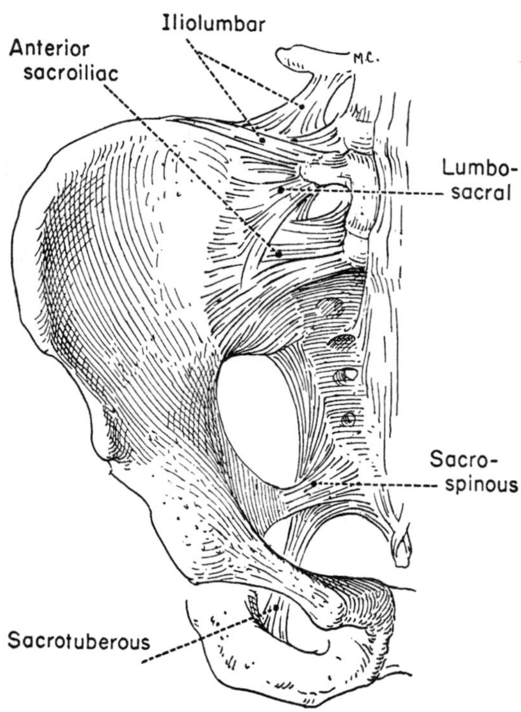

Figure 7.2 Anterior view of sacroiliac articulation showing ligaments.

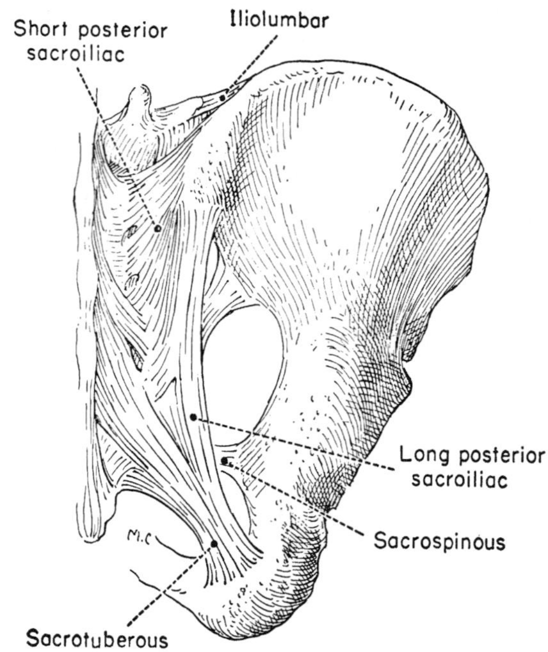

Figure 7.3 Posterior view of sacroiliac articulation showing ligaments.

Movements of the Pelvis

Changes in the position of the pelvis are brought about by virtue of the motions of the lumbar spine and the hip joints. Movements in these joints permit the pelvis to tilt forward, backward, and sideward, and to rotate horizontally.

Forward Tilt (Increased Inclination) (Figure 7.4c)

Movement of the pelvis in the sagittal plane about a bilateral axis so that the symphysis pubis turns downward and the posterior surface of the sacrum turns upward. To visualize this movement as forward tilt (increased inclination), one might consider the increase in the angle formed by the top of the pubic bone and the horizontal or the increase in deviation of the sacrum and posterior pelvis away from the vertical.

Backward Tilt (Decreased Inclination) (Figure 7.4b)

A rotation of the pelvis in the sagittal plane about a bilateral axis so that the symphysis pubis moves forward-upward and the posterior surface of the sacrum turns somewhat downward. This motion is referred to as backward tilt (decreased inclination) because the angle formed by the top of the pubic bone and the horizontal decreases and because there is a decrease in the horizontal inclination of the sacrum and posterior pelvis.

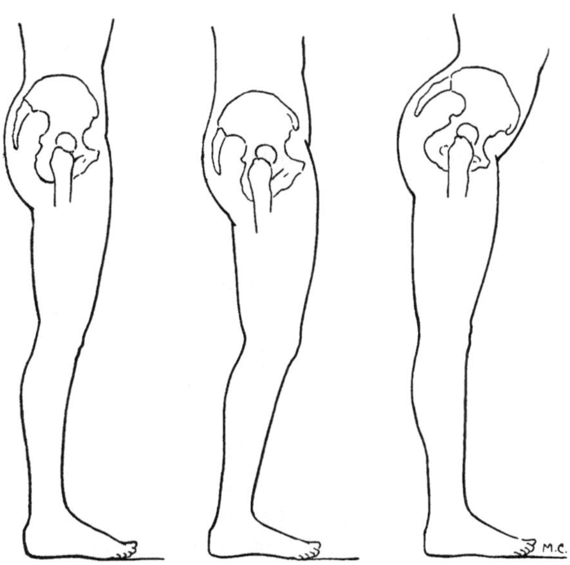

Figure 7.4 Anteroposterior inclinations of the pelvis: (a) midposition; (b) decreased inclination (backward tilt); (c) increased inclination (forward tilt).

Lateral Tilt (Figure 7.5a)

A rotation of the pelvis in the frontal plane about an anteroposterior axis so that one iliac crest is lowered and the other is raised. The tilt is named in terms of the side that moves downward. Thus, in a lateral tilt of the pelvis to the left, the left iliac crest is lowered and the right is raised.

Rotation (Lateral Twist) (Figure 7.5b)

A rotation of the pelvis in the horizontal plane about a vertical (longitudinal) axis. The movement is named in terms of the direction toward which the front of the pelvis turns.

Relationship of the Pelvis to the Trunk and Lower Extremities

Architecturally, the pelvis is strategically located. Linking the trunk with the lower extremities, it must cooperate with the motion of each yet at the same time contribute to the stability of the total structure. When the body is in the erect standing position, the pelvis receives the weight of the head, trunk, and upper extremities, divides it equally, and transmits it to the two lower extremities. The student will learn how the position of the pelvis is maintained through muscular force couples during the discussion of the biomechanics of rotary motion on pages 334–338. Whenever an individual stands on only one foot, the pelvis automatically adapts itself to this position and transmits the entire weight of the upper part of the body to one of the lower extremities. It requires a fine adjustment to do this in such a way that the balance of the total structure is preserved.

Because the pelvis depends on the joints of the lower spine and those of the hips for its movements, it is not surprising that its motion is sometimes

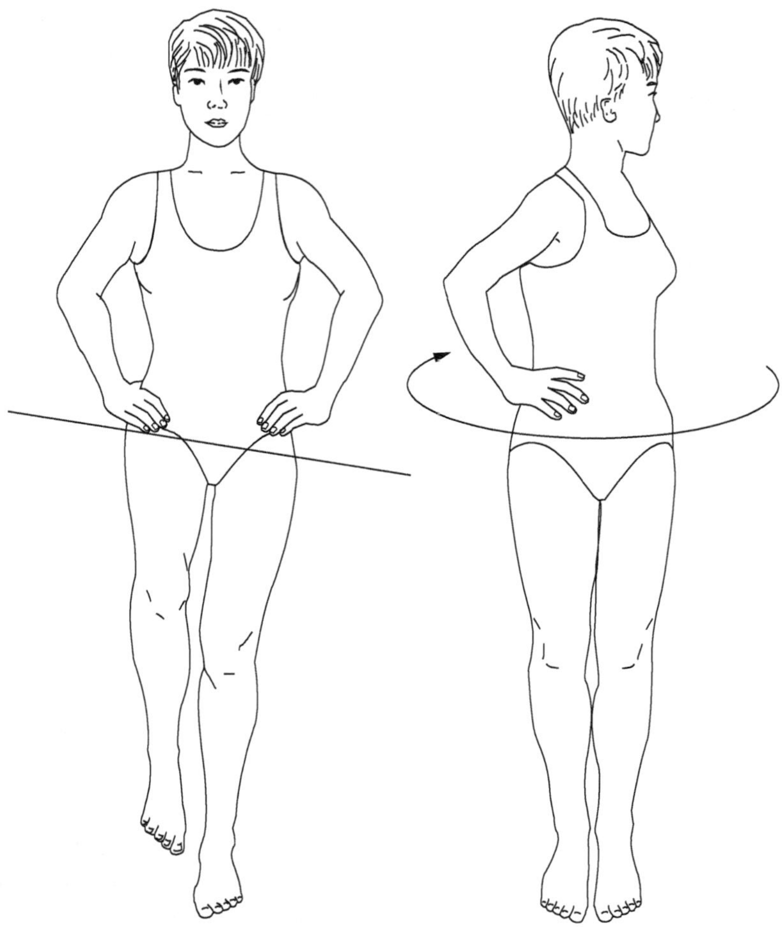

Figure 7.5 Movements of the pelvis: (a) lateral tilt to left; (b) rotation (lateral twist) to right.

associated with the motion of the trunk or spine, and sometimes with that of the thighs. In such cases the movement of the pelvis may be said to be *secondary* to that of the spine, or of the thighs, as the case may be. In fact, most movement of the pelvic girdle falls into this category. Motion of the pelvic girdle acts to change the orientation of the sacrum to facilitate movement of the trunk or to change the orientation of the acetabulum to facilitate motion in the thigh. Occasionally, however, the movement seems to be initiated in the pelvis itself, with the spine and thighs cooperating with it. In such an event, the movement of the pelvis might be considered *primary,* and that of the spine and hips secondary. One sees this type of movement when the individual "tucks the hips under" as one would have to do to change from c to b, or even from c to a, in Figure 7.4.

Posture of the pelvic girdle can most easily be analyzed through identification of key bony landmarks. The relationship between the anterior superior iliac spine and the greater trochanter of the femur provide a quick reference for the position of the pelvic girdle. It should be noted that different individuals have varying habitual angle of pelvic inclination. Habitual pelvic posture is one of the factors that might be examined when searching for the underlying causes of problems of the hip, spine, or other postural pathologies (Figure 7.6).

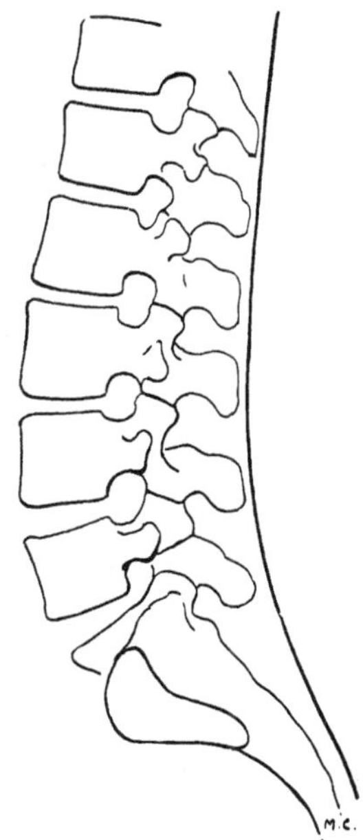

Figure 7.6 Lumbar and lumbosacral regions of the spine showing discrepancy in the lower lumbar curve as seen in the vertebral bodies and in the contour of the back. (The sketch is based on an X-ray.)

The joint analyses of the primary and secondary movements of the pelvis are given next.

Primary Movements of the Pelvis

Joint Analysis of the Primary Movements of the Pelvis as Performed from the Fundamental Standing Position

Pelvis	Spinal Joints	Hip Joints
Forward tilt	Hyperextension	Slight flexion
Backward tilt	Slight flexion	Complete extension
Lateral tilt to left	Slight lateral flexion to right	R: Slight adduction L: Slight abduction
Rotation to left (without turning the head or moving the feet)	Rotation right	R: Slight outward rotation L: Slight inward rotation

Secondary Movements of the Pelvis

Joint Analysis of Movements of the Pelvis Secondary to Those of the Spine

Spine	Pelvis
Flexion	Backward tilt
Hyperextension	Forward tilt
Lateral flexion to left	Lateral tilt to left
Rotation to left	Rotation to left

Movements of the Pelvis Secondary to Those of the Lower Extremity

Similar to the relationship between the shoulder girdle and upper extremity, the pelvis moves with the lower extremity to supplement the latter's range of motion for three types of lower extremity movements: (1) movements of both limbs acting in unison, as when swinging them forward or backward in suspension; (2) movements of both limbs acting in opposition, as when walking, running, or doing a flutter kick in swimming; and (3) movements of one limb, as when kicking or when raising one leg to the side. In double-leg swinging the pelvis tilts backward (decreased inclination) when the thigh is flexed at the hip joint, and forward (increased inclination) when the thigh is raised backward in apparent hyperextension. In opposition movements, when one leg is placed forward and the other backward, the pelvis rotates in the horizontal plane about a vertical axis. This pelvic orientation places the forward-flexed leg in slight outward rotation and the extended rear leg in slight inward rotation at the hip joint. When one thigh is moved sideward in wide abduction, the pelvis tilts laterally, lifting on the side of the abducted leg and lowering on the side of the vertical support leg. Slight abduction of the support leg at the hip joint occurs as a necessary adjustment of the tilted pelvis (Figure 7.7). In each of these

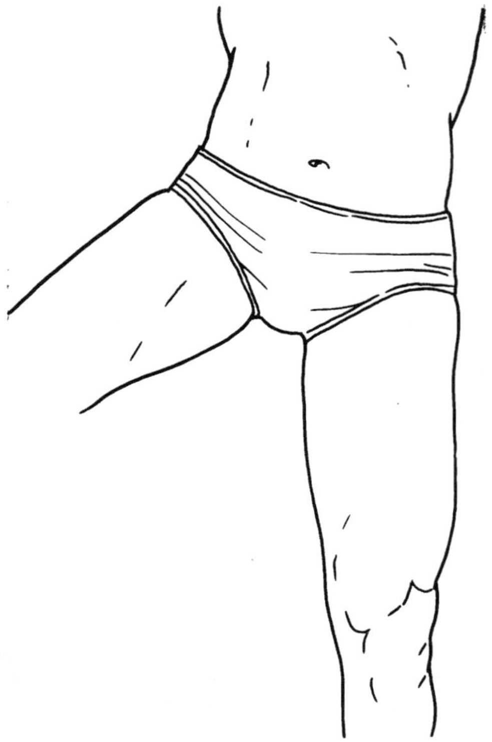

Figure 7.7 Lateral tilt of pelvis secondary to abduction of thigh at hip.

positions the pelvis positions itself so as to favor the movement of the thighs. To identify the required movement of the pelvic girdle, identify the position of the acetabulum that will most facilitate the desired motion.

Muscles of the Pelvis

All the muscles that attach to the pelvic bones or to the sacrum serve either to initiate or to control pelvic movements. As one would expect, these are all muscles either of the hip joint or of the lumbar spine, including the lumbosacral junction. The precise combination of movements at these joints depends on whether the pelvic movement is primary or whether it is secondary, supplementing either the spinal movements or those of the hip joint.

Muscles providing the force for primary movements of the pelvis when one is standing with both feet facing forward could be as follows.

Forward Tilt

Hip flexors and lumbosacral spinal extensors.

Backward Tilt

Hip extensors and lumbosacral spinal flexors.

Lateral Tilt to the Right

Left lateral lumbosacral flexors, right hip abductors.

Rotation to the Right

Left lumbosacral rotators, left hip outward rotators, and right hip inward rotators.

The Hip Joint

Structure

The hip joint (Figure 7.8), a typical ball-and-socket joint, is formed by the articulation of the spherical head of the femur with the deep cup-shaped acetabulum. The latter, formed by the junction of the three pelvic bones (ilium, ischium, and pubis), is also described as horseshoe shaped because there is a gap (the acetabular notch) at the lower part of the "cup." The entire acetabulum is lined with hyaline cartilage. This is thicker above than below, and the center is filled in with a mass of fatty tissue covered by synovial membrane. A flat rim of fibrocartilage, known as the *acetabular labrum,* is attached by its circumference to the margin of the acetabulum (Figure 7.9). It covers the hyaline cartilage, and because it is considerably thicker at the circumference than at the center, it adds to the depth of the acetabulum. Furthermore, being thicker above and behind, it serves to cushion the top and back of the acetabulum against the impact of the femoral head in forceful movements. The head of the femur also is completely covered with hyaline cartilage, except for a small pit near the center called the *fovea capitis* (see Figure 7.8). The cartilage is thicker above and tapers to a thin edge at the perimeter.

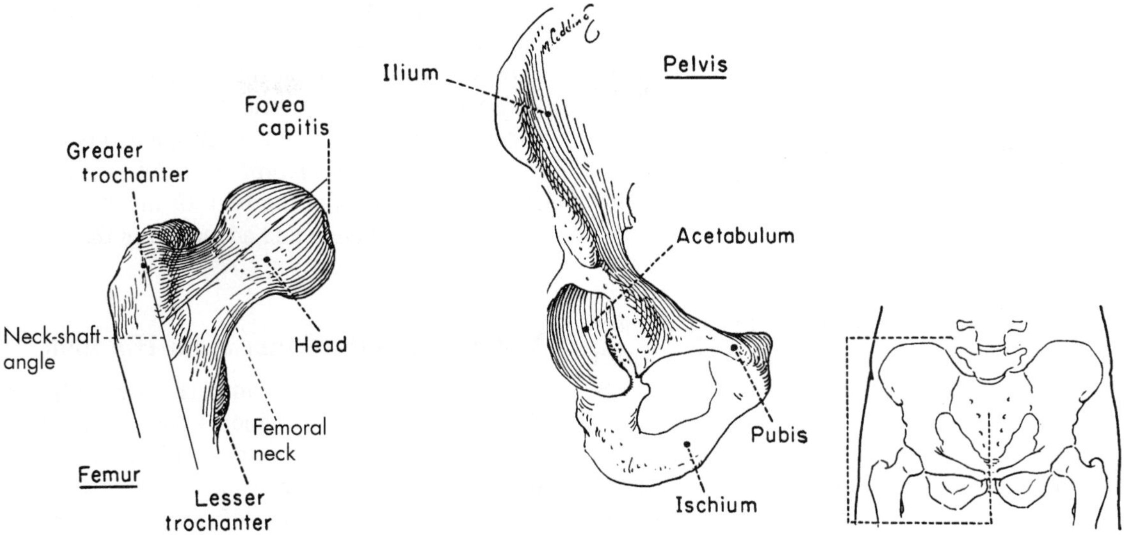

Figure 7.8 Bones of the hip joint.

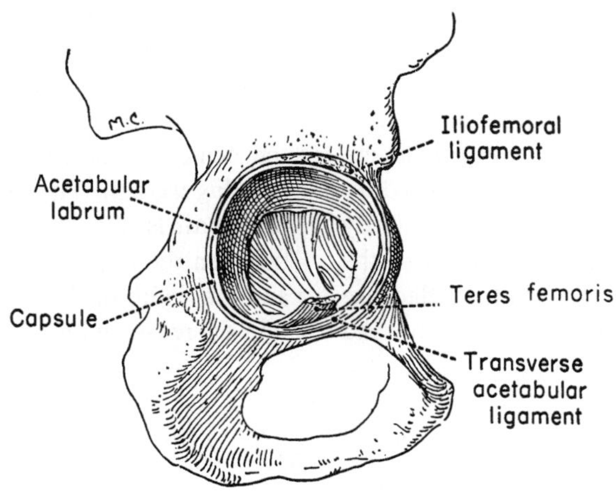

Figure 7.9 Acetabulum of right hip joint.

The head of the femur is attached to the femoral shaft by the femoral neck, which varies in length depending on body size. An obtuse angle is formed between the femoral neck and the shaft of the femur. The femoral neck–shaft angle is usually between 126 and 131 degrees in the normal adult. A greater or lesser angle is often correlated with hip injury or disease (Alonso et al., 2000; Calis et al., 2004; Nissen et al., 2005).

The femoral neck in the average person is also rotated slightly anterior to the frontal plane. This medial rotation is referred to as *femoral anteversion.* The angle of anteversion is measured as the angle between a mediolateral line through the knee and a line through the femoral head and shaft. The average range for femoral anteversion is from 15 to 20 degrees. If the angle of femoral rotation falls below this, it is referred to as *femoral retroversion*. Excessive anteversion or retroversion is associated with a number of pathologies of the hip.

Ligamentous Reinforcements

The spherical head, deep socket, and low atmospheric pressure within the joint all lend stability to the hip joint. In addition, several ligaments help limit motion at the hip joint. The *transverse acetabular* ligament is a strong, flat band of fibers continuous with the acetabular labrum, which bridges the acetabular notch and thus completes the acetabular ring.

The *teres femoris* is a flat, narrow, triangular band attached by its apex to the fovea capitis near the center of the femoral head, and by its base to the margins of the acetabular ligament (Figure 7.10). Its function is to "tie" the head of the femur to the lower part of the acetabulum and thus provide the joint with reinforcement from within.

Outer reinforcement is provided by the three ligaments of the femoral neck, one for each of the pelvic bones that unite to form the acetabulum (Figures 7.11 and 7.12). The *iliofemoral* ligament, called the Y ligament because of its supposed resemblance to an inverted Y, is an extraordinarily strong band of fibers situated at the front of the capsule and intimately blended with it. Because of its position, it serves to check extension and both outward (lateral) and inward (medial) rotation. The *pubofemoral* ligament consists of a narrow band of fibers at the medial anterior and lower portion of the capsule. It prevents excessive abduction and helps check extension and outward rotation. The *ischiofemoral* ligament is a strong triangular ligament at the back of the capsule. It limits inward rotation and adduction in the flexed position.

Movements of the Femur at the Hip Joint

The movements of the femur (Figure 7.13) are similar to those of the humerus but are not quite so free as the latter because of the deeper socket. In studying the movements of the femur, the student should first be aware of the position of the femur in the fundamental standing position. If viewed from the front, it is seen that the shaft is not vertical but slants somewhat medialward. This serves to place the center of the knee joint more nearly under the center of motion of the hip joint. Hence, the mechanical axis of the femur—a line connecting the center of the femoral head with the center of the knee joint—is almost vertical (see Figure 2.3). The degree of slant of the femoral shaft is related both to the size of the angle between the neck and shaft (angle of inclination) and the width of the pelvis. The angle of inclination decreases with age and the inner spongy or

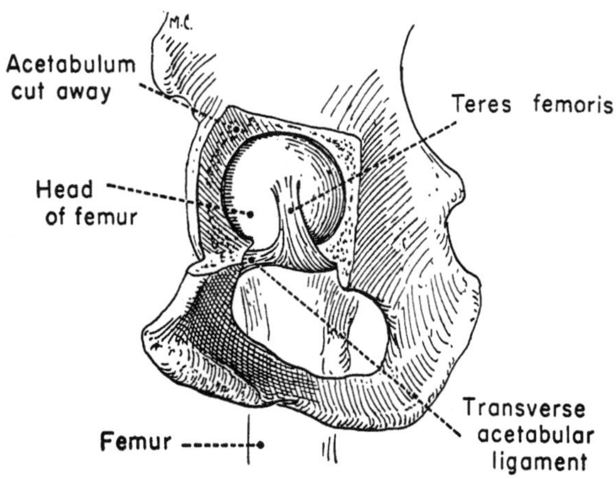

Figure 7.10 Right hip joint from within, looking toward head of femur.

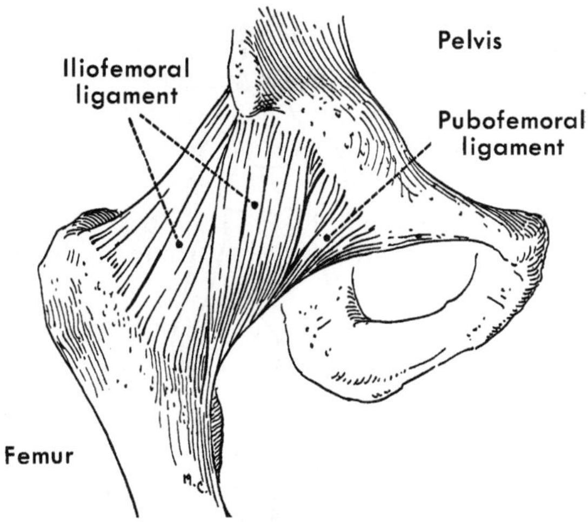

Figure 7.11 Anterior view of right hip joint.

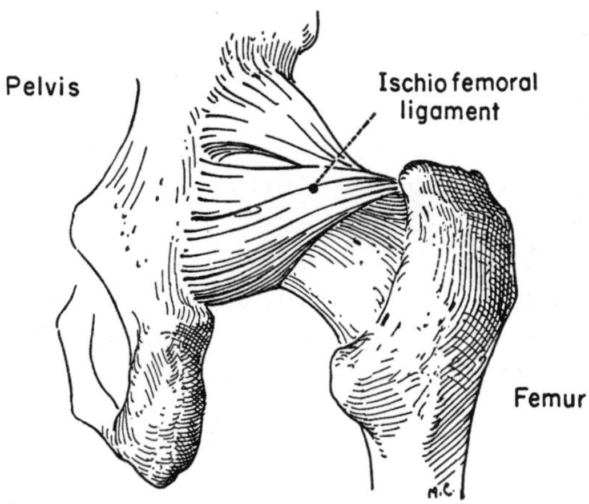

Figure 7.12 Posterior view of right hip joint.

trabecular bone becomes thinner, which makes the femur more susceptible to fracture.

As seen from the side, the shaft bows forward. This characteristic, along with the obtuse neck–shaft angle, provides resistance for the strains and stresses sustained in walking, running, and jumping and for ensuring the proper transmission of weight through the femur to the knee joint. The femur is the longest yet strongest bone of the skeletal system.

Flexion

A forward movement of the femur in the sagittal plane. If the knee is straight, the movement is restricted by the tension of the hamstring muscles. In extreme flexion the pelvis tilts backward to supplement the movement at the hip joint.

Extension

Return movement from flexion.

Hyperextension

A backward movement of the femur in the sagittal plane. This movement is extremely limited, although there may be some facilitation when the femur is rotated outward. What may appear to be hip hyperextension in many activities is instead hip extension aided by forward tilt of the pelvis. The restricting factor is the iliofemoral ligament at the front of the joint. The advantage of this restriction of movement is that it provides a stable joint for weight bearing without the need for strong muscular contraction.

Abduction

A sideward movement of the femur in the frontal plane so that the thigh moves away from the midline of the body. A greater range of movement is possible when the femur is rotated outward. Abduction is limited by the adductor muscles and the pubofemoral ligament.

Adduction

Return movement from abduction. Hyperadduction is possible only when the other leg is moved out of the way. In extreme hyperadduction, the teres femoris becomes taut.

Outward (Lateral) Rotation

A rotation of the femur around its longitudinal axis so that the knee is turned outward.

Inward (Medial) Rotation

A rotation of the femur around its longitudinal axis so that the knee is turned inward.

The range of inward and outward rotation is affected by the degree of femoral torsion (twisting

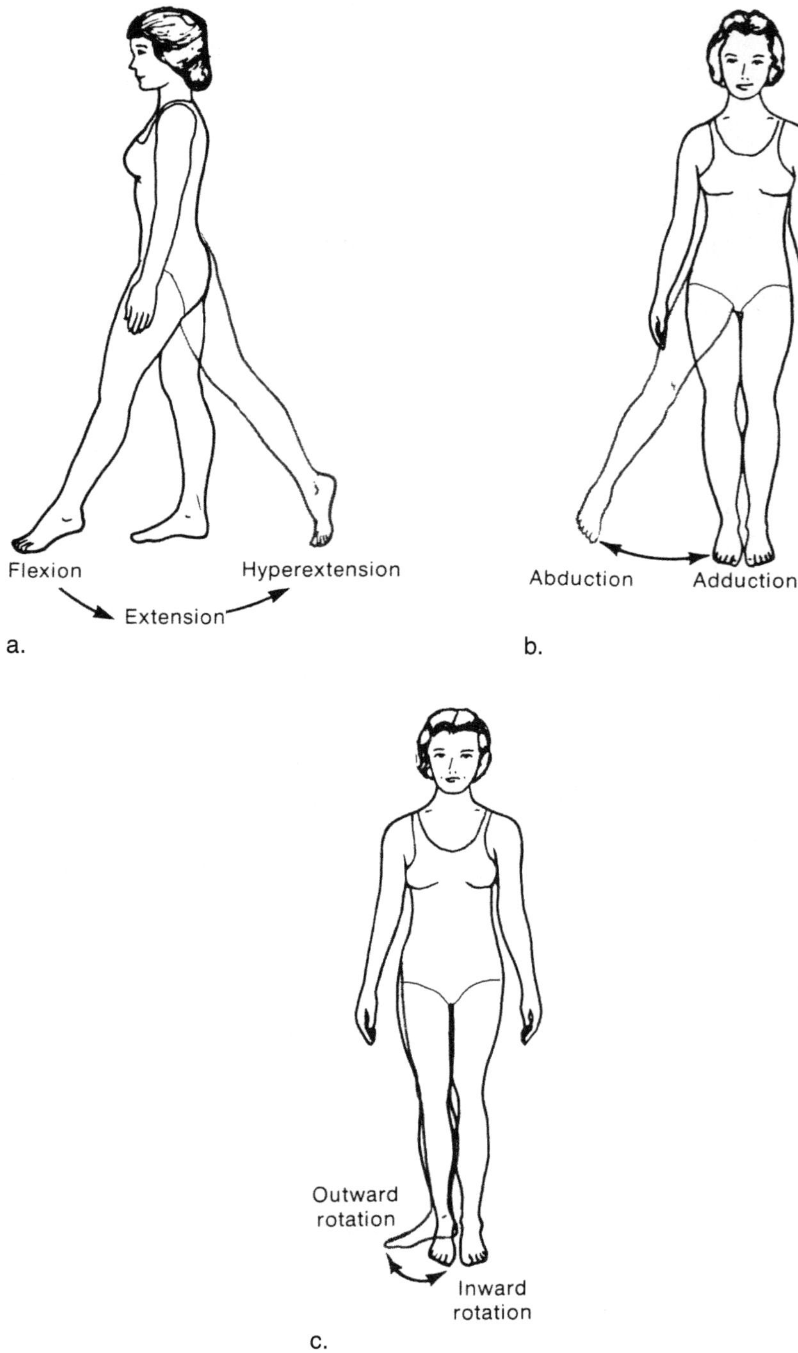

Figure 7.13 Movements of the hip joint: (a) flexion, extension, and hyperextension; (b) abduction and adduction; (c) inward and outward rotation.

of the femur on its long axis so that one end is inwardly rotated with respect to the other). The range of outward rotation usually exceeds that of inward rotation.

Circumduction

A combination of flexion, abduction, extension, and adduction performed sequentially in either direction.

Because the hip is a triaxial, ball-and-socket joint, there is also the possibility of motion in several planes simultaneously. As in the shoulder, it is possible to abduct at the hip while performing outward rotation, thus bringing the thigh to the side of the body with the foot and knee pointed upward. This motion has been variously named diagonal abduction or horizontal abduction. In this text each of the planar motions involved in any combination will be identified to avoid confusion.

MUSCLES OF THE HIP JOINT

Location

The muscles acting at the hip joint are listed here according to their position in relation to the joint. They include several muscles that act with equal or greater effectiveness at the knee joint. These are known as the two-joint muscles of the lower extremity. Only their action at the hip joint is considered in this section.

Anterior	**Posterior**
Iliopsoas	Biceps femoris
Pectineus	Semimembranosus
Rectus femoris	Semitendinosus
Sartorius	Gluteus maximus
Tensor fasciae latae	Six deep outward rotators

Medial	**Lateral**
Adductor brevis	Gluteus medius
Adductor longus	Gluteus minimus
Adductor magnus	
Gracilis	

Characteristics and Functions of Hip Joint Muscles

Iliopsoas *(Figure 7.14; Also Listed with the Spinal Muscles)*

Because the *psoas major, psoas minor,* and *iliacus* muscles share a common distal attachment and act as one muscle at the hip joint, the usual practice of treating them as one muscle is followed here. The muscle is a *strong hip flexor.* Depending on the circumstances, it will either *flex the thigh on the trunk* or it will *flex the trunk as a unit on the thighs* from a supine lying position, or in any position when the movement is performed against resistance.

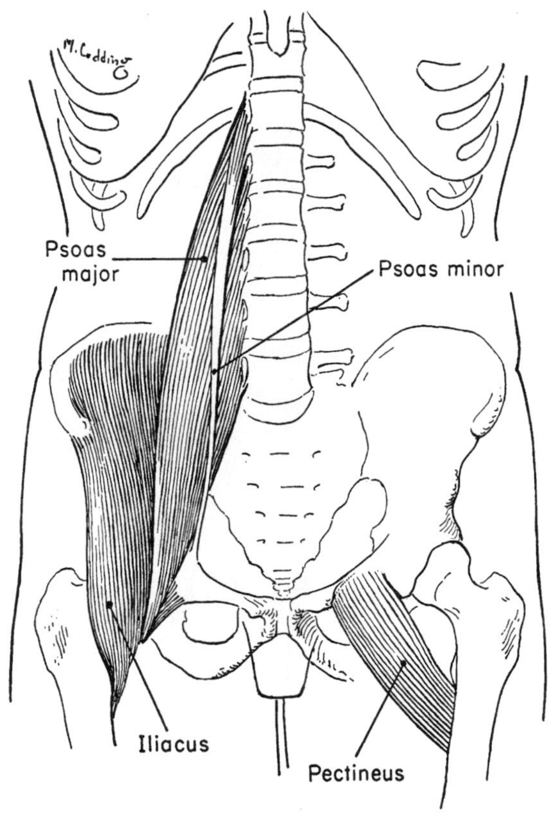

Figure 7.14 Anterior view of pelvic region showing psoas major and minor, iliacus, and pectineus.

Pectineus

This muscle (Figure 7.14) is a short, thick, quadrilateral muscle situated lateral and superior to the adductor longus and more or less parallel to it. It *flexes the thigh* and possibly *assists in adduction* when the hip is in a flexed state. Whether it also contributes to outward rotation is debatable. As a flexor it has a good angle of pull that, together with its internal structure, accounts for its ability to overcome considerable resistance. It may be palpated at the front of the pubis, just lateral to the adductor longus, but it is difficult to distinguish from the latter muscle.

Rectus Femoris (Figure 7.15; Also Listed with the Knee Muscles)

The rectus femoris muscle is the only quadriceps femoris muscle that crosses the hip joint. The muscle *flexes* the thigh and is also active during abduction and lateral rotation. It is a large bipenniform muscle, located superficially on the front of the thigh. It acts on the knee joint as well as the hip and is therefore a two-joint muscle. It shows maximum activity in single joint movements or in the countercurrent actions of hip flexion and knee extension. No activity occurs when the hip flexion is concurrent with knee flexion. It may be

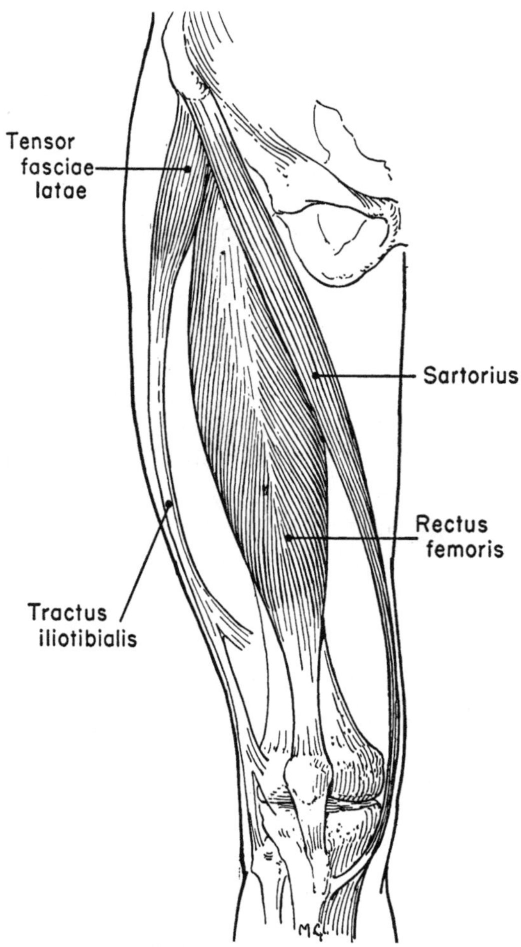

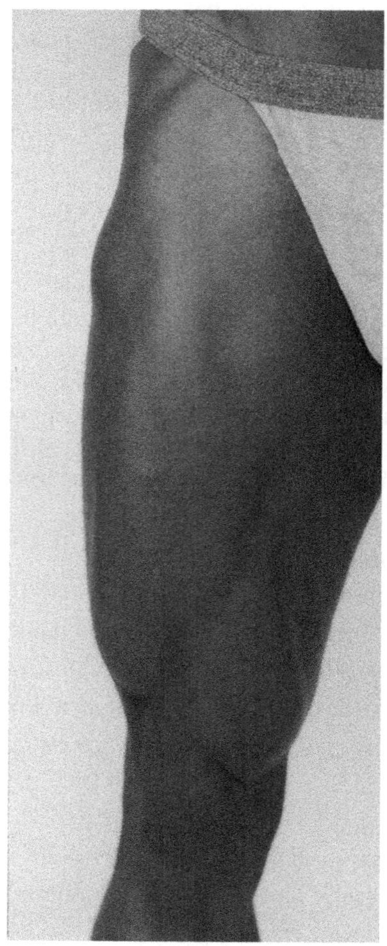

Figure 7.15 Muscles on front of right thigh.

palpated as well as seen on the anterior surface of the thigh.

Sartorius *(Figure 7.15; Also Listed with the Knee Muscles)*

This muscle is also a two-joint muscle. Its action on the thigh is *flexion*. It also shows activity in abduction when external resistance is offered, and in outward rotation while sitting.

The sartorius is a long, slender, ribbonlike muscle directed obliquely downward and medialward across the front of the thigh. The sartorius muscle is the longest muscle in the body. It is the most superficial of the anterior thigh muscles and may be readily seen and palpated on slender subjects. On others, it may be palpated at the anterior superior iliac spine. Its name derives from its alleged function of enabling one to sit with the legs crossed, "tailor" fashion.

Tensor Fasciae Latae

This muscle (Figures 7.15 and 7.18) *flexes* and *abducts the femur* and *tenses the fascia lata*. It is a small muscle located close in front of and slightly lateral to the hip joint, and it may be palpated about 2 inches anterior to the greater trochanter. Because its pull on the fascia lata is transmitted by means of the iliotibial tract down to the lateral condyle of the tibia, it helps extend the leg at the knee. Together with the gluteus maximus, which also unites with the fascia lata, it helps stabilize the knee joint in weight-bearing positions. When the lower extremities are fixed, both of these muscles help steady the pelvis and trunk on the thighs.

The Hamstrings *(Figures 7.16 and 7.17; Also Listed with the Knee Muscles)*

The three hamstring muscles—*biceps femoris, semimembranosus,* and *semitendinosus*—are situated on the back of the thigh, extending from the tuberosity of the ischium down just below the knee joint, with the biceps femoris on the lateral aspect of the posterior surface and the two "semi" muscles on the medial aspect.

The biceps femoris is the lateral hamstring muscle. Only its long head crosses the hip joint. The short head, the only one-joint muscle belonging to the hamstring group, does not cross the hip joint; therefore, it has no part in hip joint movements. The biceps femoris tendon may be palpated on the lateral aspect of the posterior surface of the knee.

Together the semimembranosus and semitendinosus constitute the medial component of the hamstring group. The semimembranosus lies anterior to the semitendinosus and has a shorter, deeper tendon that is extremely difficult to palpate. The semitendinosus tendon may easily be palpated on the medial aspect of the posterior surface of the knee when the leg is flexed against resistance from the prone lying position. It should not be confused with the gracilis tendon, which lies slightly anterior to it. All three muscles *extend the femur* or, if the thighs are bearing weight as in either the standing or long sitting position, they extend the forward flexed trunk as a unit—that is, from the hips. (Spinal action must not be confused with hip action, or vice versa.) The effectiveness of the medial hamstrings as extensors of the hip is related to knee joint action. There is maximum activity during hip extension when the knee is either stabilized or flexed simultaneously (Basmajian & DeLuca, 1985). They are inactive, however, during simultaneous hip and knee extension.

All three hamstrings, in addition to extending the hip, help stabilize it. Also, they adduct the femur from the abducted position when the movement is resisted and help rotate the extended femur. The long head of the biceps femoris rotates the femur laterally, and the inner hamstring rotates it medially.

Gluteus Maximus *(Figures 7.18, 7.19, and 7.20)*

This is the largest and most superficial of the three buttock muscles. It is a potentially *powerful hip extensor*. It also *rotates the femur outward* when the latter is extended. The *lower portion assists in adduction* from an abducted position if the movement is resisted. The *upper portion abducts*

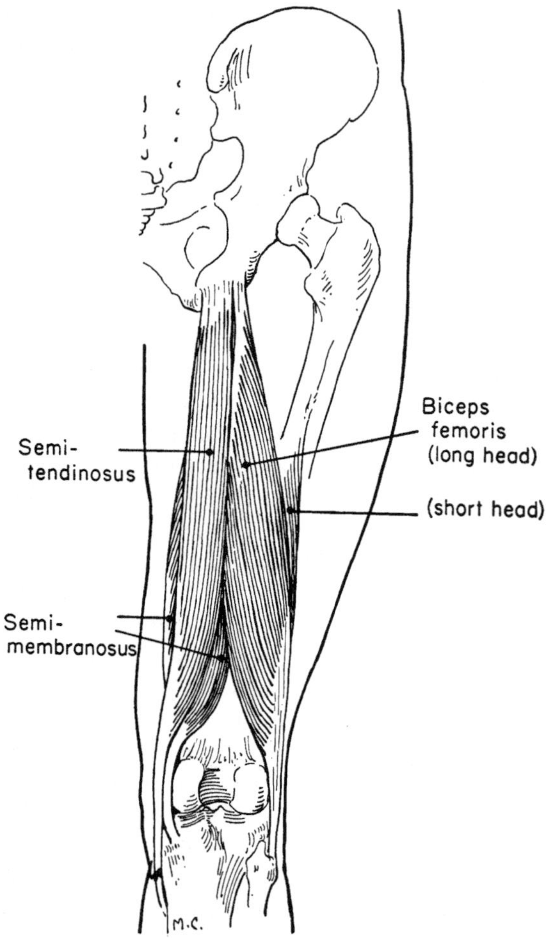

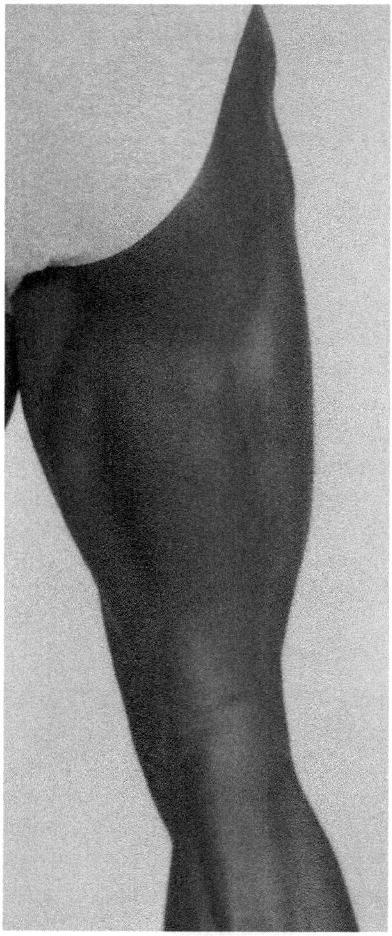

Figure 7.16 Hamstring muscles.

against strong resistance. One can understand these seemingly contradictory functions more readily after studying the relation of the muscle to the hip joint's center of motion as seen from behind. Figure 7.20 shows that roughly one-third of the muscle lies above the center of motion and two-thirds below it. This puts the uppermost fibers in a position for abducting the thigh and the lower fibers in a position for adducting the thigh, whereas the fibers lying directly behind the femoral head are not in position for doing either. The entire muscle may easily be palpated on the posterior surface of the buttock.

The gluteus maximus has been the subject of much EMG study. Contrary to what one might think because of its size and prominence, the gluteus maximus has been shown to be active during the motions named previously only when moderate to heavy resistance to the movement exists. And even though it often displays bursts of activity during brief periods of normal and fast walking, its participation is primarily as a stabilizer.

The activity of the gluteus maximus in stair climbing has been confirmed in a number of EMG studies. It has also been found to be active in walking up an inclined plane, in extending the femur against resistance, in abducting the femur, especially against resistance and when rotated outward, and in adducting the femur against resistance when in an abducted position. This muscle is also most active during the stance phase of sprint running, as opposed to push-off (Kyrolainen et al., 2005).

Gluteus maximus activity is also elicited in hyperextension movements of the thigh performed against resistance from the erect standing position, muscle setting, and vigorous hyperextension of the trunk from an erect position. In heavy lifting requiring simultaneous extension of the hips and knees, the gluteus maximus was found to be active during the middle to the last 15 to 20% of the movement (Worrell et al., 2001).

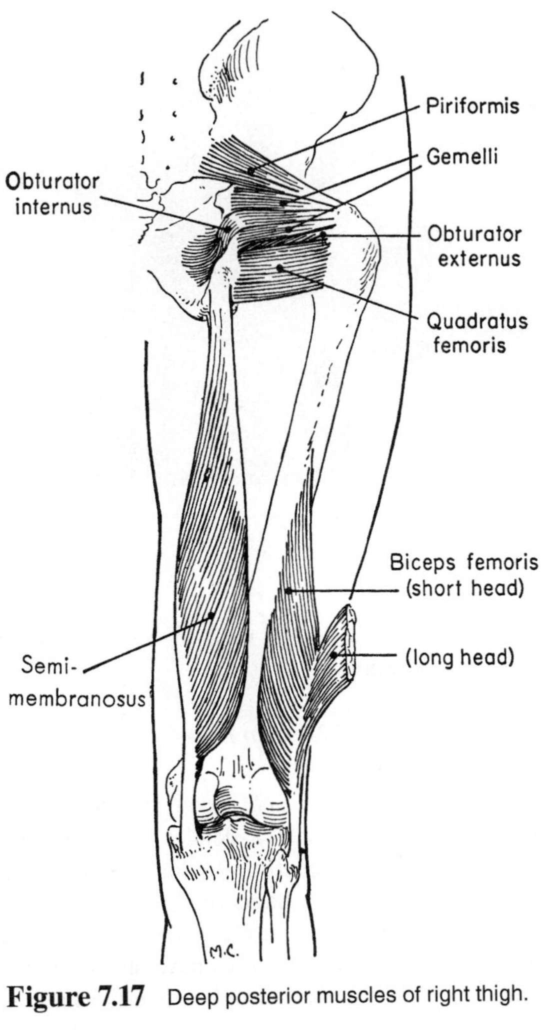

Figure 7.17 Deep posterior muscles of right thigh.

The Six Deep Outward Rotators

These six muscles (obturator externus and internus, gemellus superior and inferior, quadratus femoris, and piriformis; see Figure 7.17) form a compact group behind the hip joint. Their fibers run horizontally for the most part. The piriformis, the most superior of the group, is slightly above the joint. The quadratus femoris, the most inferior, is slightly below it. Some of the muscles have a secondary function such as abduction or adduction, but neither of these functions compares in importance with that of *outward rotation.* They are favorably situated for helping hold the femoral head in the acetabulum.

Adductor Brevis

This muscle (Figure 7.21) lies just above the adductor longus and consists of fibers that are almost horizontal when the thigh is in its normal resting or standing position. From this position it both *adducts* and *aids in flexing the femur.* If the hip is flexed to a marked degree, it combines extension with the adduction, against resistance. It is also active in inward rotation.

Adductor Longus

This muscle (Figure 7.21) *adducts* and *flexes the femur.* Steindler (1970) has pointed out that, though it ordinarily helps flex the thigh, when the flexion exceeds about 70 degrees it becomes an extensor as a result of a shift in the relationship between the muscle's line of pull and the joint's center of motion. In an EMG study in 1966, de Sousa and Vitti found that this muscle was always active during free adduction and inward rotation (Basmajian & DeLuca, 1985). The muscle may be palpated just below its proximal attachment at the medial aspect of the groin.

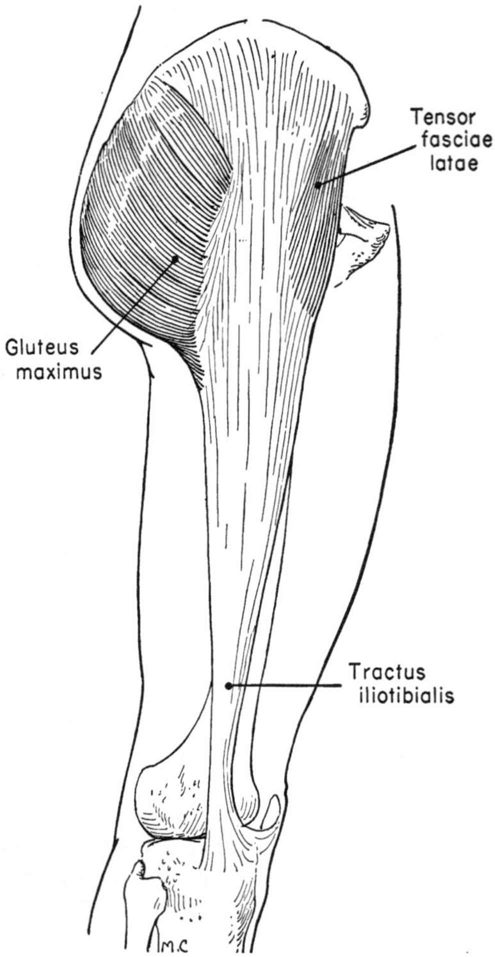

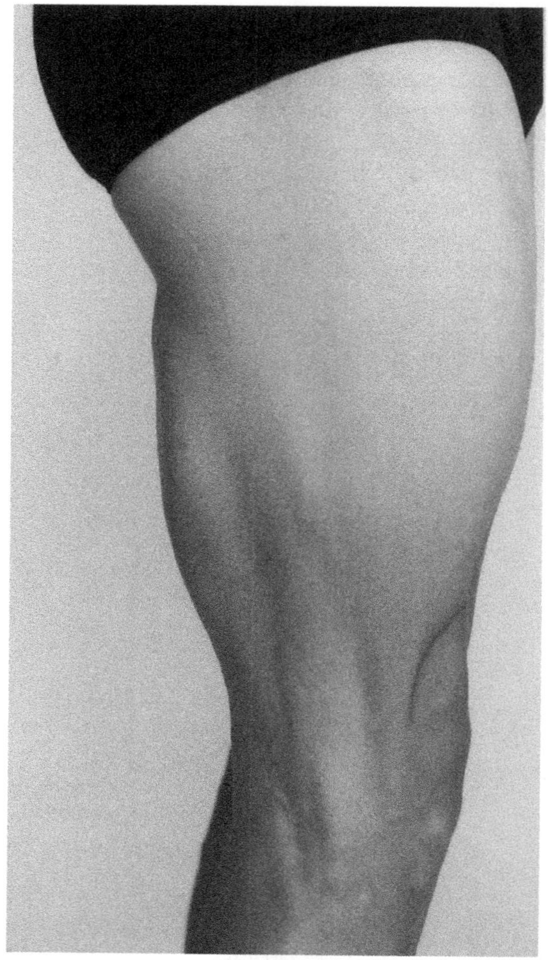

Figure 7.18 Lateral view of gluteus maximus, tensor fasciae latae, and iliotibial tract.

Adductor Magnus

This muscle (Figure 7.21) *extends the thigh as well as adducting it,* and the condyloid or *lowest portion also assists in inward rotation.* De Sousa and Vitti have noted that this muscle was not active during free adduction and extension unless the movement was performed against resistance (Basmajian & DeLuca, 1985). Like the other adductors, it was found to be active in inward rotation. The adductor magnus may be palpated on the medial aspect of the middle half of the thigh. The uppermost portion of the muscle—that is, the portion that comes from the pubis—is sometimes treated as a separate muscle called *adductor minimus.*

Gracilis (Figure 7.21; Also Listed with the Knee Muscles)

This muscle *adducts* and *flexes the femur.* As the name indicates, it is a slender muscle. Being an adductor, it is sometimes called the adductor gracilis and, like the hamstrings, sartorius, and rectus femoris, it is a muscle of the knee as well as the hip joint. EMG studies have shown that it participates in hip flexion only when the knee is extended and that it is most active during the first

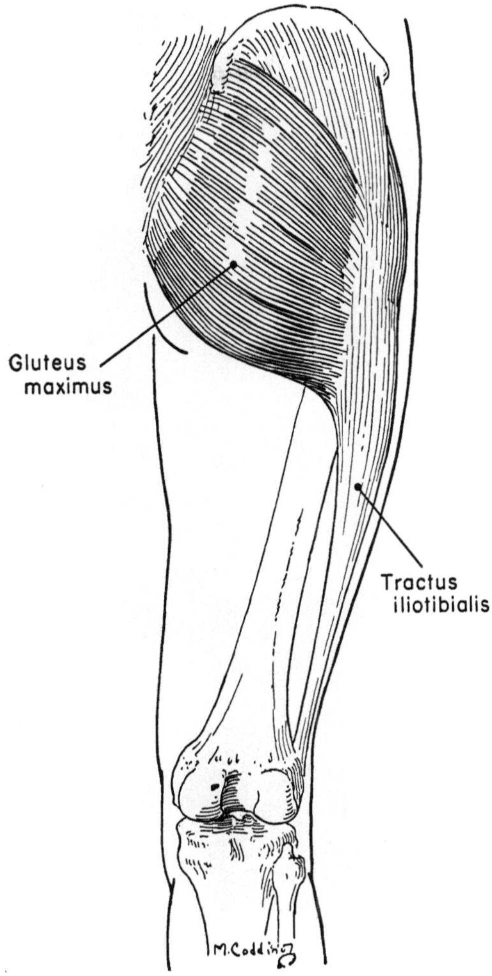

Figure 7.19 Posterior view of gluteus maximus and iliotibial tract.

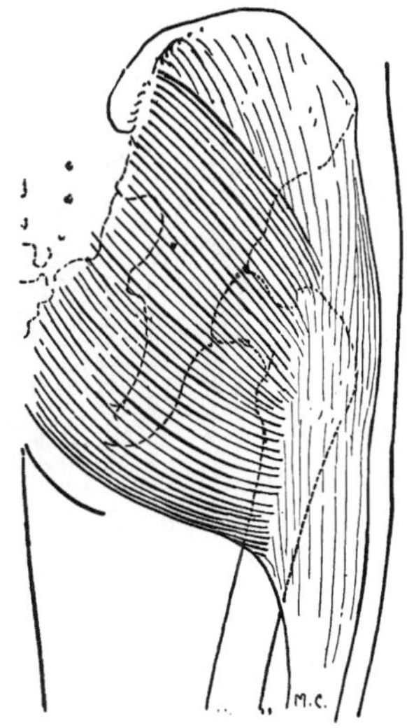

Figure 7.20 Diagram showing relation of gluteus maximus to hip joint.

part of flexion: it also helps rotate the femur medially (inward).

Gluteus Medius

This muscle (Figure 7.22a) is essentially an *abductor of the femur.* The *anterior fibers also rotate the thigh inward.* The muscle may be palpated about 2 or 3 inches above the greater trochanter.

The muscle is an important one in walking and in standing in good posture. When the weight is shifted onto one foot, tension of the gluteus medius and other abductors is an important factor in stabilization of the hip. Lack of such stabilization results in an exaggerated sideward thrust of the supporting hip and a drop of the pelvis on the opposite side, known as Trendelenburg's sign. Paralysis or weakness of this muscle causes a typical limping gait known as the Trendelenburg gait. When the weight is borne on the affected side, the trunk tilts strongly to that side and the opposite hip is thrust into prominence.

Gluteus Minimus

This muscle (Figure 7.22b) *rotates inward and abducts.* It is smaller than the gluteus medius and is situated beneath it. Whereas the medius is primarily an abductor and secondarily an inward rotator, the minimus is primarily an inward rotator and secondarily an abductor. The muscles appear to work cooperatively, each one assisting in the other's primary function.

Muscular Analysis of the Fundamental Movements of the Thigh

Flexion

This movement is performed chiefly by the tensor fasciae latae, pectineus (both of these especially during the first half of range), iliopsoas, rectus

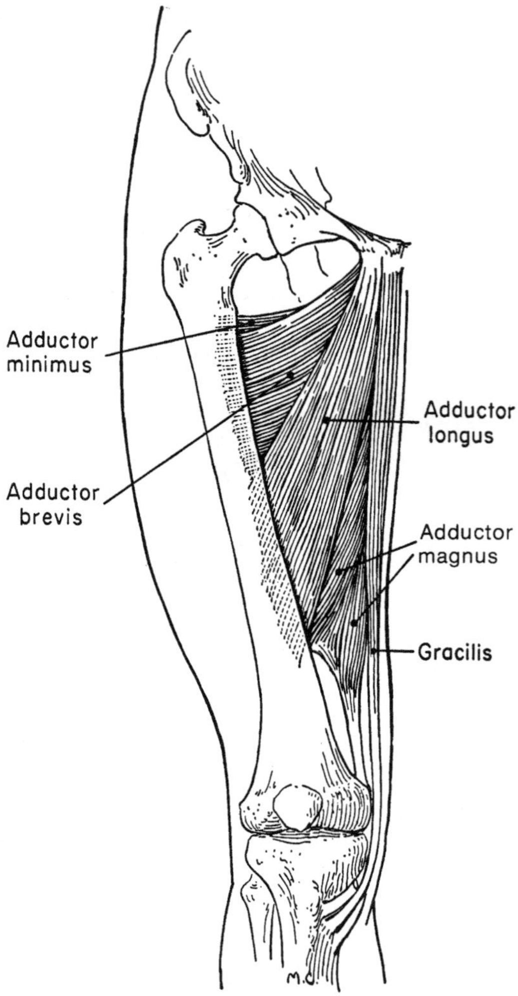

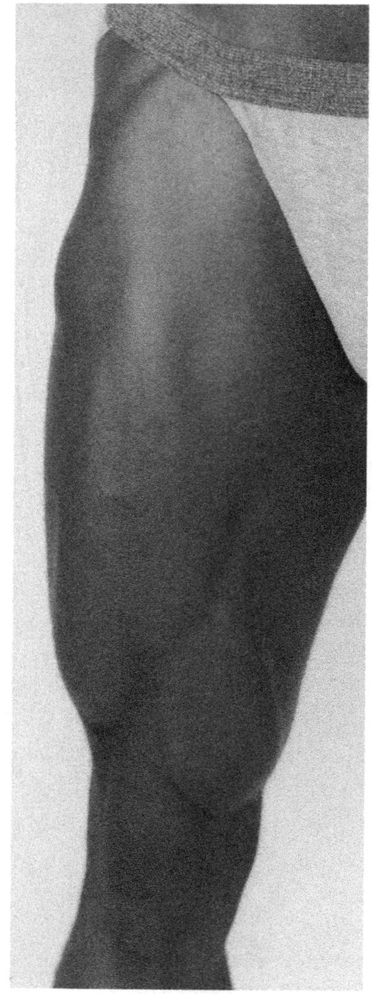

Figure 7.21 Adductor muscles of right thigh.

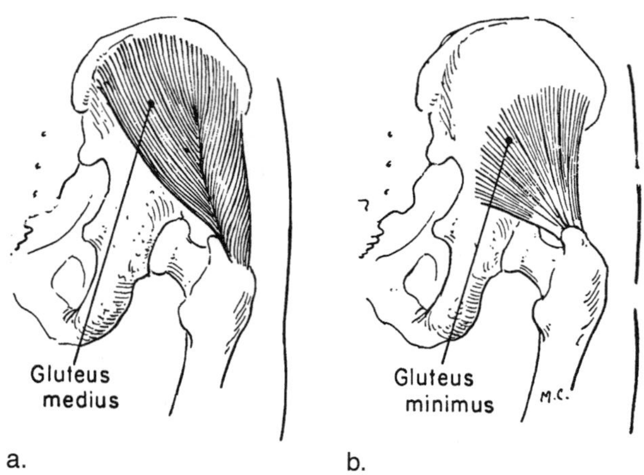

Figure 7.22 Gluteus medius and minimus.

femoris, and sartorius. The gracilis and adductors longus and brevis assist in flexion in selected positions.

Extension

The three hamstring muscles are the chief hip extensors. The gluteus maximus extends only against resistance. The three adductors also extend against resistance and when the thigh is flexed beyond a 45-degree angle.

Abduction

The chief abductors are the gluteus medius and minimus, the former being the more effective of the two. The sartorius and rectus femoris are active against resistance; the uppermost fibers of the gluteus maximus abduct against resistance during the early part of the movement, and the tensor fasciae latae abducts the thigh when it is extended.

Adduction

The adductor longus is the primary adductor. Other important adductors are the adductors magnus and brevis and the gracilis. The pectineus adducts the flexed thigh, and the lower third of the gluteus maximus assists in the movement when it is performed against resistance. The hamstrings adduct the abducted thigh against resistance.

Outward Rotation

This movement is performed by the six deep outward rotators, biceps femoris, and gluteus maximus.

Inward Rotation

The chief inward rotators are the gluteus medius and minimus, the latter being the more effective of the two. They are assisted by the semimembranosus, semitendinosus, gracilis, and adductor longus. The lower fibers of the adductor magnus rotate the thigh inward when it is extended. Some say that the tensor fasciae latae also helps, but this is debatable.

Common Injuries of the Thigh, Hip Joint, and Pelvis

Contusions

Contusions often result from a direct blow to an unprotected or inadequately protected body part. For example, participation in contact sports such as football may result in contusions to the quadriceps muscles due to blows and pinching of the quadriceps muscles between the femur and the external force. Blows to the pelvic area, including the iliac crest, may result in a contusion (hip pointer), muscle strain, or an avulsion fracture, where the muscle pulls away from the iliac crest, taking some bone with it. Landing in a sitting position or a direct blow may cause contusions to the coccyx and/or tuberosity of the ischium. All contusions are very painful, and some may be debilitating because every movement aggravates the condition. In each case accurate diagnosis is important for proper treatment. When the contusion to a muscle is not treated appropriately, or if the injury occurs repeatedly, myositis ossificans may result.

Myositis Ossificans

This is a condition in which calcification develops following repeated traumas or serious contusions to the muscle. It is likely to occur when the symptoms of muscle injury are so mild that the player insists on continuing to play. The front of the thigh and the brachialis muscle of the upper arm appear to be the most vulnerable areas so affected. The frequency with which this condition occurs is caused in large part by poor treatment such as overvigorous massage, manipulation under anesthesia, overstrenuous exercise, and too early return to participation in the activity in which a severe muscle injury has occurred.

Strains of the Hamstring Muscle Group

A high incidence of hamstring strains occurs among the very active. These tend to happen in running more than in any other activity, especially when a muscular imbalance occurs through fatigue or another condition and when there is a sudden change in direction or speed. A frequent site of the strain is the distal attachment of the biceps femoris muscle on the fibular head. Another common hamstring strain occurs in the pelvic area where the semitendinosus and the long head of the biceps femoris attach to the lower and medial impression on the tuberosity of the ischium. This is usually caused by a forceful movement of the lower extremity involving flexion of the thigh with the knees held in extension. In severe strains there may also be an avulsion fracture, especially if the ossification of the epiphysis is not yet complete.

Hip Fracture

One of the most serious injuries of the hip region is the hip fracture. Hip fractures are usually actually fractures of the neck of the femur. Due to the weight-bearing and weight-transfer functions of the hip joint, such fractures are very difficult to repair, often requiring replacement of the joint itself. Hip fractures have different etiologies at different ages. In the young person or healthy adult, this type of fracture is caused by some form of impact (a high-energy blow) in the large majority of cases (Farooq et al., 2005; Whiting & Zernicke, 1998). In the elderly, hip fractures happen more easily and are often the result of a fall. In this population, decreased bone mineral density, smaller femoral neck diameter, or increased femoral neck length all contribute to a predisposition for hip fracture.

Hip joint replacement is often the only option for the repair of a femoral neck (hip) fracture. In most hip replacements, the head and neck of the femur and a portion of the femoral shaft are manufactured from metal or plastic. The pointed shaft of the prosthetic is fitted into the bony shaft remnants, and the acetabulum is replaced with an artificial socket. A person with a hip replacement can be active, although activities with significant impact, such as jogging, are to be avoided.

References and Selected Readings

Alonso, C. G., Curiel, M. D., Carranza, F. H., Cano, R. P., & Perez, A. D. (2000). Femoral bone mineral density, neck–shaft angle and mean femoral neck width as predictors of hip fracture in men and women. *Osteoporosis International,* 11, 714–120.

Anderson, F. C., & Pandy, M. G. (2003). Individual muscle contributions to support in normal walking. *Gait and Posture,* 17(2), 159–169.

Basmajian, J. V., & Deluca, C. J. (1985). *Muscles alive* (5th ed.). Baltimore: Williams & Wilkins.

Brownbill, R. A., & Ilich, J. Z. (2003). Hip geometry and its role in fracture: What do we know so far? *Current Osteoporosis Reports,* 1, 25–31.

Calis, H. T., Eryavuz, M., & Calis, M. (2004). Comparison of femoral geometry among cases with and without hip fractures. *Yonsei Medical Journal,* 45, 901–907.

Cibulka, M. T. (2004). Determination and significance of femoral neck anteversion. *Physical Therapy,* 84, 550–558.

Croisier, J. L. (2004). Factors associated with recurrent hamstring injuries. *Sports Medicine,* 34(10), 681–695.

Dewberry, M. J., Bohannon, R. W., Tiberio, D., Murray, R., & Zannotti, C. M. (2003). Pelvic and femoral contributions to bilateral hip flexion by subjects suspended from a bar. *Clinical Biomechanics,* 18, 494–499.

Farooq, M. A., Orkazai, S. H., Okusanya, O., & Devitt, A. T. (2005). Intracapsular fractures of the femoral neck in younger patients. *Irish Journal of Medical Science,* 174(4), 42–45.

Granata, K. P., & Sanford, A. H. (2000). Lumbar-pelvic coordination is influenced by lifting task parameters. *Spine,* 25, 1413–1418.

Gupta, A., Fernihough, B., Bailey, G., Bombeck, P., Clarke, A., & Hopper, D. (2004). An evaluation of differences in hip external rotation strength and range of motion between female dancers and non-dancers. *British Journal of Sports Medicine,* 38, 178–183.

Juker, D., McGill, S., Kropf, P., & Steffen, T. (1998). Quantitative intramuscular myoelectric activity of lumbar portions of psoas and the abdominal wall during a wide variety of tasks. *Medicine and Science in Sports and Exercise,* 30(2), 301–310.

Kyrolainen, H., Avela, J., & Komi, P. V. (2005). Changes in muscle activity with increasing running speed. *Journal of Sports Sciences,* 23, 1101–1109.

Miller, M. S., Peach, J. P., & Keller, T. S. (2001). Electromyographic analysis of a human powered stepper cycle during seated and standing riding. *Journal of Electromyography and Kinesiology,* 11, 413–423.

Mohamed, O., Perry, J., & Hislop, H. (2002). Relationship between wire EMG activity, muscle length, and torque of the hamstrings. *Clinical Biomechanics,* 17(8), 569–579.

Murray, R., Bohannon, R. W., Tiberio, D., Dewberry, M. J., & Zannotti, C. M. (2002). Pelvifemoral rhythm during unilateral hip flexion in standing. *Clinical Biomechanics,* 17, 147–751.

Nguyen, N. D., Pongchaiyakul, C., Center, J. R., Eisman, J. A., & Nguyen, T. V. (2005). Identification of high-risk individuals for hip fracture: A 14-year prospective study. *Journal of Bone Mineral Research,* 20, 1921–1928.

Nissen, N., Hauge, E. M., Abrahamsen, B., Jensen, J. E., Mosekilde, L., & Brixen, K. (2005). Geometry of the proximal femur in relation to age and sex: A cross-sectional study in healthy adult Danes. *Acta Radiologica,* 46(5), 514–518.

Onishi, H., Yagi, R., Oyama, M., Akasaka, K., Ihashi, K., & Handa, Y. (2002). EMG-angle relationship of the hamstring muscles during maximum knee flexion. *Journal of Electromyography and Kinesiology,* 12(5), 399–406.

Petrofsky, J. S. (2001). The use of electromyogram biofeedback to reduce Trendelenburg gait. *European Journal of Applied Physiology,* 85(5), 491–495.

Pulkkinen, P., Partanen, J., Jalovaara, P., & Jämsä, T. (2004). Combination of bone mineral density and upper femur geometry improves prediction of hip fracture. *Osteoporosis International,* 15, 274–280.

Steindler, A. (1970). *Kinesiology of the human body.* Springfield, IL: Charles C. Thomas.

Whiting, W. C., & Zernicke, R. F. (1998). *Biomechanics of musculoskeletal injury.* Champaign, IL: Human Kinetics.

Worrell, T. W., Karst, G., Adamczyk, D., Moore, R., Stanley, C., Steimel, B., et al. (2001). Influence of joint position on electromyographic and torque generation during maximal voluntary isometric contractions of the hamstrings and gluteus maximus muscles. *Journal of Orthopedic and Sports Physical Therapy,* 31(12), 730–740.

LABORATORY EXPERIENCES

Joint Structure and Function

1. Record the essential information regarding the structure, ligaments, and cartilages of the hip joint. Study the movements both on the skeleton and the living body and explain how the joint structure affects the movements.
2. Using a protractor type of goniometer, measure the range of motion in the following joint movements on five different subjects:
   a. Hip flexion, with straight knee
   b. Hip flexion, with flexed knee
   c. Total abduction of both thighs
3. From an erect standing position with the feet together, take a fairly long step forward with the right foot, stopping with weight mostly over the right foot and with the left foot still in place but with the heel raised and the ball of the foot bearing just enough weight to

maintain balance. Analyze the joint action that has taken place at each hip joint and in the pelvic girdle.

4. Analyze the joint action of each hip joint in each phase of riding a bicycle.

Muscular Action

Identify as many muscles as possible in the following experiments.

5. **Decrease of Pelvic Inclination**
   Subject: Lie on back with knees drawn up and feet resting on floor. Tilt pelvis in such a manner that lumbar spine flexes and therefore flattens.
   Assistant: Kneeling at subject's head and facing subject's feet, place thumbs on the anterior superior iliac spines and fingers under the lower back. Resist movement by pushing iliac spines toward subject's feet.
   Observer: Palpate rectus abdominis and gluteus maximus.
6. **Increase of Pelvic Inclination**
   Subject: In erect standing position, stiffen the knees and push the buttocks as far back as possible.
   Observer: Palpate tensor fasciae latae, sartorius, pectineus, and iliocostalis. Does the adductor longus or gracilis contract?
7. **Lateral Tilt of Pelvis**
   Subject: Stand on one foot on a stool with other leg hanging free. Pull free hip up as far as possible.
   Assistant: Give slight resistance by holding down ankle.
   Observer: Palpate oblique abdominals, iliocostalis, adductor magnus, adductor longus, and gracilis on side of free leg.
8. **Hip Flexion**
   a. *Subject:* Sit on a table with legs hanging over edge. Flex the thigh at the hip joint.
   Assistant: Resist movement slightly by pressing down on knee.
   Observer: Palpate pectineus, tensor fasciae latae, sartorius, rectus femoris, and adductor longus. Does the gracilis contract?
   b. *Subject:* Lie on one side, rolled toward face. Flex thigh of top leg, allowing knee to flex passively.
   Assistant: Resist movement by pushing against knee.
   Observer: Palpate iliopsoas.
9. **Hip Extension**
   a. *Subject:* Stand facing table with trunk flexed forward until it rests on table. Grasp sides of table. Extend one thigh by raising one leg, keeping the knee extended.
   Assistant: Resist movement by pushing down on thigh close to knee. Second time, give resistance at heel.
   Observer: Palpate gluteus maximus, adductor magnus, and hamstrings.
   b. *Subject:* Lieface down on table and extend lower extremity at the hip joint, keeping the knee extended.
   Assistant: Resist movement by pushing down on knee.
   Observer: Palpate same muscles as in a.
10. **Hip Abduction**
    Subject: Lie on one side and abduct the top lower extremity at the hip joint.
    Assistant: Resist movement by pushing down on knee.
    Observer: Palpate gluteus maximus, gluteus medius, and tensor fasciae latae.
11. **Hip Adduction**
    Subject: Lie on one side with the top lower extremity abducted; then adduct it.
    Assistant: Resist movement by pressing up against knee.
    Note: Unless resistance is applied, the action will be performed by means of the eccentric contraction of the abductors.
    Observer: Palpate three adductors and name them.
12. **Outward Rotation of Thigh**
    Subject: Stand on one foot with the other leg flexed at the knee so that the lower leg extends horizontally backward. Rotate the free thigh outward by swinging the foot medially.
    Assistant: Steady subject's knee and resist movement of leg at ankle.
    Observer: Palpate gluteus maximus.
13. **Inward Rotation of Thigh**
    Subject: Stand on one foot with other leg flexed at the knee so that the lower leg extends

horizontally backward. Rotate the free thigh inward by swinging the foot laterally.

Assistant: Steady subject's knee and resist movement of leg at ankle.

Observer: Palpate gluteus medius, tensor fasciae latae, and lower adductor magnus.

Kinesiological Analysis

14. Choose a simple motor skill from Appendix G. Do a complete anatomical analysis of the hip region, following the format shown in Table 1.2.

CHAPTER 8

The Lower Extremity

The Knee, Ankle, and Foot

OUTLINE

OBJECTIVES

At the conclusion of this chapter, the student should be able to:

1. Name, locate, and describe the structure and ligamentous reinforcements of the articulations of the knee, ankle, and foot.
2. Name and demonstrate the movements possible in the joints of the knee, ankle, and foot, regardless of starting position.
3. Name and locate the muscles and muscle groups of the knee, ankle, and foot, and name their primary actions as agonists, stabilizers, neutralizers, or antagonists.
4. Analyze the fundamental movements of the lower leg and foot with respect to joint and muscle actions.
5. Describe the common injuries of the leg, knee, and ankle.
6. Perform an anatomical analysis of the lower extremity in a motor skill.

The Knee Joint

The knee joint is the largest and most complex joint in the human body. It is a masterpiece of anatomical engineering. Placed midway down each supporting column of the body, it is subject to severe stresses and strains in its combined functions of weight bearing and locomotion. To take care of the weight-bearing stresses, it has massive condyles; to facilitate locomotion, it has a wide range of motion; to resist the lateral stresses due to the tremendous lever effect of the long femur and tibia, it is reinforced at the sides by strong ligaments; to combat the downward pull of gravity and to meet the demands of such violent locomotor activities as running and jumping, it is provided with powerful musculature. It would be difficult, indeed, to find a mechanism better adapted for meeting the combined requirements of stability and mobility than the knee joint.

Structure

Although the knee is classified as a hinge joint, its bony structure resembles two condyloid or ovoid joints lying side by side, yet not quite parallel (Figure 8.1). The lateral flexion permitted in a single ovoid joint is not possible in the knee joint because of the presence of the second condyle. The two rockerlike condyles of the femur rest on the two slightly concave areas on the top of the tibia's broad head. These articular surfaces of the tibia are separated by a roughened area, called the intercondyloid eminence, which terminates both anteriorly and posteriorly in a slight hollow but rises at the center to form two small tubercles like miniature twin mountain peaks (Figure 8.2). During knee extension, the intercondyloid tubercles enter the intercondyloid fossa of the femur. The medial articular surface of the tibia is oval; the lateral is smaller and more nearly round. Each is overlaid by a somewhat crescent-shaped fibrocartilage, known as a semilunar cartilage, or meniscus.

The lower end of the femur terminates in the two rockerlike condyles already mentioned. The lateral condyle is broader and more prominent than the medial. The medial condyle projects downward farther than the lateral. This is evident, however, only when a disarticulated femur is held vertically. In its normal position in the body, the femur slants inward from above. This slant is known as the obliquity of the femoral shaft. Observation of the mounted skeleton will show that the downward projection of the medial condyle compensates for the obliquity of the femoral shaft.

Another interesting feature of the condyles is that they are not quite parallel. Whereas the

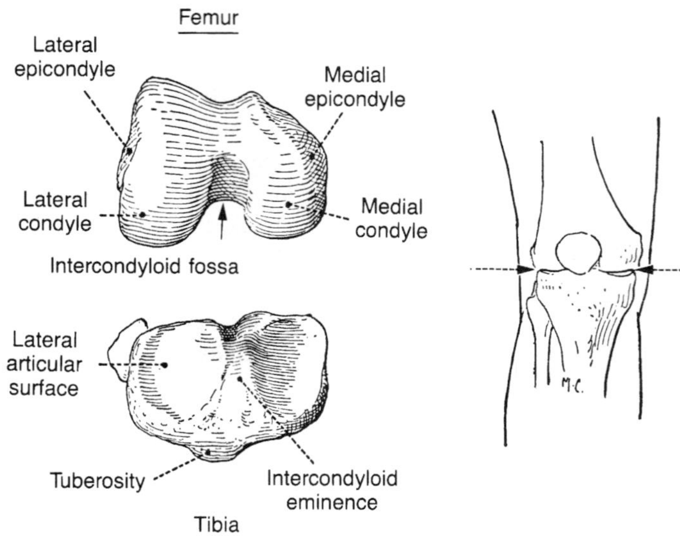

Figure 8.1 Articulating surfaces of knee joint.

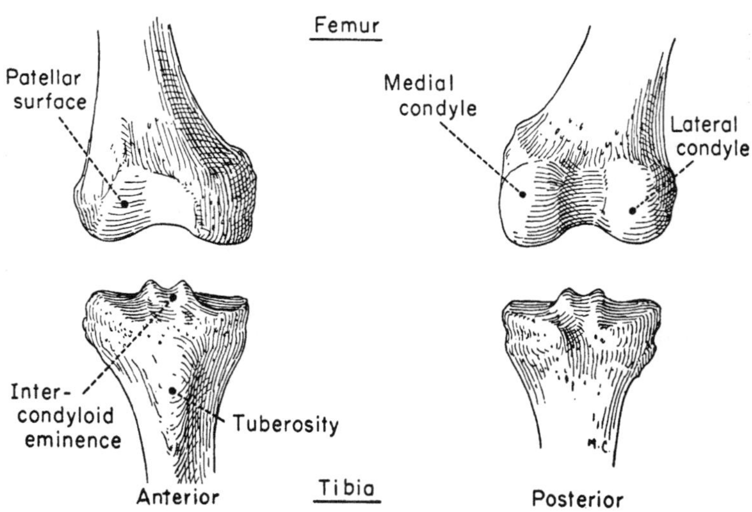

Figure 8.2 Anterior and posterior views of bones of knee joint.

lateral condyle lies in the sagittal plane, the medial condyle slants slightly medially from front to back. This is an important factor in the movements of the knee.

Anteriorly, the two condyles are continuous with the smooth, slightly concave surface of the patellar facet for the articulation of the patella. The patella, or kneecap, is a large sesamoid bone located slightly above and in front of the knee joint. It is held in place by the quadriceps tendon above, by the patellar ligament below, and by the intervening fibers that form a pocket for the patella (Figure 8.3).

The articular cavity is enclosed within a loose membranous capsule that lies under the patella and folds around each condyle but excludes the

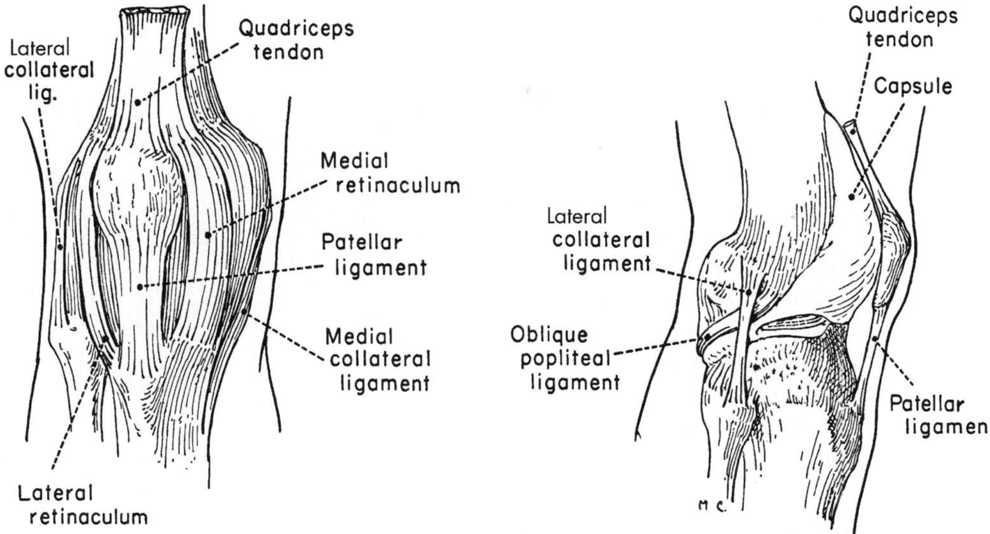

Figure 8.3 (a) Anterior and (b) lateral views of knee joint showing ligaments.

intercondyloid tubercles and cruciate ligaments. It is supplemented by expansions from the fascia lata, iliotibial tract, and various tendons. The oblique popliteal ligament covers the posterior surface of the joint completely, shielding the cruciate ligaments and other structures not enclosed within the capsule.

The synovial membrane of the knee joint is the most extensive of any in the body. It folds in and around the joint in a manner far too complicated to attempt to describe here. There are numerous bursae in the vicinity of the knee joint. The largest and most important of these bursae are the prepatellar, infrapatellar, and suprapatellar bursae.

Menisci

The menisci (Figure 8.4) are circular rims of fibrocartilage situated on the articular surfaces of the head of the tibia. They are relatively thick at their peripheral borders but taper to a thin edge at their inner circumferences. Thus they deepen the articular facets of the tibia and, at the same time, serve in a shock-absorbing capacity. The inner edges are free, but the peripheral borders are attached loosely to the rim of the head of the tibia by fibers from the inner surface of the capsule.

The lateral meniscus forms an incomplete circle, conforming closely to the nearly round articular facet. Its anterior and posterior horns, which almost meet at the center of the joint, are attached to the intercondyloid eminence.

The medial cartilage is shaped like a large letter *C*, broader toward the rear than in front. Its anterior horn tapers off to a thin strand attached to the anterior intercondyloid fossa. It is not as freely movable as the lateral cartilage, because of

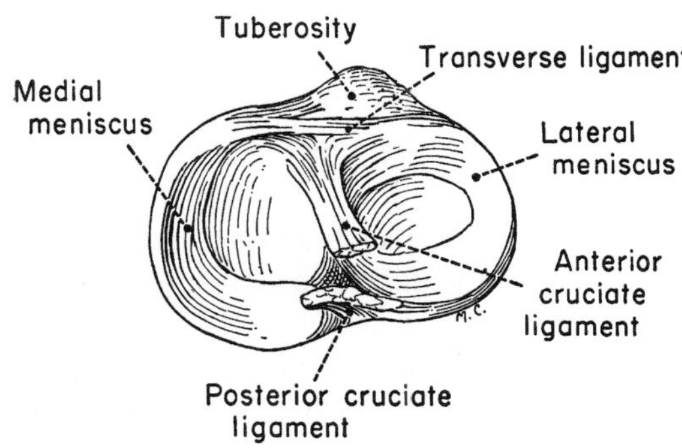

Figure 8.4 The menisci of the knee joint.

its secure anchorage to the medial collateral ligament at the medial side of the knee and the semimembranosus muscle posteriorly. Largely because of these points of attachment, the medial cartilage is more frequently injured than the lateral.

Patellofemoral Joint

The patella is the largest sesamoid bone in the body. Located on the anterior side of the femur at the knee joint, the patella has several functions. The depth of the patella serves as a pulley to increase the angle of pull of the quadriceps muscles. Because all four of these muscles converge at the patella, through the quadriceps tendon, the patella functions to direct the force of the quadriceps through the patellar ligament.

The posterior surface of the patella articulates with the femur at the patellar surface, or patellar groove. As the knee flexes, the patella slides in this groove in a motion referred to as patellar tracking. As the quadriceps muscles exert a pull on the patella, the patella is pulled against the femur, increasing both contact area and contact forces. As the patella tracks downward over the femur during knee flexion, it will tilt inferiorly and slightly medially, returning during extension (Patel et al., 2003).

Ligaments of the Knee

Patellar Ligament (*Figure 8.3*)

This is a strong, flat ligament connecting the lower margin of the patella with the tuberosity of the tibia. Passing over the front of the patella, the superficial fibers are continuations of the central fibers of the quadriceps femoris tendon.

Medial Collateral Ligament
(*Figures 8.3a and 8.5*)

This is a broad, flat, membranous band on the medial side of the joint. It is attached above to the medial epicondyle of the femur below the adductor tubercle and below to the medial condyle of the tibia. It is firmly attached to the medial meniscus. This fact should be noted because of its

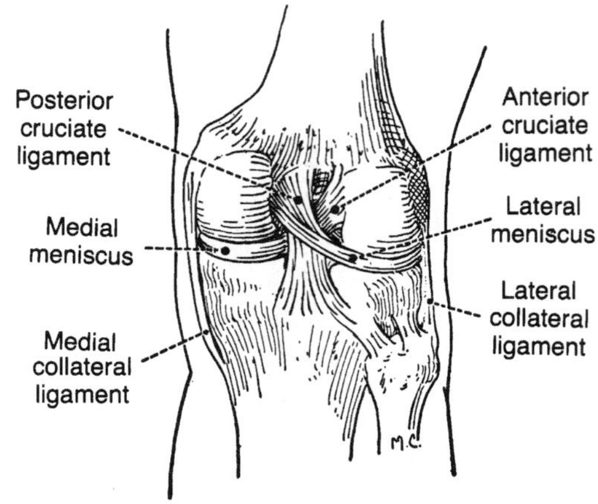

Figure 8.5 Posterior view of knee joint showing cruciate ligaments.

significance in knee injuries. It serves to check extension and to prevent motion laterally.

Lateral Collateral Ligament
(*Figures 8.3 and 8.5*)

This is a strong, rounded cord attached above to the back of the lateral epicondyle of the femur and below to the lateral surface of the head of the fibula. It serves to check extension and to prevent motion medially.

Oblique Popliteal Ligament (*Figure 8.3b*)

This is a broad, flat ligament covering the back of the knee joint. It is attached above to the upper margin of the intercondyloid fossa and posterior surface of the femur and below to the posterior margin of the head of the tibia. Medially it blends with the tendon of the semimembranosus muscle, and laterally with the lateral head of the gastrocnemius. It too protects against hyperextension.

The Cruciate Ligaments (*Figure 8.5*)

These are two strong, cordlike ligaments situated within the knee joint, although not enclosed within the joint capsule. They are called cruciate because they cross each other. They are further designated anterior and posterior, according to their attachments to the tibia. They serve to check certain movements at the knee joint. They limit extension and prevent rotation in the extended position. They also check the forward and backward sliding of the femur on the tibia, thus safeguarding the anteroposterior stability of the knee.

Anterior cruciate ligament *(Figure 8.5)* This passes upward and backward from the anterior intercondyloid fossa of the tibia to the back part of the medial surface of the lateral condyle of the femur.

Posterior cruciate ligament *(Figure 8.5)* This is a shorter and stronger ligament than the anterior. It passes upward and forward from the posterior intercondyloid fossa of the tibia to the lateral and front part of the medial condyle of the femur.

Transverse Ligament (Figure 8.4)

This is a short, slender, cordlike ligament connecting the anterior convex margin of the lateral meniscus to the anterior end of the medial meniscus.

The Iliotibial Tract (Figures 7.18 and 7.19)

The iliotibial tract is said to act like a tense ligament that connects the iliac crest with the lateral femoral condyle and the lateral tubercle of the tibia. At the knee joint the tract serves as a stabilizing ligament between the lateral condyle of the femur and the tibia.

Movements

The movements that occur at the knee joint are primarily flexion and extension. A slight amount of rotation can take place when the knee is in the flexed position and the foot is not supporting the weight or during the initial stages of flexion and the final stages of extension (Figure 8.6).

Flexion and Extension

The movements of flexion and extension at the knee are not as simple as those of a true hinge joint. This can be demonstrated in the classroom

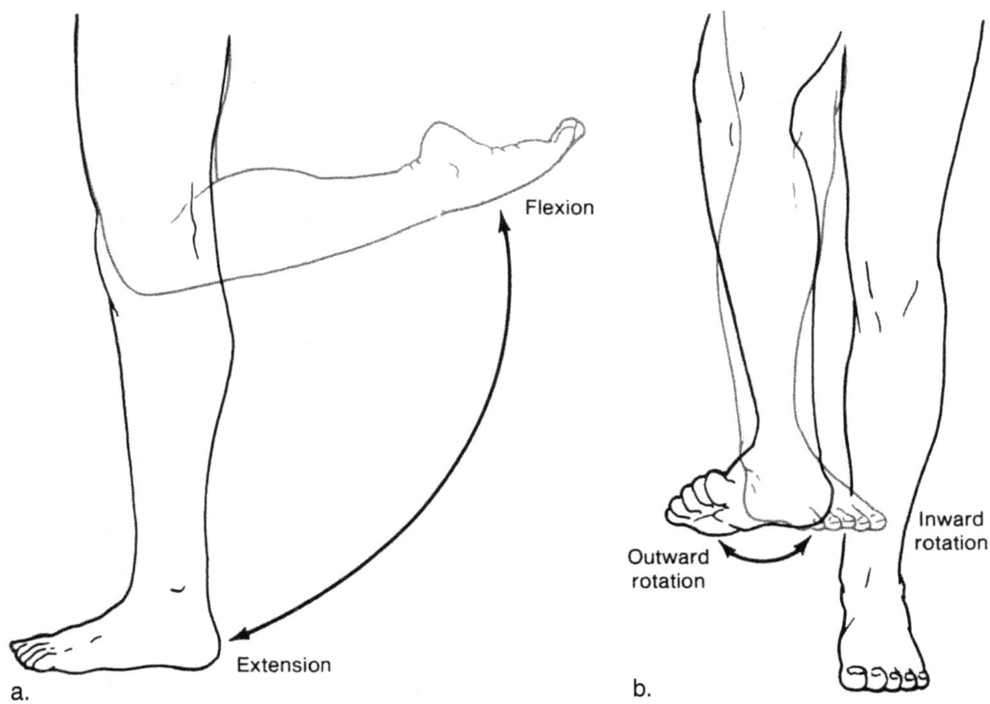

Figure 8.6 Movements of the knee joint: (a) flexion and extension; (b) inward and outward rotation (in flexed, non-weight-bearing position).

by holding a disarticulated femur and tibia together in a position of extension and then, holding the tibia stationary, flexing the femur on the tibia as though the individual were assuming a squat or sitting position. If no other adjustment is made, the femoral condyles will roll back completely off the top of the tibia. What prevents this from happening in real life is the fact that, as the condyles roll backward, they simultaneously glide forward and thus remain in contact with the menisci throughout each phase of the movement. In addition, the anterior cruciate becomes taut and prevents further backward translation. Conversely, when the femur extends on the tibia, the forward roll of the femoral condyles is accompanied by both a backward glide and the pull of the posterior cruciate to help prevent forward dislocation.

Because the femoral condyles are not quite parallel and the medial condyle is slightly longer, a slight degree of rotation occurs during the initial phase of flexion and the final phase of extension. This can be seen readily on the living subject who stands with the knees slightly flexed and then extends them completely. The patellae turn slightly medialward, indicating slight inward rotation of the thighs. Because of the inequality of the two condyles, the medial condyle continues to roll forward after the lateral condyle has ceased its movement. The inward rotation of the femur that accompanies the completion of extension is commonly known as the "locking" or "screw home" mechanism of the knees. In persons who tend to hyperextend their knees habitually, the rotation is more pronounced.

When the leg is flexed or extended in a non-weight-bearing position, the tibia rotates on the femur, instead of vice versa. The final phase of extension is accompanied by slight outward rotation of the tibia. At the beginning of flexion the tibia rotates inward until the midposition is attained.

The rotation that occurs in the final stage of extension and the initial phase of flexion is an inherent part of these movements and should not be confused with the voluntary rotation that can be performed when the leg is not bearing weight and the knee is in a flexed position.

Inward and Outward Rotation in the Flexed Position

In spite of the fact that the knee joint is classified as a hinge joint, its condylar structure accommodates movement other than just flexion and extension under certain conditions. When the leg has been flexed at the knee, the collateral ligaments become slack and it is possible to rotate the leg on the thigh through a total range of about 50 degrees. This can occur, however, only when the leg is not bearing the body weight. It is impossible, for instance, to rotate either the leg or the thigh in this manner when the body is in a stooping position. A good way to demonstrate rotation of the tibia is to sit on a chair with the heel resting lightly on the floor. In this position, with the knee and thigh held motionless, the foot should be turned first in and then out. The action will be that of inward and outward rotation of the tibia. The movement taking place within the foot itself should be discounted. Taut collateral and cruciate ligaments prevent rotation when the leg is extended at the knee, either in a weight-bearing or non-weight-bearing position. Inward or outward movements of the foot in the extended position are due to rotation at the hip joint.

MUSCLES OF THE KNEE JOINT

Location

The muscles acting on the knee joint are classified as anterior or posterior according to the relation of their distal tendons to the transverse axis of the joint.

Anterior	**Posterior**
Quadriceps femoris group	Hamstring group
Rectus femoris	Biceps femoris
Vastus intermedius	Semimembranosus
Vastus lateralis	Semitendinosus
Vastus medialis	Sartorius
	Gracilis
	Popliteus
	Gastrocnemius

Characteristics and Functions of Individual Muscles

Quadriceps Femoris Group

This group (Figures 8.3, 8.7, and 8.8) consists of the rectus femoris and the vasti: vastus intermedius, vastus lateralis, and vastus medialis. Of these, only the rectus femoris, the most superficial of the four, crosses the hip joint. The vastus intermedius lies posterior to the rectus and is completely covered by it. The distal portions of the four muscles unite to form a single broad, flat tendon that attaches to the base of the patella, the base being the upper border. The patellar ligament connecting the patella with the tuberosity of the tibia is a vital part of the quadriceps femoris. Actually, the patella is a sesamoid bone encased within the quadriceps tendon, with the patellar ligament being but a continuation of this and the tibial tuberosity the true distal point of attachment of the muscle group. All four muscles extend the leg at the knee joint and function as a unit in doing so.

The vastus lateralis and vastus medialis, with their fibers converging toward the patella, act with the vastus intermedius and rectus femoris, with their longitudinal approach, to steady the knee joint in weight-bearing positions and to maintain a balanced

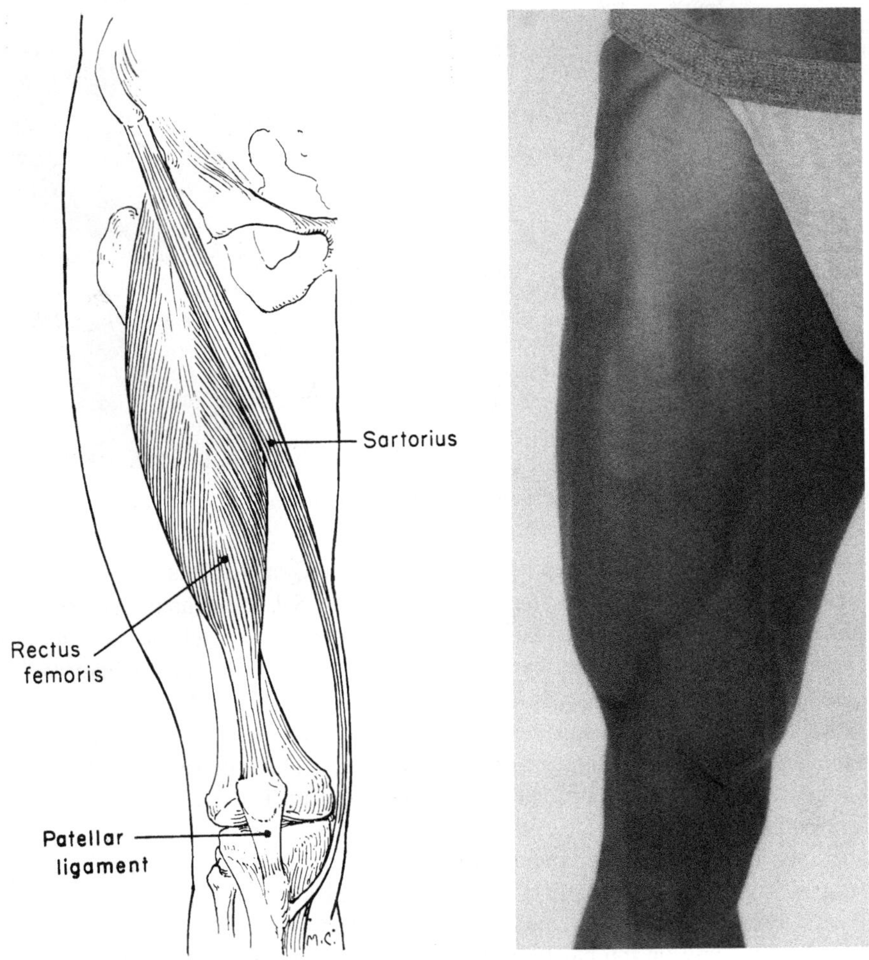

Figure 8.7 Front of thigh showing rectus femoris and sartorius muscles.

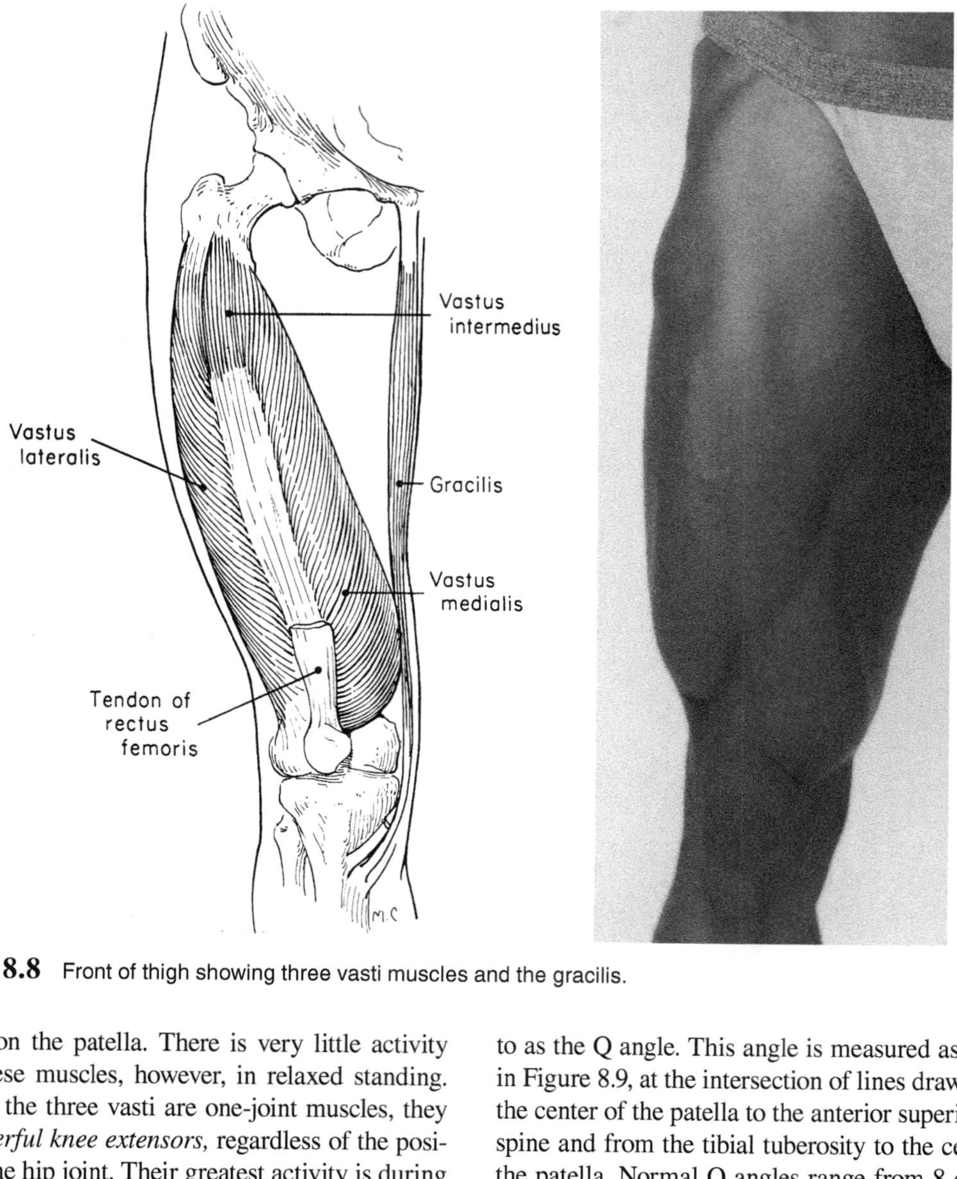

Figure 8.8 Front of thigh showing three vasti muscles and the gracilis.

tension on the patella. There is very little activity from these muscles, however, in relaxed standing. Because the three vasti are one-joint muscles, they are *powerful knee extensors,* regardless of the position of the hip joint. Their greatest activity is during the last part of knee extension. The vastus medialis is the most active of the three throughout the greatest range of knee extension. Its lower portion is also important in preventing lateral dislocation of the patella. When the knee is fully extended, static contraction of the quadriceps serves to pull up or "set" the patella, a mild exercise used in rehabilitation of the injured knee. This pull on the patella is not directly vertical but is at an angle to the femur. The pull angle of the quadriceps is commonly referred to as the Q angle. This angle is measured as shown in Figure 8.9, at the intersection of lines drawn from the center of the patella to the anterior superior iliac spine and from the tibial tuberosity to the center of the patella. Normal Q angles range from 8 degrees to 17 degrees, usually slightly higher in females than in males. The influence of Q angle on patellofemoral problems is still a matter of debate. Research on this topic has produced conflicting results, and the final word has yet to be written (Hand & Spalding, 2004; Heiderscheit et al., 2000; Mizuno et al., 2001).

The two-joint *rectus femoris* (also listed with the hip muscles) is of bipenniform structure with all except the lowest fibers slanting obliquely downward and sideward from the central tendon and the lowest fibers being approximately vertical (see Figure 8.7). The upper three-quarters of the muscle consists of the muscle fibers, with the last quarter, down to the base of the patella, being the muscle's distal tendon. The entire muscle contracts regardless of whether it is producing movement at the hip joint or knee joint. It is most effective at the knee joint when the hip joint is extended. The muscle may be palpated on the central-anterior surface of the thigh.

The majority of the *vastus lateralis* fibers slant downward and medialward to the tendon. The muscle may be palpated on the anterolateral aspect of the thigh, lateral to the rectus femoris.

Most of the fibers of the *vastus medialis* slant downward and lateralward to the tendon, with the lowest ones almost horizontal in direction. If the lateralis and medialis were looked upon as one muscle, it would be considered to be of bipenniform construction, with the fibers slanting in direct opposition to those of the rectus femoris. The fleshy part of both the medialis and lateralis extends down almost to the level of the base of the patella. The vastus medialis may be palpated on the anteromedial aspect of the lower third of the thigh, medial to the rectus femoris.

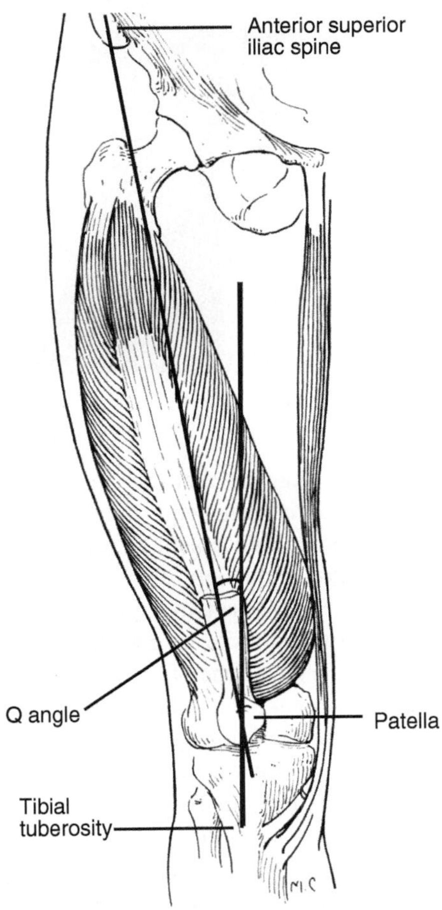

Figure 8.9 Q angle.

Hamstring Group (Also Listed with the Hip Muscles)

The hamstrings (Figures 8.10 and 8.11), so named from their large, cordlike tendons behind the knee joint, consist of the biceps femoris, semimembranosus, and semitendinosus muscles. Although the biceps femoris constitutes the lateral hamstring, its long head lies approximately along the midline of the posterior aspect of the thigh, as far down as the popliteal space. The long head comes from the tuberosity of the ischium, and the short head originates from the linea aspera on the posterior surface of the thigh. The two join at the distal tendon close to the lateral condyle of the femur, not far above the tendon's attachment to the head of the fibula. It is an important *flexor of the knee.* When the knee is flexed and not bearing weight, the biceps femoris can rotate the lower leg outward. Its tendon may be palpated behind the knee on its lateral aspect. The long head is fusiform in construction; the short head is penniform.

The *semimembranosus* and *semitendinosus* constitute the medial hamstrings. The former lies deeper than the latter and attaches higher on the tibia. The semitendinosus is attached to the medial surface of the tibia, below the head, just below the attachment of the gracilis and behind that of the sartorius. Like the biceps femoris, they *flex* the knee joint. Unlike the biceps femoris, the semimembranosus and semitendinosus medially rotate the unweighted and flexed tibia. The semitendinosus may be palpated on the medial aspect of the posterior surface of the knee. The tendon of the semimembranosus is almost impossible to palpate successfully because it is shorter than its partner and is partially covered by the latter, as well as by the gracilis tendon.

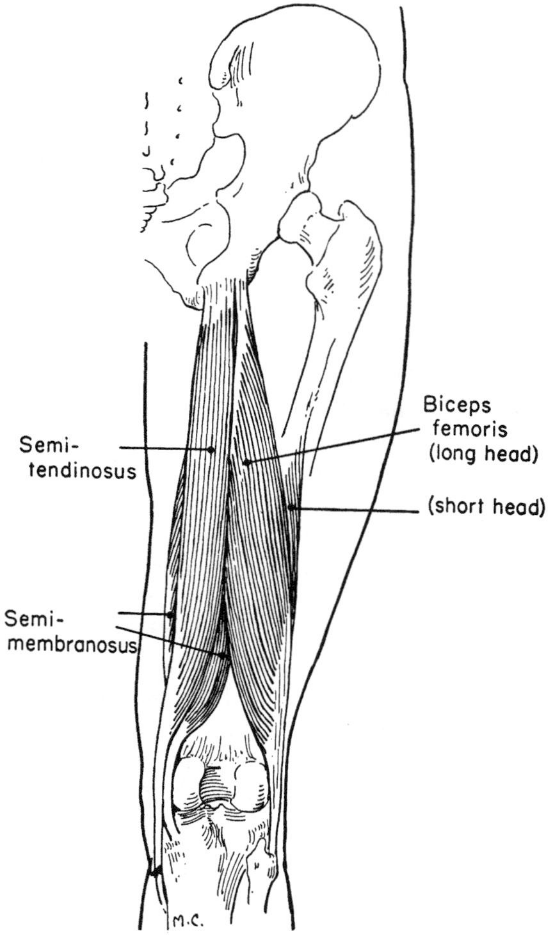

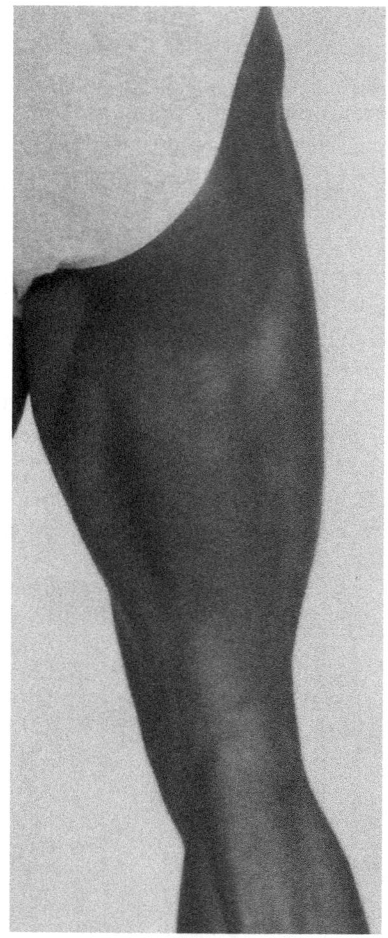

Figure 8.10 Hamstring muscles.

Nearly everyone is familiar with the limiting effect of the hamstrings. Many experience difficulty in touching the toes with the fingers without bending the knees and in sitting erect on the floor with the legs extended straight forward because the hamstrings are frequently not long enough to permit such extreme stretching at the hips and knees simultaneously.

Hamstrings-Quadriceps Ratio

Since most lower extremity motions involve cocontraction of the hamstrings and quadriceps muscle groups, the relative strength of these two sets of muscles can have an impact on the knee joint. This coactivation helps stabilize the knee against anterior displacement as well as against some abduction-adduction stress. In examining the lines of pull of these two large muscle groups, one can see two opposite facing triangles, a very stable arrangement. If one of these muscle groups is excessively weak, this stable structure is impaired, opening the knee up to injury. A normal hamstring-to-quadriceps ratio (H/Q) is around 55–60%. Interestingly, females often show a lessening of this ratio at maturity, which may explain (to some degree) the higher incidence of knee injuries in females (Hewett, et al., 2009).

Sartorius *(Also Listed with the Hip Muscles)*

This is a long, slender, ribbonlike muscle (see Figure 8.7) superficially located and directed obliquely downward and medialward across the front of the thigh. On its way to its distal attachment, it curves around behind the bulge of the medial condyles in such a way that its line of pull is posterior to the axis of the knee joint. Thus, even though at least two-thirds of the muscle, including both its proximal and distal attachments, lies on the anterior aspect of the lower extremity, its action at the knee joint is generally *flexion,* not extension. It also assists in inward rotation of the tibia when the leg is flexed at the knee and *is not bearing weight.* The line of pull of the sartorius is determined by the direction of its distal tendon, between the latter's point of contact with the medial condyle of the tibia and its attachment to the upper anteromedial surface of the tibial shaft, almost as far forward as the anterior crest. It may be palpated at the anterior superior iliac spine, as well as along its entire length, where it is clearly visible on a thin, well-muscled subject.

Gracilis *(Also Listed with the Hip Muscles)*

This is a long, slender muscle (see Figures 8.8 and 8.11) situated on the medial aspect of the thigh. Its action at the knee joint is *flexion.* It also is slightly active in *inward rotation of the tibia when the knee is in a flexed position and the foot is not bearing weight.* It may be palpated on the medial aspect of the posterior surface of the knee, anterior to the semitendinosus tendon but close to it.

Popliteus

This muscle (see Figure 8.11) *rotates the tibia inward* and *helps flex the knee.* In structure and function it resembles the pronator teres muscle of the elbow. In a subject who is standing, it "unlocks" the knee joint preliminary to flexion. It also helps protect and stabilize the knee joint from forward dislocation of the femur when a squatting position is assumed and maintained. During walking, it is active throughout most of the weight-bearing phase (Basmajian & DeLuca, 1985).

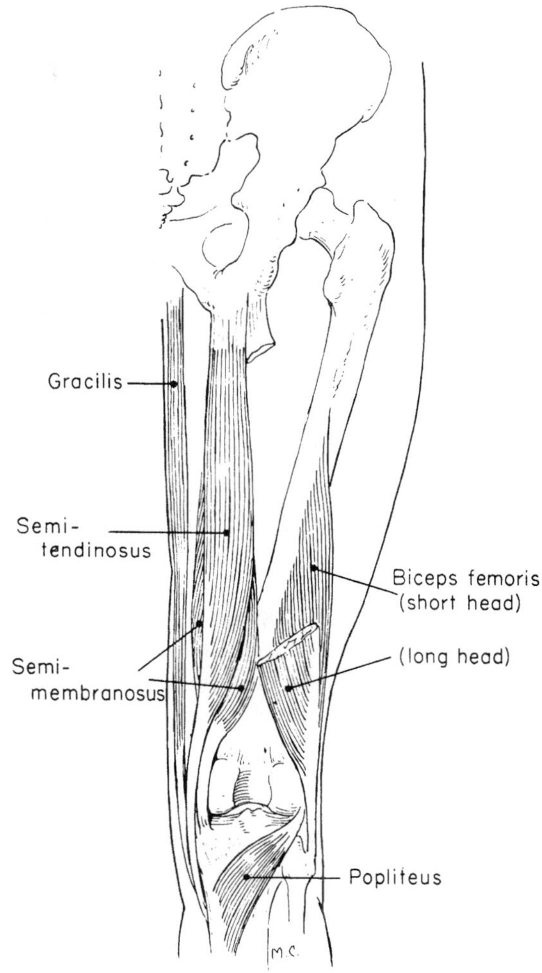

Figure 8.11 Posterior muscles of thigh and knee.

Gastrocnemius *(Also Listed with the Ankle Muscles)*

This large calf muscle (see Figure 8.23), although primarily a muscle of the ankle joint, has an important function at the knee joint. It is in a position to help *flex* the knee and does so when the leg is not bearing weight. It also functions at the knee as a *posterior ligament* to protect the joint in movements involving violent extension, as in running and jumping.

When the foot is fixed in weight bearing, *the gastrocnemius can help maintain knee extension.*

It does this when the hip and knee are in strong extension and when plantar flexion of the ankle is inhibited, such as when the line of gravity passes in front of the knee and ankle joints. Under these circumstances, the gastrocnemius is able to pull back and down on the femoral condyles, thus contributing to knee extension. Its activity in "relaxed standing at ease" was found in three-fourths of subjects tested barefooted. The wearing of high heels increased the frequency of subjects whose muscles were active. The muscle is easy to palpate, including both the muscle belly in the calf and the tendon behind the ankle.

Muscular Analysis of the Fundamental Movements of the Leg at the Knee Joint

Flexion

The knee joint has five important flexors, namely the three hamstring muscles (biceps femoris, semimembranosus, and semitendinosus), the sartorius, and the gracilis; the latter is especially important during the early part of flexion, provided that the hip is not flexing simultaneously. Two additional muscles that help with flexion are the popliteus and gastrocnemius.

It should be remembered that when the weight is borne by the feet and the knees are allowed to flex, as in stooping, the knee flexors are not responsible for the movement. The flexion is produced by the force of gravity and is controlled by the extensor muscles that are contracting eccentrically, that is, in lengthening contraction.

The three adductors have also been shown to be active in most children during flexion and extension of the knee with or without external resistance. They were also active under the same conditions in most adults during knee flexion, but activity of these muscles during extension occurred only when resistance was applied (Basmajian & DeLuca, 1985).

Extension

This action is performed by the four muscles that make up the quadriceps femoris group: the rectus femoris, the vastus intermedius, the vastus lateralis, and the vastus medialis.

Outward Rotation of the Tibia

This action is performed by the biceps femoris. It can occur only when the knee is flexed in a non-weight-bearing situation.

Inward Rotation of the Tibia

This action is performed chiefly by the semimembranosus, semitendinosus, and popliteus, with possible help from the gracilis and sartorius. As with outward rotation, it can occur only when the knee is flexed and the foot is not bearing weight.

The Ankle and the Foot

The foot has two functions of great importance: support and propulsion. In studying the structure of the foot, one should keep these functions in mind. Only by seeing the foot in terms of the combined static and dynamic demands made upon it can one fully appreciate its intricate mechanism.

The foot is united with the leg at the ankle joint. Within the foot itself are the seven tarsal bones. Two of the joints in this region are of sufficient importance to the kinesiologist to merit special attention. These are the subtalar and midtarsal joints, the latter including the talonavicular and calcaneocuboid articulations. The movements within the foot occur mainly at these two joints.

The structure of the ankle, tarsal joints, and toes will be described separately, but the muscles of these three regions will be discussed together because many of them act on more than one joint.

Structure of the Ankle

The ankle (talocrural) joint (Figures 8.12, 8.13, and 8.14) is a hinge joint. It is formed by the articulation of the talus (astragalus) with the malleoli of the tibia and the fibula. The malleolus of the fibula lies more posterior and extends more distally than that of the tibia. The malleoli of the tibia and fibula, bound together by the transverse tibiofibular ligament, the anterior and posterior ligaments of the lateral malleolus, and the interossei, constitute a mortise into which the upper, rounded portion of the talus fits. The transverse tibiofibular ligament secures the

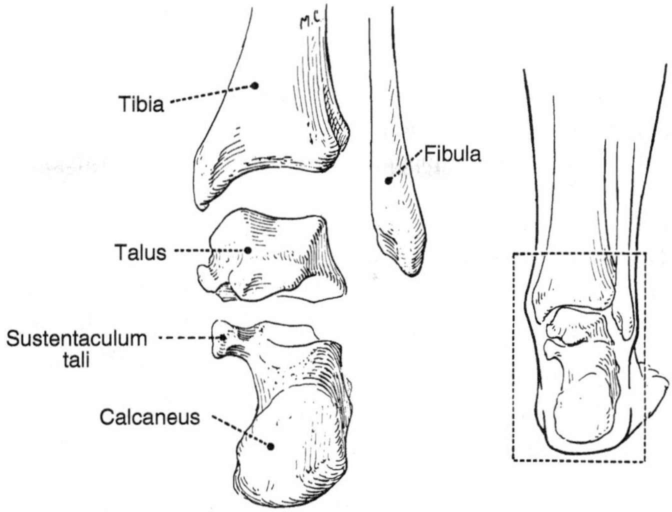

Figure 8.12 Bones of ankle and subtalar joints, posterior view.

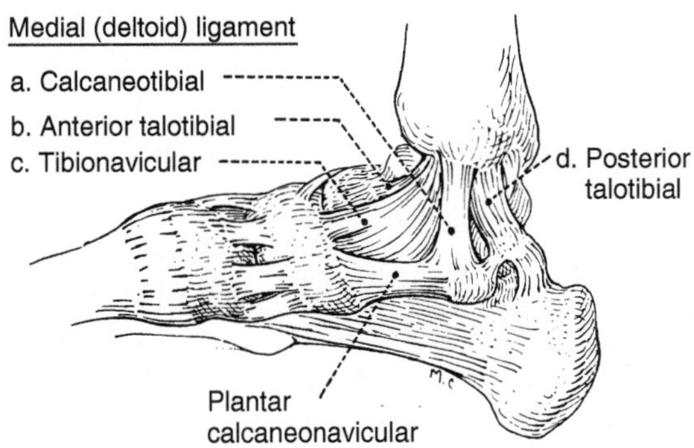

Figure 8.13 Medial ligaments of ankle joint.

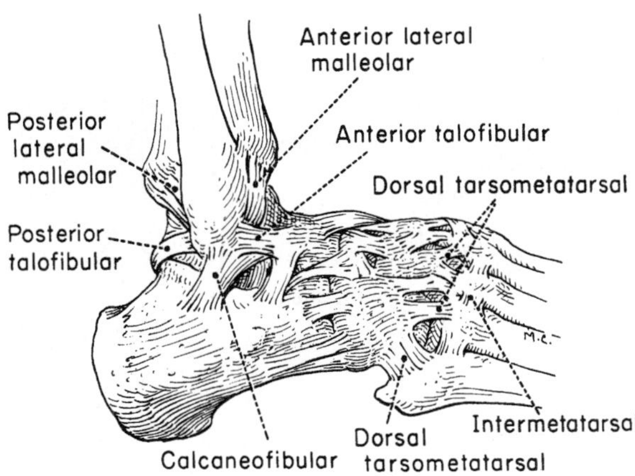

Figure 8.14 Lateral ligaments of ankle joint.

lateral and medial malleoli and the back surface of the talus. The ankle joint is surrounded by a thin, membranous capsule that is thicker on the medial side of the joint. In the back it is a thin mesh of membranous tissue and is not continuous, as are most capsules. It is reinforced by several strong ligaments.

Ligamentous Reinforcement

The medial side of the ankle joint is protected by five strong, ligamentous bands (see Figure 8.13), four of them connecting the medial malleolus of the tibia with the posterior tarsal bones, the calcaneus, talus, and navicular. These four ligaments are known collectively as the deltoid ligament. Individually they are the calcaneotibial, the anterior talotibial, the tibionavicular, and the posterior talotibial ligaments. The fifth band (plantar calcaneonavicular) provides a horizontal connection between the navicular bone and the sustentaculum tali projection on the medial aspect of the calcaneus. It is also known as the spring ligament.

The lateral side of the ankle is reinforced (see Figure 8.14) by three ligaments collectively called the lateral collateral ligament. These connect the lateral malleolus with the upper lateral aspect of the calcaneus and with anterior and posterior portions of the talus. The components of the lateral collateral ligament are named the calcaneofibular and anterior and posterior talofibular ligaments, respectively. The lateral ligaments are weaker than the medial ligaments, and the anterior talofibular ligament is the weakest of all. Inspection of Figures 8.13 and 8.14 gives one the impression that the lateral side of the ankle is less protected than the medial. These facts help explain the high incidence of lateral ankle sprains.

Structure of the Foot

The foot as a whole (Figures 8.15 and 8.16) is usually described as an elastic arched structure, the keystone of the arch being the talus. This bone has several marks of distinction. Aside from being

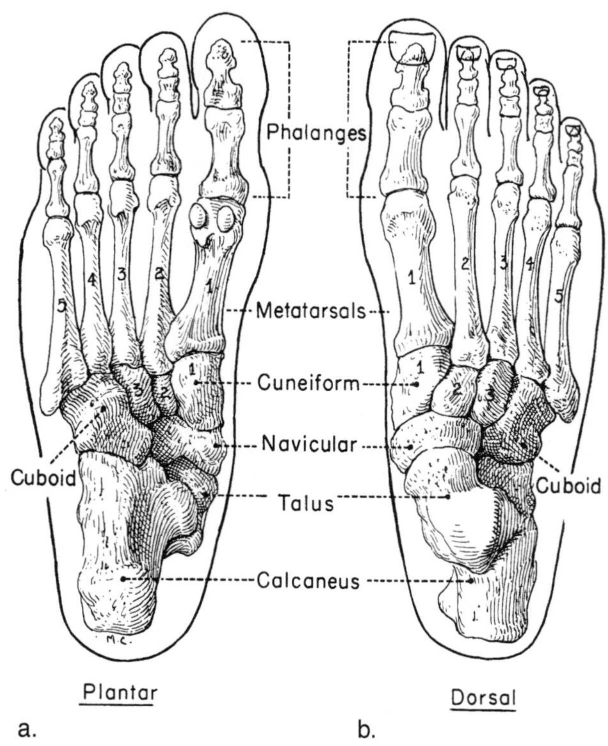

Figure 8.15 Bones of the foot: plantar and dorsal views.

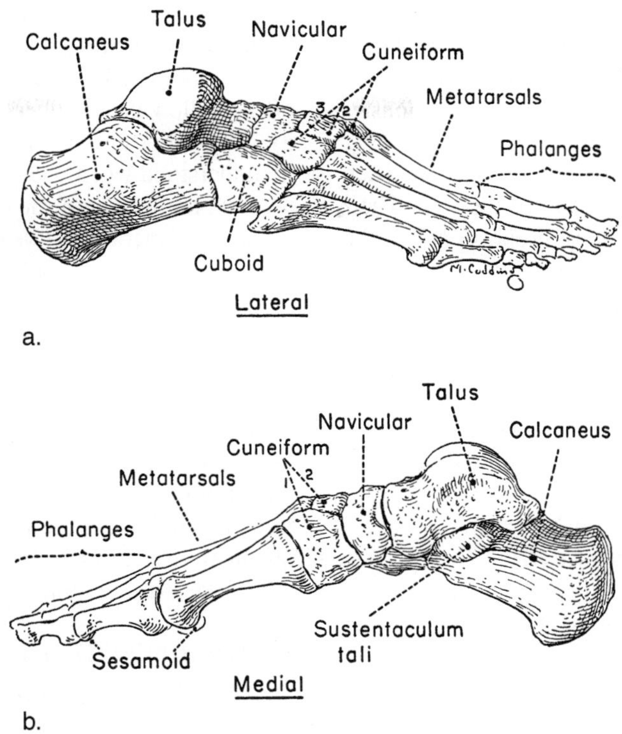

Figure 8.16 Bones of the foot: lateral and medial views.

the connecting link between the foot and the leg, it is distinguished by having no muscles attached to it and by receiving and transmitting the weight of the entire body (with the exception of the foot itself), a function that requires great strength and firm support.

The foot has two arches, a longitudinal and a transverse. The longitudinal arch extends from the heel to the heads of the five metatarsals. It is sometimes described as being made up of a medial and a lateral component. The lateral component includes the calcaneus, cuboid, and fourth and fifth metatarsals (Figure 8.16a). The medial component consists of the calcaneus, talus, navicular, three cuneiforms, and the three medial metatarsals (Figure 8.16b). The lateral component has a nearly flat contour and lacks mobility; hence, it is better adapted to the function of support. The medial component, with its greater flexibility and its curving arch, is adapted to the function of shock absorption, so important in all forms of locomotion. The longitudinal arch is strongly supported by the plantar fascia. The fascia is a relatively strong sheet of tissue attached to the calcaneous, each of the metatarsal heads, and several of the tarsal bones (cuneiform and navicular) as well as the base of the first and fifth metatarsals. The plantar fascia helps maintain the arch of the foot. It also transmits forces from the Achilles tendon to the forefoot. These loads can be as much as 92% of the body weight (Cheung et al., 2004; Erdemir et al., 2004). Contrary to popular opinion, the height of the longitudinal arch is not indicative of the strength of the arch. Thus, a low arch is not necessarily a weak one, *provided it is not associated with a pronated (i.e., abducted and everted) foot.*

The transverse arch is the side-to-side concavity on the underside of the foot formed by the anterior tarsal bones and the metatarsals. The anterior boundary of this arch under the metatarsal heads is known as the metatarsal arch. There is some disagreement as to whether this should be called an arch, because it flattens completely when bearing weight. The metatarsal arch exists, therefore, only in non-weight-bearing situations. The toes, especially the large and powerful "big toes," are largely responsible for propulsion. They provide the push-off at the end of the step. Their use in locomotion is directly proportional to the vigor and speed of the walk or run.

The strength and elasticity of the foot, which is comprised of twenty-six bones, are due largely to the ligaments that bind the bones together and to the muscles that work to preserve the balance of the foot. Thus, both ligaments and muscles share the responsibility for maintaining the integrity of the feet.

Subtalar Joint (Talocalcaneal)

This is the joint (Figure 8.17) between the underside of the talus and the upper and anterior aspects of the calcaneus, or heel, bone. It is reinforced by four small talocalcaneal ligaments. A fifth ligament, the *plantar calcaneonavicular,* is probably the most important of all. It is a broad, thick ligament that connects the sustentaculum tali projection of the calcaneus with the underside of the navicular bone. It passes under the talus and aids in supporting it. It is actually part of the subtalar joint, because it contains a fibrocartilaginous facet that is lined with synovial membrane. This is commonly called the *spring ligament* because of the yellow elastic fibers that give it its elasticity. The importance of this ligament can be readily understood when one remembers that the talus receives the weight of the entire body. The shock-absorbing function of this elastic support is obvious. It is probably equally obvious that excessive prolonged pressure on this ligament through improper use of the feet will cause it to stretch permanently and thus result in a lowered arch.

Unfortunately, Figure 8.17b gives a somewhat misleading picture of this ligament. Although it looks like a cord-shaped ligament on the medial aspect of the ankle, the part that shows in the picture is actually just the medial border of a broad ligament that extends beneath the head of the talus, like a taut hammock.

Midtarsal Joint (Transverse Tarsal; Chopart's Joint)

The midtarsal joint consists of two articulations, the lateral one being the calcaneocuboid joint and the medial one the talonavicular. Viewed from above, the continuous line of articulation—the talonavicular and calcaneocuboid—forms a somewhat shallow letter *S* (Figures 8.15b and 8.18). The talonavicular

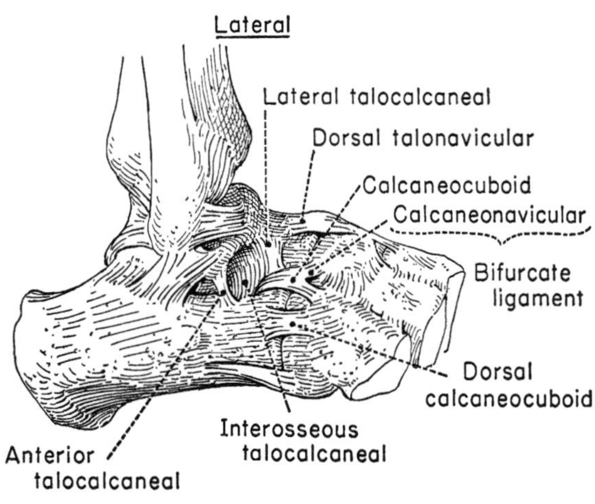

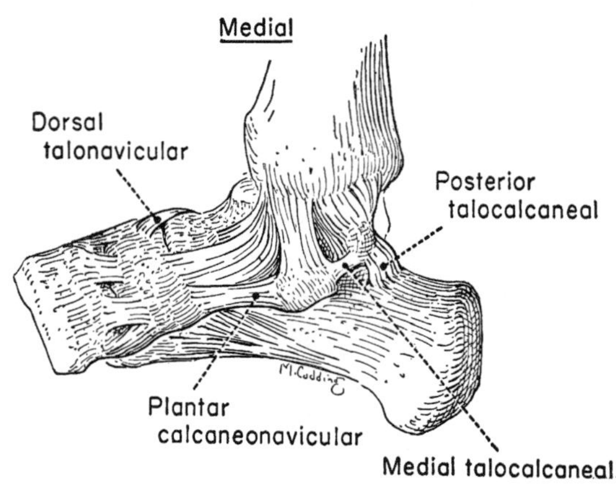

Figure 8.17 Ligaments of tarsal joints.

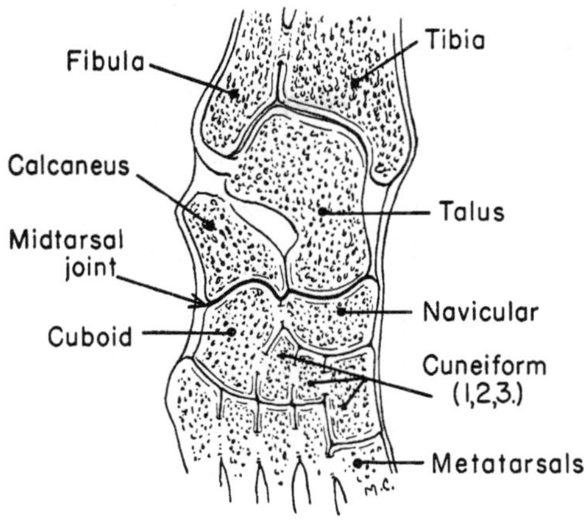

Figure 8.18 Oblique section of tarsal bones showing midtarsal joint.

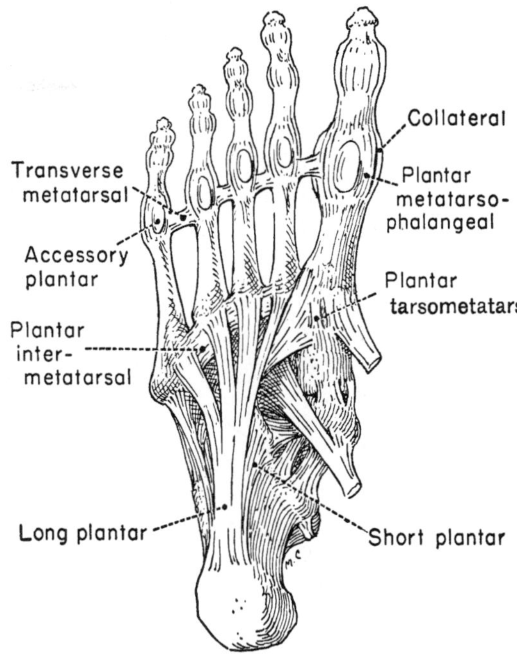

Figure 8.19 Plantar ligaments of foot.

joint is a modified ball-and-socket joint and permits somewhat restricted movements about three axes. The calcaneocuboid joint is nonaxial and permits only slight gliding motions. These seem to be supplementary or secondary to the freer motions of the talonavicular joint. Several ligaments reinforce these joints, but the ones that give the most support are the *long and short plantar (calcaneocuboid) ligaments.* These are both wide, thick ligaments of great strength.

Tarsometatarsal Joints

These joints (Figures 8.15 and 8.19) are nonaxial, with the possible exception of the great toe joint, which looks slightly like a saddle joint. The movements are of a gliding nature that resembles a restricted form of flexion, extension, abduction, and adduction.

Intermetatarsal Joints

These joints (see Figures 8.14 and 8.19) include two sets of side-by-side articulations, those between the bases and those between the heads of the metatarsal bones. They are all nonaxial joints. The articulations between the heads of the metatarsal bones are an important part of the metatarsal arch. The total result of the movements occurring there is a spreading or flattening of the arch when the weight is on it and a return to its plantar concavity when the weight is taken off it.

Metatarsophalangeal Joints

These joints (see Figures 8.15 and 8.19) may best be described as a modified form of condyloid joint. The joint of the great toe differs from the others in that it is larger and has two sesamoid bones beneath it.

Interphalangeal Joints

As is true of the fingers, these are all hinge joints (see Figures 8.15 and 8.19).

Movements of the Foot at the Ankle, Tarsal, and Toe Joints

Ankle Joint

The movements of the ankle joint occur about an axis that is usually described as bilateral but is actually slightly oblique, as evidenced by the

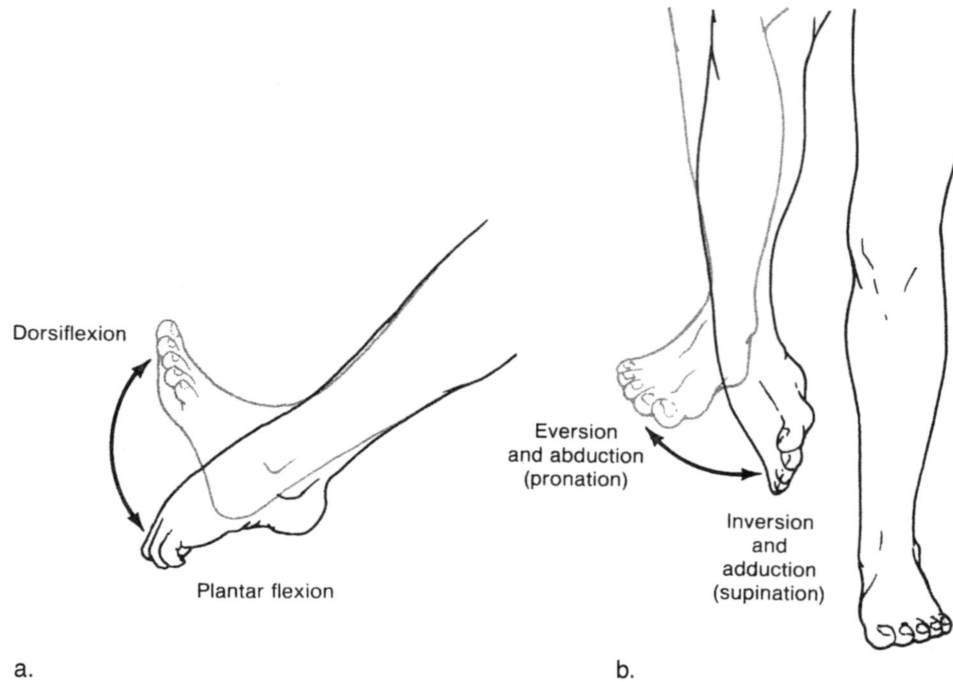

Figure 8.20 Movements of the foot at the ankle and tarsal joints: (a) dorsiflexion and plantar flexion; (b) supination and pronation (tarsal joint only).

slightly posterior position of the lateral malleolus relative to the medial. This is of minor significance, but it explains the tendency of the foot to turn out when it is fully dorsiflexed and to turn in when fully plantar flexed (Figure 8.20).

Dorsiflexion (flexion) A forward-upward movement of the foot in the sagittal plane, so that the dorsal surface of the foot approaches the anterior surface of the leg.

Plantar flexion (extension) A forward-downward movement of the foot in the sagittal plane, so that the dorsal surface of the foot moves away from the anterior surface of the leg.

Tarsal Joints

The movements that take place at the *midtarsal, subtalar,* and other *tarsal* joints occur together and are usually closely related to the ankle joint movements. Except for the talonavicular joint, which belongs to the ball-and-socket category, they are all nonaxial joints and therefore permit only slight gliding movements (Figure 8.20).

Dorsiflexion Slight decrease in convexity of dorsal surface and in concavity of plantar surface of tarsal region. Accompanies dorsiflexion of ankle.

Plantar flexion Increase in convexity of dorsal surface and in concavity of plantar surface of tarsal region. Accompanies plantar flexion of ankle.

Inversion and adduction (supination) A lifting of the medial border of the arch combined with a medial bending of the front of the foot.

Eversion and abduction (pronation) A slight raising of the lateral border of the foot combined with a slight lateral bending of the front of the foot.

Tarsometatarsal and Intermetatarsal Joints

These joints have a slight gliding motion. The first metatarsal bone has a slightly greater degree of motion at these joints than do the other metatarsals because of the absence of any ligament between its base and the base of the second metatarsal.

Metatarsophalangeal Joints

Flexion, extension, and limited abduction and adduction.

Interphalangeal Joints

Flexion and extension; also hyperextension, especially of the great toe.

MUSCLES OF THE ANKLE AND FOOT

Location

Eleven of the twenty-two muscles of the ankle and foot are intrinsic; that is, they are located entirely within the foot. The other eleven are extrinsic; they have distal tendon attachments on the foot but are otherwise located outside it (Table 8.1). A twelveth extrinsic muscle, the plantaris, has been omitted because it is a vestige often absent in human beings. When present it assists the ankle extensor muscles.

Characteristics and Functions of Individual Muscles

Tibialis Anterior

This muscle (Figure 8.21a) lies along the full length of the anterior surface of the tibia from the lateral condyle down to the medial aspect of the tarsometatarsal region. Approximately one-half to two-thirds of the way down the leg, it becomes tendinous. The tendon passes in front of the medial malleolus on its way to the first cuneiform. The muscle *dorsiflexes the ankle and foot,* and *supinates (inverts and adducts) the tarsal joints* when the foot is dorsiflexed. In EMG studies it was found that one-half the subjects in free standing had activity in the tibialis anterior that went away when the subjects leaned forward. The muscle is also active during the initial contact phase of walking, allowing the foot to be lowered to the ground in a controlled manner. The muscle may be palpated on the anterior surface of the leg just lateral to the tibia.

TABLE 8.1 Ankle and Foot Muscles

Extrinsic Muscles	Intrinsic Muscles
Anterior Aspect of Leg	Extensor digitorum brevis
Tibialis anterior	Flexor digitorum brevis
Extensor digitorum longus	Quadratus plantae
Extensor hallucis longus	Lumbricales
Peroneus tertius	Abductor hallucis
Lateral Aspect of Leg	Flexor hallucis brevis
Peroneus longus	Adductor hallucis
Peroneus brevis	Abductor digiti minimi
Posterior Aspect of Leg	Flexor digiti minimi brevis
Gastrocnemius	Dorsal interossei
Soleus	Plantar interossei
Tibialis posterior	
Flexor digitorum longus	
Flexor hallucis longus	

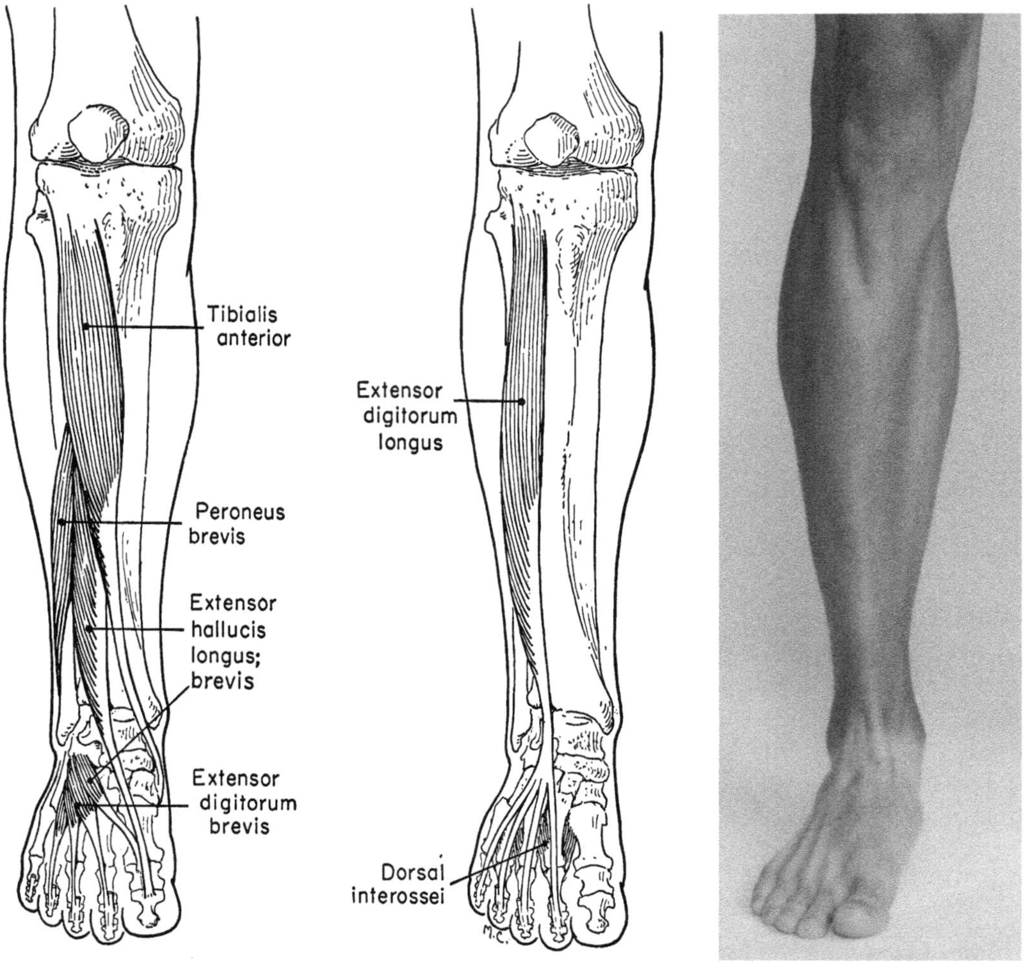

Figure 8.21 Anterior muscles of the leg.

Extensor Digitorum Longus

This muscle (Figures 8.21b and 8.22) *extends the four lesser toes.* It also *dorsiflexes both the ankle and the tarsal joints* and *helps evert and abduct the latter.* It is a penniform muscle, situated lateral to the tibialis anterior muscle in the upper part of the leg and lateral to the extensor hallucis longus in the lower part. Just in front of the ankle joint the tendon divides into four tendons, one for each of the lesser toes. The muscle may be palpated on the anterior surface of the ankle and the dorsal surface of the foot, lateral to the tendon of the extensor hallucis longus.

Extensor Hallucis Longus

This muscle (see Figure 8.21a) *extends and hyperextends the great toe.* It also *dorsiflexes the ankle and the tarsal joints.* Like the preceding muscle, it is penniform in structure. Its upper portion lies beneath the tibialis anterior and extensor digitorum longus, but about halfway down the leg the tendon emerges between these two muscles, thus becoming superficial. After it reaches the ankle, the tendon slants medially across the dorsal surface of the foot to the top of the great toe. It may be palpated on the dorsal surface of the foot and great toe.

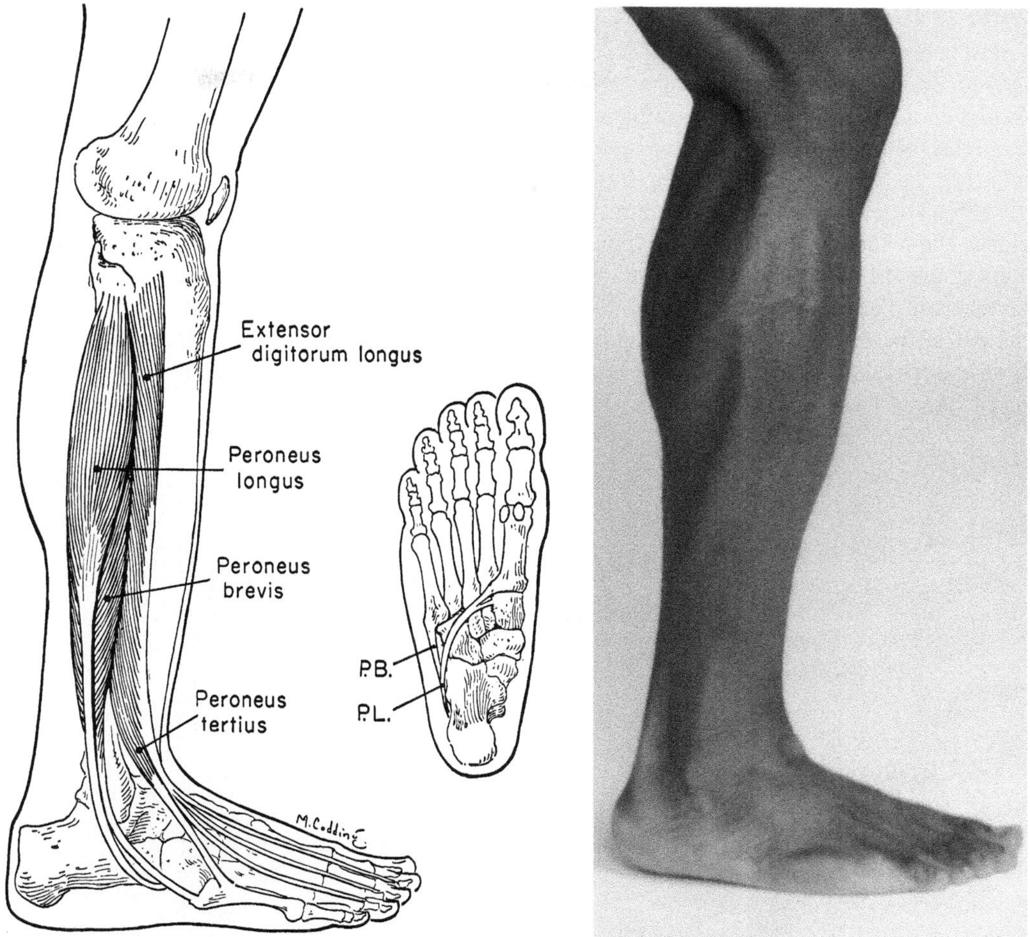

Figure 8.22 Lateral muscles of the leg. (P.B. = peroneus brevis; P.L. = peroneus longus.)

Peroneus Tertius

This muscle (see Figure 8.22) *dorsiflexes and pronates (everts and abducts) the tarsal joints* and *dorsiflexes the ankle.* It is a small muscle that lies lateral to the extensor digitorum longus, sometimes described as the fifth tendon of the latter muscle. It may be palpated on the dorsal surface of the foot close to the base of the fifth metatarsal.

Peroneus Longus

This muscle (see Figure 8.22) *plantar flexes, everts, and abducts the tarsal joints,* and *plantar flexes the ankle.* It also is most active during the propulsive phase of walking. It is situated superficially on the lateral aspect of the leg with its distal tendon passing behind the lateral malleolus and proceeding forward and downward to the margin of the foot, where it passes behind the tuberosity of the fifth metatarsal. At this point it turns under the foot, passes through the peroneal groove of the cuboid, and slants forward across the plantar surface of the foot to its attachment at the base of the first metatarsal and first cuneiform, not far from the attachment of the tibialis anterior. The muscle belly may be palpated on the lateral surface of the lower half of the leg and just above and behind the lateral malleolus.

Peroneus Brevis

This muscle (see Figures 8.21a and 8.22) *plantar flexes and everts and abducts the tarsal joints* and *helps plantar flex the ankle.* It is a penniform muscle, lying beneath the peroneus longus on the lower half of the lateral aspect of the leg. Its tendon passes behind the lateral malleolus immediately anterior to the tendon of longus and continues forward just above the longus tendon to its attachment on the tuberosity of the fifth metatarsal, below the attachment of the peroneus tertius. It may be palpated on the lateral margin of the foot, just posterior to the base of the fifth metatarsal.

Gastrocnemius (Also Listed with the Knee Muscles)

This is a powerful fast-twitch fiber muscle (Figure 8.23) for *plantar flexing the foot at the ankle joint.* It is the most superficial muscle on the back of the leg and can be seen as two bulges in the upper part of the calf when it is well developed. Its two heads, together with the soleus, constitute the triceps surae. The lateral and medial portions of the muscle remain distinct from each other as far down as the middle of the back of the leg. Then they fuse to form the broad tendon of Achilles.

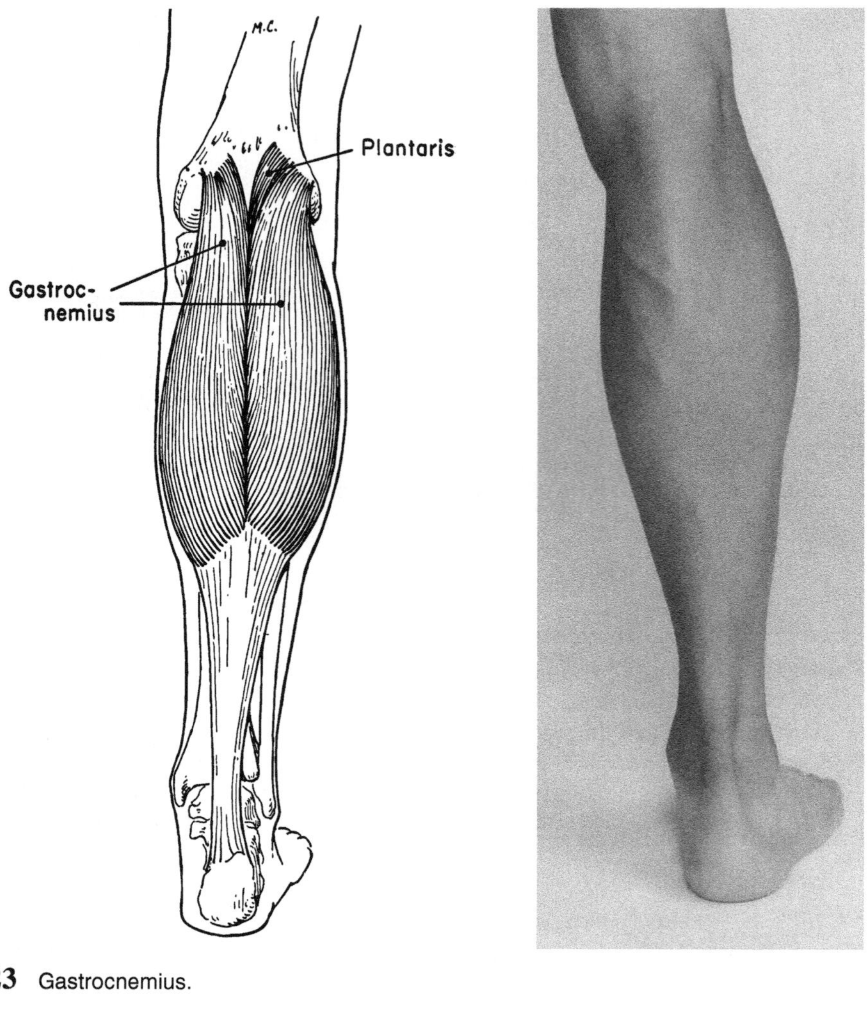

Figure 8.23 Gastrocnemius.

The most familiar function of this muscle is to *enable one to rise on the toes.* It has also been shown to be active in most individuals during normal relaxed standing. The muscle has a large angle of pull, approximately 90 degrees when the foot is in its fundamental position. Its internal structure and its leverage combine to make it an exceedingly powerful muscle. The gastrocnemius is more active with the knee extended than with a flexed knee. It is most active in closed kinetic chain activity in the standing position but shows a moderate level of activity when resisted in seated, prone, and supine positions (Carlsson et al., 2001; Tamaki et al., 1997). It may be palpated in the calf of the leg and on the back of the ankle.

Soleus

Like the gastrocnemius, this muscle (Figure 8.24) *plantar flexes the foot at the ankle joint.* It lies beneath the gastrocnemius, except along the lateral aspect of the lower half of the calf where a portion of it lies lateral to the upper part of the Achilles tendon. Its fibers are inserted into the Achilles tendon in a bipenniform manner. It is predominantly comprised of slow-twitch fibers. In an EMG study of the leg muscles, when the subjects balanced on one foot, the soleus was consistently more active than the gastrocnemius. In another study the soleus was most active in minimal contractions and when the foot was in a dorsiflexed position. This seems to imply that it was especially active in the reduction of dorsiflexion. Campbell and coworkers, using fine wire electrodes, have shown that the medial part of the soleus is a strong dynamic and static plantar flexor, whereas the lateral part is primarily a stabilizer (Basmajian & DeLuca, 1985). The muscle may be palpated slightly lateral to and below the lateral bulge of the gastrocnemius.

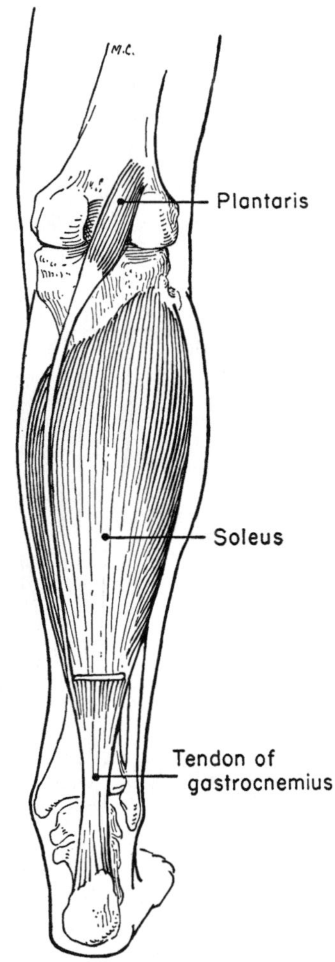

Figure 8.24 Posterior muscles of the leg, middle layer.

Tibialis Posterior

This muscle (Figure 8.25) *plantar flexes the tarsal joints and helps plantar flex the ankle.* It participates in *supination (inversion and adduction)* when the foot is plantar flexed. It is the deepest muscle on the back of the leg. The main part of the muscle covers the intermuscular septum between the tibia and the fibula. In the lower front of the leg its tendon slants across the medial side of the ankle, passes behind the medial malleolus and above the sustentaculum tali, and then turns under the foot around the medial margin of the navicular bone to insert into its underside. The muscle is penniform in structure. Because of its direction of pull and its numerous attachments on the plantar surface of the tarsal bones, an important function of this muscle appears to be maintenance of the

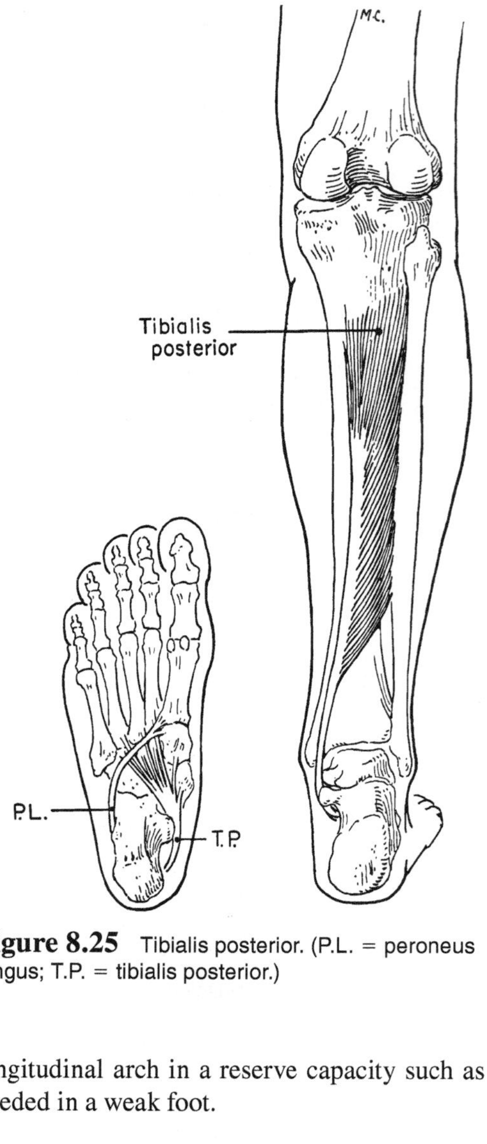

Figure 8.25 Tibialis posterior. (P.L. = peroneus longus; T.P. = tibialis posterior.)

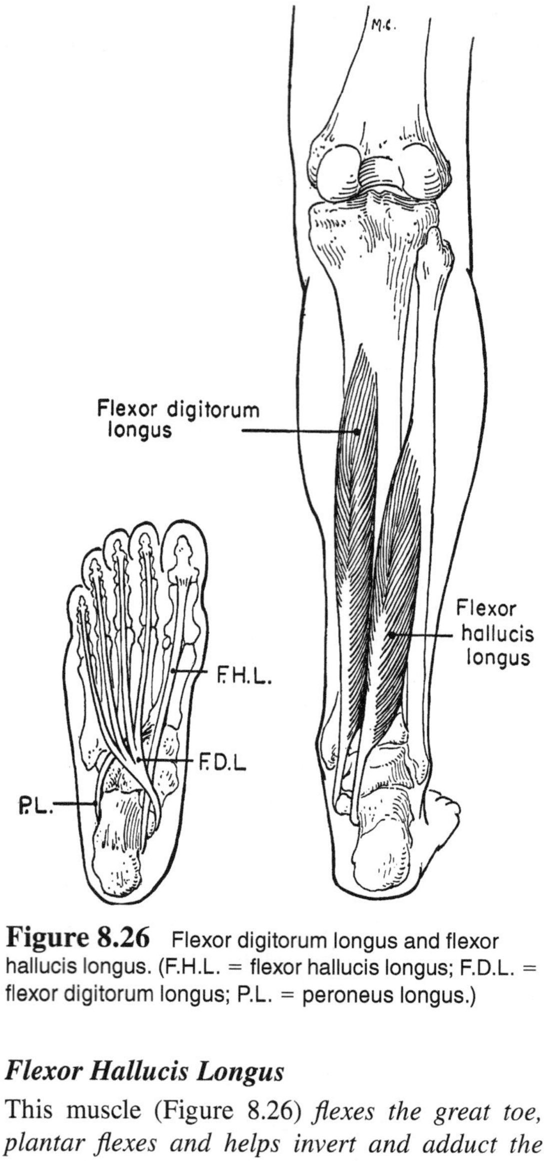

Figure 8.26 Flexor digitorum longus and flexor hallucis longus. (F.H.L. = flexor hallucis longus; F.D.L. = flexor digitorum longus; P.L. = peroneus longus.)

longitudinal arch in a reserve capacity such as is needed in a weak foot.

Flexor Digitorum Longus

This muscle (Figure 8.26) *flexes the four lesser toes, plantar flexes and helps invert and adduct the tarsal joints, and helps plantar flex the ankle.* It is situated on the medial side of the back of the leg behind the tibia. Penniform in structure, its distal tendon passes behind the medial malleolus between the tendons of the tibialis posterior and flexor hallucis longus. Beneath the tarsal bones it divides into four tendons that go to the distal phalanx of each of the four lesser toes.

Flexor Hallucis Longus

This muscle (Figure 8.26) *flexes the great toe, plantar flexes and helps invert and adduct the tarsal joints, and helps plantar flex the ankle.* It is situated on the lateral side of the back of the leg, behind the fibula and the lateral portion of the tibia. The fibers unite with the distal tendon in a penniform manner. The tendon crosses behind the ankle to the medial side, passes behind and beneath the sustentaculum tali, and runs forward under the medial margin of the foot to the distal phalanx of the great toe. It is the most posterior of the three tendons that pass behind the medial malleolus. One of its important functions is to provide the push-off in walking, running, and jumping. It may be palpated on the medial border of the calcaneal tendon close to the calcaneus.

Intrinsic Muscles of the Foot

These muscles (Figures 8.27, 8.28, and 8.29) will be treated as a group rather than individually. There are eleven of these small muscles or muscle groups. All but one, the extensor digitorum brevis, are on the plantar surface and are usually described as being arranged in four layers. The dorsal interossei muscles, although included in the deepest layer, are situated between the metatarsal bones rather than on either surface (see Figure 8.21b). The extensor digitorum brevis, which includes the hallucis although the latter is sometimes described as a separate muscle, is situated on the dorsal surface of the foot (see Figure 8.21a). With the exception of the *lumbricales* and the *quadratus plantae,* which help flex the lesser toes, the names of these muscles indicate their functions. As one might expect, these intrinsic muscles are much more highly developed

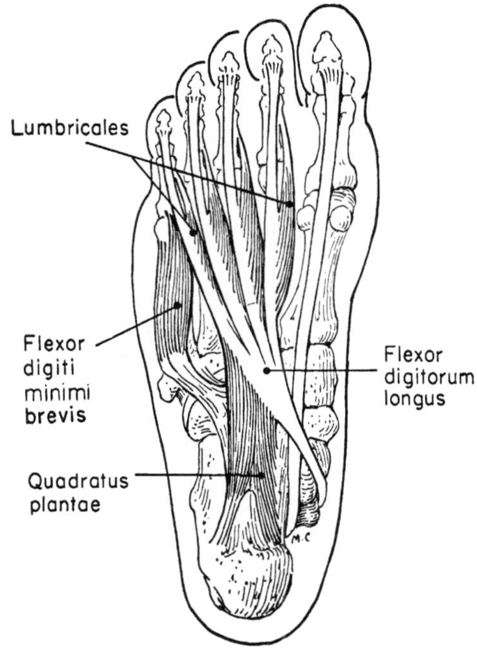

Figure 8.28 Plantar muscles of the foot, middle layer.

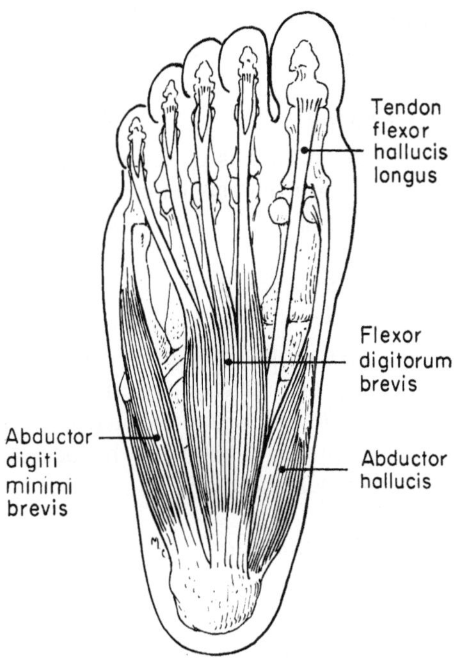

Figure 8.27 Plantar muscles of the foot, superficial layer.

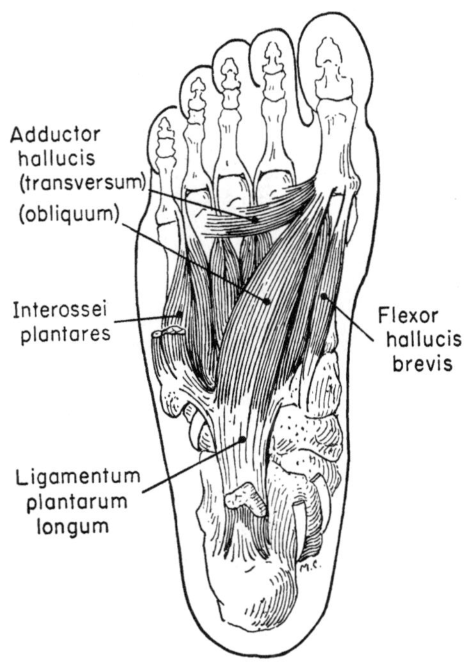

Figure 8.29 Plantar muscles of the foot, deep layer.

in primitive people than in people who habitually wear shoes.

Various research investigations have shown that the intrinsic muscles act as a functional unit, have a significant role in stabilization of the foot during propulsion, and tend to show more activity in feet that are habitually pronated. They do not show activity during relaxed standing in either normal or pronated feet and are not active in the normal *static* support of the longitudinal arches. They do, however, show definite activity in voluntary attempts to increase the height of the arches. They are also definitely active in the movement of rising on the toes.

Plantar Fascia

On the plantar surface of the foot the muscles are covered by fascia (Figure 8.30), divided into medial, central, and lateral portions. The central portion, known as the plantar aponeurosis, is particularly strong and fibrous. It extends under the whole length of the foot, connecting the tuberosity of the calcaneus with the bases of the proximal phalanges of the five toes. This is an exceedingly strong band that serves as an effective binding rod for the longitudinal arch.

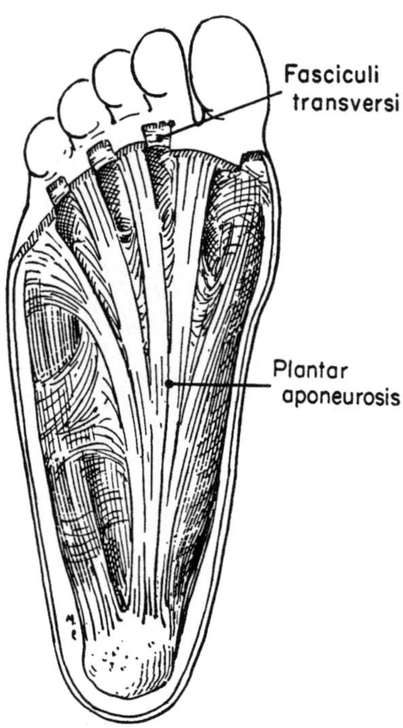

Figure 8.30 Plantar fascia of the foot (superficial).

Muscular Analysis of the Fundamental Movements of the Ankle and Foot (Tarsal Joints and Toes)

The Ankle

Dorsiflexion

Performed by the tibialis anterior, peroneus tertius, extensor digitorum longus, and extensor hallucis longus.

Plantar Flexion

Performed by the gastrocnemius, soleus, and peroneus longus, with possible help from the tibialis posterior, peroneus brevis, flexor digitorum longus, and flexor hallucis longus.

The Tarsal Joints

Dorsiflexion

The same as for dorsiflexion of the ankle.

Plantar Flexion

Performed by the tibialis posterior, flexor digitorum longus, flexor hallucis longus, and peroneus longus and brevis.

Supination (Inversion and Adduction) (Figure 8.31b)

Performed by the tibialis anterior (when the foot is dorsiflexed) and tibialis posterior (when the foot is plantar flexed), with possible help from the flexor digitorum longus and flexor hallucis longus (Basmajian & DeLuca, 1985).

Pronation (Eversion and Abduction) (Figure 8.31a)

Performed by the peroneus longus, brevis, and tertius, with possible help from the extensor digitorum longus.

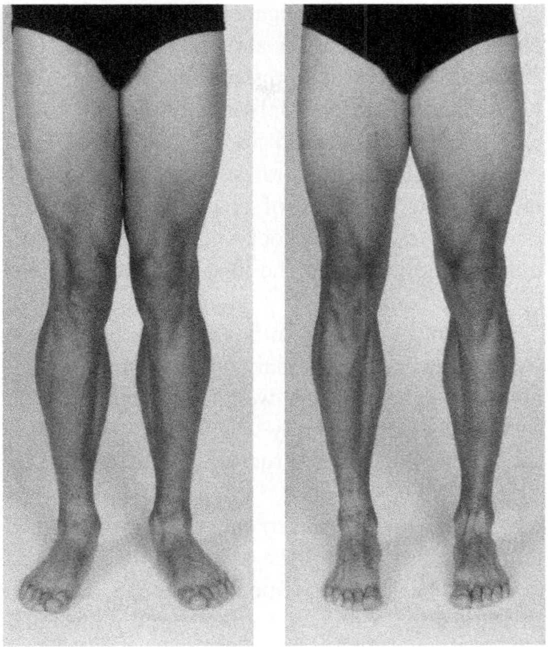

a. b.

Figure 8.31 The feet and legs in weight-bearing position: (a) in eversion and abduction; (b) in inversion and adduction.

The Toes (Exclusive of the Intrinsic Muscles)

Flexion

Performed by the flexor digitorum longus and flexor hallucis longus.

Extension

Performed by the extensor digitorum longus and extensor hallucis longus.

Maintenance of the Arches

The arches of the foot are maintained by a combination of bony structure, aponeuroses, ligaments, and tendons. The irregular tarsal bones fit together to form the basic structure of the longitudinal arch. The plantar fascia and the tendons of the deep plantar flexors act as a cable holding the arch shape. The spring ligament, the deltoid ligament, and the interosseus ligaments provide stability within the tarsal region and between the tarsal bones and the talus.

In a strong foot, muscle activity is involved for balance, adjusting the foot when encountering uneven surfaces, during locomotion, and when incurring other stresses such as standing on tiptoes. In a weak foot, such as with flat feet, muscles play a greater role. However, it has been demonstrated consistently that bones and ligaments are the primary structures for maintaining the arches.

Common Injuries of the Leg, Knee, Ankle, and Foot

The Leg

Shin Contusions

These injuries are very common because of the exposed position of the tibia and its lack of protection. A direct blow may cause an injury that varies in severity all the way from a simple bruise to a severe traumatic tibial periostitis, a condition in which the periosteum may be seriously damaged. Unlike the femur, the tibia has no anterior muscles to cushion it against sharp blows. It is important, therefore, to make every effort to protect the bone by the use of shin guards or other forms of padding in activities where there is a high risk of shin bruising.

Tibial Stress Injuries

Conditions associated with overuse or repeated stress to the tibia, the fascia, and the anterior compartment of the shank have often been lumped under the catch-all term "shin splints." In reality, pain or discomfort in the medial anterior region of the shank may be the result of any number of conditions. Micro tears of muscle or fascia, increased pressure in the various soft tissue compartments, stress fractures of the tibia, and inflammation of the fascia (fasciitis) can all lead to symptoms of pain and tenderness. The onset is gradual, and the condition may be due to repeated tiny tears where the tibialis posterior or anterior attaches to the tibia or to tears or sprains in the interosseous membrane. Softer surfaces and supporting the arches may be helpful in relieving the symptoms, but rest is often necessary for recovery.

Leg Fracture

Fractures of the tibia, the fibula, or both are most common among young people. The severity of the fracture is usually determined by the degree to which bone segments are displaced. A nondisplaced fracture of the fibula is a much less severe injury than a displaced fracture of both the tibia and the fibula. In any case, fractures should be treated as serious injuries, as there may be a concomitant injury to the epiphysis and to other soft tissue structures that will lead to permanent instability or dysfunction.

The Knee

Vulnerability of the Knee Joint

There can be no question as to the vulnerability of the knee. It is probably the most susceptible to injury of any of the joints in the body. Two factors appear to be responsible for this: its complicated structure and its position midway between the hip and the sole of the foot. Superficially, it looks like a hinge joint, but its action combines the movements of a hinge with the gliding of an irregular joint. Furthermore, when it is flexed it is capable of a slight degree of medial and lateral rotation. Several writers have called attention to the strains and stresses to which the knee is subject and have emphasized the need to be aware of these forces for knee function. Additionally, misalignments that cause the unequal or off-center transmission of forces through the knee joint are predisposing factors contributing to knee injuries. Common examples of these conditions are knock-knees (genu valgum) and bowlegs (genu varum). In knock-knees (genu valgum) the knees are closer to the midline of the body than is normal. In the standing position the knees are closer together than the feet, so that when the feet are placed side by side, the knees are either pressed together or are slightly overlapping with one behind the other. Mechanically, the condition means that the weight-bearing line of the lower extremity passes lateral to the center of the knee joint. This puts the medial ligament (tibial collateral) under increased tension and subjects the lateral meniscus to increased pressure and friction. Such a joint is unstable. Not only is it more prone to injury than a well-aligned joint, but in all weight-bearing positions postural strains are constantly present. The condition of bowlegs (genu varum) is just the reverse of knock-knees, with the additional complication of the long bones themselves being curved laterally.

When the knee is in flexion, it is in an open position, with stability maintained by muscle, tendon, and ligament. In a weight-bearing situation, such as a squat, the body weight is borne primarily by the soft tissue structures, with little bony support.

In downward movement, the hip and knee joints are flexing and the ankle joints are dorsiflexing. The joint movements are *caused* by the force of gravity; they are *controlled* by the muscles that normally cause the opposite movements but that, for this purpose, are engaged in *eccentric contraction.* In the return movement—that is, the return to the erect standing position—the same muscles are working, but this time in *concentric contraction.*

The demands placed on the muscles and ligaments of the knee joint during deep squats are severe. These factors should be considered when contemplating the assignment of exercises involving repeated full squats or long-held squat positions.

Contusion

This condition occurs frequently among athletes and can be caused either by a fall or by a blow against the front or side of the knee. The problem presented by a contusion of the knee is that it often masks a more serious injury, such as ligament damage. Therefore, if there is uncertainty, this injury should be treated as the more serious injury to prevent further deterioration.

Collateral Ligament Sprain

This is doubtless one of the most, if not *the most,* frequently reported knee injury, at least in the world of sports (Arnheim & Prentice, 1998).

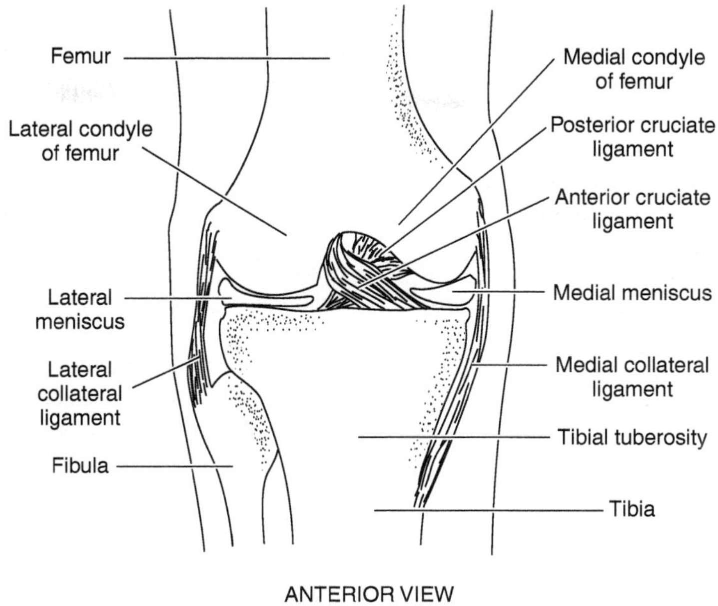

Figure 8.32 Anterior view of the right knee joint. *Source:* From *Modern Principles of Athletic Training* (7th ed.), by D. D. Arnheim (p. 567). Copyright © 1989, Mosby College Publishing, St. Louis, MO. Reprinted by permission.

To understand the reason for this, a thorough knowledge of the structure of the joint is essential (pp. 179–183 and Figure 8.32). Although classified as a hinge joint, it is by no means a typical one like the interphalangeal finger joints, for instance. In flexion and in the return from flexion, a certain amount of gliding occurs. When the knee is flexed, it is capable of a slight amount of voluntary rotation. When it receives a blow from the side or when it is subjected to severe wrenching in the weight-bearing position, it can easily be forced beyond its normal range of rotary motion. Furthermore, although abduction and adduction are not normal knee motions—that is, one cannot voluntarily perform them—the leg can be passively abducted or adducted by an outside force. A slight degree of this probably does no harm, but a severe lateral blow or violent wrenching is likely to tear the ligament on the opposite side.

Because the knee is protected medially, the majority of knee sprains are caused by a blow from the lateral side toward the medial side or by a severe medialward twist (Arnheim & Prentice, 1998). This means that the leg has been violently adducted and medially rotated at the knee joint. The stress is primarily on the ligaments on the inner side of the knee. If the force is great enough to be transmitted to the deep layer of the medial collateral ligament, it is likely to affect the medial meniscus, which is attached to the ligament. Injuries to the lateral side are much less common. Cruciate ligament sprain and rupture are often encountered when forces cause the tibia to move forward or backward.

Strengthening of the muscles that cross the knee joint is an important part of the rehabilitation of injured knee joints. The muscles and their tendons help stabilize the joint and provide support that may be compromised because of the damaged ligaments. Moreover, it is important to maintain the strength of these muscles for their stabilizing role in sustaining the integrity of the joint and preventing injuries to it.

Chondromalacia

Chondromalacia of the patella most often occurs among young adults and affects the cartilage on the articulating surface of the patella. The etiology of this degenerating disease is unknown, but it is conjectured that an incongruence between the patella and the femur may contribute to it. Common symptoms include pain upon movement, swelling, and a grating sensation. Treatment includes doing isometric exercises, wearing a band (brace) for support, and limiting certain activities.

Osgood-Schlatter Disease

Osgood-Schlatter disease, affecting adolescents, is caused by repeated usage of the knee extensors, resulting in a tearing or avulsion at the epiphysis of the tibial tuberosity, the point for attachment of the patellar tendon. Symptoms include swelling, hemorrhage, and pain when running, jumping, or kneeling. Treatment includes ice therapy, rest, and subsequent isometric strengthening exercises.

The Ankle

Of all the injuries to which the lower extremity is prone, those affecting the ankle joint have the highest incidence. One reason for this is thought to be the arrangement of the muscles. The long tendons cross the ankle in a way that makes for a lack of bulk and for good leverage but contributes little to stabilization (Arnheim & Prentice, 1998). Consequently, this joint is unusually susceptible to strains, sprains, dislocations, and fractures.

Strains

A strain is a muscle injury. This includes the muscle tendon and the connective tissue by means of which the muscle is attached to the bone. Landing from jumping exposes the tendons of the ankle and foot muscles to the danger of strain. The impact of landing may force the ankle joints beyond their normal range of motion. This gives the Achilles tendon a sudden wrench that may cause tearing, either at the point of the tendon's attachment to the bone or at the junction between the tendon and the muscle belly. This is potentially a very debilitating injury requiring expert treatment.

The distal tendons of both the anterior and posterior tibial muscles are also subject to strain. The aftereffects of each of these can be quite troublesome because they are both inverters (supinators) of the foot, in addition to which the posterior tibial helps support the longitudinal arch in weak feet or under exceptional stress.

Sprains

A sprained ankle is all too familiar. It results from a sudden wrench or twist and is usually associated with forced inversion of the foot with the lateral ligaments being stretched or torn and sometimes ruptured or pulled off of the bone. The affected ligaments are any of those on the lateral aspect of the ankle—the calcaneofibular, anterior talofibular, and posterior talofibular. The interosseous talocalcaneal ligament, although not strictly an ankle ligament, may also be affected.

Fractures

Ankle fractures are usually caused by a sudden wrenching or twisting, the same factors that cause sprains but, whereas sprains are the result of excessive inversion of the foot, fractures result from excessive eversion. The majority of ankle fractures occur to the malleoli, especially the lateral malleolus. In the more serious fractures, some dislocation as the result of a separation between the tibia and fibula is also likely, with a consequent widening of the socket or mortise. Prompt and adequate treatment to restore the joint integrity is all important if permanent damage is to be avoided.

The Foot

Plantar Fasciitis

Plantar fasciitis is a broad term used to describe pain and tenderness along the sole of the foot. This condition may be due to inflammation of the plantar fascia, micro tears of the fascia, or a complete rupture. Plantar fasciitis is generally an overuse injury, but lack of flexibility in the muscles of the lower extremity may also be a contributing factor. Tension in the muscles of the lower leg will produce tension in the plantar fascia, and over the long term, the plantar fascia will be damaged. Stretching has been shown to be helpful in both prevention and treatment of plantar fasciitis (Whiting & Zernicke, 1998).

References and Selected Readings

Ahmed, A. M., & McLean, C. (2002). In vitro measurement of the restraining role of the anterior cruciate ligament during walking and stair ascent. *Journal of Biomechanical Engineering,* 124(6):768–779.

Arnheim, D. D., & Prentice, W. E. (1998). *Essentials of athletic training* (4th ed.). St. Louis, MO: McGraw-Hill.

Basmajian, J. V., & Deluca, C. J. (1985). *Muscles alive* (5th ed.). Baltimore: Williams & Wilkins.

Besier, T. F., Draper, C. E., Gold, G. E., Beaupre, G. S., & Delp, S. L. (2005). Patellofemoral joint contact area increases with knee flexion and weight-bearing. *Journal of Orthopedic Research,* 23(2), 345–350.

Buford, W. L. Jr., Ivey, F. M., Nakamura, T., Patterson, R. M., & Nguyen, D. K. (2001). Internal/external rotation moment arms of muscles at the knee: Moment arms for the normal knee and the ACL-deficient knee. *Knee,* 8(4), 293–303.

Carlsson, U., Lind, K., Moller, M., Karlsson, J., & Svantesson, U. (2001). Plantar flexor muscle function in open and closed chain. *Clinical Physiology,* 21(1), 1–8.

Cheung, J. T., Zhang, M., & An, K. N. (2004). Effects of plantar fascia stiffness on the biomechanical responses of the ankle-foot complex. *Clinical Biomechanics,* 19(8), 839–846.

Erdemir, A., Hamel, A. J., Fauth, A. R., Piazza, S. J., & Sharkey, N. A. (2004). Dynamic loading of the plantar aponeurosis in walking. *Journal of Bone and Joint Surgery* [American Volume], 86-A(3), 546–552.

Freeman, M.A.R., & Pinskerova, V. (2005). The movement of the normal tibiofemoral joint. *Journal of Biomechanics,* 38, 197–208.

Gefen, A. (2003). The in vivo elastic properties of the plantar fascia during the contact phase of walking. *Foot and Ankle International,* 24(3), 238–244.

Griffin, N. L., & Richmond, B. G. (2005). Cross-sectional geometry of the human forefoot. *Bone,* 37(2), 253–260.

Hand, C. J., & Spalding, T. J. (2004). Association between anatomical features and anterior knee pain in a "fit" service population. *Journal of the Royal Naval Medical Service,* 90(3), 125–134.

Heiderscheit, B. C., Hamill, J., & Caldwell, G. E. (2000). Influence of Q-angle on lower-extremity running kinematics. *Journal of Orthopedic and Sports Physical Therapy,* 30(5), 271–278.

Hewett, T. E., Myer, G. D., & Zazulak, B. T. (2009). Hamstrings to quadriceps peak torque ratios diverge between sexes with increasing isokinetic angular velocity. *Journal of Science and Medicine in Sport,* 11, 452–459.

Hunt, A. E., & Smith, R. M. (2005). Mechanics and control of the flat versus normal foot during the stance phase of walking. *Clinical Biomechanics,* 19(4), 391–397.

Kitaoka, H. B., Ahn, T. K., Luo, Z. P., & An, K. N. (1997). Stability of the arch of the foot. *Foot and Ankle International,* 18(10), 644–648.

Kura, H., Luo, Z. P., Kitoaka, H., & An, K. N. (1997). Quantitative analysis of the intrinsic muscles of the foot. *Anatomy Record,* 249, 143–151.

Luger, E. J., Nissan, M., Karpf, A., Steinberg, E. L., & Dekel, S. (1999). Patterns of weight distribution under the metatarsal heads. *Journal of Bone and Joint Surgery* [European Volume], 81(2), 199–202.

Mesfar, W, & Shirazi-Adl, A. (2005). Biomechanics of the knee joint in flexion under various quadriceps forces. *Knee,* 12(6), 424–434.

Mizuno, Y., Kumagai, M., Mattessich, S. M., Elias, J. J., Ramrattan, N., Cosgarea, A. J., et al. (2001). Q-angle influences tibiofemoral and patellofemoral kinematics. *Journal of Orthopedic Research,* 19, 834–840.

Nakagawa, S., Johal, P., Pinskerova, V., Komatsu, T., Sosna, A., Williams, A., et al. (2004). The posterior cruciate ligament during flexion of the normal knee. *Journal of Bone and Joint Surgery* [Eur.], 86(3), 450–456.

Nyland, J., Lachman, N., Kocabey, Y., Brosky, J., Altun, R., & Caborn, D. (2005). Anatomy, function, and rehabilitation of the popliteus musculotendinous complex. *Journal of Orthopedic and Sports Physical Therapy,* 35(3), 165–179.

Patel, V. V., Hall, K., Ries, M., Lotz, J., Ozhinsky, E., Lindsey, C., et al. (2004). A three-dimensional MRI analysis of knee kinematics. *Journal of Orthopedic Research,* 22, 283–292.

Patel, V. V., Hall, K., Ries, Lindsey, C., Ozhinsky, E., Lu, Y., et al. (2003). Magnetic resonance imaging of patellofemoral kinematics with weight-bearing. *Journal of Bone and Joint Surgery* [Am.], 85-A(12), 2419–2424.

Powers, C. M., Ward, S. R., Fredericson, M., Guillet, M., & Shellock, F. G. (2003). Patellofemoral kinematics during weight-bearing and non-weight-bearing knee extension in persons with lateral subluxation of the patella: A preliminary study. *Journal of Orthopedic and Sports Physical Therapy,* 33(11), 677–685.

Riddle, D. L., Pulisic, M., Pidcoe, P., & Johnson, R. E. (2003). Risk factors for plantar fasciitis: A matched case-control study. *Journal of Bone and Joint Surgery* [Am.], 85-A(7), 1338.

Ridola, C., & Palma, A. (2001). Functional anatomy and imaging of the foot. *Italian Journal of Anatomy and Embryology,* 106(2), 85–98.

Ruohola, J. P., Kiuru, M. J., & Pihlajamaki, H. K. (2006). Fatigue bone injuries causing anterior lower leg pain. *Clinical Orthopedics and Related Research,* 444, 216–223.

Shelburne, K. B., Pandy, M. G., Anderson, F. C., & Torry, M. R. (2004). Pattern of anterior cruciate ligament force in normal walking. *Journal of Biomechanics,* 37(6), 797–805.

Smith, P. N., Refshauge, K. M., & Scarvell, J. M. (2003). Development of the concepts of knee kinematics. *Archives of Physical Medicine and Rehabilitation,* 84(12), 1895–1902.

Tamaki, H., Kitada, K., Akamine, T., Sakou, T., & Kurata, H. (1997). Electromyogram patterns during plantarflexions at various angular velocities and knee angles in human triceps surae muscles. *European Journal of Applied Physiology and Occupational Physiology,* 75(1), 1–6.

Tecklenburg, K., Dejour, D., Hoser, C., & Fink, C. (2006). Bony and cartilaginous anatomy of the patellofemoral joint. *Knee,* 14(3), 235–240.

Whiting, W. C., & Zernicke, R. F. (1998). *Biomechanics of musculoskeletal injury.* Champaign, IL: Human Kinetics.

Williams, A., & Logan, M. (2004). Understanding tibio-femoral motion. *Knee,* 11(2), 81–88.

LABORATORY EXPERIENCES

Knee Joint: Joint Structure and Function

1. Record the essential information regarding the structure, ligaments, and cartilages of the knee joint. Study the movements both on the skeleton and on the living body and explain how the joint structure affects movements.

Muscular Action

Identify as many muscles as possible in the following experiments.

2. **Flexion at Knee**
   Subject: Lie facedown and flex leg at knee by raising foot.
   Assistant: Steady subject's thigh and resist movement by pushing down on ankle.
   Observer: Palpate biceps femoris, semitendinosus, gracilis, sartorius, and gastrocnemius.
3. **Extension at Knee**
   a. *Subject:* Rise from a squat position.
      Observer: Palpate quadriceps femoris.
   b. *Subject:* Sit on table with legs hanging over edge. Extend leg.
      Assistant: Steady subject's thigh and resist movement by holding ankle down.
      Observer: Palpate quadriceps femoris.
4. **Outward Rotation of Leg with Knee in Flexed Position**
   Subject: Sit on table with legs hanging over edge. Rotate foot laterally as far as possible without moving thigh.
   Assistant: Steady subject's thigh and give slight resistance by holding foot.
   Observer: Palpate biceps femoris.
5. **Inward Rotation of Leg with Knee in Flexed Position**
   Subject: Sit on table with legs hanging over edge. Rotate foot medially as far as possible without moving thigh.
   Assistant: Steady subject's thigh and give slight resistance by holding foot.
   Observer: Palpate semitendinosus, gracilis, and sartorius.

Ankle and Foot: Joint Structure and Function

6. Record the essential information regarding the structure, ligaments, and cartilages of the ankle, subtalar, and midtarsal joints. Study the movements of these joints both on the skeleton and on the living body and explain how the joint structures affect the movements.
7. Using a goniometer, compare the total range of plantar and dorsiflexion of the ankle in a group of five or more subjects (a) with extension at the knee and (b) with flexion at the knee.
8. Make a similar comparison between two groups, one consisting of three to five varsity-level swimmers and the other of the same number of recreational swimmers, or make a similar comparison between ballet and nonballet dancers.

Ankle and Foot: Muscular Action

Identify as many muscles as possible in the following experiments.

9. **Plantar Flexion**
   Subject: Perform each of the following actions:
   a. Stand and rise on the toes. b. Hold one foot off the floor and extend it vigorously.
   Observer: Compare the muscular action of the leg in a and b.
10. **Dorsiflexion**
    Subject: Sit on a table with the legs straight and with the feet over the edge. Dorsiflex one foot as far as possible.
    Assistant: Resist the movement by holding the foot.
    Observer: Identify the tibialis anterior, peroneus tertius, extensor digitorum longus, and extensor hallucis longus.
11. **Pronation (Eversion and Abduction)**
    Subject: In same starting position as in Experience 10, pronate one foot without extending it.
    Assistant: Steady the leg at the ankle and resist the movement by holding the foot.
    Observer: Identify the muscles that contract.
12. **Supination (Inversion and Adduction)**
    Subject: In same position as in Experience 10, supinate one foot as far as possible.
    Assistant: Steady the leg at the ankle and resist the movement by holding the foot.
    Observer: Identify the muscles that contract.

Kinesiological Analysis

13. Choose a simple motor skill from Appendix G. Do a complete anatomical analysis of the lower extremity following the analysis outline in Table 1.2.

CHAPTER 9

The Spinal Column and Thorax

OUTLINE

OBJECTIVES

At the conclusion of this chapter, the student should be able to:

1. Name, locate, and describe the structures and ligamentous reinforcements of the articulations of the spinal column and thorax.
2. Name and demonstrate the movements possible in joints of the spinal column and thorax, regardless of starting position.
3. Name and locate the muscles and muscle groups of the spinal column and thorax and name their primary actions as agonists, stabilizers, neutralizers, or antagonists.
4. Analyze the fundamental movements of the spinal column and thorax with respect to joint and muscle actions.
5. Describe the common injuries of the spinal column and thorax.
6. Perform an anatomical analysis of the movements of the spinal column in a motor skill.

STRUCTURE AND ARTICULATIONS OF THE SPINAL COLUMN

If you were faced with the problem of devising a single mechanism that would simultaneously (1) give stability to a collapsible cylinder, (2) permit movement in all directions and yet always return to the fundamental starting position, (3) support three structures of considerable weight (a globe, a yoke, and a cage), (4) provide attachment for numerous flexible bands and elastic cords, (5) transmit a gradually increasing weight to a rigid basinlike foundation, (6) act as a shock absorber for cushioning jolts and jars, and (7) encase and protect a cord of extreme delicacy, you would be staggered by the immensity of the task. Yet the spinal column fulfills all these requirements with amazing efficiency. It is at the same time an organ of stability and mobility, of support and protection, and of resistance and adaptation. It is an instrument of great precision, yet of robust structure. Its architecture and the manner in which it performs its many functions are worthy of careful study. From the kinesiological point of view, we are interested in the spine chiefly as a mechanism for maintaining erect posture and for permitting movement of the head, neck, and trunk.

To understand these functions of the spine, it is necessary to have a clear picture, first, of the spinal column as a whole and, second, of the distinguishing characteristics of the different regions. The spinal column, consisting of seven cervical, twelve thoracic, and five lumbar vertebrae, the sacrum (five fused sacral vertebrae), and the coccyx (three to five fused vertebrae), presents four curves as seen from the side (Figure 9.1). At birth, the vertebral column is convex backward. The thoracic and sacrococcygeal curves remain convex to the rear and are considered primary curves. The cervical and lumbar curves reverse direction of the curvature during infancy and early childhood and are referred to as secondary curves. The curvature at the cervical region develops when the infant raises its head; the lumbar region develops its anterior convexity when the infant assumes an upright posture and begins to walk. The curves are a response to gravity and continue to develop through puberty.

An exaggerated curve in the thoracic region is referred to as a kyphosis, and one in the lumbar region is referred to as a lordosis. Kyphotic curves have a backward convexity. Lordotic curves have a forward convex curve. A lateral deviation of the spine is called a scoliosis. Any significant deviation from the expected gradual curves as well as misalignments among the vertebrae may seriously affect an individual's movement capabilities or predispose a person to injury.

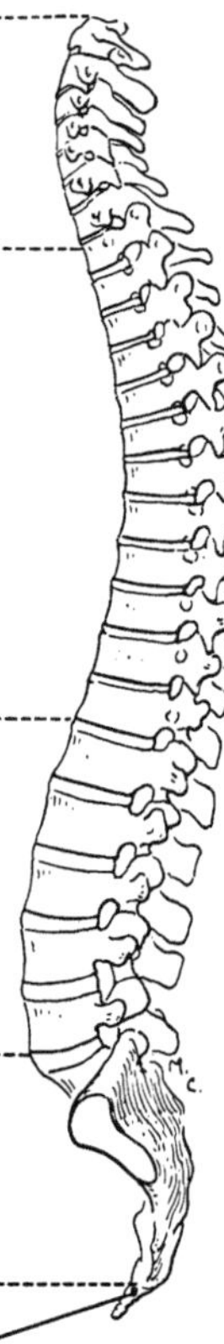

Figure 9.1 Lateral view of the spinal column showing anteroposterior curves.

From the first cervical to the fifth lumbar vertebra, the vertebral bodies become increasingly larger. This is an important factor in fulfilling the weight-bearing role of the spine. The vertebral bodies decrease in size from the first sacral through the coccygeal region. The sacral vertebrae complete the pelvic girdle, which transmits the weight of the head and trunk onto both femoral heads.

There are two sets of interspinal articulations, those between the vertebral bodies and those between the vertebral arches. The latter are in pairs, with one on either side of each vertebra. The articulations of the first two vertebrae are atypical and will be described separately.

Such a close relationship exists between the structure of the spinal column and the movements that take place in its different regions that the student will find it well worth the effort to acquire a thorough grasp of the structure, particularly of the joints, before proceeding to the movements. If possible, both a skeleton and a strung set of vertebrae should be referred to frequently while studying spinal structure.

Articulations of the Vertebral Bodies

These joints (Figure 9.2) are classified as synchondroses or cartilaginous joints. The bodies of the vertebrae are united by means of fibrocartilages, otherwise known as intervertebral discs. These correspond to the surfaces of the adjacent vertebral bodies, except in the cervical region, where they are smaller from side to side. They adhere to the hyaline cartilage both above and below, with no articular cavity in this type of joint. In thickness they are fairly uniform in the thoracic region, but in the cervical and lumbar regions they are thicker in front than in back. Altogether, they constitute one-fourth the length of the spinal column. Each disc consists of two parts, an outer fibrous rim and an inner pulpy nucleus known as the nucleus pulposus. This is a ball of firmly compressed elastic material, a little like the center of a golf ball. It constitutes a center of motion and permits compression in any direction, as well as torsion. The intervertebral discs are also important as shock absorbers, resisting compressive forces.

The discs consist of a large percentage (80 to 90%) of water. With advancing age, this fluid is absorbed and the discs shrink and become brittle. This change is noticeable in the reduced height and a significant increase in disc problems in older people.

Ligamentous Reinforcement

The joints of the spinal column are reinforced by several ligaments (Figures 9.3 and 9.4). The vertebral bodies are held together by two long ligaments, one in front and one in back. The anterior longitudinal ligament starts as a narrow band and widens as it descends from the occipital bone to the sacrum. The posterior longitudinal ligament, descending from the occipital bone to the coccyx, is relatively narrow throughout but has lateral expansions opposite each intervertebral fibrocartilage. Both ligaments are stronger in the thoracic region than in either the cervical or the lumbar region (Table 9.1 on page 218).

Articulations of the Vertebral Arches

The articulations (Figure 9.5) between the facets of the vertebral arches are nonaxial diarthrodial joints. Each of these joints has an articular cavity and is enclosed within a capsule. A slight amount of gliding motion is permitted. The resultant movement of each vertebra is determined largely by the direction in which the articular facets face. In any given region of the vertebral column, motion between two adjacent vertebrae is only a few degrees. It is the cumulative effect of motion in all of the involved vertebrae that produces the large range of motion seen in the spine. For example, each of the lower five pairs of cervical vertebrae are capable of between 4 and 6 degrees of rotation. Adding the cumulative rotation of these segments to the approximately 40-degree rotation permitted between C1 and C2 gives a total range of motion

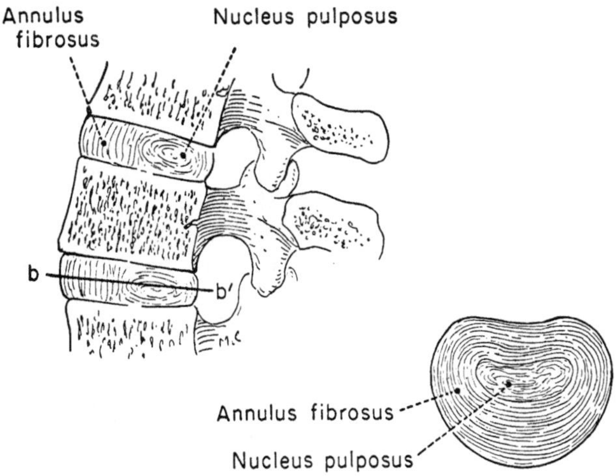

Figure 9.2 (a) Sagittal section of lumbar vertebrae and intervertebral fibrocartilages. (b) Transverse section of intervertebral fibrocartilage, through b–b′.

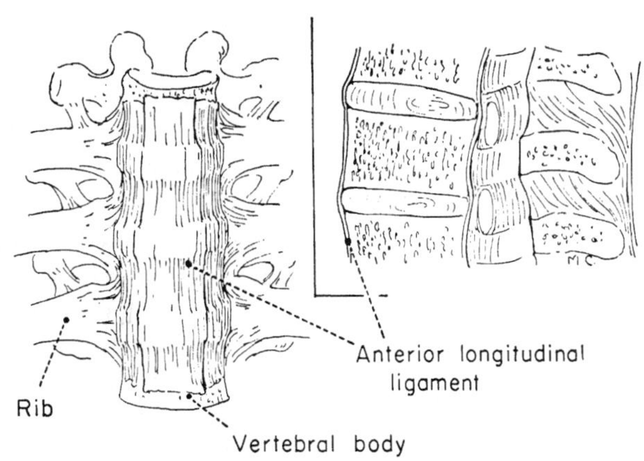

Figure 9.3 Anterior longitudinal ligament of the spine: (a) anterior view; (b) sagittal section of vertebrae showing lateral view of ligament.

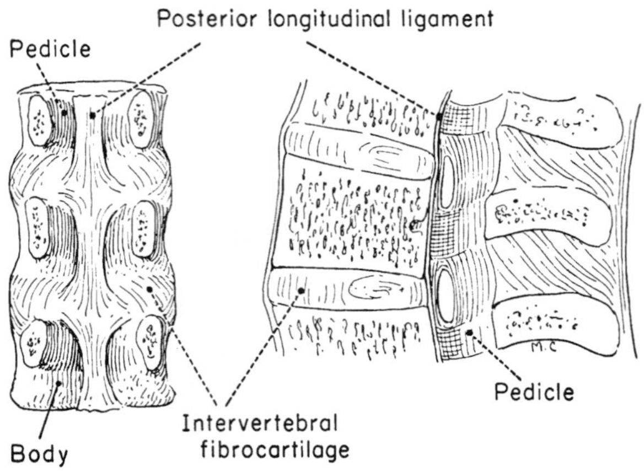

Figure 9.4 Posterior longitudinal ligament of spine: (a) frontal section of vertebrae showing posterior view of ligament; (b) sagittal section of vertebrae showing lateral view of ligament.

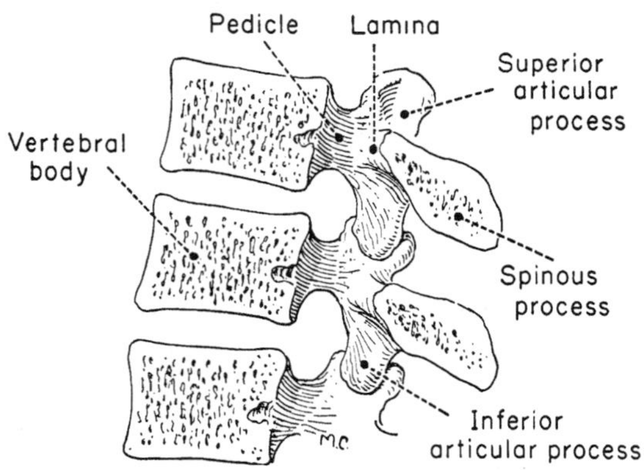

Figure 9.5 Sagittal section of vertebrae showing articulations of the vertebral arches.

of 70 degrees (Bogduk & Mercer, 2000). The facets in the cervical region slant at about a 45-degree angle, lying halfway between the horizontal and the frontal planes (Figure 9.6a). Such a slant would seem to favor rotation and lateral flexion and to be unfavorable to flexion and hyperextension. Yet these latter movements occur as freely as does lateral flexion, whereas rotation from the second cervical vertebra down can be rated as only moderate. In the thoracic region they lie slightly more in the frontal and less in the horizontal plane than do the cervical articulations, and they have a slight inward and outward slant (Figure 9.6b). The upper facets face backward, slightly upward, and lateralward; the lower facets face forward, slightly downward, and medialward. They are adapted equally well to rotation and to lateral bending. In the lumbar region, except at the lumbosacral articulation, the articular facets lie more nearly in the sagittal plane (Figure 9.6c). The upper facets face inward and slightly backward; the lower facets face outward and slightly forward. Furthermore, the upper facets present slightly concave surfaces and the lower facets convex. By this arrangement of the facets, the lumbar vertebrae are virtually locked against rotation. The slight amount of rotation that does occur is made possible by the looseness of the capsules. At the lumbosacral articulation, the facets lie somewhat more in the frontal plane than is true of the other lumbar joints.

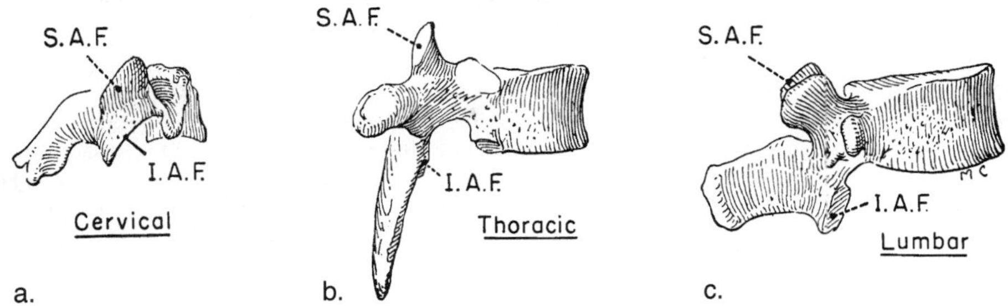

Figure 9.6 Articular facets of vertebrae: (a) cervical; (b) thoracic; (c) lumbar. (S.A.F. = Superior articular facet. I.A.F. = Inferior articular facet.)

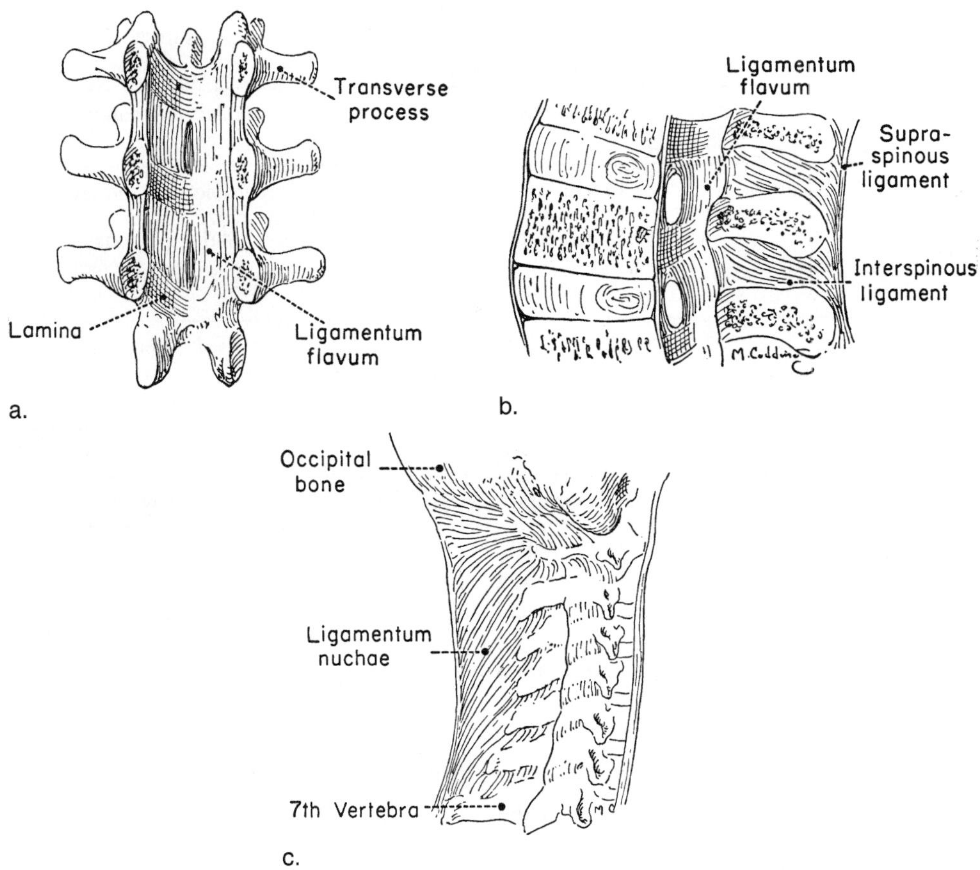

Figure 9.7 Ligaments of vertebral articulations: (a) frontal section of three lumbar vertebrae showing anterior view of vertebral arches and ligamentum flavum; (b) sagittal view of lumbar vertebrae showing ligaments of vertebral arches; (c) side view of cervical spine showing ligamentum nuchae.

The ligaments reinforcing these joints may be identified in Figure 9.7. The ligamenta flava and the interspinous and supraspinous ligaments are all thickest and strongest in the lumbar region. There remain two rather thin ligaments, the intertransverse, connecting the transverse processes of adjacent vertebrae, and the ligamentum nuchae, which is the continuation of the supraspinous ligament in the cervical region (see Table 9.1).

TABLE 9.1 Ligaments of the Vertebral Column

Ligaments	Function	Region
Anterior longitudinal	Limits extension. Reinforces anterior portion of annulus fibrosus.	Axis to sacrum well developed in lumbar and thoracic
Anterior atlantoaxial (continuation of anterior longitudinal ligament)	Limits extension.	Axis and atlas
Posterior longitudinal	Limits flexion. Reinforces posterior portion of annulus fibrosus.	Axis to sacrum
Ligamentum flavum	Limits flexion, especially in lumbar area.	Axis to sacrum
Ligamentum nuchae (continuation of the supraspinous ligaments)	Limits flexion.	Cervical region
Supraspinous*	Limits flexion.	Thoracic and lumbar
Posterior atlantoaxial* (continuation of ligamentum flavum)	Limits flexion.	Atlas and axis
Tectorial membrane* (continuation of posterior longitudinal ligament)	Limits flexion.	Axis to occipital bone
Interspinous	Limits flexion.	Primarily lumbar
Intertransverse*	Limits lateral flexion.	Primarily lumbar
Alar*	Limits rotation of head to same side and lateral flexion to opposite side.	Axis to skull

*Not pictured.

Source: From *Joint Structure and Function: A Comprehensive Analysis,* by C. Norkin & P. Levangie (p. 128). Copyright © 1983, F. A. Davis, Philadelphia. Reprinted by permission.

Atlanto-Occipital Articulation

This is the articulation (Figure 9.8) between the head and the neck. It consists of a pair of joints, one on each side. Each condyle of the occipital bone of the skull articulates with the corresponding superior articular fossa of the first vertebra, known as the atlas. Each articulation by itself belongs to the condyloid (ovoid) classification, but the movement that occurs in the two joints together is more like that of a hinge joint. The rigid relationship between the two joints results in a restriction of the lateral motion that would normally occur in an ovoid joint. The movements that take place at the atlanto-occipital articulation are chiefly flexion and extension, with a slight amount of lateral flexion (Figure 9.10a and b). Combining these four motions results in limited circumduction. There is no rotation.

Atlantoaxial Articulation

This is a perfect example of a pivot joint—a joint whose sole function is rotation (Figure 9.9). The toothlike peg (odontoid process, or dens) that projects

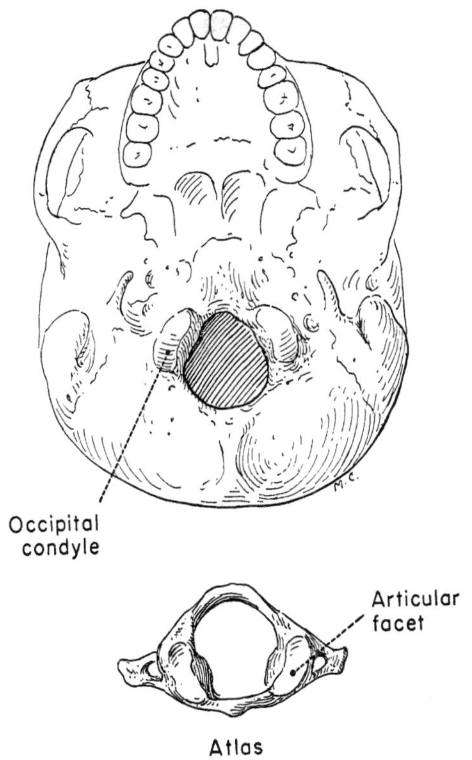

Figure 9.8 Bones forming atlanto-occipital articulation.

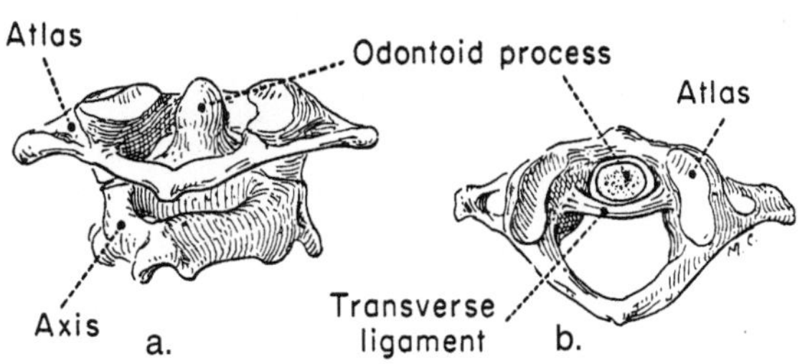

Figure 9.9 Atlantoaxial articulation: (a) posterior view; (b) superior view.

upward from the second cervical vertebra, otherwise known as the axis, or epistropheus, fits into the ring formed by the inner surface of the anterior arch of atlas and the transverse ligament that bridges across the tips of the arch. Because no rotation occurs at the atlanto-occipital joint, rotation of atlas on axis will carry the head with it; thus the movement occurring at the atlantoaxial joint contributes to the movement of the head on the trunk (Figure 9.10c).

MOVEMENTS OF THE SPINE AS A WHOLE

Individual Movements

The movements of the spinal column, which resemble those of a ball-and-socket joint, are described as follows.

Flexion

This is a forward-downward bending in the sagittal plane about a bilateral axis (Figure 9.11a). It involves a compression of the anterior parts of the intervertebral discs and a gliding motion of the articular processes. It occurs more freely in the cervical, upper thoracic, and lumbar regions. The cervical curve may be reduced to a straight line and the lumbar curve, in flexible individuals, may be reversed. The greatest anteroposterior motion in the lumbar spine usually occurs between the fifth lumbar vertebra and the sacrum.

Extension and Hyperextension

Extension is the return movement from flexion (Figure 9.11b). Hyperextension is a backward-downward movement in the sagittal plane. It occurs most freely in the cervical and lumbar regions, and particularly at the lumbosacral junction. In the thoracic region, hyperextension is limited by the overlapping of the spinous processes.

Lateral Flexion

This is a sideward bending in the frontal plane about an anteroposterior axis (Figure 9.11c). It is freest in the cervical region and quite free in the lumbar region and at the thoracolumbar junction, but it is limited in the thoracic region by the presence of the ribs. Each rib (except the 1st, 10th, 11th, and 12th) articulates with two adjacent vertebrae and the intervening disc, and each rib (except the 11th and 12th) articulates with the transverse process of the lower of the two vertebrae (Figure 9.12). Thus the ribs serve as splints, restricting lateral flexion of the thoracic spine to a marked degree. It is amazing that any motion can take place there at all.

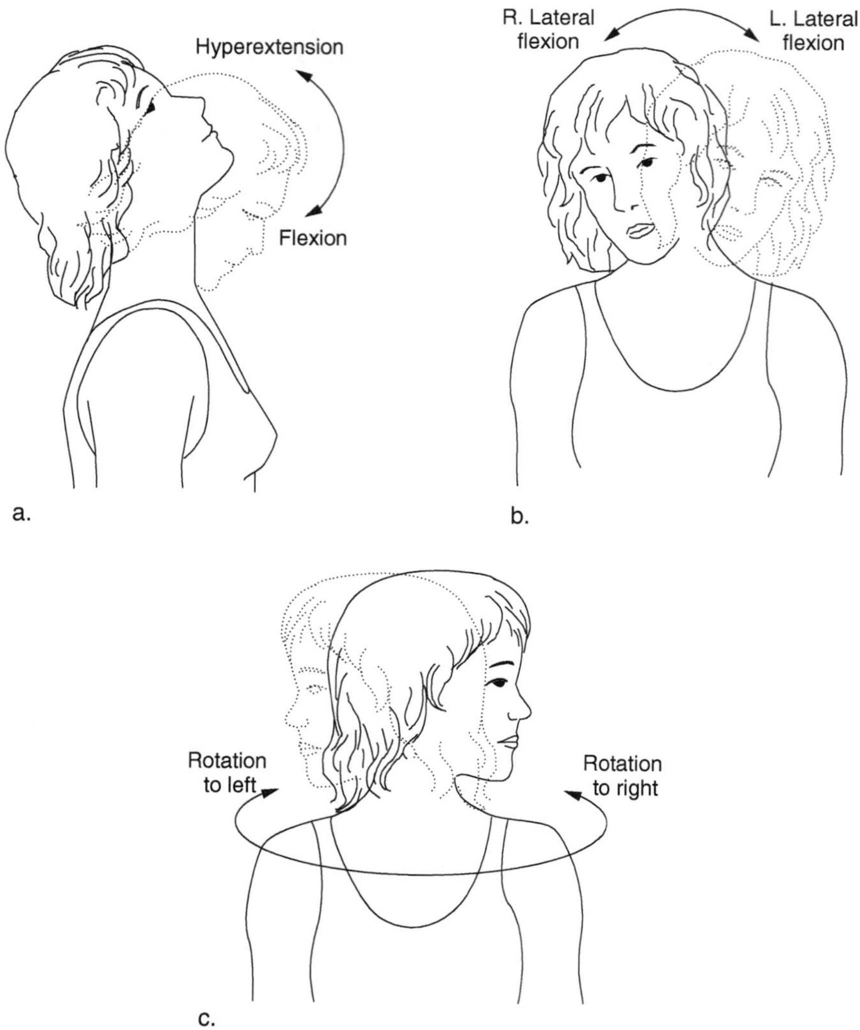

Figure 9.10 Movements of the head and neck: (a) flexion, extension, and hyperextension; (b) lateral flexion; (c) rotation.

For several reasons—the slant of the articular processes, the presence of the anteroposterior curves of the spine, and muscular and ligamentous tensions—lateral flexion is always accompanied by a certain amount of torsion. When lateral flexion is performed from the erect position, the maximum movement occurs in the lumbar region and at the thoracolumbar junction, with only slight involvement of the lower thoracic spine. The torsion occurs in the same part of the spine and consists in a turning of the vertebral bodies toward the side of the lateral flexion. Thus, if the spine bends to the right (forming a curve concave to the right), the vertebral bodies turn slightly to the right, with the spinous processes, therefore, turning to the left.

If the lateral flexion of the trunk is performed from a position of hyperextension, and the hyperextension is maintained throughout the movement, the lateral flexion moves lower in the spine,

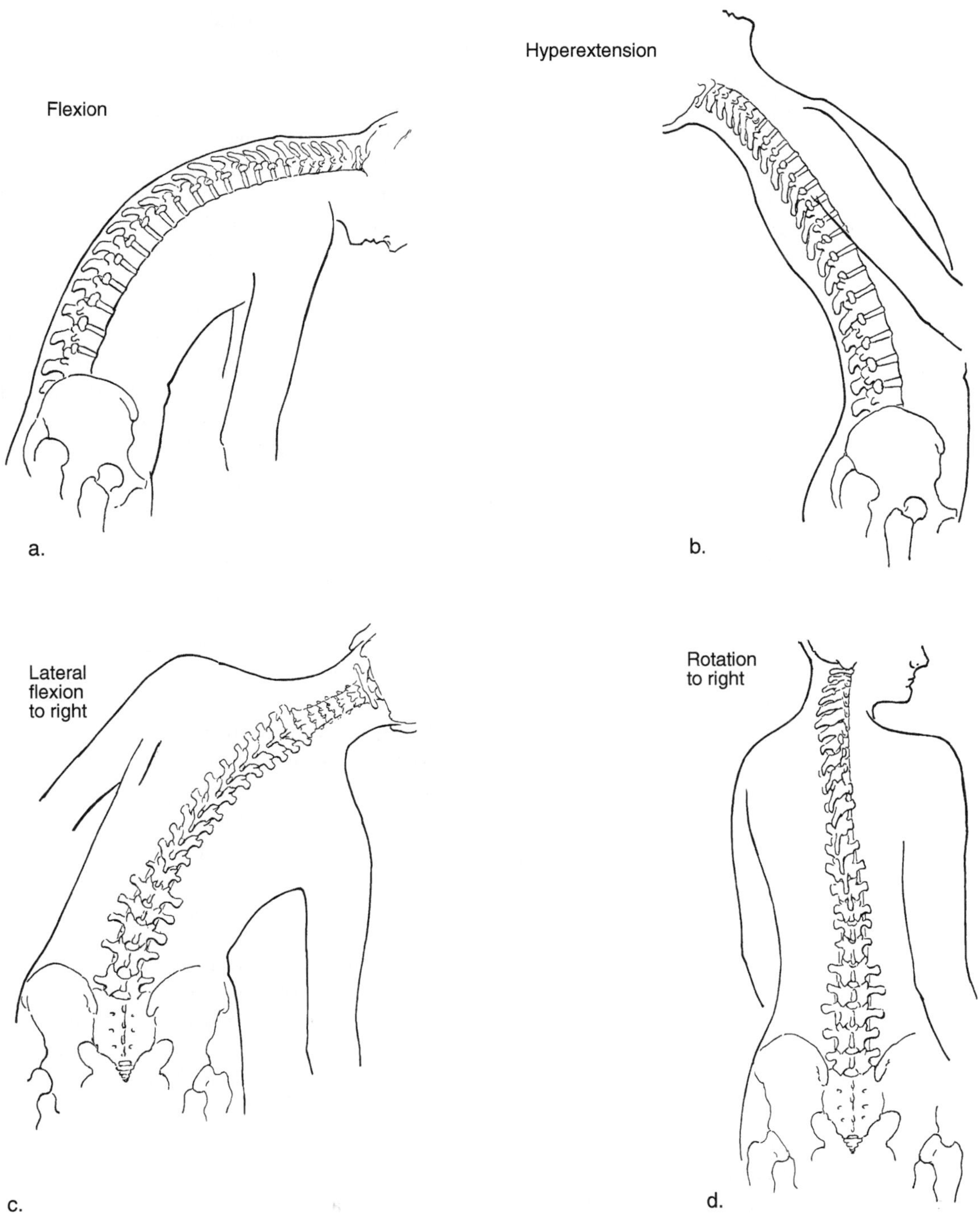

Figure 9.11 Movements of the spinal column.

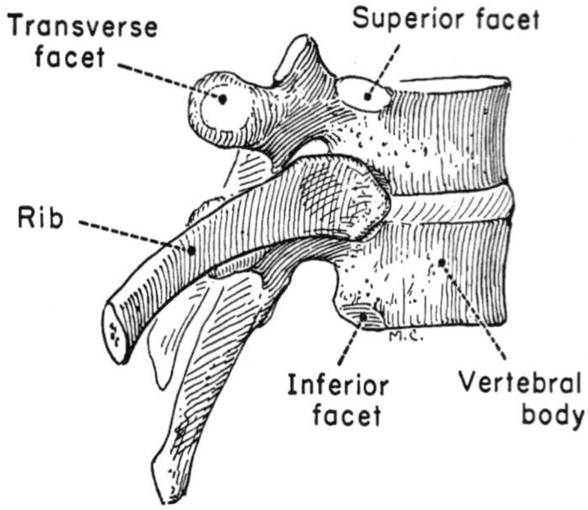

Figure 9.12 Articulation of a rib with two adjacent vertebrae.

occurring almost entirely below the eleventh thoracic vertebra. The torsion occurs in this same region and in the same manner that it does when the lateral flexion is performed from the erect position. The position of hyperextension seems to lock the thoracic spine against lateral movements.

If the lateral flexion is performed from a position of forward flexion, the movement occurs higher in the spine than ordinarily, the greatest deviation being at the level of the eighth thoracic vertebra. The torsion in this case reverses itself. Thus, in a side bend to the right, the vertebral bodies turn to the left and the spinous processes to the right. This reversal is not inconsistent. It is directly related to the anteroposterior curves of the spine. In the first two examples—that is, when the lateral flexion is performed either from the erect or from the hyperextended position—most of the movement takes place in the lower part of the spine, the part that is concave to the rear. The rotation that accompanies the side bend in these two cases is called concave side rotation because the bodies turn in the direction of the concave, or inner, side of the laterally curved spine. When the side bend is performed from the flexed position, most of the movement takes place in the thoracic spine, the region that is convex to the rear. The rotation that accompanies the lateral flexion in this case is called convex side rotation because the vertebral bodies turn in the direction of the convex, or outer, side of the laterally curved spine.

Rotation

This is a rotary movement of the spine in the horizontal plane about a vertical (longitudinal) axis (see Figure 9.11d). Spinal rotation is named by the way the front of the upper spine turns with reference to the lower part. Thus, a turning of the head and shoulders to the right constitutes rotation to the right. A turning of the legs and pelvis to the left, without turning the upper part of the body, also constitutes rotation of the spine to the right because the anatomical relationships are the same as in the former example. The movement of rotation is freest in the cervical region, with 90% of the movement being attributed to the atlantoaxial joint. It is next freest in the thoracic region and at the thoracolumbar junction. Owing to the interlocking of the articular processes, it is extremely limited in the lumbar region, there being only about 5 degrees of rotation to each side. In the cervical region there is no rotation between the atlas and the skull, but free rotation at the pivot joint between atlas and axis. Whenever rotation occurs in the spine, it is accompanied by a slight amount of unavoidable lateral flexion to the same side.

When performed from the erect position, rotation of the spine (below the seventh cervical vertebra) occurs almost entirely in the thoracic region. When performed from the position of hyperextension, the movement shifts lower in the spine, occurring in the vicinity of the thoracolumbar junction. When performed from the flexed position, the rotation is higher than usual, occurring in the upper thoracic spine. Regardless of the position in which the rotation is performed—whether erect, flexed, or hyperextended—the slight lateral flexion that accompanies it is always to the same side as the rotation. Thus if the spine rotates to the left, it flexes slightly to the left. This movement is very slight, however, and can scarcely be detected.

Circumduction

This is a circular movement of the upper trunk on the lower, a combination of flexion, lateral flexion, and hyperextension, but not including rotation.

Summary of Spinal Movements

Flexion; extension; hyperextension
- Free in all three regions
- Cervical and thoracic curves may be reduced to straight lines
- Limited hyperextension in thoracic region due to downward orientation of spinous processes
- Lumbar curve may be reversed in flexible subjects

Lateral flexion
- Free in cervical and lumbar regions
- Limited in thoracic region by rib attachments
- Accompanied by torsion

Rotation
- Freest at top of spine, least free at bottom
- Limited in lumbar region due to superior and inferior articular surfaces oriented in sagittal plane
- Accompanied by slight lateral flexion

Circumduction
- Sequential combination of flexion, lateral flexion, and hyperextension

Regional Classification of Spinal Movements

Atlanto-occipital joint
- Flexion and extension
- Hyperextension
- Slight lateral flexion

Atlantoaxial joint
- Rotation

Remaining cervical joints
- Free flexion and extension
- Free hyperextension
- Free lateral flexion
- Free rotation

Thoracic region
- Moderate flexion
- Slight hyperextension (inhibited by spinous processes)
- Moderate lateral flexion (inhibited by ribs)
- Free rotation

Lumbar region
- Moderate to free flexion and extension
- Free hyperextension
- Free lateral flexion
- Slight rotation (inhibited by orientation of articular surfaces)

Summary of Factors Influencing Stability and Mobility of the Spine

Before considering the muscular analysis of the spinal movements, it is advisable to review some of the special characteristics that contribute to the spine's stability and modify its mobility in one way or another.

Active

Muscle activity plays a large role in stability of the spine. Anyone who has fallen asleep while seated knows the feeling of having the spine collapse when the muscles relax. Maintaining muscle stiffness in the spinal muscles is truly a dynamic activity. The tension in the postural muscles must constantly adapt to changes in position, load, and even breathing pattern. There is no one muscle that acts to produce stability in the spine. Instead, all the muscles of the trunk region act together, much like the guy wires supporting a large radio antenna. According to McGill and colleagues (2003), the important factor here is the learned pattern of muscle contraction and the endurance of those muscles.

The coordination and activation of the muscles that contribute to spine stability is based on several motor control, strategies. Without going into detail on motor control, it can be stated that the neuromuscular base for stability is dependent on voluntary control, reflex activity, and feedback responses. The patterns of activation of these systems vary with situational demands.

Passive

The tendency of the compressed intervertebral discs to push the vertebrae apart, combined with the tendency of the ligaments to press them together, is an important factor in the stability of the spinal column. Throughout life the discs are the main shock-absorbing mechanisms in the vertebral column.

There is a direct relationship between the thickness of the discs and the degree of movement permitted, with greater freedom of motion where the discs are thick.

Anteroposterior Curves

The alternating anteroposterior curves of the spinal column influence the nature and the degree of movements that occur in the different regions. Individual variations from the so-called normal curves cause variations in the movement patterns. The anteroposterior curves are said to serve as a safeguard against the development of abnormal lateral curves (curvature of the spine, scoliosis).

Thickness and Strength of the Ligaments

These differ in the different regions and have a corresponding influence on the motions permitted in each region (see Table 9.1).

Direction and Obliquity of the Articular Facets

These are characteristic for each region and play an important part in determining the type of motion permitted in each.

Size and Obliquity of the Spinous Processes

These overlap like shingles in the thoracic region, hence limiting hyperextension. In the lumbar region they are horizontal and, although they are wide, they do not restrict motion.

Articulations of the Ribs with the Vertebrae

These limit lateral flexion in the thoracic region.

MUSCLES OPERATING THE SPINAL COLUMN

Location

The muscles responsible for the movements of the spine, with the exception of two groups, have at least one attachment on the spinal column or the skull. The exceptions are the abdominal and the hyoid muscles. Both groups are superficially located on the front of the body. Nevertheless, both groups, the abdominal muscles in particular, are effective movers or stabilizers of the spine. The muscles are listed according to aspect and region.

Anterior Aspect

- Cervical Region
  - Prevertebral muscles (longus capitis and colli, rectus capitis anterior, and lateralis)
  - Hyoid muscles (suprahyoids and infrahyoids)
- Thoracic and Lumbar Regions
  - Abdominal muscles
    - Obliquus externus abdominis
    - Obliquus internus abdominis
    - Rectus abdominis
    - Transversus abdominis

Posterior Aspect

- Cervical Region Only
  - Splenius capitis and cervicis
  - Suboccipitals (rectus capitis posterior major and minor, obliquus capitis superior and inferior)
- Cervical, Thoracic, and Lumbar Regions
  - Erector spinae (iliocostalis, longissimus, and spinalis)
  - Deep posterior spinal muscles (multifidi, rotatores, interspinales, intertransversarii, and levatores costarum)
  - Semispinalis thoracis, cervicis, and capitis

Lateral Aspect

- Cervical Region
  - Scalenus anterior, posterior, and medius (commonly called the three scalenes)
  - Sternocleidomastoid
  - Levator scapulae
- Lumbar Region
  - Quadratus lumborum
  - Psoas major

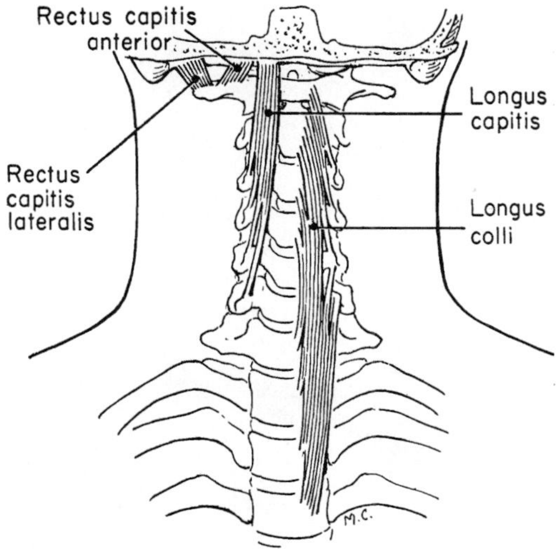

Figure 9.13 Prevertebral muscles of cervical spine (anterior view).

Characteristics and Functions of Individual Spinal Muscles

Anterior Aspect

Prevertebral muscles As Figure 9.13 shows, the longus colli and capitis extend vertically up the front of the vertebrae, the colli from the upper three thoracic to the first cervical (atlas) and the capitis from the lower cervical to the occipital bone. The rectus capitis muscles pass obliquely upward from the atlas to the skull, the anterior slanting medially and the lateralis laterally. With the exception of the longus colli, these muscles flex the head and neck when the left and right muscles act together. Acting separately, they flex the head and neck laterally or rotate it to the opposite side. The longus colli acts only on the neck and is active in resisted forward flexion, resisted lateral flexion, and rotation to the same side. It also stabilizes the neck during coughing, talking, and swallowing.

Hyoid muscles Also called the strap muscles, these are small anterior muscles in the cervical region (Figure 9.14). There are four suprahyoids and four infrahyoids. Together they flex the head and neck. They are primarily muscles of some phase of swallowing, but they contract in cervical flexion whenever the movement is performed against

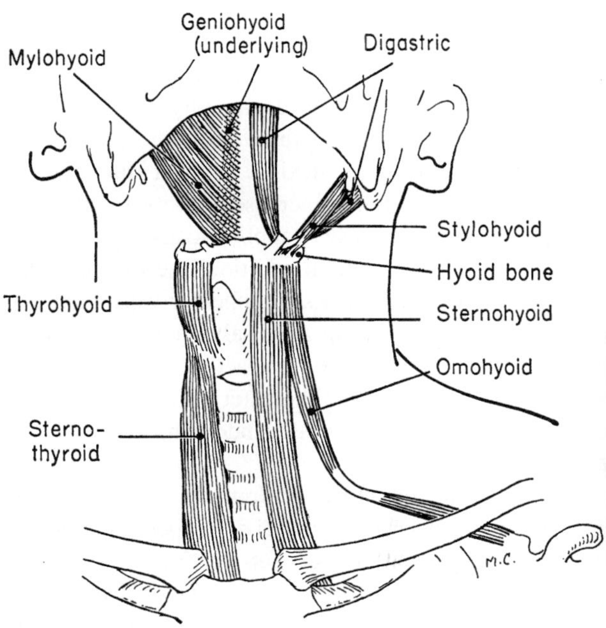

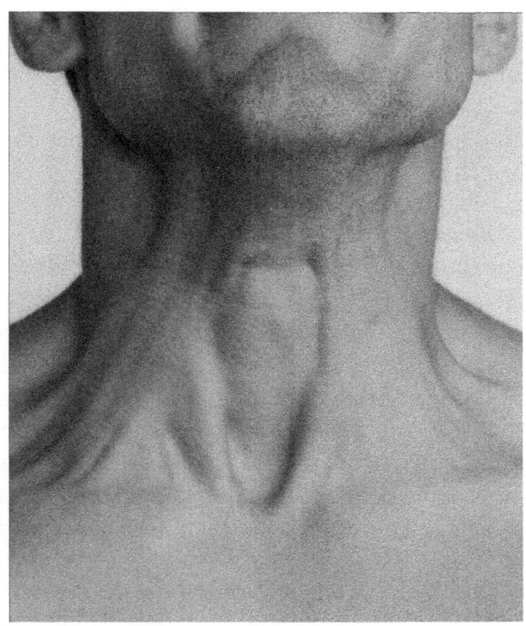

Figure 9.14 Hyoid muscles (anterior view).

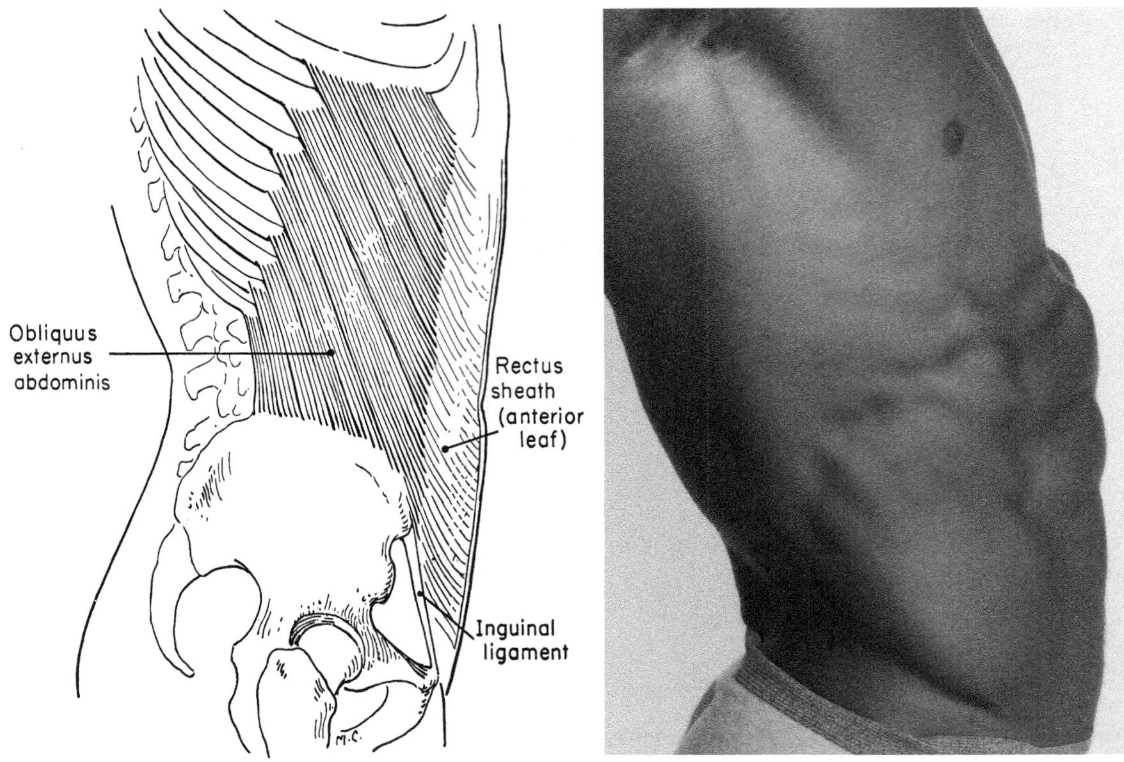

Figure 9.15 External oblique abdominal muscle (obliquus externus abdominis).

resistance. By neutralizing one another's pull on the hyoid bone, their action is transferred to the head and thence to the cervical spine. They may be palpated just below the jawbone.

Abdominal Muscles

Obliquus externus abdominis The fibers of this muscle (Figure 9.15) run diagonally upward and outward from the lower part of the abdomen, the two muscles together forming an incomplete letter *V,* as seen from the front. When both sides contract, they flex the thoracic and lumbar spine against gravity or other resistance. When only one side contracts in combination with other anterior, lateral, and posterior muscles on the same side, it *flexes the spine laterally.* When it combines with other spinal rotators, it rotates the spine to the opposite side—that is, the right muscle *rotates the spine to the left.*

Investigators have found that external obliques show the greatest activity in movements performed from the supine position such as forward and/or lateral flexion. Both of the obliques have been found to increase activity to stabilize the spine in response to applied loads or to support lower-limb motion. In addition, the external and internal obliques working together were found to show activity during a Valsalva maneuver (holding the breath while contracting the abdominal muscles forcefully). The external oblique may be palpated at the side of the abdomen.

Obliquus internus abdominis This muscle (Figure 9.16) lies beneath (i.e., deeper than) the external oblique. Its fibers fan out from the crest of the ilium, most of them passing diagonally forward and upward toward the rib cartilages and sternum, some horizontally forward toward the linea alba,

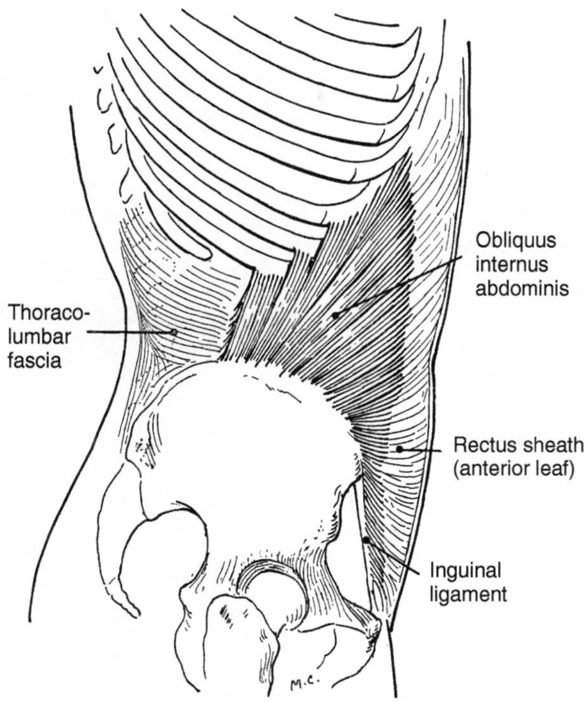

Figure 9.16 Internal oblique abdominal muscle (obliquus internus abdominis).

and some diagonally forward and downward toward the crest of the pubis. EMG experiments have also shown it to have marked activity in leaning backward and in decreasing the pelvic tilt from the supine position during leg raising and lowering (hip flexion/extension). In summary, the internal oblique *flexes the lumbar and thoracic spine, flexes the spine laterally, and rotates the spine to the same side.* It may be palpated at the side of the abdomen, below the external oblique. It may also be palpated through the external oblique when the latter is relaxed, as in rotation.

Rectus abdominis This is the most superficial of the abdominal muscles (Figure 9.17). It is situated on the anterior surface of the abdomen on either side of the linea alba. It is a long, flat band of muscle fibers extending longitudinally between the pubis and the lower part of the chest. At three different levels, transverse fibrous bands known as tendinous inscriptions cross the muscle fibers. The muscle is enclosed within a sheath formed by the aponeuroses of the other muscles making up the abdominal wall. The upper rectus was found to be more active in exercises involving the upper part of the body, such as spine flexion from the supine position. The lower rectus was found to be more active in moments involving a decrease of pelvic tilt, such as in the supine position bending the knees and lifting them toward the face until the fifth lumbar vertebra is raised approximately 5 inches above the supporting surface (Sarti et al., 1996). In brief, the rectus abdominis *flexes the lumbar and thoracic spine,* and *one side working alone helps flex the spine laterally.* The muscle may be palpated on the front of the abdomen about 2 or 3 inches from the midline, from the pubis to the sternum.

Transversus abdominis This muscle (Figure 9.18) is made up of a broad sheet of fibers that run horizontally from the thoracolumbar fascia and

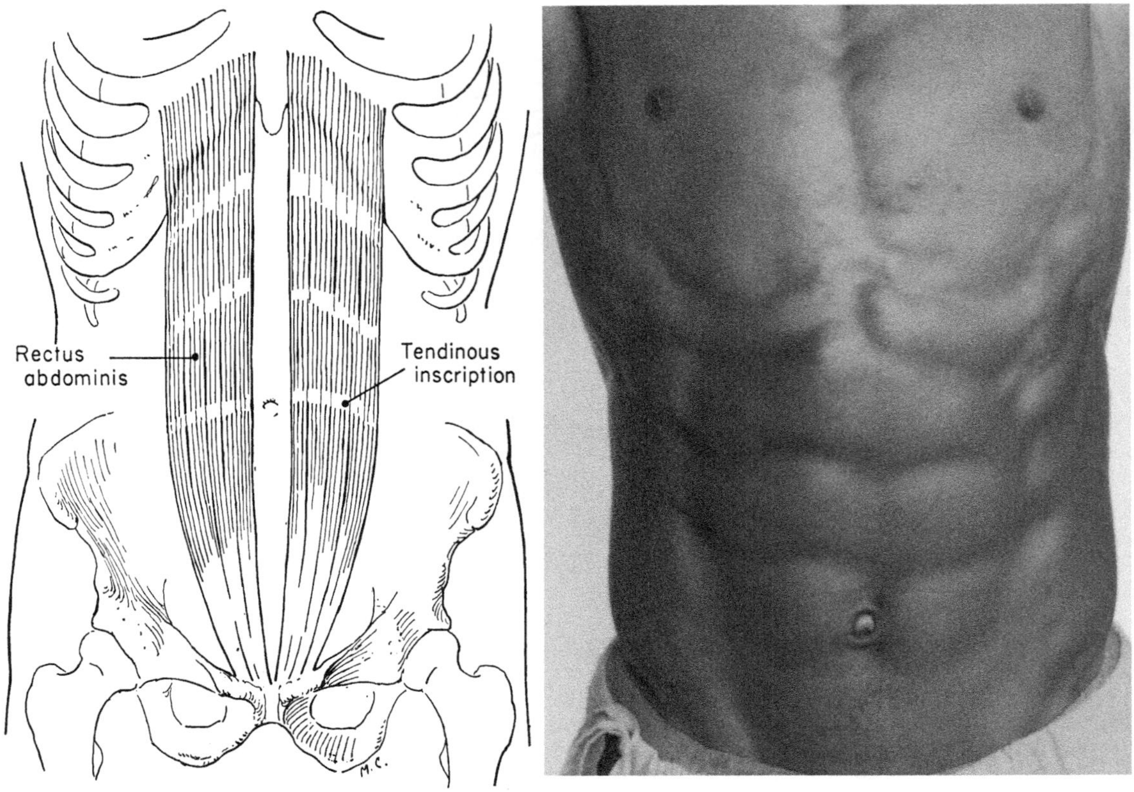

Figure 9.17 Rectus abdominis.

cartilages of the lower ribs forward to the linea alba. Its primary pull is inward against the abdominal viscera, hence it is a strong muscle of exhalation and expulsion. It does, however, help *stabilize the trunk* when acts requiring great effort are performed and may be primarily responsible for the maintenance of intra-abdominal pressure during lifting. Portions of this muscle are also active during rotation to the same side; other portions contribute to opposite-side rotation (Urquhart & Hodges, 2005).

The Abdominal Muscles as Spinal Flexors

The rectus abdominis and the external and internal obliques work together to flex the lumbar and thoracic spine. They play a small part, however, in flexing the spine from an erect position. This movement is produced by the force of gravity and controlled by the extensors in eccentric contraction. The only circumstance that would necessitate continued contraction of the abdominal muscles would be if the spine were being flexed against resistance, such as would occur if a person were lifting a weight by pulling down on a pulley rope and supplementing arm strength by flexing the spine instead of by the more efficient method of bending the knees and using the body weight.

The abdominal muscles are markedly active when the spine is being flexed from a supine position, especially at the beginning of this movement before the hips start to flex. Their activity is increased if a weight is held against the chest or on top of the head. (Obviously, the head and neck flexors are also working hard.) Once the hips start to flex, the abdominal muscles play a double role—namely, as movers in flexing the spine and as stabilizers of the pelvis against the pull of the hip flexors. When a straight spine sit-up is performed,

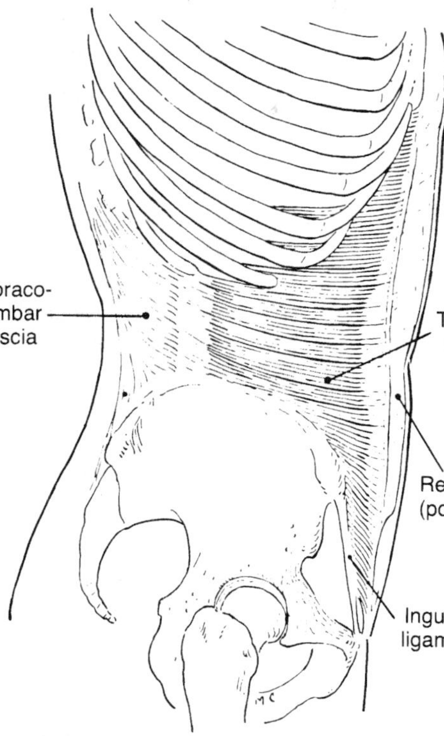

Figure 9.18 Transversus abdominis.

the abdominal muscles do not act as movers at all. In this exercise, the trunk as a whole is flexing at the hip joints on the lower extremities. As the hip flexors are attached to the movable pelvis, the latter needs to be stabilized against their pull, and this is done by means of the static contraction of the abdominal muscles. If the latter are not strong enough to prevent the tilting of the pelvis, the abdominal action then becomes an involuntary eccentric or lengthening contraction. If the student is thoroughly familiar with the attachments of the abdominal muscles, he or she will know that these muscles cannot be movers in this exercise because they *do not cross the hip joints.*

The abdominal wall The abdominal wall consists of the four abdominal muscles. Together, these muscles form a strong anterior support for the abdominal viscera. They are subject to considerable stress from the pressure of the latter against their inner surface. The more stretched they become, as in the case of a protruding abdomen, the more heavily the organs rest upon the abdominal wall, subjecting it to direct gravitational stress. Thus a vicious circle is set in motion. The pressure against the lower abdominal wall stretches it still more, causing its protrusion to increase and subjecting it to ever-increasing gravitational stress. As is so often the case, correction of this postural fault is much more difficult than its prevention. A strong abdominal wall is greatly to be desired.

Trunk stability The abdominal wall acts to stabilize the trunk during extension and some postural adjustments. Cocontraction of the abdominal muscles produces an increase in intra-abdominal pressure, which acts to increase the stiffness of the trunk. Increased trunk stiffness provides for an increased ability to adjust to loading. Without the stiffness provided by muscle cocontraction, the spine can tolerate only about 90 N (20 lbs) of compressive load before it buckles (McGill et al., 2003). In many lifting tasks, trunk stiffness is necessary to avoid undue motion of the individual vertebrae as the result of external forces. Excessive loading without trunk stability may predispose one to disc rupture or other injuries of the spine.

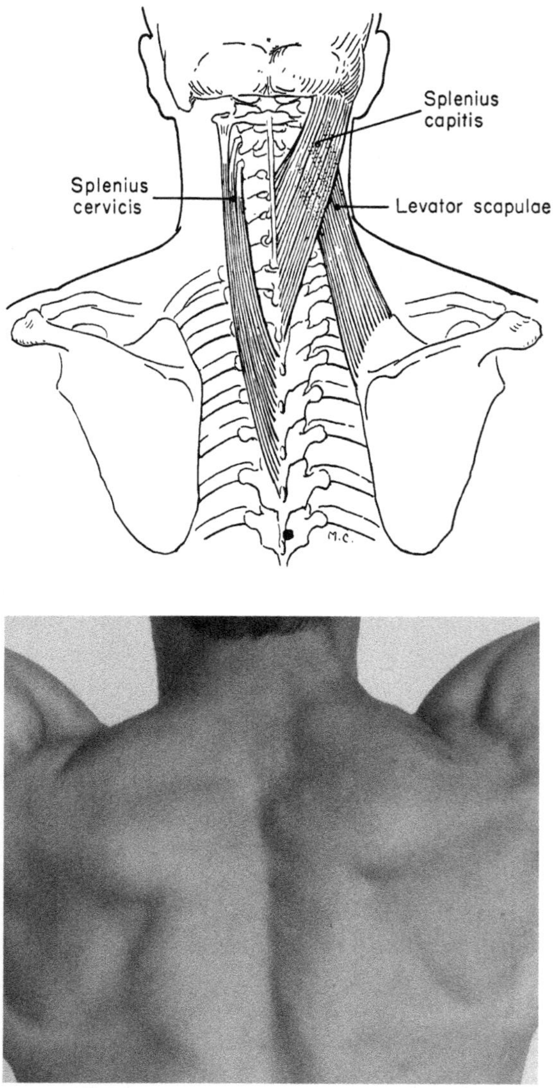

Figure 9.19 Posterior and lateral muscles of cervical spine.

Posterior Aspect

Splenius capitis and cervicis These two muscles consist of bands of parallel fibers, slanting outward as they ascend from their centrally located lower attachments to their more laterally located upper attachments. The capitis is much broader than the cervicis. Figure 9.19 clearly shows the left cervicis and the right capitis muscles. The viewer should try to visualize both muscles on both sides. When the left and right sides contract together, they serve to *extend and hyperextend the head and neck.* They also help support the head in erect posture. One side contracting alone can *flex the head and neck laterally and also rotate them to the same side.* The muscles may be palpated on the back of the neck just lateral to the trapezius and posterior to the sternocleidomastoid above the levator scapulae, especially if the head is extended against resistance in the prone position and the shoulders are kept relaxed. It is difficult to identify these muscles, however.

Suboccipital group This is a group of four short muscles (Figure 9.20) situated at the back of the lower skull (occipital bone) and upper two vertebrae (atlas and axis). It includes the obliquus capitis superior and inferior and the rectus capitis posterior major and minor. Acting together on both sides, this group extends and hyperextends the head. When one side acts alone, it *flexes the head laterally or rotates it to the same side.*

Erector spinae The muscle (Figure 9.21) commences as a large mass in the lumbosacral region but soon divides into three branches.

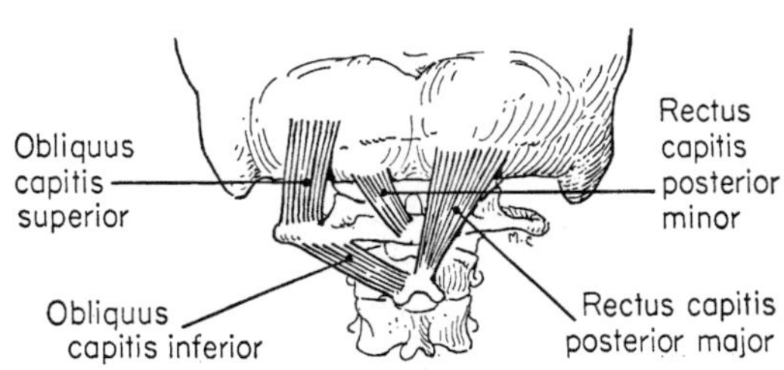

Figure 9.20 Suboccipital muscles (posterior view).

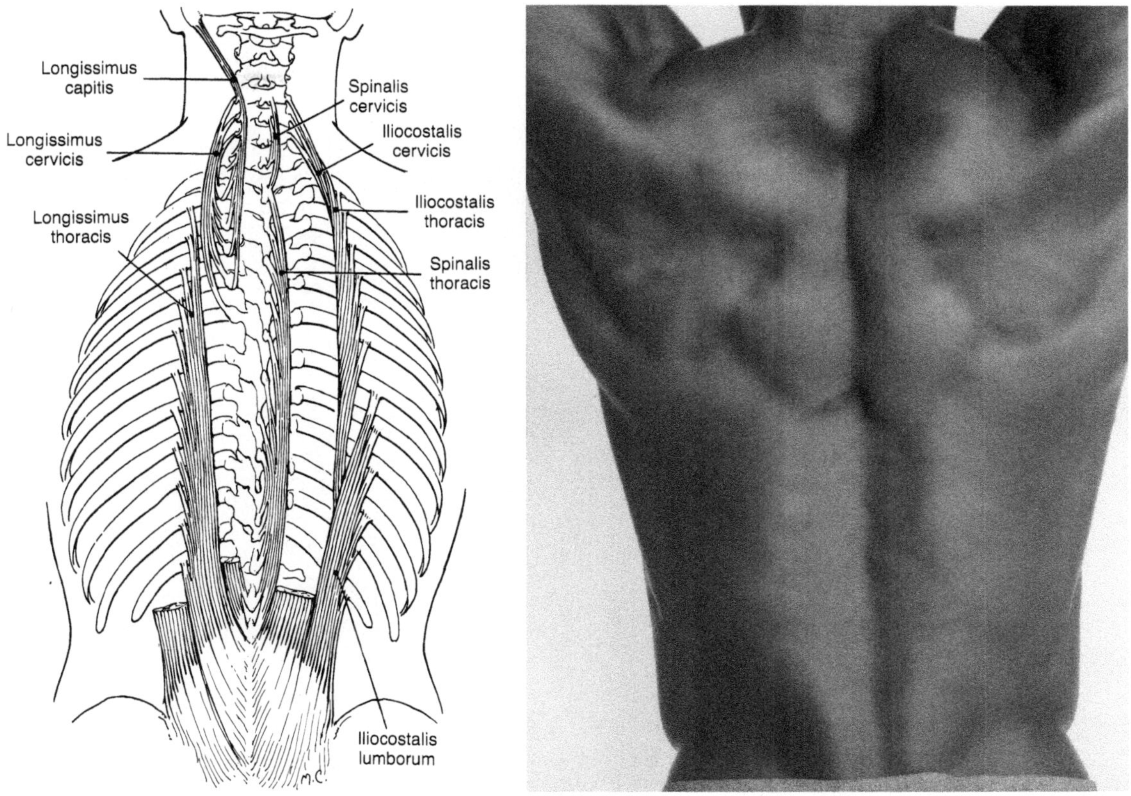

Figure 9.21 The erector spinae.

The *iliocostalis* branch consists of lumbar, thoracic, and cervical portions that are named *lumborum, thoracis,* and *cervicis,* respectively. It receives an additional tendon of origin from each rib throughout the thoracic region and gives off small slips to insert into the ribs in the thoracic region and into the transverse processes of the vertebrae in the cervical region.

The *longissimus* branch consists of three distinct portions that, in fact, appear to be three separate muscles (Figure 9.21). *Longissimus thoracis* is a broad band lying against the angles of the ribs; *longissimus cervicis* is narrower and lies slightly closer to the spine, connecting the transverse processes of the upper thoracic vertebrae with those of the lower cervical vertebrae; and *longissimus capitis* is a thin strand that lies against the vertebrae for its lower two-thirds and then slants outward and upward to the mastoid process of the temporal bone.

The *spinalis* branch lies against the vertebrae and is attached by separate slips to the spinous processes. It is of significance in the thoracic region only.

Electromyographic studies have shown that the erector spinae contributes little to the maintenance of erect posture unless a deliberate effort is made to extend the thoracic spine more completely or unless the weight is carried forward over the balls of the feet, in which case some static contraction of the muscle is required. In ordinary standing, the level of activity is quite low.

In forward flexion from the standing position, the erector spinae undergoes eccentric contraction until the weight of the trunk is supported by the ligaments in a flexion–relaxation response.

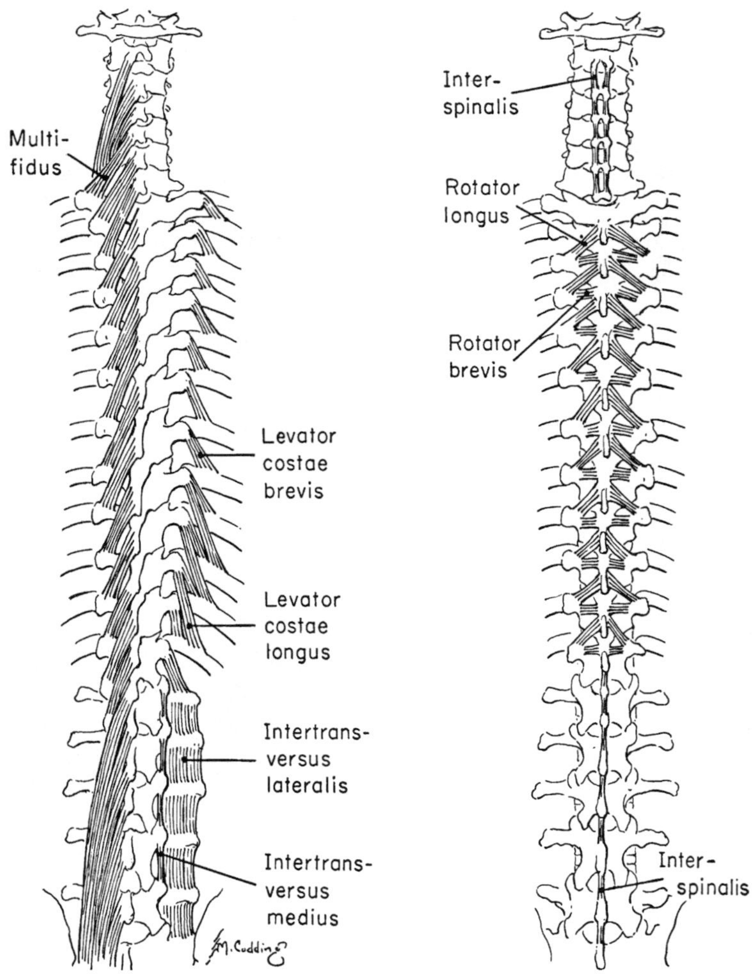

Figure 9.22 Deep posterior muscles of the spine including part of the transversospinalis (multifidus, rotators, and semispinalis).

When the trunk returns from this position, the muscle contracts concentrically until the body is again erect and balanced. However, many times the lumbar region of this muscle does not become active to initiate the return from full flexion, and often there are moments when this muscle is quiet during continued extension.

In almost all vigorous exercises performed from the standing position, the most active part of the erector spinae was the spinalis and the least active was the iliocostalis lumborum. The muscle engages most forcefully in its functions of extension, hyperextension, and lateral flexion when these movements are performed against gravity or other resistance. Hyperextension from the prone lying position while lifting both arms and legs is considered the best exercise for strengthening the erector spinae (Plamondon et al., 2002).

In brief, when the two sides of the muscle contract with equal force, the erector spinae *extends the head and spine* (assuming that all of its branches are contracting). When one side contracts alone, especially in conjunction with lateral and anterior muscles of the same side, it causes lateral flexion. And when one side alone contracts in a certain precise combination with lateral and

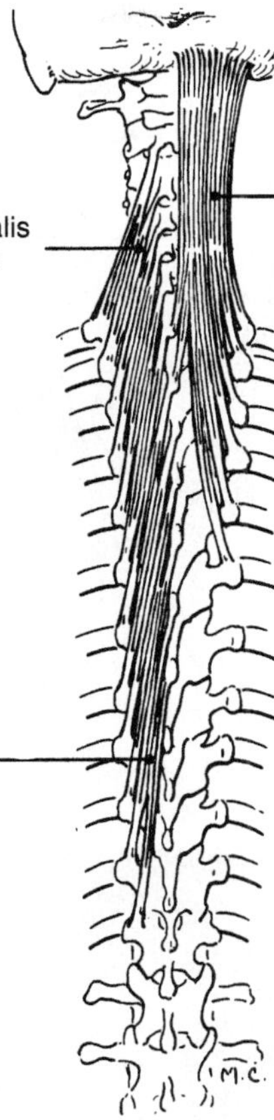

Figure 9.23 Semispinalis (posterior view), including part of the transversospinalis (multifidus and rotators).

anterior muscles—some on the same side, some on the opposite side—it rotates the head and spine to its own side. The lumbar and lower thoracic portions of the muscle may be palpated in the two broad ridges on either side of the spine.

Deep posterior spinal muscles This group (Figure 9.22) includes the multifidi, rotatores, interspinales, intertransversarii, and levatores costarum. The latter is primarily a muscle of the thorax but is included here as a possible assistant in extension and lateral flexion. These muscles consist of small slips, in most cases inserting into the vertebrae immediately above their lower attachments. Some of the fibers run vertically, and some slant medially as they ascend. The former are best developed in the cervical and lumbar regions, where their action is that of extension. The latter are best developed in the thoracic region, where they either extend or rotate. It has been suggested that the muscles in this group are responsible for localized movements. It seems likely that they also help stabilize the spine. In brief, acting symmetrically, they *extend and hyperextend the spine,* and acting asymmetrically, they *rotate the spine to the opposite side and assist in lateral flexion.*

Semispinalis thoracis, cervicis, and capitis These muscles (Figure 9.23) lie close to the vertebrae beneath the erector spinae. The thoracis and cervicis portions consist of small bundles of fibers that slant medially as they ascend to the spinous processes several vertebrae above. The lower portion of the semispinalis capitis—that is, the portion starting from the upper thoracic vertebrae—has a slight medial slant, but the bundles in the cervical region attaching to the occipital bone are vertical. Like the muscles in the preceding group, they extend and hyperextend the thoracic and cervical spine when both sides contract together, and when only one side contracts, they cause *lateral flexion and rotation to the opposite side.*

Transversospinalis This is not a different muscle from those already listed but represents a different organization of the deep muscles of the back. Some texts use this term for the three spinal muscles whose fibers slant medially as they ascend, namely the *semispinalis, multifidi,* and *rotatores* (see Figures 9.22 and 9.23).

Thoracolumbar fascia Although not a muscle, the thoracolumbar fascia (see Figure 9.18) is described here because of its importance to the deep muscles of the spine and erector spinae. It binds these muscles together, holding them close to the skeletal structure and separating them from the more superficial muscles of the back. In the lumbar region, it curves around the lateral margin of the erector spinae and folds in front of it to attach to the tips of the transverse processes of the vertebrae and to the intertransverse ligaments. Its lateral portion provides attachment for the transverse abdominis (see Figure 9.18), and its posterior

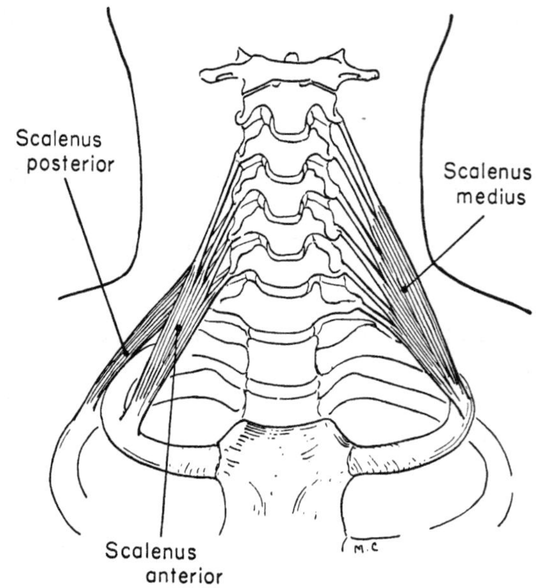

Figure 9.24 The scalenes: anterior, posterior, and medius (anterior view).

portion blends with the aponeurosis of the latissimus dorsi (see Figure 5.14).

Lateral Aspect

Scalenus anterior, posterior, and medius The three scalenes (Figure 9.24) run diagonally upward from the sides of the two upper ribs to the transverse processes of the cervical vertebrae. Acting together, they flex the cervical spine and, acting on one side at a time, they *flex the neck laterally and assist in extension.* They also serve to elevate the upper ribs in forced inspiration. They may be palpated on the side of the neck between the sternocleidomastoid and the upper trapezius but are difficult to identify.

Sternocleidomastoid This muscle (Figure 9.25) arises from two heads, one from the top of the sternum and the other from the top of the clavicle about 2 inches lateral to the first. They unite to attach to bones of the skull close below and behind the ear. Acting together, they flex the head and neck. Acting on one side at a time, they flex the head and neck laterally; they also rotate them to the opposite side (see Figure 9.27a). They may be easily palpated, as well as seen, on the side of the neck from just under the ear to the front of the neck on either side of the sternoclavicular joint.

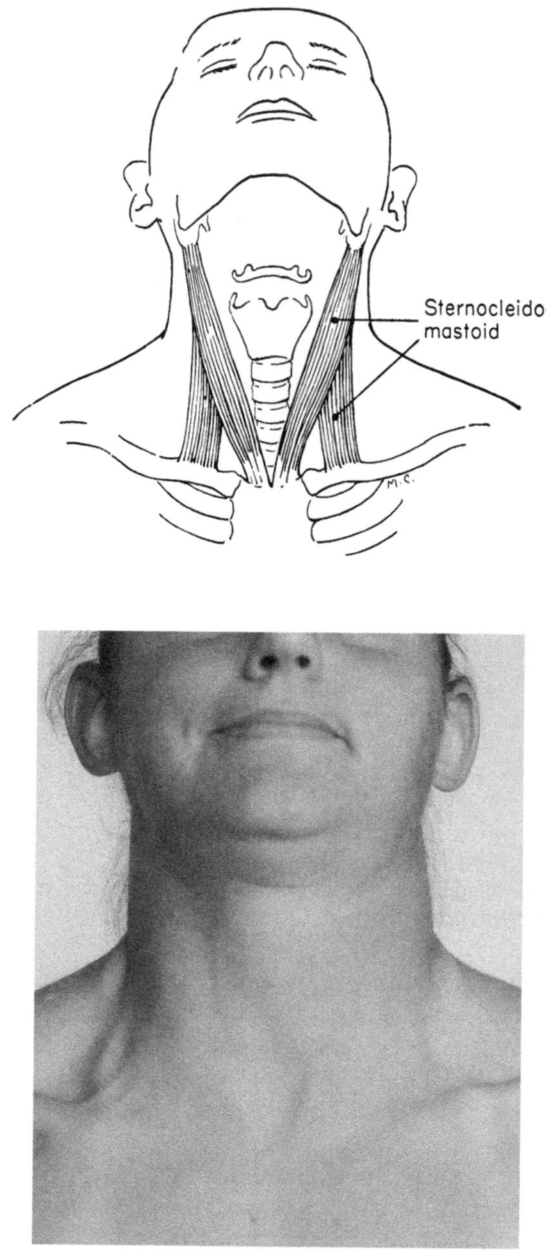

Figure 9.25 Sternocleidomastoid muscle.

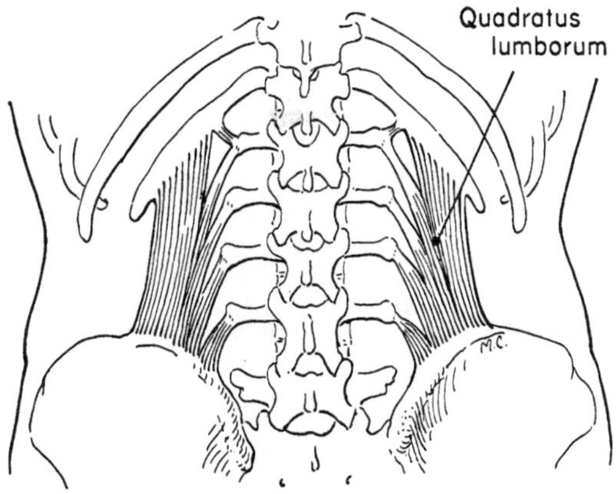

Figure 9.26 Quadratus lumborum (posterior view).

Levator scapulae (Figure 9.19, also listed with the Muscles of the Shoulder Girdle) When one scapula is fixed, the muscle on that side will help flex the cervical spine laterally. If both muscles contract at the same time when both scapulae are fixed, they neutralize each other without effecting any movement. This action may possibly help stabilize the neck, especially when the body is in the prone position, supported on "all fours."

Quadratus lumborum This flat muscle (Figure 9.26) is situated behind the abdominal cavity at the side of the lumbar spine. It extends from the crest of the ilium to the lowest rib and has slips branching medially to attach to the tips of the transverse processes of the upper four lumbar vertebrae. Acting bilaterally, it is credited with stabilizing the pelvis and lumbar spine. Acting unilaterally, it flexes the lumbar spine to the same side (lateral flexion). In a 1972 EMG study, Waters and Morris found that together with other posterior spinal muscles, as well as with the abdominal muscles, it contracted regularly in each cycle of walking. According to the electromyogram reproduced in *Muscles Alive* (Basmajian & DeLuca, 1985), its action appears to coincide with the moment of heel contact. The muscle may be palpated on a thin, muscular subject just lateral to the erector spinae in the lumbar region.

Psoas (Also listed with the Muscles of the Hip). Like the quadratus lumborum, the psoas (see Figure 7.14) is situated at the back of the abdominal cavity. Together, these two form the posterior abdominal wall. Although the psoas is primarily a muscle of the hip joint, its action on the lower spine and pelvis is of interest. Because the psoas major muscle at its promixal end attaches to the sides of the bodies to the front and lower borders of the transverse processes of all the lumbar vertebrae, it has been thought to be a mover of the lumbar portion of the spinal column.

Although there appear to be diverse opinions regarding such muscular actions, it seems likely that the differences are not of great importance. Frequently, when there is lack of agreement regarding movement, one may safely assume that the true function of the muscular contraction, with reference to the joints in question, is more likely to be stabilization or balance than purposeful movement. In their edition of *Brunnstrom's Clinical Kinesiology,* Lemkuhl and Smith (1983) described this type of action with unusual clarity. They liken the muscles that are situated near the spinal column (erector spinae, psoas major, and so on) to guy ropes supporting an upright pole. When the pole starts to tip, the tension of the ropes on the opposite side increases. In like manner, if a person starts to lean backward, possibly to favor weak posterior muscles, the muscles on the front of the spine spring into action. Thus it would appear that the most important role of the psoas is *stabilization or balancing of the spine* in response to other forces acting on the latter. In addition, unilateral contraction contributes to *lateral flexion* of the lumbar spine.

MUSCULAR ANALYSIS OF THE FUNDAMENTAL MOVEMENTS OF THE HEAD AND SPINE

In general, the muscles situated anterior to the spine flex it, those posterior to it extend it, and those lateral to it, when acting on one side only, either flex it laterally or rotate it, depending on the

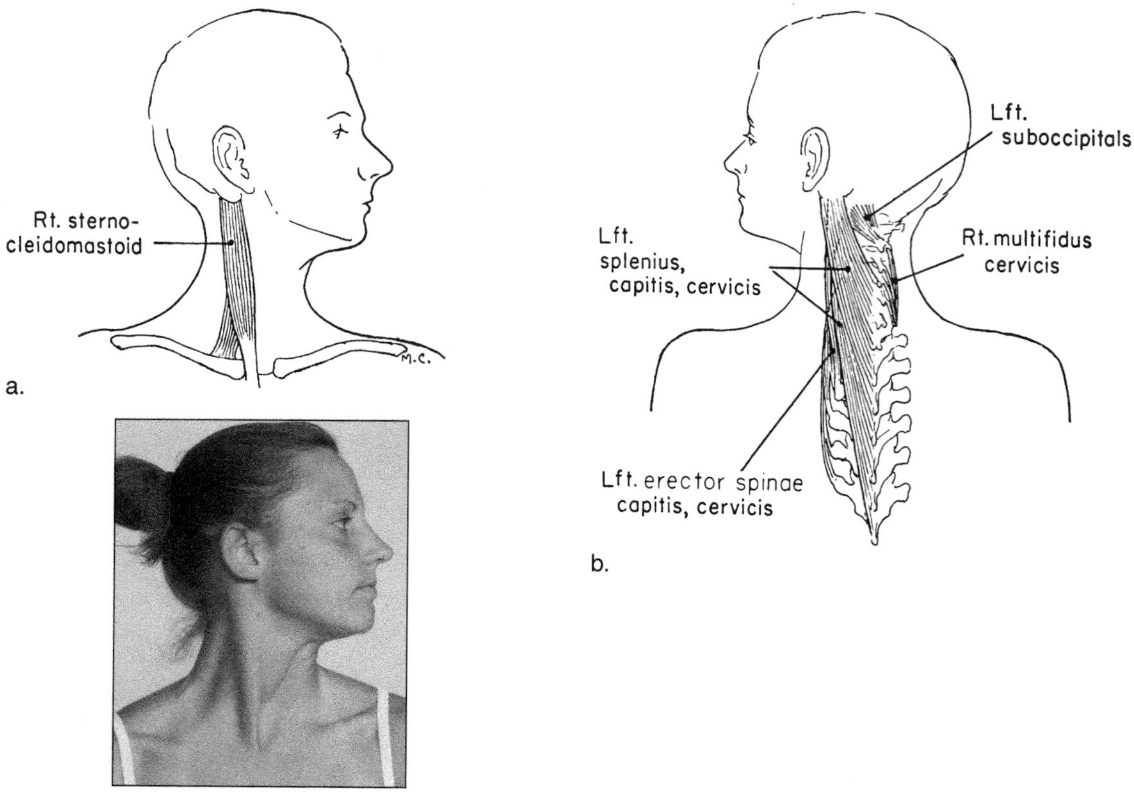

Figure 9.27 Muscles that contract to rotate the head and neck to the left.

requirements of the intended movement. *Because of the effect of gravity, however, the anterior muscles fulfill their function as flexors most successfully when the body is supine, the posterior muscles as extensors when the body is prone, and the lateral muscles as lateral flexors when the body is resting on the side.* These facts should be kept in mind when one is analyzing the muscular actions of the fundamental movements.

Cervical Spine and Atlanto-Occipital Joint

Flexion

This movement is performed chiefly by the sternocleidomastoid, the three scalenes, and the prevertebral muscles. The supra- and infrahyoid muscles, whose chief function is to move the hyoid bone up or down in movements related to swallowing and vocalizing, give added force to cervical flexion when they contract together, and movements of the mouth are prevented.

Extension and Hyperextension

Many muscles contribute to these movements: the splenius capitis and cervicis, the capitis and cervicis portions of the erector spinae, semispinalis, deep posterior spinal muscles, and the suboccipitalis. When the left and right sides of trapezius I contract together, they also help extend the head and neck.

Lateral Flexion

This movement is performed by the simultaneous contraction of the extensors and flexors of the same side. Specifically, the chief lateral flexors include the capitis and cervicis portions of the splenius, erector spinae, semispinalis, three scalenes, and sternocleidomastoid. The suboccipitals, cervical portions of the deep posterior spinal muscles, and levator scapulae are in a position to aid in lateral flexion when they are needed.

Rotation

The sternocleidomastoid and deep posterior spinal muscles rotate the head and neck to the opposite side and the splenius, erector spinae, and occipitals rotate them to the same side (Figure 9.27).

Thoracic and Lumbar Spine

The muscles that produce motion in the trunk are arranged in such a way that their effectiveness depends heavily on their distance from the vertebral column. Both the relative size of the trunk muscles and their arrangement in the body play a role in producing trunk motion and in the etiology of injuries to the vertebral areas. Figure 9.28 shows both the relative sizes and the locations of the various muscles of this region.

Flexion

This movement is performed by the three abdominal muscles: the rectus abdominis and external and internal obliques. As an aid to their effective action, the pelvis must often be stabilized by the hip flexors, especially when the movement is performed from the supine position.

Extension and Hyperextension

The thoracic and lumbar portions of the erector spinae and the semispinalis thoracis are the chief extensors, but the deep posterior spinal muscles also have a significant role. When hyperextension is performed from the prone lying position, the erector spinae is particularly active.

Lateral Flexion

Many muscles are active in this movement—the erector spinae, internal and external oblique abdominals, and quadratus lumborum in particular, with the semispinalis thoracis, rectus abdominis, deep posterior spinal muscles, psoas, and latissimus dorsi supplying additional force if needed. When the trunk is flexed to the right from a sidelying position on the left, the working muscles are those on the right side of the trunk.

Rotation

Rotation to the left (Figure 9.29) is effected by the left internal oblique abdominal muscle and the thoracic and lumbar portions of the left erector

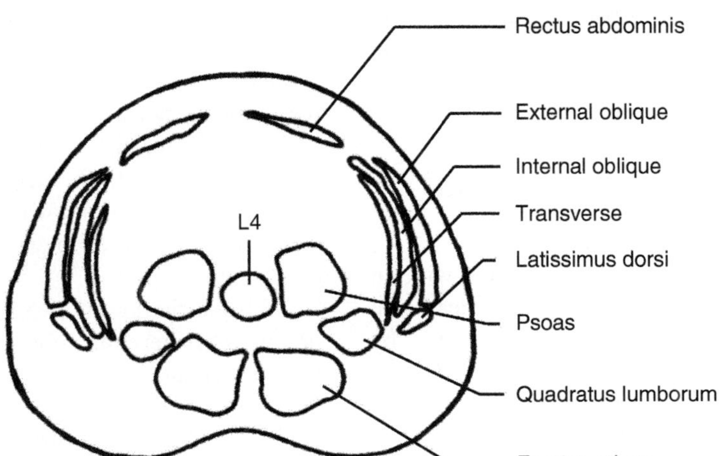

Figure 9.28 Relative positions of the trunk muscles as shown by magnetic resonance imaging.

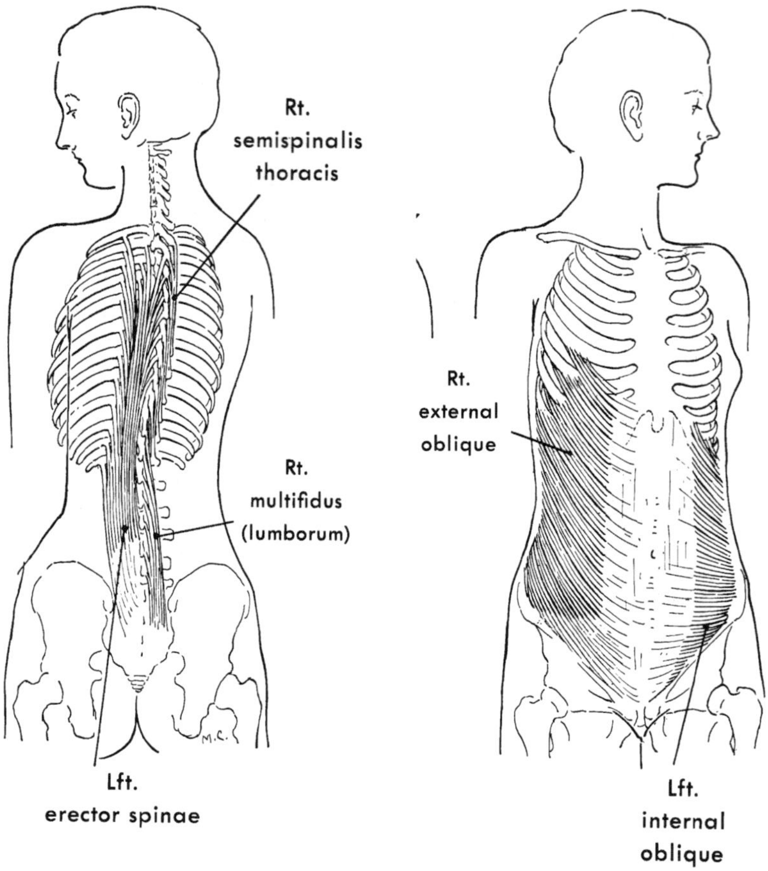

Figure 9.29 Muscles that contract to rotate the trunk to the left.

spinae, especially the iliocostalis thoracis branch, the right external oblique abdominal muscle, right latssimus dorsi, semispinalis thoracis, multifidus, and other deep posterior spinal muscles.

Structure and Articulations of the Thorax

The thorax is a bony cartilaginous cage with an inverted V-shaped opening in front beneath the sternum (Figure 9.30). It is formed mainly by the ribs and their cartilages but also includes the sternum, which constitutes the anterior base of attachment for the ribs, and the thoracic portion of the spine, which provides the posterior base of attachment. The upper seven ribs whose cartilages articulate directly with the sternum are called true ribs and the remaining five, false ribs. This is a misleading term, the only difference being that the latter do not articulate with the sternum. In each case the cartilages of the eighth, ninth, and tenth ribs unite with the cartilage above; the eleventh and twelfth ribs, known as the "floating ribs," have no anterior attachment but end anteriorly in cartilaginous tips.

All but the lowest two ribs articulate anteriorly with the sternum, either directly or indirectly, and all articulate posteriorly with the vertebrae. More specifically, with the exception of the first, tenth, eleventh, and twelfth ribs, the head of each rib articulates with two adjacent vertebrae, thus spanning the disc between (Figure 9.31). The first,

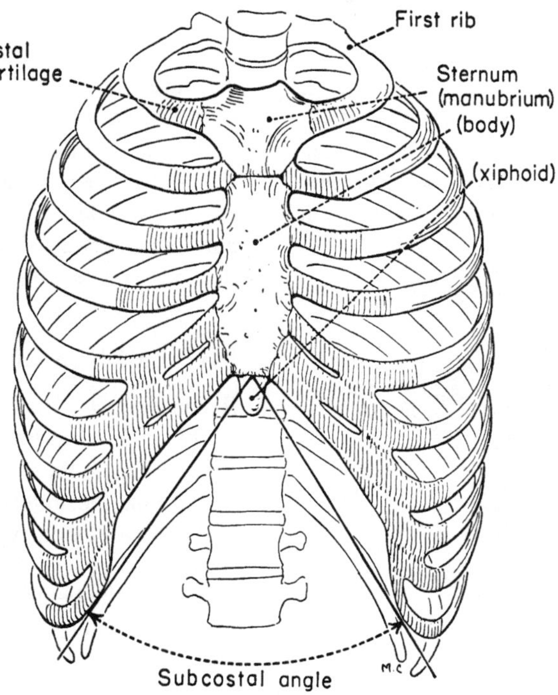

Figure 9.30 Anterior view of thorax.

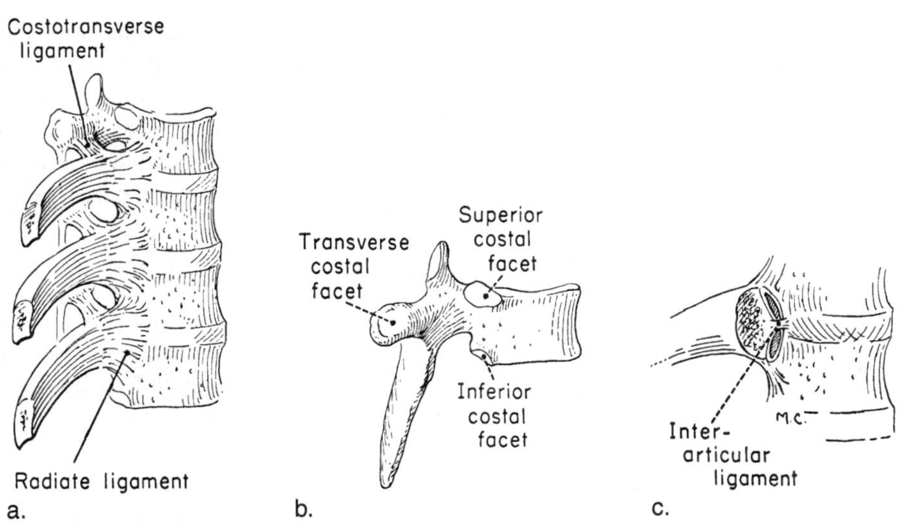

Figure 9.31 Anterior and lateral views of costovertebral articulations.

tenth, eleventh, and twelfth ribs articulate with a single vertebra. Except in the case of the last two ribs, each rib has an additional vertebral articulation between the tubercle of the rib and the adjacent transverse process of the vertebra (Figure 9.32). All of these articulations are nonaxial, diarthrodial joints and permit only a slight gliding action.

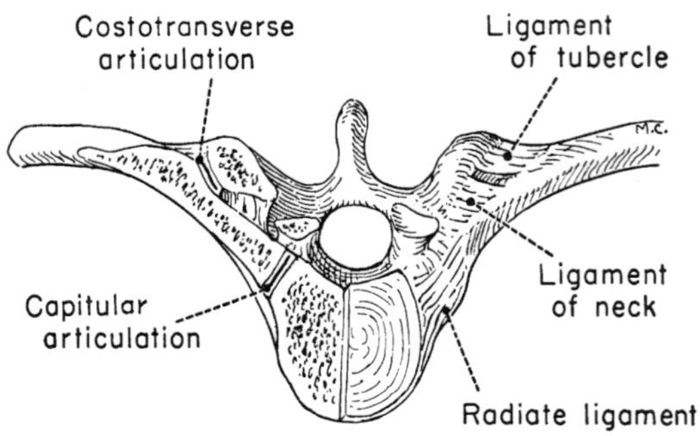

Figure 9.32 Superior view of costovertebral articulations.

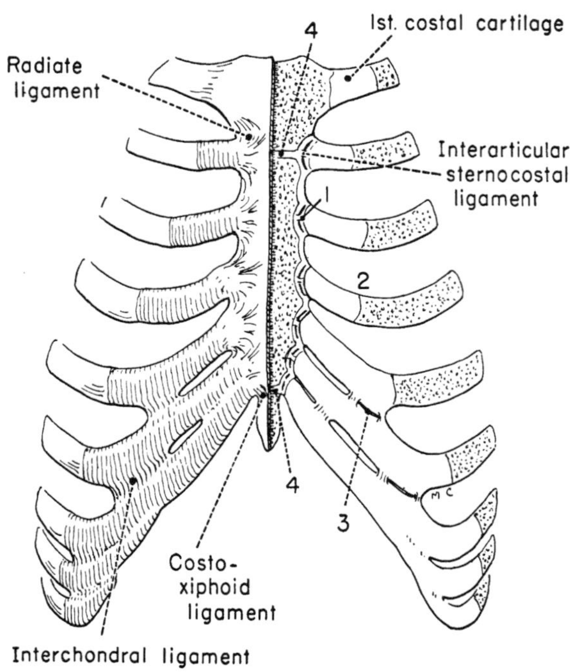

Figure 9.33 Sternocostal articulations (1 = sternocostal; 2 = costochondral; 3 = interchondral; 4 = intersternal).

There are four groups of sternocostal articulations: (1) the sternocostal joints between the costal cartilages and the sternum; (2) the joints between each rib and its cartilage, known as the costochondral joints; (3) the joints between one costal cartilage and another, called the interchondral joints; and (4) the two intersternal joints, one between the manubrium and body of the sternum, the other between the body and the xiphoid process (Figure 9.33).

Movements of the Thorax

Because most of the ribs are attached both posteriorly and anteriorly, their movement is extremely limited. In the thoracic expansion associated with inhalation, the anterior ends of the ribs are elevated in a flexion type of movement. This is accompanied by a slight eversion in which the lower margin of the central portion of the rib turns upward and lateralward, the inner surface being made to face somewhat downward. As the anterior ends of the upper ribs move upward, they also push forward, carrying the sternum forward and upward with them. In the case of the lower ribs, the anterior ends move laterally, thus "opening" the chest and widening the subcostal angle.

Although expansion of the thorax is ordinarily associated with inhalation for the purpose of providing the body with oxygen, there is another purpose: Whenever one exerts maximal muscular effort of short duration, a deep breath is taken and held while exerting the effort. This action stabilizes the ribs and sternum and thus provides firm anchorage for the upper extremity and trunk muscles that are used in forceful lifting, pushing, and pulling (Figure 9.34).

Phases of Respiration

Based on their own findings as well as on those of several other investigators, Basmajian and DeLuca (1985) recognize four phases of respiration. In brief, these are as follows.

Preinspiration

This is a brief static phase that precedes the intake of air.

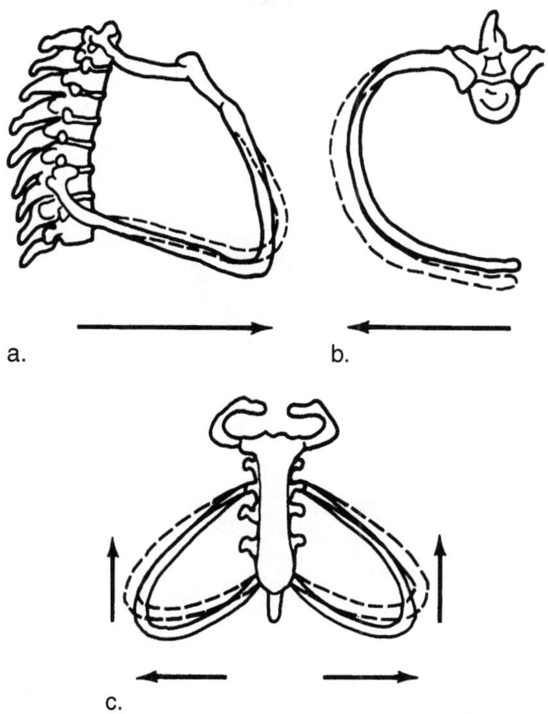

Figure 9.34 Expansion of thorax during inhalation: (a) lateral view; (b) superior view; (c) anterior view.

Inspiration

This phase is characterized by expansion of the thorax and the taking in of air.

Pre-expiration

This is a brief static phase that follows inspiration and precedes expiration.

Expiration

This phase is characterized by an outflow of air accompanying a decrease in thoracic volume.

Muscles of Respiration

The muscles associated with respiration may be divided into two groups. The first group consists of the muscles of the thorax and includes those muscles associated with the ribs whose primary function is respiration. The second group consists of those muscles of the spine and shoulder girdle whose functions in respiration, although important, are not their primary functions. Because only their activity in respiration is described here, the reader is directed to other sections of the text for additional information on the muscles included in this latter group.

Muscles with Primary Function of Respiration

Diaphragm
Intercostales, externi and interni
Serratus posterior inferior
Serratus posterior superior
Transversus thoracis

Muscles with Secondary Function of Respiration

Abdominals
Erector spinae
Extensors of cervical and thoracic spine
Pectoralis major and minor
Quadratus lumborum
Scalenes, anterior, posterior, and medius
Sternocleidomastoid

Characteristics of Individual Muscles with Primary Function in Respiration

Diaphragm

This muscle (Figure 9.35) is a dome-shaped sheet that separates the thoracic and abdominal cavities from each other. Its contraction causes depression of its central tendon, and this increases the vertical dimension of the thorax. It also has a tendency to lift the lower ribs, but this appears to be resisted by the quadratus lumborum and iliocostalis lumborum. As the diaphragm moves downward, it presses against the abdominal organs which, in turn, push forward against the relaxed abdominal wall. By increasing the intra-abdominal pressure, these actions help in defecation, vomiting, and other forms of expulsion as well as supporting posture.

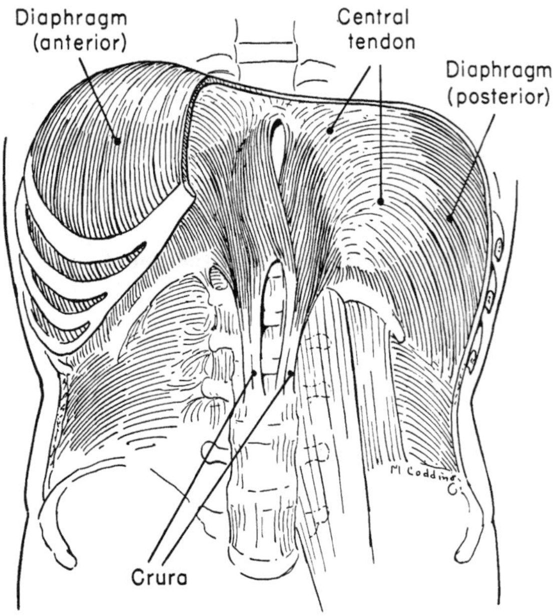

Figure 9.35 The diaphragm.

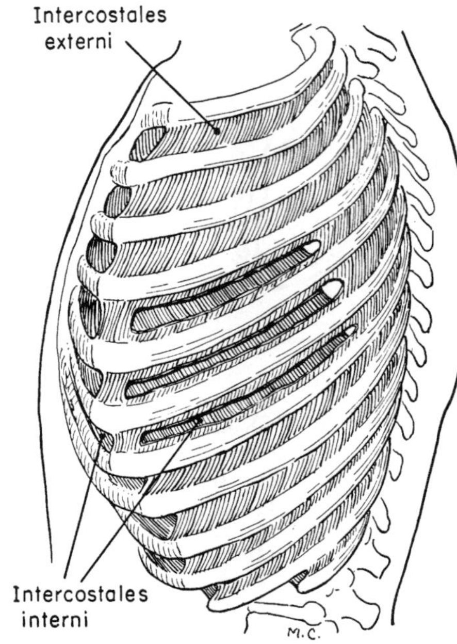

Figure 9.36 The intercostal muscles.

Intercostales, Externi and Interni

These muscles (Figure 9.36) are two layers of similar sets of muscles, each set consisting of short parallel fibers that connect adjacent ribs. The fibers of the outer set slant downward and forward from one rib to the rib below, and those of the inner set slant in the reverse direction, that is, downward and backward. Both sets extend dorsally as far as the angles of the ribs. Ventrally, the external layer extends only as far forward as the costal cartilages, whereas the internal extends to the sternum. Hence the anterior portion of the internal intercostals is not covered by the external layer.

In a computer tomography scan of these muscles (Wilson et al., 2001), it was found that the dorsal external intercostals are active during inspiration. The ventral portion of the external intercostals is quiet unless a forced inhalation is performed. The lower ventral external intercostals may have some expiratory action.

Serratus Posterior Inferior

Like four chevrons, these broad bands (Figure 9.37) connect the lower borders of the lowest four ribs with the spinous processes and ligaments of lower vertebrae (lower two thoracic and upper two or three lumbar). They are assumed to *depress the four ribs and to stabilize them* against the pull of the diaphragm. They are too deep to palpate or to test electromyographically by present techniques.

Serratus Posterior Superior

Like four steeply slanted, inverted chevrons, these bands (Figure 9.37) connect the upper borders of the second, third, fourth, and fifth ribs with the spinous processes and ligaments of the lower two or three cervical and the upper two thoracic vertebrae. They are assumed to help *elevate the four ribs* and in so doing to *expand the upper thorax.* Like the inferior, this muscle is too deep to palpate or to check by present EMG means.

Transversus Thoracis

This muscle (Figure 9.38) connects the lower half of the inner surface of the sternum and adjoining costal cartilages with the lower borders and inner surfaces of the costal cartilages of the second, third, fourth, fifth, and sixth ribs. It consists of flat

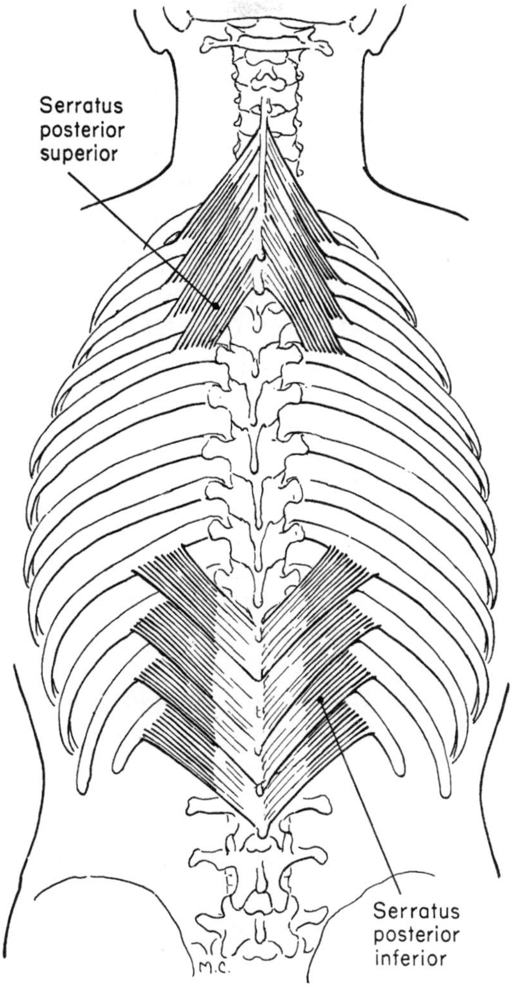

Figure 9.37 Serratus posterior superior and inferior.

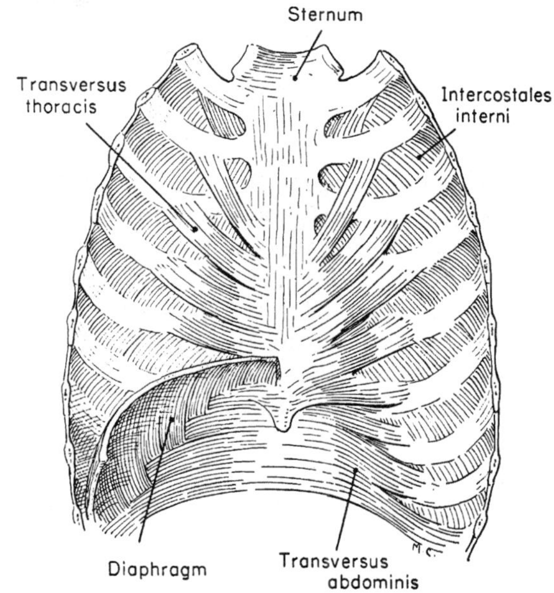

Figure 9.38 Posterior (inner) view of anterior wall of thorax.

bands that radiate upward and outward from the inner surface of the sternum to the ribs, the lowest fibers being continuous with those of the transversus abdominis. It acts during expiration.

Characteristics of Individual Muscles with Secondary Function in Respiration

Abdominals

The abdominals (see Figures 9.15, 9.16, and 9.17) are considered to be the most important muscles for expiration, becoming more active when the expiration is forced. Normal quiet breathing is considered passive, and very little muscular activity occurs during it. The transversus abdominis and the internal and external obliques, in that order, have been found to be the most important muscles of forced expiration (Abe et al., 1996; Cresswell et al., 1992).

Erector Spinae

This extensive muscle (see Figure 9.21) of the back serves to *stabilize the spine and pelvis* against the pull of the abdominal muscles. By resisting the tendency of the latter to flex the spine, it forces them to concentrate their activity on abdominal compression.

Quadratus Lumborum

An EMG study conducted in 1965 by Boyd and coworkers confirms the assumption that this muscle (see Figure 9.26) anchors the last rib against the pull of the diaphragm, which would otherwise tend to lift it and, in so doing, lose some of the force for depressing its central tendon (Basmajian & DeLuca, 1985).

Scalenes, Anterior, Posterior, and Medius

These three muscles (see Figure 9.24) connect the transverse processes of the cervical vertebrae with the first two ribs. They were formerly thought to be primarily lateral flexors of the neck and secondarily accessory or stabilizing muscles of respiration, their function being to anchor the first two ribs for the intercostals. Currently, the scalenes are thought to be active but delayed during quiet inspiration, although there seems to be some amount of individual variation (Hug et al., 2006). These muscles may be palpated on the side of the neck between the sternocleidomastoid and upper trapezius muscles.

Sternocleidomastoid

As an accessory muscle of respiration, this muscle (see Figure 9.25) shows marked electrical activity in forced inspiration. It helps elevate the sternum and clavicle. In vigorous inspiration the head is usually held firmly erect, and, instead of flexing the head and neck, the sternocleidomastoid has a slight lifting effect on the sternum and sternal end of each clavicle. It may be palpated on the side of the neck just below the ear and on the front of the neck at the junction of the clavicle and sternum.

Muscular Analysis of Respiration

Inspiration

The action of the diaphragm accounts for about one-third of the air exchanged in normal breathing. Action in the scalenes and the intercostals (especially the external) also occurs in quiet inspiration. With forced inspiration, these major muscles of inspiration, as well as the sternocleidomastoid, serratus posterior superior, levatores costarum, quadratus lumborum, erector spinae, and pectoralis major and minor, are active.

Expiration

Quiet expiration is generally considered to be a passive act. However, some activity has been recorded in the intercostals, serratus posterior muscles, diaphragm, and quadratus lumborum. The major muscles of forced expiration are the transversus abdominis and oblique abdominals. The erector spinae are active as stabilizers against the pull of the abdominals. Other participants include the transversus thoracic and intercostals. The diaphragm has been found to be quiet during vigorous expiration.

Common Injuries of the Neck, Back, and Thorax

Neck Injuries

Although these, fortunately, are not common except in severe falls, blows, or accidents, they are of prime concern. If there is the slightest suspicion of serious injury, it is literally of vital importance that the individual not be moved at all until having been examined by a physician, and then only under the physician's close supervision. *The danger of death or paralysis from the neck down cannot be overemphasized.*

Whiplash

A whiplash is a cervical sprain resulting from a violent motion. In a whiplash injury the neck is violently moved through an S-curve, with the upper portion of the cervical spine undergoing flexion while the lower portion of the cervical region is hyperextending or fixed. The pain often occurs one day after the injury and involves muscle strains and tears to ligaments. It may also include a herniated disc in the cervical region.

Muscle and Ligament Injuries

Strains (injuries to muscles) and sprains (injuries to ligaments) are both common injuries, largely because there are so many muscles and ligaments in the region of the spine. In the early stages of these injuries it is often difficult to distinguish between them. The strain is usually the result of either a violent contraction, a movement in more than one plane, or poor posture. A sprain may be caused by the same kind of movements that cause a strain, but in sprains the damage is a tearing of the ligaments.

In trunk bending motions, the ligamentous structures and the muscles of the spine bear a substantial portion of the load. The vertebral articular facets are not structured for weight bearing other than under compressive loads. The loading that occurs at an angle to the longitudinal axis of the spine is more likely to produce tension in the muscles and ligaments, as well as in the intervertebral discs.

Vertebral Fracture

Fractures of the vertebrae may affect the vertebral body, the vertebral arches, spinous processes, or the articular facets. The severity of the fracture is determined by the location of the fracture and the extent to which bone is displaced. In severe fractures it is possible that the spinal cord may be compromised or severed. Fractures of the vertebrae are often the result of impact. Motor vehicle accidents produce a large number of impact fractures. Sports-related injuries to the spine are also a consideration. High-impact sports such as football or high-impact landing sports such as snowboarding and pole vault carry risks of vertebral injury (Gerbino & d'Hemecourt, 2002; Yamakawa et al., 2001).

The risk of vertebral fracture increases with age. Older people with osteoporosis or osteoarthritis are much more likely to suffer fractures of the vertebrae than are younger adults. Vertebral fracture is the most common fracture in older adults due to the increased brittleness of bones as bone mineral is lost. Compressive forces on the spine are much more likely to cause failure in this population. In addition, women are much more likely to suffer a fracture than are men (Ferguson & Steffen, 2003; Johnell & Kanis, 2005).

Disc Problems

Intervertebral discs are subject to repeated stresses throughout the activities of daily living, work, and sports. Two of the most common pathologies of the disc are disc degeneration and disc herniation. Disc degeneration is a condition in which the annulus fibrosus deteriorates, perhaps to the point where it can no longer withstand the stresses produced by compression of the nucleus pulposa. Such degeneration may be due to a decrease in hydration with age, tissue stiffening, overuse, and repetitive loading (Whiting & Zernicke, 1998).

The conditions that cause a herniated disc—namely, the compression of two adjacent vertebrae with such magnitude that the annulus fibrosus is ruptured—are often brought about by repeated heavy lifting with the body in poor alignment. If this has happened to an athlete, participation in athletics is unwise until the rupture can be repaired. Otherwise the nucleus pulposus is likely to protrude through the break in the disc and press on the spinal cord or a spinal nerve. The area most likely to be affected is the lumbar spine, especially between the fourth and fifth lumbar vertebrae. This condition can be, but does not have to be, painful.

Rib Fractures

These injuries are fairly common in contact sports such as football and wrestling, or in traumatic blows to the chest. The usual causes are either direct blows or forceful compressions. Sudden, violent, muscular contraction may also be a cause. In most fracture injuries, two or more ribs are likely to be involved. A fracture should be suspected if breathing is accompanied by severe pain. A possible serious complication of rib fractures is damage to the soft tissues when the broken ends of the bone are pushed inward (Arnheim & Prentice, 1998).

Low Back Pain

Nonspecific low back pain has become a frequent complaint, estimated to affect up to 85% of the population. At any given time, up to 33% of the population suffers from low back pain (Woolf & Pfleger, 2003). Low back pain can have a number of causal factors. Some of the most common are inefficient or asymmetrical lifting, restricted postures, whole body vibration, repetitive stress and overuse, and prolonged sitting. Children have been found to be at risk for low back pain from the asymmetrical carrying of backpacks (Korovessis et al., 2005; Mackenzie et al., 2003). Athletes in many sports, especially those requiring endurance, impact, or heavy resistance, have a higher risk of low back pain than does the nonathlete population (Baker & Patel, 2005; Bono, 2004). Osteoporosis and osteoarthritis can also be causative factors in low back pain. Low back pain may be a symptom of an underlying condition such as disc herniation, strain or sprain, irregularities in bone structure, or pinched nerves. Pain should be taken seriously until the cause is identified. Much low back pain has no identifiable underlying etiology. Back pain is often treated with stretching, postural exercise, or other forms of therapy. Strengthening the muscles of the abdominal region and the low back and hips has also been shown to have some effectiveness in treating pain without surgery. It is important to maintain mobility.

REFERENCES AND SELECTED READINGS

Abe, T., Kusuhara, N., Yoshimura, N., Tomita, T., & Easton, P. A. (1996). Differential respiratory activity of four abdominal muscles in humans. *Journal of Applied Physiology,* 80, 1379–1389.

Adams, M. A., & Dolan, P. (2005). Spine biomechanics. *Journal of Biomechanics,* 38, 1972–1983.

Andersson, E. A., Grundstrom, H., & Thorstensson, A. (2002). Diverging intramuscular activity patterns in back and abdominal muscles during trunk rotation. *Spine,* 27(6), E152–E160.

Arnheim, D. D., & Prentice, W. E. (1998). *Essentials of athletic training* (4th ed.). St. Louis, MO: McGraw-Hill.

Bahr, R., Andersen, S. O., Loken, S., Fossan, B., Hansen, T., & Holme, I. (2004). Low back pain among endurance athletes with and without specific back loading—a cross-sectional survey of cross-country skiers, rowers, orienteerers, and nonathletic controls. *Spine,* 29(4), 449–454.

Baker, R. J., & Patel, D. (2005). Lower back pain in the athlete: Common conditions and treatment. *Primary Care,* 32(1), 201–229.

Basmajian, J. V., & Deluca, C. J. (1985). *Muscles alive* (5th ed.). Baltimore: Williams & Wilkins.

Bogduk, N., & Mercer, S. (2000). Biomechanics of the cervical spine. I. Normal kinematics. *Clinical Biomechanics,* 15(9), 633–648.

Bono, C. M. (2004). Low-back pain in athletes. *Journal of Bone Joint Surgery,* 86-A(2), 382–396.

Cholewicki, J., & VanVliet, J. J. (2002). Relative contribution of trunk muscles to the stability of the lumbar spine during isometric exertions. *Clinical Biomechanics,* 17(2), 99–105.

Cresswell, A. G., Grundstrom, H., & Thorstensson, A. (1992). Observations on intra-abdominal pressure and patterns of abdominal intramuscular activity in man. *Acta Physiologica Scandinavica,* 144, 409–418.

Ferguson, S. J., & Steffen, T. (2003). Biomechanics of the aging spine. *European Spine Journal,* 12(Suppl 2), S97–S103.

Ferrario, V. F., Sforza, C., Serrao, G., Grassi, G., & Mossi, E. (2002). Active range of motion of the head and cervical spine: A three-dimensional investigation in healthy young adults. *Journal of Orthopedic Research,* 20(1), 122–129.

Feuerstein, M., Marcus, S. C., & Huang, G. D. (2004). National trends in nonoperative care for nonspecific back pain. *Spine Journal,* 4(1), 56–63.

Gabriel, D. A., Matsumoto, J. Y., Davis, D. H., Currier, B. L., & An, K. N. (2004). Multidirectional neck strength and electromyographic activity for normal controls. *Clinical Biomechanics,* 19(7), 653–658.

Gerbino, P. G., & d'Hemecourt, P. A. (2002). Does football cause an increase in degenerative disease of the lumbar spine? *Current Sports Medicine Reports,* 1(1), 47–51.

Haughton, V. M., Rogers, B., Meyerand, M. E., & Resnick, D. K. (2002). Measuring the axial rotation of lumbar vertebrae in vivo with MR imaging. *American Journal of Neuroradiology,* 23(7), 1110–1116.

Hug, F., Raux, M., Prella, M., Morelot-Panzini, C., Straus, C., & Similowski, T. (2006). Optimized analysis of surface electromyograms of the scalenes during quiet breathing in humans. *Respiratory Physiology and Neurobiology,* 150(1), 75–81.

Ishii, T., Mukai, Y., Hosono, N., Sakaura, H., Fujii, R., Nakajima, Y., et al. (2004). Kinematics of the subaxial cervical spine in rotation in vivo three-dimensional analysis. *Spine,* 29(24), 2826–2831.

Johnell, O., & Kanis, J. (2005). Epidemiology of osteoporotic fractures. *Osteoporosis International,* 16(Suppl 2), S3–S7.

Korovessis, P., Koureas, G., Zacharatos, S., & Papazisis, Z. (2005). Backpacks, back pain, sagittal spinal curves and trunk alignment in adolescents: A logistic and multinomial logistic analysis. *Spine,* 30(2), 247–255.

Kumar, S., Narayan, Y., & Garand, D. (2003). An electromyographic study of isokinetic axial rotation in young adults. *Spine Journal,* 3(1), 46–54.

Kumar, S., Zedka, M., & Narayan, Y. (1999). EMG power spectra of trunk muscles during graded maximal voluntary isometric contraction in flexion-rotation and extension-rotation. *European Journal of Applied Physiology,* 80, 527–541.

Lee, P. J., Roger, E. L., & Granata, K. P. (2006). Active trunk stiffness increases with co-contraction. *Journal of Electromyography and Kinesiology,* 16(1), 51–57.

Lemkuhl, L. D., & Smith, L. K. (1983). *Brunnstrom's clinical kinesiology* (4th ed.). Philadelphia: F. A. Davis.

Lundon, K., & Bolton, K. (2001). Structure and function of the lumbar intervertebral disk in health, aging, and pathologic conditions. *Journal of Orthopedic and Sports Physical Therapy,* 31(6), 291–303.

Mackenzie, W. G., Sampath, J. S., Kruse, R. W., & Sheir-Neiss, G. J. (2003). Backpacks in children. *Clinical Orthopedics and Related Research,* 409, 78–84.

Masharawi, Y., Rothschild, B., Dar, G., Peleg, S., Robinson, D., Been, E., et al. (2004). Facet orientation in the thoracolumbar spine: Three-dimensional anatomic and biomechanical analysis. *Spine,* 29(16), 1755–1763.

McGill, S. M. (2004). Linking latest knowledge of injury mechanisms and spine function to the prevention of low back disorders. *Journal of Electromyography and Kinesiology,* 14, 43–47.

McGill, S. M., Grenier, S., Kavcic, N., & Cholewicki, J. (2003). Coordination of muscle activity to assure stability of the lumbar spine. *Journal of Electromyography and Kinesiology,* 13(4), 353–359.

Moorhouse, K. M., & Granata, K. P. (2009). Role of reflex dynamics in spinal stability: Intrinsic muscle stiffness alone is insufficient for stability. *Journal of Biomechanics,* 40(5), 1058–1065.

Ong, A., J. Anderson, & Roche, J. (2009). A pilot study of the prevalence of lumbar disc degeneration in elite athletes with lower back pain at the Sydney 2000 Olympic Games. *British Journal of Sports Medicine,* 37(3), 263–266.

O'Sullivan, P. B., Grahamslaw, K. M., Kendell, M., Lapenskie, S. C., Moller, N. E., & Richards, K. V. (2002). The effect of different standing and sitting postures on trunk muscle activity in a pain-free population. *Spine,* 27(11), 1238–1244.

Plamondon, A., Serresse, O., Boyd, K., Ladouceur, D., & Desjardins, P. (2002). Estimated moments at L5/S1 level and muscular activation of back extensors for six prone back extension exercises in healthy individuals. *Scandinavian Journal of Medicine and Science in Sports,* 12(2), 81–89.

Pope, M. H., Goh, K. L., & Magnusson, M. L. (2002). Spine ergonomics. *Annual Review of Biomedical Engineering,* 4, 49–68.

Reeves, N. P., Narendrac, K. S., & Cholewicki, J. (2007). Spine stability: The six blind men and the elephant. *Clinical Biomechanics* [Bristol, Avon], 22(3), 266–274.

Roy, A. L., Keller, T. S., & Colloca, C. J. (2003). Posture-dependent trunk extensor EMG activity during maximum isometrics exertions in normal male and female subjects. *Journal of Electromyography and Kinesiology,* 13(5), 469–476.

Sarti, M. A., Monfort, M., Fuster, M. A., & Villaplana, L. A. (1996). Muscle activity in upper and lower rectus abdominis during abdominal exercises. *Archives of Physical Medicine and Rehabilitation,* 77, 1293–1297.

Sjolie, A. N. (2004). Associations between activities and low back pain in adolescents. *Scandinavian Journal of Medicine and Science in Sports,* 14(6), 352–359.

Urquhart, D. M., & Hodges, P. W. (2005). Differential activity of regions of transversus abdominis during trunk rotation. *European Spine Journal,* 14(4), 393–400.

Whiting, W. C., & Zernicke, R. F. (1998). *Biomechanics of musculoskeletal injury.* Champaign, IL: Human Kinetics.

Wilson, T. A., Legrand, A., Gevenois, P. A., & De Troyer, A. (2001). Respiratory effects of external and internal intercostal muscles in humans. *Journal of Physiology,* 530, 319–330.

Woolf, A., & Pfleger, B. (2003). Burden of major musculoskeletal conditions. *Bulletin of the World Health Organization,* 81(9), 646–656.

Yamakawa, H., Murase, S., Sakai, H., Iwama, T., Katada, M., Niikawao, S., et al. (2001). Spinal injuries in snowboarders: Risk of jumping as an integral part of snowboarding. *Journal of Trauma,* 50(6), 1101–1105.

LABORATORY EXPERIENCES

Joint Structure

1. Study the bones of the spinal column. Classify the structure for each of the following joints, including the articulations of both the bodies and the arches. Explain how the structure of each joint affects its function.
   a. Atlanto-occipital
   b. Atlantoaxial
   c. A middle cervical joint
   d. The joint between the seventh cervical and the first thoracic vertebrae
   e. A middle thoracic joint
   f. The joint between the twelfth thoracic and the first lumbar vertebrae
   g. A middle lumbar joint
   h. The lumbosacral joint

Joint Action

2. Have a subject sit tailor fashion on a table and flex the spine as completely as possible. Observe the shape of the spine as seen from the side. Compare the three regions of the spine as to forward flexibility.
3. Have a subject sit astride a chair, facing its back, and hyperextend the spine as completely as possible. Observe the shape of the spine, as in Experience 2.
4. Have a subject sit astride a bench and laterally flex the spine as far as possible, first to one side and then to the other. Observe from the rear.
5. Have a subject sit astride a bench with the hands at the neck, then rotate the trunk as far as possible, first to one side, then to the other. Observe and compare the regions of the spine as to rotating ability.
6. Observe flexion, hyperextension, lateral flexion, and rotation of the spine in several subjects, preferably subjects representing different body builds, and note individual differences.
7. Have a subject lie facedown on a table with the legs and pelvis supported on the table, the trunk extending forward beyond the table, and the hands clasped behind the neck.
   a. Have the subject flex the spine laterally. Compare the thoracic and lumbar regions. Note the torsion accompanying the lateral flexion.
   b. Have the subject flex the spine and then flex it laterally. Observe as in a.
   c. Have the subject hyperextend the spine (with someone helping support the elbows) and then flex laterally. Observe as in a.
   d. Have the subject rotate the trunk to one side as far as possible. Compare the thoracic and lumbar regions. Is any lateral flexion apparent in the spine?
   e. Have the subject flex the spine and then rotate it. Observe as in a.
   f. Have the subject hyperextend the spine and then rotate it. Observe as in d.
8. **Movement of the Thorax in Respiration**
   Subject: Breathe naturally for a while, then as deeply as possible.
   Observer: (a) Place the hands on the sides of the thorax and note the movement in the lateral diameter. (b) Place one hand on the ribs at the subcostal angle (just below the sternum) and the other hand against the back at the same level. Note the movement in the anteroposterior diameter. (c) Place the fingers on the sternum. Can you detect any movement in normal respiration? In deep respiration?

Muscular Action

The purpose of these exercises is not to test the strength of the muscles but to enable the observer to study the action of the muscles in simple movements of the body.

The procedure, therefore, is quite different from that followed by the physical therapist in testing muscle strength. It is suggested that students work in groups of three: one acting as the subject, one as an assistant helping support or steady the stationary part of the body and giving resistance to the moving part, and one palpating the muscles and recording the results. The procedures in Appendix B may be used for this purpose. They may also be used for the analysis of other movements.

9. **Flexion of the Neck**
   a. *Subject:* Lie on the back and lift the head, bringing the chin toward the chest.
      Observer: Palpate and identify as many of the contracting muscles as possible.
   b. *Subject:* Lie on the back and lift the head, leading with the chin.
      Observer: Compare the action of the sternocleidomastoid in b with its action in a.
10. **Extension and Hyperextension of the Neck**
    a. *Subject:* Lie facedown on a table with the head over the edge. Raise the head as far as possible, hyperextending both the head and the neck.
       Assistant: May resist the movement if stronger muscular action is desired.
       Observer: Palpate and identify as many of the contracting muscles as possible.
    b. *Subject:* Lie facedown on a table with the head over the edge. Raise the head as far as possible with the chin tucked in.
       Assistant: Resist the retraction of the chin.
       Observer: Compare the muscular action in b with that in a.
11. **Lateral Flexion of the Head and Neck**
    Subject: Lie on one side and raise the head toward the shoulder without turning the head or tensing the shoulder.
    Assistant: Give slight resistance at the temple.
    Observer: Palpate and identify as many muscles as possible.
12. **Rotation of the Head and Neck**
    Subject: Sit erect and rotate the head to the left as far as possible.
    Assistant: Give fairly strong resistance to the side of the jaw.
    Observer: Palpate the sternocleidomastoids. Which one contracts?
13. **Flexion of the Thoracic and Lumbar Spine**
    Subject: Lie on the back with the arms folded across the chest. Flex the head, shoulders, and upper back from the table, keeping the chin in. There is no need to come to a sitting position, because this is intended as a movement of spinal, not hip, flexion.
    Assistant: Hold the thighs down.
    Observer: Palpate the rectus abdominis and the external oblique abdominal muscle.
14. **Extension and Hyperextension of the Thoracic and Lumbar Spine**
    Subject: Lie facedown with the hands on the hips. Hyperextend the head and trunk as far as possible.
    Assistant: Hold the feet down.
    Observer: Palpate the erector spinae and the gluteus maximus. What is the function of the latter muscle in this movement?
15. **Lateral Flexion of the Thoracic and Lumbar Spine**
    Subject: Lie on one side with the bottom arm placed across the chest and the hand resting on the opposite shoulder, and with the hand of the top arm resting on the hip. Laterally flex the trunk.
    Assistant: Hold the legs down. If necessary, help the subject by pulling at the elbow.
    Observer: Palpate the rectus abdominis, external oblique abdominal muscle, erector spinae, and latissimus dorsi.
16. **Rotation of the Thoracic and Lumbar Spine**
    Subject: Sit astride a bench with the hands placed behind the neck. Rotate to one side as far as possible without leaving the bench.
    Assistant: Resist the movement by grasping the subject's arms close to the shoulders and pushing (or pulling) in the opposite direction.
    Observer: Palpate as many of the spinal and abdominal muscles as possible. Disregard the muscles of the scapula and arm.
17. **Muscular Action in Forced Inhalation**
    a. *Subject:* Inhale through a small rubber tube, pinching it slightly in order to furnish resistance.
       Observer: Note the action of the sternocleidomastoid, cervical and thoracic extensors, and upper trapezius. Can any other muscular action be detected? If so, explain.
    b. *Subject:* Run in place or around the room until short of breath. Hang from a horizontal bar.
       Observer: Can you detect any action of the pectoralis major accompanying inhalation?

(By stabilizing the arms, the hanging position causes the pectoralis major to act on the ribs.)

18. **Muscular Action in Vigorous Exhalation**
    Subject: Blow through a small rubber tube, pinching it slightly or holding a finger loosely over the end, or blow into a spirometer, flarimeter, or toy balloon.
    Observer: Note the action of the abdominal muscles and the erector spinae. Explain.

Action of the Muscles Other Than the Movers

19. **Sit-Up**
    Subject: Lie on the back and come to a sitting position, keeping the spine as rigid as possible.
    Assistant: Hold the feet down.
    Observer: Palpate the abdominal muscles, erector spinae, and sternocleidomastoid. Explain the function of each.
20. **Double Leg Lowering**
    Subject: Lie on the back. Raise both legs, then slowly lower them halfway.
    Observer: Palpate the abdominal muscles and erector spinae. Explain the function of each.
21. **Trunk Flexion**
    Subject: Stand with the feet slightly separated. Flex forward from the hips, keeping the back flat.
    Observer: Palpate the erector spinae. Explain its function.
22. **Push-Up**
    Subject: Assume a front-leaning rest position on the hands and toes with the body straight. Let the arm flex at the elbows until the chest almost touches the floor, then push up again, keeping the body straight the entire time. Do not let the body sag or hump.
    Observer: Palpate the abdominal muscles. Explain their function.

Kinesiological Analysis

23. Choose a simple motor skill from Appendix G. Do a complete anatomical analysis of the motions of the spinal column while following the analysis outline in Table 1.2.

PART II

Fundamentals of Biomechanics

Introduction to Part II

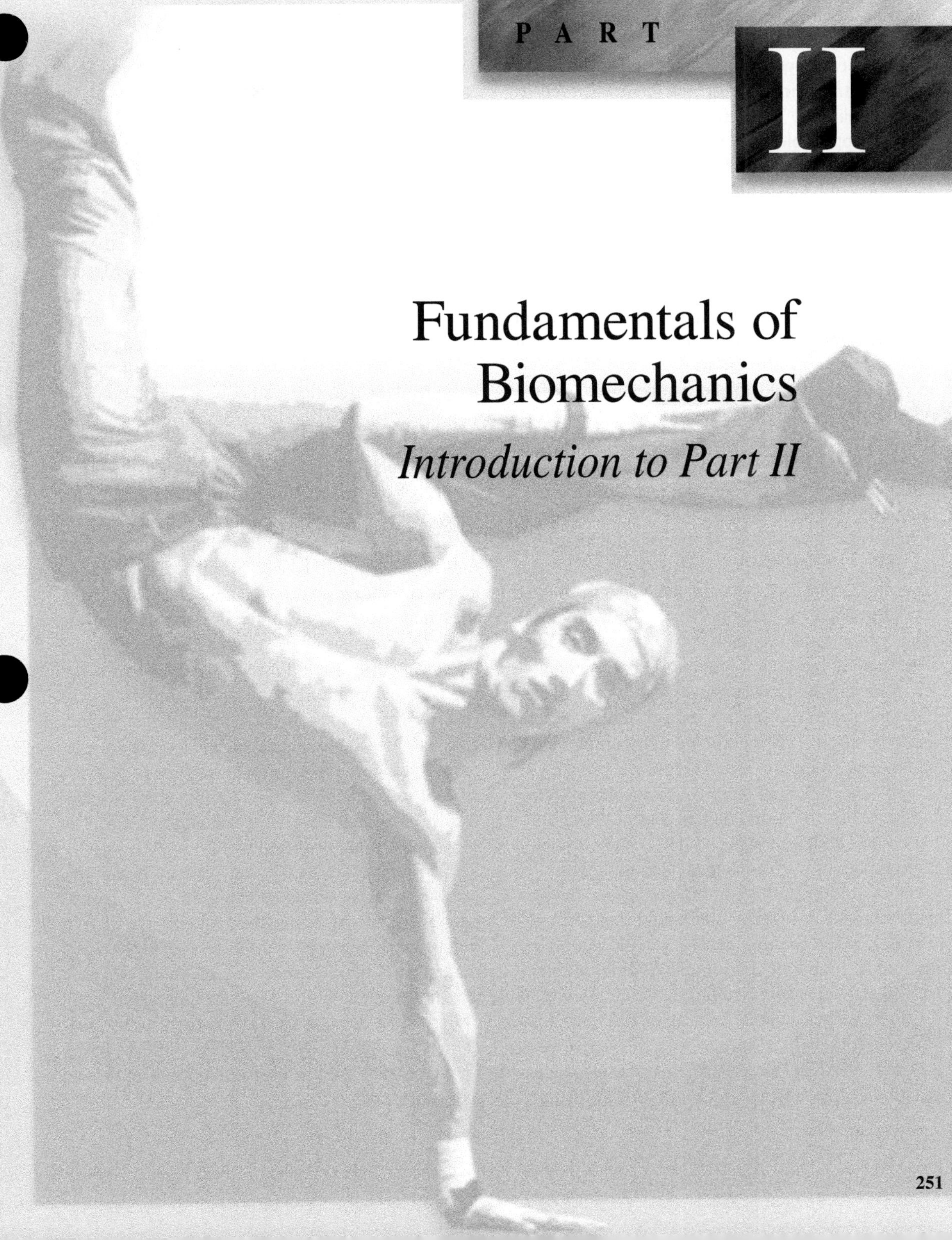

As seen by the kinesiologist, the human body is a highly complex machine constructed of living tissue. As such it is subject to the laws and principles of mechanics as well as those of biology. The principles of mechanics are directly applicable both to the movements of the human body and to the implements it handles. Principles of balance and equilibrium, motion, and the application of forces apply equally to people in motion as they do to rockets and wheels, gears and missiles. A study of the fundamental principles of mechanics as they apply to movement skills will aid the teacher, therapist, and coach in the analysis of skills for the intelligent evaluation of technique and correction of error. Applications in research can lead to the determination of the relative merits of existing techniques as well as to the development of techniques yet unknown.

In the branch of science called biomechanics, the principles and methods of mechanics are applied to the structure and function of biological systems. Because biology is concerned with all living things, biomechanics is a very broad branch of science, and the biomechanics of sport is only one of the applied areas in which applications are made of the same common core of knowledge and fundamental research found in physics, mathematics, anatomy, and physiology. Other fields of applied biomechanics include industrial engineering and ergonomics, physical rehabilitation, medicine and biomedical physics, and aerospace science.

Of the fields of applied biomechanics, the biomechanics of sport, dance, and physical education are the least advanced, but increased availability and use of advanced technology in the form of digital and real-time recording devices have resulted in research and study that formerly was almost prohibitive because of the agonizing amount of time they consumed. Additional impetus has also been supplied through the founding in 1973 of the International Society of Biomechanics (ISB) and, in 1977, the American Society of Biomechanics (ASB). The influence of these societies in stimulating study and disseminating knowledge through international meetings has done much to advance knowledge in this fascinating field of applied biomechanics, the biomechanics of sport and physical education.

Part II introduces the student to some elementary concepts necessary for understanding the biomechanics of sport and physical education. Chapter 10 presents mechanical concepts and terminology basic to the study of mechanics as an aspect of kinesiology. The need to understand basic mathematical concepts in order to use appropriate formulas and understand basic principles is also set forth in this chapter. The level of mathematics needed for this and subsequent chapters is relatively elementary and, with the aid of the examples given and the mathematics review in Appendix D, the average kinesiology student should have no difficulty. Under no circumstances, however, should the student become so involved with juggling numbers in this part that the sight of the forest is lost for the trees.

Part II continues with a chapter on the fundamentals of motion description, with particular emphasis placed on an understanding of projectiles and "free flight." Specific applications are made to sport and physical education activities. A similar approach is followed in subsequent chapters on the conditions of linear motion, the conditions of rotary motion, and the center of gravity and stability. Each chapter concludes with a variety of problems and exercises designed to help the student understand the direct application of principles of mechanics to the execution of skills in sport and physical education.

Throughout Part II, the student is encouraged to think in terms of applying newly gained knowledge of the biomechanical aspects of motion to the analysis of familiar motor skills. Using the analysis outline presented in Table 1.1, each new mechanical concept should be applied to an evaluation of a motor skill. Such practice in using knowledge for analysis will help build a strong foundation for the growing practitioner in human movement analysis.

Assumption:

- Students have a working knowledge of basic three-term equation algebra.

Review:

- Appendix D offers a review of the mathematics skills required.

References

Atwater, A. E. (1980). Kinesiology/biomechanics: Perspectives and trends. *Research Quarterly for Exercise and Sport,* 51, 193–218.

National Association for Sport and Physical Education. (2003). Guidelines for undergraduate biomechanics. AAHPERD. www.aahperd.org/naspe/publications/teachingTools/guidance.cfm.

Nelson, R. C. (1971). Biomechanics of sport: An overview. In *Selected topics in biomechanics,* edited by J. M. Cooper (pp. 31–37). Chicago: The Athletic Institute.

Wartenweiler, J. 1979. The manifold implications of biomechanics. In *Biomechanics IV* edited by R. C. Nelson and C. A. Morehouse, 11–14. Baltimore: University Park Press.

CHAPTER

10 TERMINOLOGY AND MEASUREMENT IN BIOMECHANICS

OUTLINE

- ***Introduction to Terminology***
  - Mechanics
  - Biomechanics
- ***Quantities in Biomechanics***
  - The Language of Science
  - Units of Measurement
  - Scalar and Vector Quantities
- ***Vector Analysis***
  - Vector Representation
  - Combination of Vectors
  - Resolution of Vectors
  - Location of Vectors in Space
  - Trigonometric Resolution and Combination of Vectors
  - Value of Vector Analysis
- ***Laboratory Experiences***

OBJECTIVES

At the conclusion of this chapter, the student should be able to:

1. Define the terms *mechanics* and *biomechanics,* and differentiate between them.
2. Define the terms *kinematics, kinetics, statics,* and *dynamics,* and state how each relates to the structure of biomechanics study.
3. Convert the units of measurement employed in the study of biomechanics from the U.S. system to the metric system, and vice versa.
4. Describe the nature of scalar and vector quantities, and identify such quantities as one or the other.
5. Demonstrate the use of the trigonometric method for the combination and resolution of two-dimensional vectors.
6. Identify the scalar and vector quantities represented in individual motor skills and describe the vector quantities using vector diagrams.

INTRODUCTION TO TERMINOLOGY

In the context of this text, kinesiology is an area of study concerned with the musculoskeletal analysis of human motion and the study of mechanical principles and laws as they relate to the study of human motion. Students of human motion capable of accurately analyzing the musculoskeletal actions occurring in the execution of a movement are well on their way toward knowing what is happening during that movement. Those who have taken the further step of acquiring a working knowledge of how human motion is governed by physical laws and principles have added an additional dimension to their understanding of how and why the motion occurs as it does. Together, all this information provides a scientific foundation upon which to make appropriate decisions concerning the safest, most effective, and most efficient execution of any movement pattern. It is only through such study that definitive answers may be found concerning the "best" way for an individual to perform a skill and the reasons the method selected is indeed the best. In sport, for example, the record-breaking "form" of one athlete may or may not be appropriate for another of different body build and size. In fact, although they break records, top performers' techniques may include actions that, if eliminated, would result in even greater performance. Unless subjected to scientific scrutiny, discrimination between the success factors and deterrent factors may be confused or not even identified.

Mechanics

Where *forces* and *motion* are concerned, the area of scientific study that provides accurate answers to what is happening, why it is happening, and to what extent it is happening is called *mechanics.* It is that branch of physics concerned with the effect that **forces** have on bodies and the motion produced by those forces. The study of mechanics is engaged in by those people whose occupations or professions require an understanding of force, matter, space, and time. Engineers, to a large extent, are involved with the application of mechanics. Navigation, astronomy, space, and communications experts all study mechanics. The same is true of individuals concerned with the study of human motion and the forces causing it. The laws and principles used to explain the motion of planets or the strength of buildings and bridges apply equally to humans. *All* motion, including motions of the human body and its parts, is the result of the application of forces and is subject to the laws and principles that govern force and motion.

Biomechanics

When the study of mechanics is limited to living structures, especially the human body, it is called *biomechanics*. **Biomechanics** is an interdisciplinary science based on many of the fundamental disciplines found in the physical and life sciences. Generally, biomechanics is considered to be that aspect of the science concerned with the basic laws governing the effect forces have on the state of rest or motion of any living system, whereas the applied areas of biomechanics deal with solving practical problems. Anatomists, orthopedists, space engineers, industrial engineers, biomedical engineers, physical therapists, physical educators, dancers, and coaches all have an interest in biomechanics and in applying its principles to the improvement of human movement. Professional applications may differ, but the same basic laws of biomechanics provide a common foundation for all. In this context the part of biomechanics that applies to sport, dance, and physical education may be considered to be that part of kinesiology that involves the mechanics of human motion.

As the name implies, biomechanics is concerned with the study of biological systems using the techniques of the branch of physics called mechanics. Figure 10.1 illustrates the framework for the study of biomechanics. The frames inside Figure 10.1 are the tools in a biomechanics laboratory that are used to study the related quantities. For example, EMG stands for electromyography and is used to study muscle activity. Motion capture is usually thought of as taking video of someone wearing reflective markers and is used to measure position, velocity, acceleration, joint angles, and so on. Force platforms are used to measure how hard something is pushing or pulling.

Statics and Dynamics

The study of mechanics is divided into two areas, statics and dynamics. **Statics** covers situations in which all forces acting on a body are balanced, and the body is in equilibrium. A body in a static situation would exhibit either no motion or a constant, unchanging motion. With a knowledge of the principles of statics, one may have a better understanding of levers and a greater ability to solve problems such as locating the body's center of gravity or center of buoyancy.

The branch of biomechanics dealing with bodies subject to *unbalance* is called **dynamics**. The principles of dynamics explain circumstances in which an excess of force in one direction or a turning force causes an object to change speed or direction. In this situation an object might move from a static position to one of motion or might undergo some change in the motion state. Principles of work, energy, and accelerated motion are included in the study of dynamics.

Kinematics and Kinetics

The terms *kinematics* and *kinetics* are also part of the vocabulary of the study of mechanics. **Kinematics** has been referred to as the geometry of motion. It describes the motion of bodies in terms of time, displacement, velocity, and acceleration. The motion occurring may be in a straight line (linear kinematics) or rotating about a fixed point (angular kinematics). Kinematics is concerned only with the analytical and mathematical descriptions of all kinds of motion and *not* with the forces that cause the motion. The branch of mechanics that considers the *forces* that produce or change motion is called **kinetics**. Linear kinetics is concerned with the causes of linear motion, and angular kinetics deals with the forces that cause angular motion.

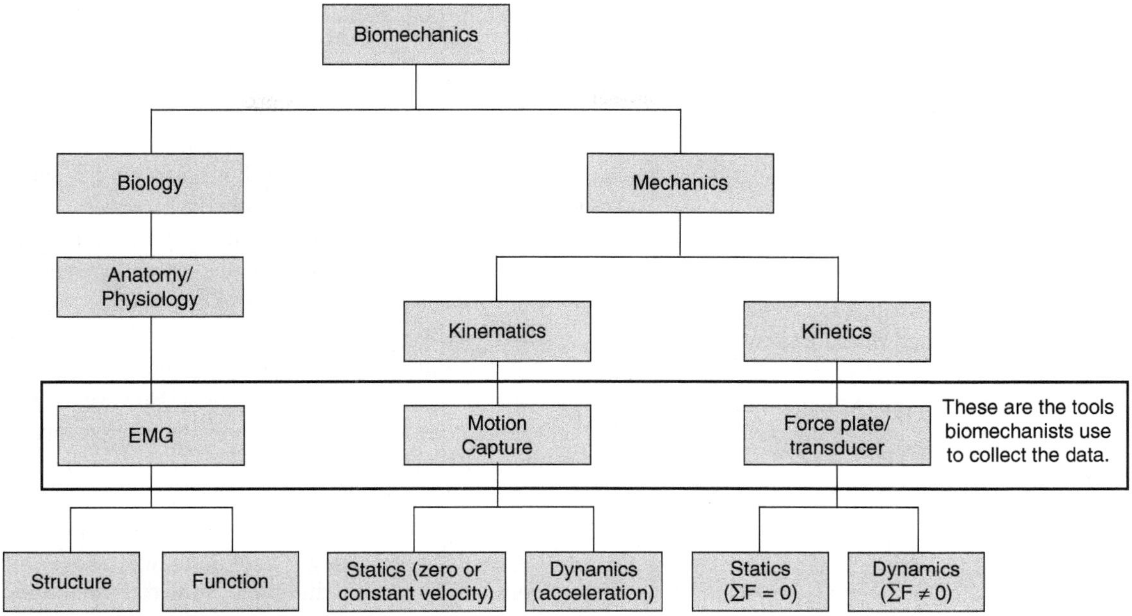

Figure 10.1 The study of biomechanics.

Quantities in Biomechanics

The Language of Science

Mathematics is the language of science. It enables us to express relationships quantitatively rather than merely descriptively. It provides objective evidence of the superiority of one technique over another and thus forms the basis for developing effective measures for improving both the safety and the effectiveness of performance. Furthermore, it makes possible continuing advancement of knowledge through research. Had it not been for the use of mathematics, the contributions of great scientists like Archimedes, Galileo, and Newton would not have been possible.

In the biomechanical aspects of kinesiology, as in all mechanics, the depth of understanding of the principles and laws that apply to it is greatly increased through experimental and mathematical evidence. Hence, it is to the student's advantage to become conversant with appropriate mathematical concepts and techniques. The mathematics needed for the quantitative treatment of the simple mechanics discussed in this text is not difficult. It consists of elementary algebra and right triangle trigonometry. A review of these essential mathematical concepts is presented in Appendix D.

Units of Measurement

The units of measurement employed in the study of biomechanics are expressed in terms of space, time, and mass. Currently in the United States, there are two systems of unit measurement for these quantities, the U.S. system and the metric system. Although the metric system is currently used in research and literature, a comparison of equivalent values is helpful. Appendix F presents some common units used in biomechanics study and their U.S. and metric equivalents.

Length

In the metric or decimal system, all units differ in size by a multiple of 10. In ascending order, linear units are millimeters, centimeters, meters, and kilometers. In the U.S. system the basic unit of length is the foot. Other possible units are inches, yards, and miles.

Mass and Force (Weight)

Mass is the quantity of matter a body contains. The **weight** of a body depends on its quantity of matter and the strength of the gravitational attraction acting on it. The measure of gravitational *force* is called weight. The mass of an object will not change even if taken to the moon, but its weight will. The kilogram, equal to the mass of a liter of water, is the unit of mass in the metric system. The unit of force (weight) is the newton (N), and for most of the United States a mass of 1 kilogram weighs approximately 9.80 newtons. In the U.S. system, the pound is the basic unit of force (weight).

Time

The basic unit of time for both systems of measurement is the second.

Scalar and Vector Quantities

Quantities that are used in the description of motion may be classified as either scalar or vector in nature.

Scalar quantities are single quantities. They possess only size or amount. This size or amount is referred to as magnitude and completely describes the scalar quantity. The units of measure described in the previous section are primarily scalar quantities because they are described only by magnitude. Examples of scalar quantities would be such things as a speed of 8 kilometers per hour, a temperature of 70 degrees, an area of 2 square kilometers, a mass of 10 kilograms, or a height of 2 meters.

There are also double quantities that cannot be described by magnitude alone. These double quantities are called **vector** quantities. A vector quantity is described by both magnitude and direction. Examples of vector quantities would be a velocity of 8 kilometers per hour in a northwest direction, 10 newtons of force applied at a 30-degree angle, a displacement of 100 meters from the starting point. The importance of clearly designating vector quantities can be seen if the direction component of the double quantity is altered. Consider, if two people on opposite sides of a door push with equal magnitudes (amounts) of force, the door will not move. If, on the other hand, they both push on the same side of the door, thus changing the *direction* of one of the forces, the result will be very different. The nature of the movement of the door depends on both the *amount* and *direction* of the force. Force, therefore, is a vector quantity. If the individual who ran 8 kilometers runs 8 more kilometers, the total distance run will be 16 kilometers. However, if the runner goes 8 kilometers in one direction, reverses, and runs back to the starting point, the change in position, or **displacement**, is zero. The runner is 0 kilometers from the starting point. Displacement, then, is also a vector quantity possessing both magnitude and direction. Numerous quantities in biomechanics are vector quantities. In addition to force, displacement, and velocity already mentioned, some other examples are momentum, acceleration, friction, work, and power. Vector quantities exist whenever *direction* and *amount* are inherent characteristics of the quantities.

VECTOR ANALYSIS

Vector Representation

A vector is represented by an arrow whose length is proportional to the magnitude of the vector. The direction in which the arrow points indicates the direction of the vector quantity. Figure 10.2 shows examples of arrows indicating the vector quantities of displacement, force, and velocity.

Vector quantities are equal if magnitude and direction are the same for each vector. Although all of the following vectors are of the same length (magnitude), only two are equal vector quantities. They are the two that also have the same direction (d and f).

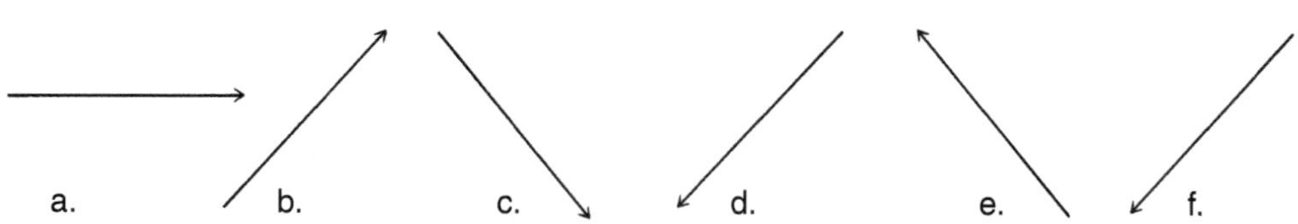

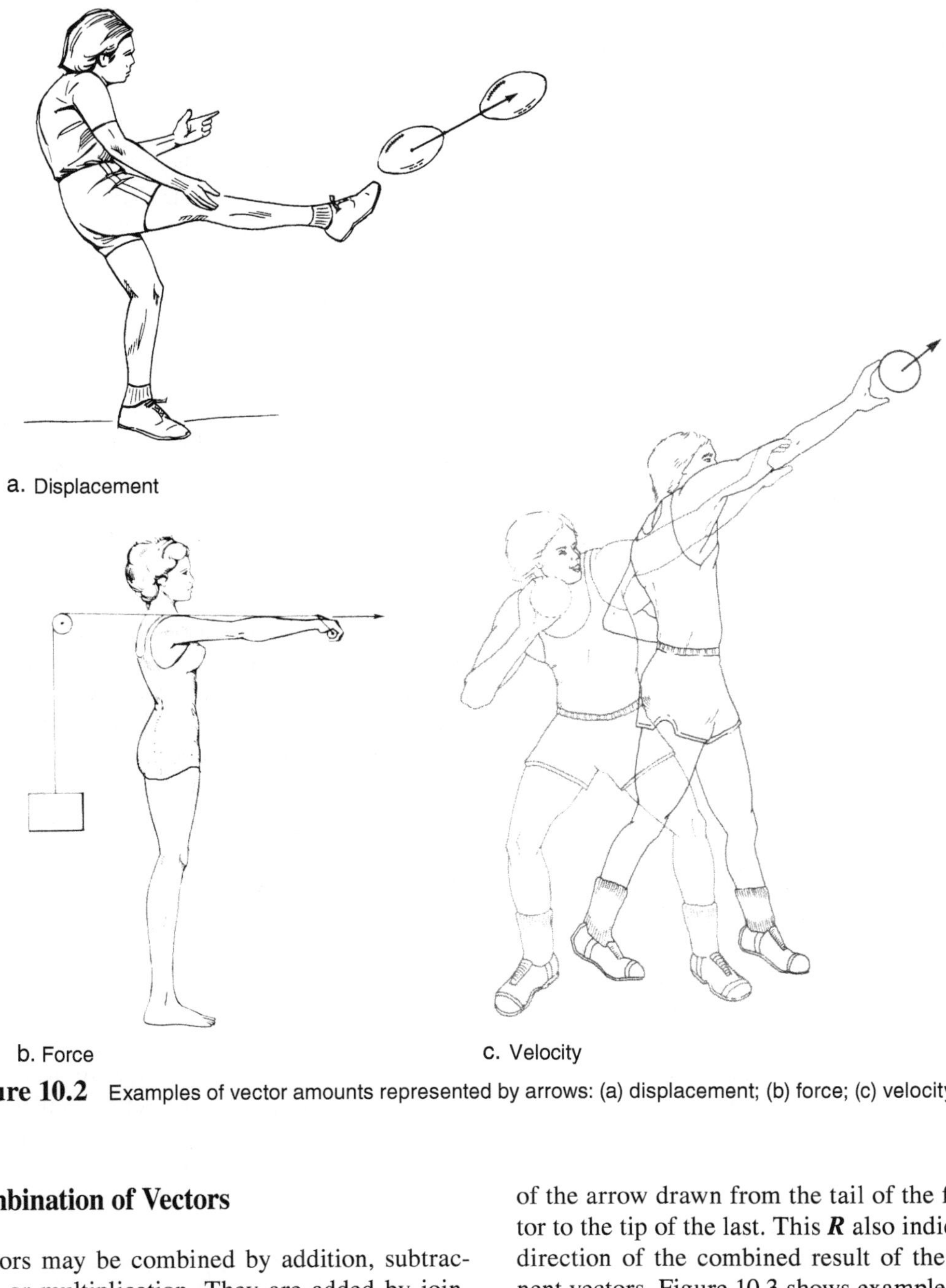

Figure 10.2 Examples of vector amounts represented by arrows: (a) displacement; (b) force; (c) velocity.

Combination of Vectors

Vectors may be combined by addition, subtraction, or multiplication. They are added by joining the head (the arrow end or tip of the vector) of one with the tail of the next while accounting for magnitude and direction. The combination results in a new vector called the **resultant (*R*)**. The resultant vector is represented by the length of the arrow drawn from the tail of the first vector to the tip of the last. This ***R*** also indicates the direction of the combined result of the component vectors. Figure 10.3 shows examples of vectors that have been combined by addition. Note that the head of the resultant ***R*** meets the *head* of the last component vector. These drawings also show that very different component vectors may produce the same resultant.

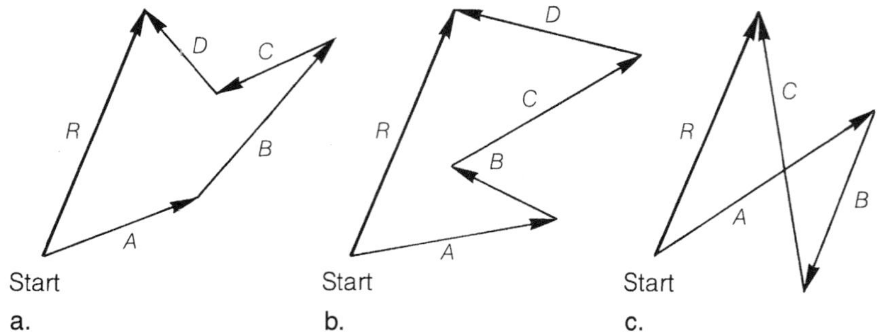

Figure 10.3 Vectors are added by joining the head of one with the tail of the next. The same resultant vector ***R***, in examples (a), (b), and (c), may be obtained from the combination of dissimilar components.

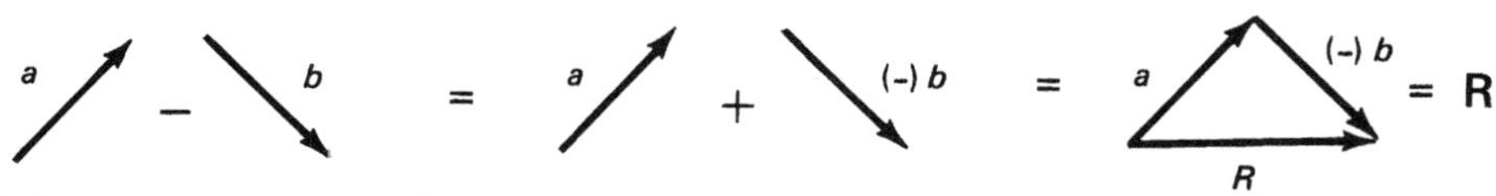

Figure 10.4 Vectors may be combined by subtraction.

The subtraction of vectors is done by changing the sign of one vector (multiply by –1) and then adding as before (Figure 10.4).

Resolution of Vectors

As just explained, the combination of two or more vectors results in a new vector. Conversely, any vector may be broken down or resolved into two component vectors acting at right angles to each other. The vector in Figure 10.2c represents the velocity with which the shot was put. Should one wish to know how much of that velocity was in a horizontal direction and how much in a vertical direction, the vector must be resolved into horizontal and vertical components. In Figure 10.5, ***A*** and ***B*** are the vertical and horizontal *components* of resultant ***R***. The vector addition of these components once again would result in the resultant vector ***R***. The arrows over ***A, B,*** and ***R*** indicate that they are vector quantities.

Location of Vectors in Space

In describing motion, it is helpful to have a frame of reference within which one can locate a position in space or change in position. Frame of reference describes the orientation of objects in a given space. When discussing movement of the whole body, the term *global reference frame* is often used. The global reference frame in this case could be described in terms of the cardinal planes as presented in Chapter 2, or it could be broadened to include the position of the body in relation to some external frame of reference such as a room, a playing field, or an external observer. A *local reference frame* is more finite and may be used to describe individual joint motions in terms of their individual axes. As an example, flexion of the shoulder joint might be described globally as being in the sagittal plane, while locally the motion might be described as it relates to the plane of the scapula. In mechanics, frame of reference is used to describe motion. Consider someone riding down a river on a boat. The person tosses a ball straight up and then catches it as it lands. The person on the boat (local frame of reference) will see the ball as traveling only in a vertical direction. However, someone standing on the shore observing (global reference) will see the ball travel horizontally as well as vertically. It is possible to locate an object in three dimensions, but to simplify understanding, the description that follows is limited to motion in two dimensions, that is, one plane.

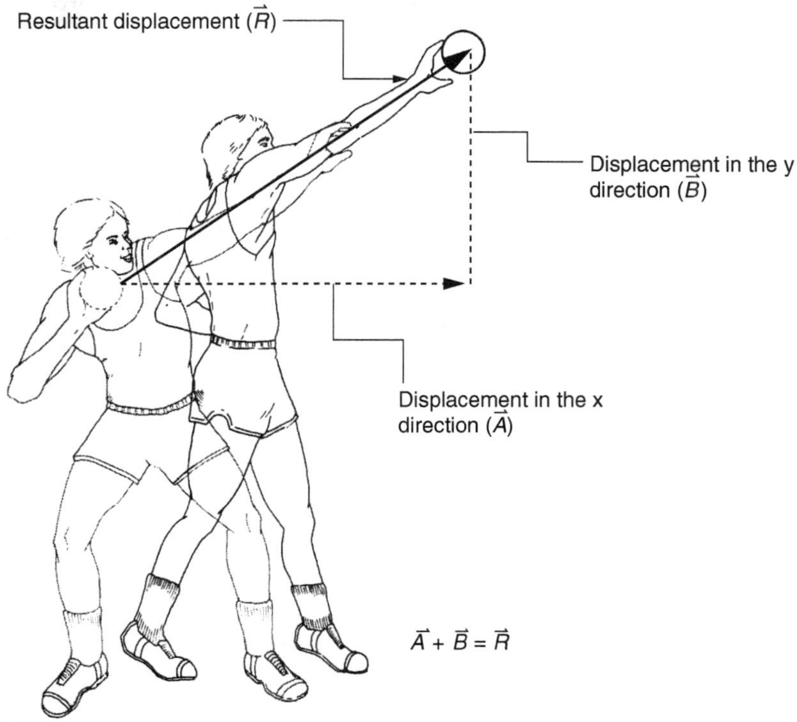

Figure 10.5 A resultant vector may be resolved or broken down into two component vectors acting at right angles to each other. The velocity vector *R* has a horizontal component *B* and a vertical component *A*.

The position of a point *P* can be located using either *rectangular* coordinates or *polar* coordinates. In the two-dimensional rectangular coordinate system, the plane is divided into four quadrants by two perpendicular intersecting lines. The horizontal line is the *x*-axis, and the vertical line is the *y*-axis. Values along either axis are measured from the point of intersection of the two axes, where *x* and *y* are both equal to zero (0, 0). The location of point *P* is represented by two numbers, the first equal to the number of *x* units and the second to the number of *y* units away from the intersection or origin. In Figure 10.6, the rectangular coordinates for point *P* are (*x*, *y*) in a and (13, 5) in b. In this latter example, point *P* is at the head of vector ***R*** and the location of the vector tail is at the origin. This vector's location in space is established. The tail is at (0, 0), and the head is at (13, 5).

Point *P* may also be described using polar coordinates. These consist of the distance (*r*) of point *P* from the origin and the angle (θ) that the line *r* makes with the *x*-axis. The polar coordinates for point *P* in Figure 10.6c are (r, θ). If *P* is the vector head, *r* equals the vector's magnitude, and θ is equal to its direction. In polar terms the vector's description is (r, θ).

In these coordinate systems, degrees are customarily measured in a counterclockwise direction. Also, by convention, *x* values to the right of the *y*-axis are positive (+) and those to the left are negative (−). The *y* values above the *x*-axis are positive and those below are negative. Point *A* in Figure 10.7 has (*x*, *y*) coordinates of (4.3, 2.5) and (r, θ) coordinates of (5, 30°). The (*x*, *y*) coordinates for point *B* are (−1.5, −3) and the polar coordinates are (3.4, 240°).

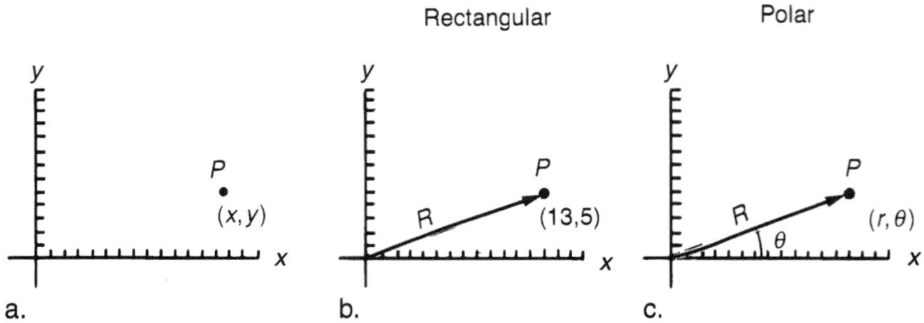

Figure 10.6 A point in space may be located in two dimensions using an *x*-and *y*-axis as a frame of reference. In (a) point *P* is *x* units from the *y*-axis and *y* units from the *x*-axis. In (b) point *P* is 13*x* units from the *y*-axis and 5*y* units from the *x*-axis. In (c) point *P* is *r* units from the *x*, *y* intersection and *θ* degrees from the *x*-axis.

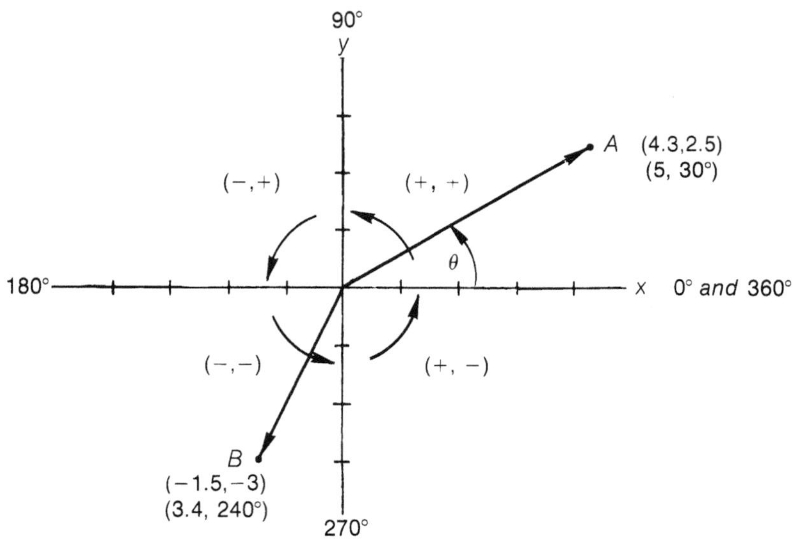

Figure 10.7 Coordinate quadrants. Values of *x* and *y* are positive in the upper right quadrant and negative in the lower left; *x* is negative in the upper left, and *y* is negative in the lower right.

Trigonometric Resolution and Combination of Vectors

Any vector may be resolved into horizontal and vertical components if the trigonometric relationships of a right triangle are employed. Let us use the example of a headed soccer ball with a velocity at impact of 9.6 m/sec in the direction of 18 degrees with the horizontal. To find the horizontal velocity (V_x) and vertical velocity (V_y) at takeoff a right triangle is constructed. With the velocity (*R*) as the hypotenuse of the triangle, the vertical and horizontal components of velocity become the vertical and horizontal sides of the triangle (Figure 10.8). To obtain the values of V_x and V_y the sine and cosine functions are used as shown in Figure 10.8. The horizontal velocity of the ball V_x turns out to be 9.1 m/sec and the vertical velocity V_y is 3.0 m/sec.

The combination of vectors is also possible with the use of right triangle trigonometric

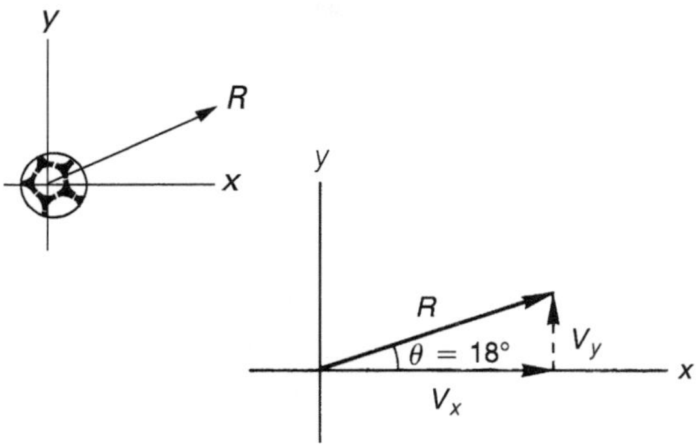

Given: $R = 9.6$ m/sec

$\theta = 18°$

To find: Value of V_y

$$\sin \theta = \frac{\text{opp}}{\text{hyp}} = \frac{V_y}{R}$$

$$V_y = \sin 18° \times 9.6 = .3090 \times 9.6$$

$$\boxed{V_y = 3.0 \text{ m/sec}}$$

To find: Value of V_x

$$\cos \theta = \frac{\text{adj}}{\text{hyp}} = \frac{V_x}{R}$$

$$V_x = \cos 18° \times 9.6 = .9511 \times 9.6$$

$$\boxed{V_x = 9.1 \text{ m/sec}}$$

Figure 10.8 Resolution of a vector using the trigonometric method. Horizontal and vertical components are determined by using cosine and sine functions. The vector shown here represents the velocity of the headed soccer ball.

relationships. If two vectors are applied at right angles to each other, the solution should appear reasonably obvious because it is the reverse of the example just explained. If a volleyball is served with a vertical velocity of 15 m/sec and a horizontal velocity of 26 m/sec, the velocity of the serve and the angle of release may be determined as shown in Figure 10.9. The resultant velocity—that is, the velocity of the serve—is 30 m/sec and the angle of projection is 30 degrees.

If more than two vectors are involved or if they are not at right angles to each other as shown in previous examples, the resultant may be obtained by determining the *x* and *y* components for each individual vector and then summing these individual components to obtain the *x* and *y* components of the resultant. Once the *x* and *y* components are known, the magnitude and direction of *R* may be obtained. If we were interested in determining the composite force of the two muscles and the resultant direction or angle of pull, then to solve this problem trigonometrically, the horizontal and vertical components for each muscle must first be determined, as in Figure 10.10 on the next page.

Next, to obtain the *y* component of the resultant effect of the *two* muscles, the *y* values for muscles *J* and *K* are summed ($\Sigma y = 173.6 + 514.2$; $\Sigma y = 687.8$ N). Similarly, the *x* component for *R* is the sum of the *x* values for *J* and *K* ($\Sigma x = 984.8 + 612.8$; $\Sigma x = 1597.6$ N).

As we have seen before, a knowledge of the horizontal (*x*) and vertical (*y*) components makes it possible to determine the resultant vector. A triangle is formed and the unknown parts are found. Figure 10.10 presents the solution once the *x* and *y* values for muscles *J* and *K* have each been summed. The summed F_y and F_x values form the two sides of the triangle, and the unknown resultant force is the hypotenuse. Using the tangent relationship between the two sides, the resultant angle of pull of the two muscles was calculated to be 23.3 degrees. With this additional information, the composite or resultant force of 1,739 newtons was found using the $\sin \theta$ = opposite/hypotenuse relationship.

In the explanation of coordinate systems, it was shown that values of *x* and *y* may be negative and that values of θ may exceed 90 degrees

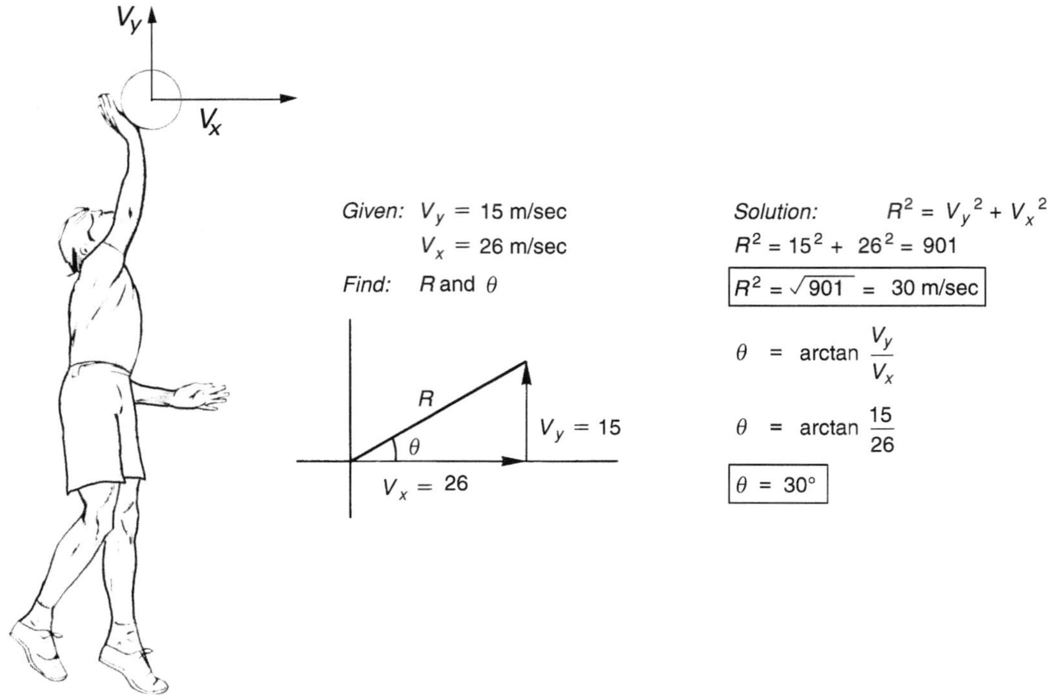

Figure 10.9 Trigonometric solution to combination of two vectors applied at right angles.

(see Figure 10.7). An example of a problem with these additional factors is that of the hiker who plots the stated course and then must determine the resultant displacement at the completion of the course:

A hiker walks the following course: 2,000 meters at 30 degrees, 1,000 meters at 100 degrees, and 500 meters at 225 degrees. What is her resultant displacement? The solution is presented in Figure 10.11.

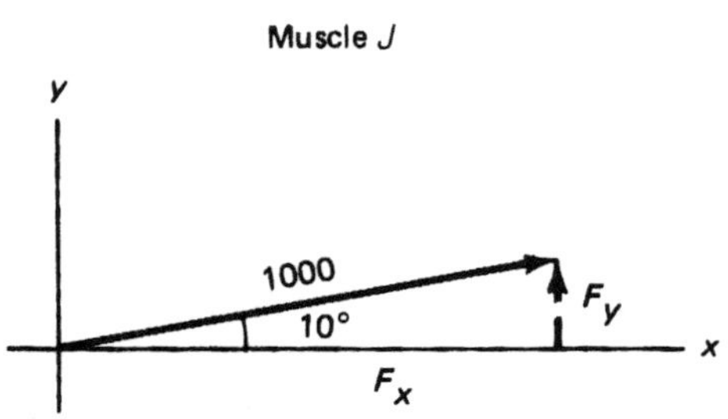

Muscle J: $r = (1000 \text{ N}, 10°)$
$y = r \sin \theta$
$y = (1000)(.1736)$
$\boxed{y = 173.6 \text{ N}}$ = vert. component for muscle J

$x = r \cos \theta$
$x = (1000)(.9848)$
$x = 984.8$ N = horiz. component for muscle J

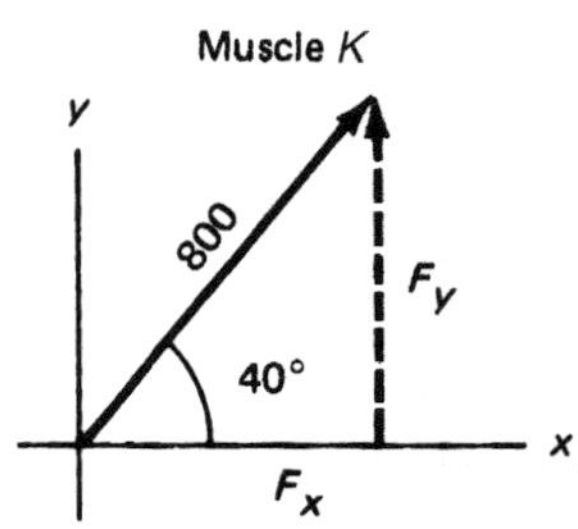

Muscle K: $r = (800 \text{ N}, 40°)$
$y = r \sin \theta$
$v = (800)(.6428)$
$\boxed{y = 514.2 \text{ N}}$ = vert. component for muscle K

$x = r \cos \theta$
$x = (800)(.7660)$
$x = 612.8$ N = horiz. component for muscle K

Given: $\Sigma y = 687.8$ N
$\Sigma x = 1597.6$ N

Find: θ and r

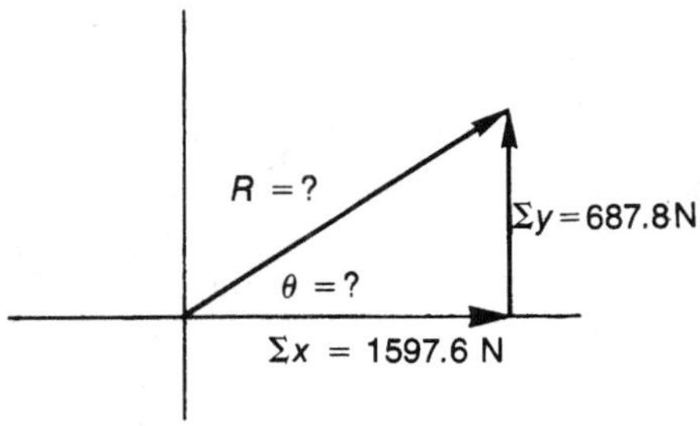

Solution: $\theta = \arctan \dfrac{\Sigma y}{\Sigma x}$

$$\theta = \arctan \frac{687.8}{1597.6} = .4305$$

$$\boxed{\theta = 23.3^\circ}$$

$$R = \frac{687.8}{\sin 23.3^\circ} = \frac{687.8}{.3955}$$

$$\boxed{R = 1739 \text{ N}}$$

Figure 10.10 Trigonometric combination of summed vectors. The sum of all x components becomes the horizontal vector component; the sum of all y components becomes the vertical vector component. ***R*** and θ are determined by combining Σx and Σy.

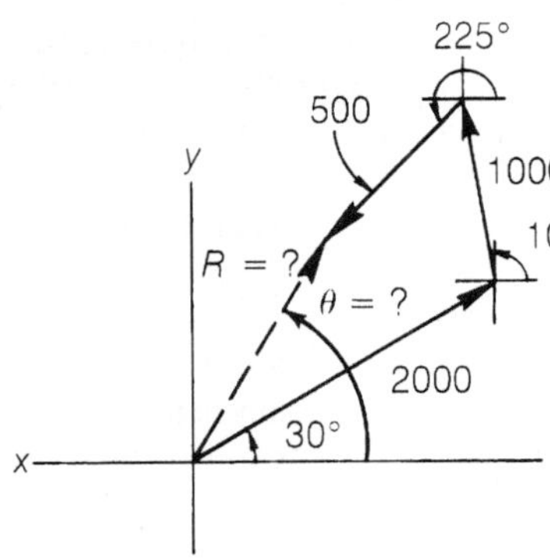

Resolution of Individual Vectors:

For 2000 m at 30°:

$x = 2000$ m cos 30°	$y = 2000$ m sin 30°
$x = 2000$ m × .866	$y = 2000$ m × .500
$x = 1732$ m	$y = 1000$ m

For 1000 m at 100°:

$\theta = 100^\circ - 90^\circ$	$\theta = 10^\circ$
$x = -1000$ m sin 10°	$y = 1000$ m cos 10°
$x = -1000$ m × .174	$y = 1000$ m × .985
$x = -174$ m	$y = 985$ m

For 500 m at 225°:

$\theta = 225^\circ - 180^\circ$	$\theta = 45^\circ$
$x = -500$ m cos 45°	$y = -500$ m sin 45°
$x = -500$ m × .707	$y = -500$ m × .707
$x = -353.5$ m	$y = -353.5$ m

$x = 1732 + (-174) + (-353.5) = 1204.5$ m
$y = 1000 + 985 + (-353.5) = 1631.5$ m

$$R = \sqrt{x^2 + y^2} = \sqrt{1204.5^2 + 1631.5^2} = \boxed{2028 \text{ m}}$$

$$\theta = \arctan \quad \frac{y}{x} = \frac{1631.5}{1204.5} = 1.354 \quad \boxed{\theta = 53.6}$$

Figure 10.11 Combination of vectors involving negative values of x and y and values of θ larger than 90 degrees.

Value of Vector Analysis

The ability to handle variables of motion and force as vector or scalar quantities should improve one's understanding of motion and the forces causing it. The effect that a muscle's angle of pull has on the force available for moving a limb is better understood when it is subjected to vector analysis. Similar study of the direction and force of projectiles improves one's understanding of the effect of gravity, angle of release, and force of release upon the flight of a projectile. The effect of several muscles exerting their combined forces on a single bone is also clarified when treated quantitatively as the combination of vector quantities to obtain a *resultant*. Indeed, the effect that a change in any variable may produce becomes much more apparent. Without the use of a vector relationship, it would be difficult if not impossible to describe motion and forces in meaningful, quantitative terms.

REFERENCES AND SELECTED READINGS

Ireson, G. (2001). Beckham as physicist? *Physics Education,* 36, 10–13.

Özkaya, N., Nordin, M., & Frankel, V. H. (1999). *Fundamentals of biomechanics: Equilibrium, motion, and deformation* (2nd ed.). New York: Springer.

Pendrill, A. M., & Williams, G. (2005). Swings and slides. *Physics Education,* 40, 527–533.

Trizeren, A. (2000). *Human body dynamics: Classical mechanics and human movement.* New York: Springer.

LABORATORY EXPERIENCES

1. Define the following key terms:
   Statics
   Dynamics
   Kinematics
   Kinetics
   Scalar
   Vector
   Component vector
2. Express the following units in metric terms:
   a. A force of 25 pounds
   b. A mass of 5 slugs
   c. A distance of 11 inches
   d. A velocity of 20 feet per second
   e. A volume of 3 quarts
3. Determine the distance between each set of points (scale: 1 unit = 10 cm).
   a. (2, 3); (5, 7)
   b. (1, 2); (3, 3)
   c. (1.5, 3.0); (6, 6)
   d. (0, 0); (6.2, 3.6)
4. Find the x and y component for each of the following vectors:
   a. 45 m/sec at 25°
   b. 85 N at 135°
   c. 118 kg at 310°
   d. 25 m/sec^2 at 210°
5. A basketball official runs 20 meters along the sideline in one direction, reverses, and runs 8 meters. What is the distance run? What is the displacement? Draw a vector diagram.
6. The muscular force of a muscle is 650 N and the muscle is pulling on the bone at an angle of 15 degrees. What are the vertical and horizontal components of this force?
7. At the moment of release, a baseball has a horizontal velocity component of 25 meters per second and a vertical velocity component of 14 meters per second. At what angle was it released, and what was its initial velocity in the direction of the throw in m/sec? In ft/sec?
8. A child is being pulled in a sled by a person holding a rope that has an angle of 20 degrees with the horizontal. The total force being used to move the sled at a constant forward speed is 110 N. How much of the force is horizontal? Vertical?
9. An orienteer runs the following course: 1,000 meters at 45°, 1,500 meters at 120°, 500 meters at 190°.

a. Draw the course to scale accurately.
b. Determine the resultant displacement trigonometrically.
c. Express the orienteer's position at the end of the course in terms of rectangular coordinates; polar coordinates.

10. A football lineman charges an opponent with a force of 175 pounds in the direction of 310 degrees. The opponent charges back with a force of 185 pounds in the direction of 90 degrees. What is the resultant force, and in what direction will it act?
11. Referring to Figures 2.3 and 7.21, make a tracing of the femur and adductor longus muscle. Draw a straight line to represent the mechanical axis of the femur and another to represent the muscle's line of pull.
    a. Using a protractor, determine the angle of pull of the muscle (angle formed by muscle's line of pull and mechanical axis of bone).
    b. Assuming a total muscle force of 900 N, calculate the force components.
12. Muscle *A* has a force of 450 N and is pulling on a bone at an angle of 15 degrees. Muscle *B* has a force of 600 N and is pulling on the same bone at the same spot, but at an angle of 30 degrees. Muscle *C* has a force of 325 N and is pulling at the same spot with an angle of pull of 10 degrees. What is the composite effect of these muscles in terms of amount of force and direction?
13. Name as many vector and scalar quantities you can think of that are part of the games of football, tennis, or golf.
14. Choose one of the following sports:
    Volleyball
    Soccer
    Ice hockey
    a. For that sport, make a list of the individual motor skills represented and classify each skill according to the classification model presented in Chapter 1 (p. 6–7).
    b. Name the underlying mechanics objective for each skill identified (Chapter 1, p. 12–13).
    c. Identify the scalar and vector quantities that are a part of each skill identified. For each skill, draw and label a vector diagram for *one* of the vector quantities named.

CHAPTER

11

THE DESCRIPTION OF HUMAN MOTION

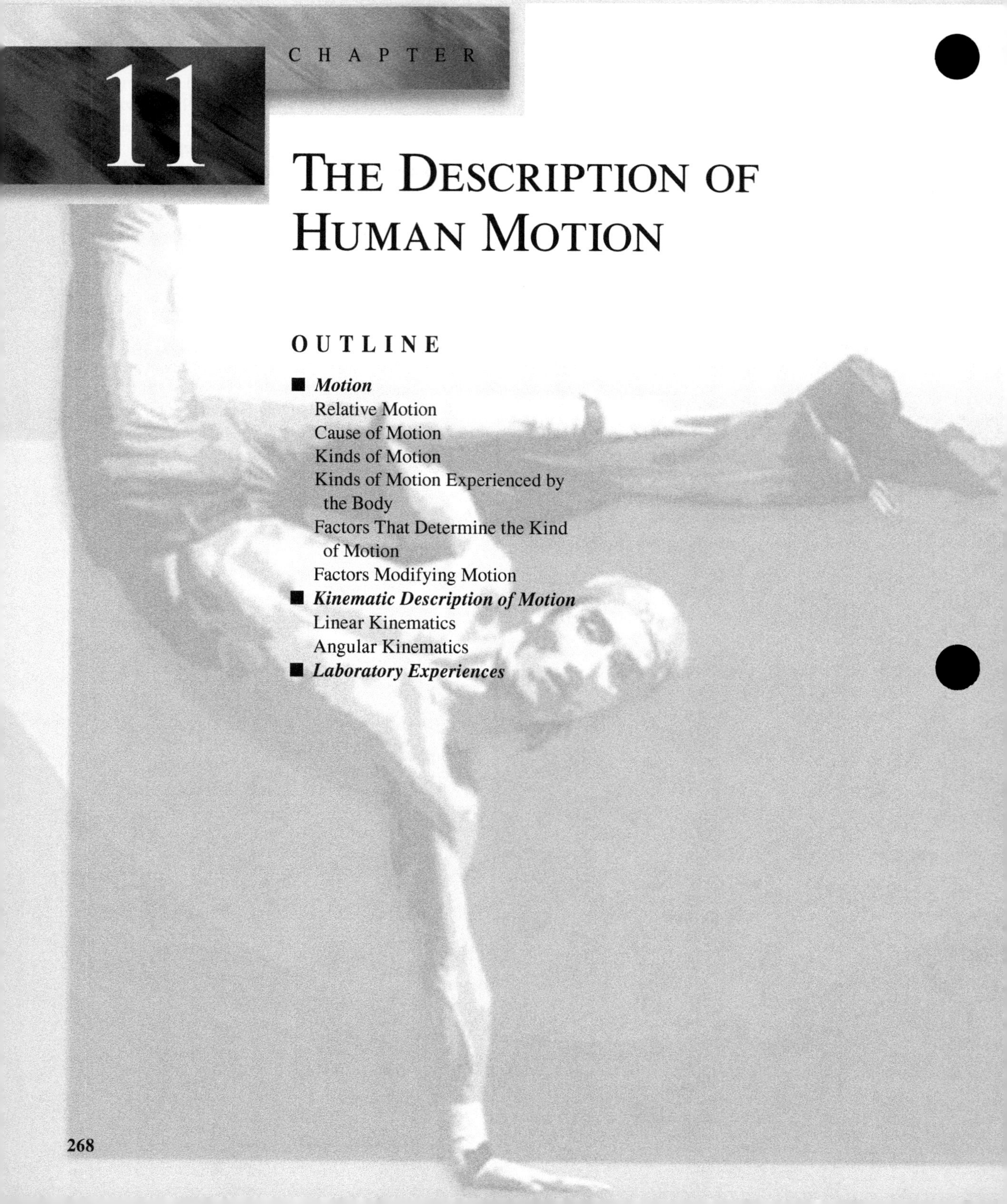

OUTLINE

OBJECTIVES

At the conclusion of this chapter, the student should be able to:

1. Name the kinds of motion experienced by the human body, and describe the factors that cause and modify motion.
2. Name and properly use the terms that describe linear and rotary motion: *position, displacement, distance, speed, velocity,* and *acceleration.*
3. Explain the interrelationships that exist among displacement, velocity, and acceleration, and use the knowledge of these interrelationships to describe and analyze human motion.
4. Describe the behavior of projectiles, and explain how angle, speed, and height of projection affect that behavior.
5. Describe the relationship between linear and rotary movement, and explain the significance of this relationship to human motion.
6. Identify the critical kinematic components that would be used to fully describe the skillful performance of a selected motor task.

MOTION

If we are to understand the movements of the human musculoskeletal system and the objects put into motion by this system, we need first to turn our thoughts to the concepts of motion itself. What is motion? What determines the kind of motion that will result when an object or a part of the human body is made to move? How is motion described in mechanical terms? How do these generalities about motion apply to movements of the musculoskeletal system? Indeed, how does one know that motion is occurring?

Relative Motion

Motion is the act or process of changing place or position with respect to some reference object. Whether a body is at rest or in motion depends totally on the reference, global or local. When a person is walking down the street or riding a bicycle or serving a tennis ball, it seems obvious that movement is involved. Less obvious is the motion status of the sleeping passenger in a smoothly flying plane or of an automobile parked at a curb. If the earth is the reference point, all but the parked car are in motion relative to the earth, and even the parked car is in motion if the reference point is the sun. On the other hand, if the bicycle is the reference point, the person riding it is at rest relative to the bicycle, and the sleeping passenger is at rest with respect to anything in the plane. The relative motion of each is defined in relation to the specific reference object or point. It is possible, therefore, to be at rest and in motion at the same time relative to different reference points. The sleeping passenger is at rest relative to the plane and in motion relative to the earth. The relative motion of two bodies depends entirely on their relative velocities through space. Two joggers running at 8 km/hr in the same direction are at rest with respect to each other. However, if one jogs at 8 km/hr and the other at 10 km/hr, the faster jogger would appear to be traveling at 2 km/hr to the slower jogger and at 10 km/hr to the earth.

Cause of Motion

It is difficult to think of motion without visualizing a specific object in the act of moving. If we did not actually see how it changed from a stationary condition to a moving one, we might wonder what caused it to be set in motion. Did someone pull on it, or push against it, or perhaps blow on it or even attract it with a magnet? What are these assumed causes of motion? Without exception, each cause of motion is a form of force. Force is the instigator of movement. If we see an object in motion, we know that it is moving because a force has acted on it. We know, too, that the force must have been sufficiently great to overcome the object's inertia, or resistance to motion, for unless a force is greater than the resistance offered by the object, it cannot produce motion. We can push against a stone wall all day without moving it so much as 1 millimeter, but a bulldozer can knock down the wall at the first impact. The magnitude of the force relative to the *magnitude of the resistance* is the determining factor in causing an object to move.

Kinds of Motion

What are the ways in which an object may move? The hand moves in an arc when the forearm turns at the elbow joint and the neighboring joints are held motionless. A hockey puck may slide across the ice without turning. On the other hand, it may revolve as it slides. A figure skater spins in place. Arrows, balls, and jumpers move through the air in an arc known as a parabola. As we note the different ways in which objects move, we are impressed with the almost limitless variety in the patterns of movement. Objects move in straight paths and in curved paths; they roll, slide, and fall; they bounce; they swing back and forth like a pendulum; they rotate about a center, either partially or completely; and they frequently rotate at the same time that they move as a whole from one place to another. Although the variety of ways in which objects move appears to be almost limitless, careful consideration of these ways reveals that there are, in actuality, only two major classifications of movement patterns. These are linear or translatory and angular or rotary. Either an object moves in its entirety from one place to another, or it turns about a center of motion. Sometimes it does both simultaneously.

Linear (Translatory) Movement

This kind of movement is termed translatory because the object is translated as a whole from one location to another. Translatory movement is commonly called linear motion and is further classified as rectilinear or curvilinear. *Rectilinear motion* is the straight-line progression of an object as a whole with all its parts moving the same distance in the same direction at a uniform rate of speed. The child on the sled in Figure 11.1, a water skier pulled by a boat, or a bowling ball moving in a straight path are examples of rectilinear motion.

Curvilinear motion refers to all curved translatory movement; that is, the object moves in a curved pathway. The paths of a ball or any other projectile in flight, the wrist during the force phase in bowling (Figure 11.2), or a skier in a sweeping turn are all examples of curvilinear motion.

A special form of curvilinear motion, which on the surface does not appear to be translatory, is that called *circular motion*. This type of motion occurs when an object moves along the circumference

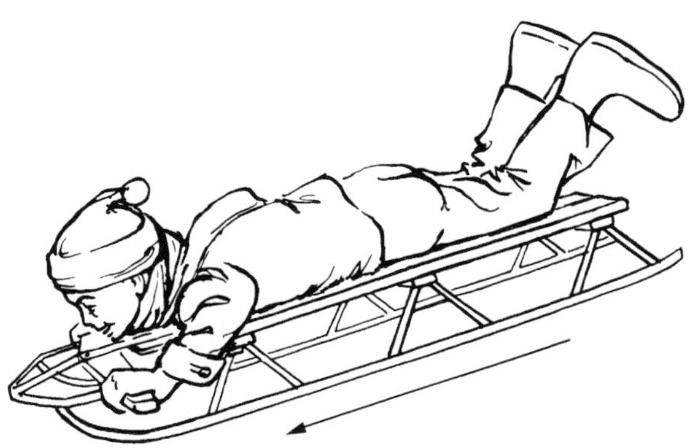

Figure 11.1 An example of rectilinear motion.

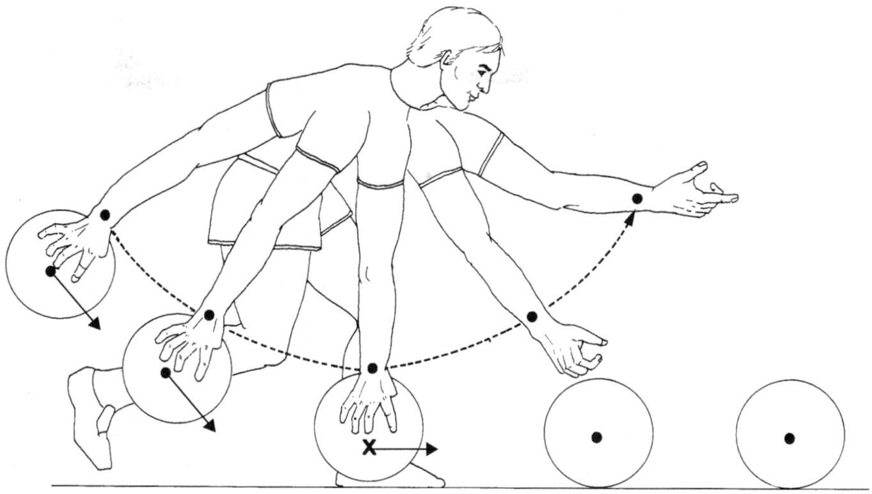

Figure 11.2 The wrist follows a curvilinear path during the delivery of a bowling ball. The arrows indicate the direction the ball would travel if it was released at that moment.

of a circle, that is, a curved path of constant radius. The logic for calling this type of motion linear relates to the fact that it occurs when an unbalanced force acts on a moving body to keep it in a circle. If that unbalanced force stops acting on the object and the object is free to move, it will move in a linear path tangent to the direction in which it is moving at the moment of release. A classic example is an object tied to the end of a string and swung in circles around the head. When the object is released, it will fly off in a straight line. The hammer in the hammer throw follows a circular path until it is released, at which time it flies along a curvilinear path until it lands. The path of a ball held in the hand as the arm moves around in windmill fashion is another example of circular motion. If the ball is released during the motion, it will fly off at a tangent and continue in a straight line until gravity forces it into a curved path (Figure 11.2). Other examples of bodies in circular motion are the gondola on a moving Ferris wheel or the knot on the ring of a spinning lariat.

Angular (Rotary) Motion

This kind of motion is typical of levers and of wheels and axles. Angular, or rotary, motion occurs when any object acting as a radius moves about a fixed point. The distance traveled may be a small arc or a complete circle and is measured as an angle, in degrees. Most human body segment motions are angular movements in which the body part moves in an arc about a fixed point. The axial joints of the skeleton act as fixed points for angular motion in the segments. The arm engages in angular motion when it moves in windmill fashion about a fixed point or axis in the shoulder. The head's motion in the act of indicating "no," the lower leg in kicking a ball, or the hand and forearm in turning a doorknob are all examples of angular motion. In each instance the moving body segment may be likened to the radius of a circle. The arm moving in windmill fashion and the lower leg and foot in kicking are the radii (Figure 11.3). In the "no" action of the head and in the doorknob being turned by the forearm and hand, the radius is perpendicular to the long axis running vertically through the middle of the head and lengthwise through the middle of the forearm and hand, respectively. These movements are not to be confused with circular motion. Circular motion describes the motion of any point on the radius, whereas angular motion is descriptive of the motion of the entire radius. When a ball is held in the hand as the arm moves in a windmill fashion,

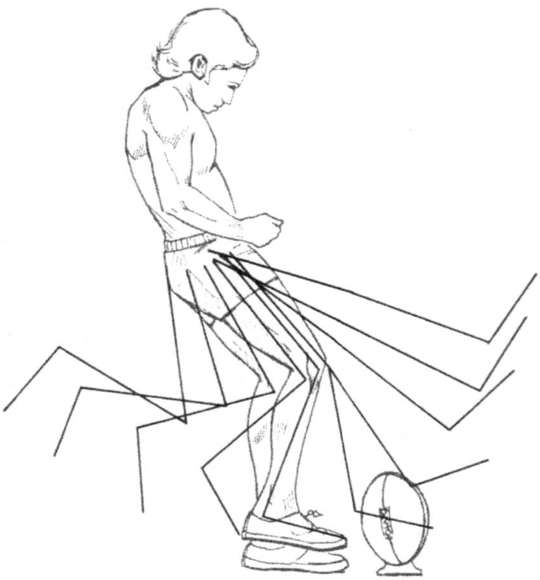

Figure 11.3 Example of angular motion. The lower leg rotates about an axis in the knee joint. Similarly, the thigh engages in rotary motion moving about an axis in the hip joint.

the ball is moving with circular motion, while the arm acts as a radius moving with angular motion about the fixed point of the shoulder.

Other Movement Patterns

Reciprocating motion denotes repetitive movement. The use of the term is ordinarily limited to repetitive translatory movements, as illustrated by a bouncing ball or the repeated blows of a hammer, but technically it includes all kinds. The term *oscillation* refers specifically to repetitive movements in an arc. Familiar examples of this type of movement are seen in the pendulum, metronome, and playground swing.

Often an object displays a combination of rotary and translatory movement. This is sometimes referred to as general motion. The bicycle, automobile, and train move linearly as the result of the rotary movements of their wheels. Likewise, people, as they walk or run down the street, experience translatory motion because of the angular movement of their body segments. The angular motions of several segments of the body are frequently coordinated in such a way that a single related segment will move linearly. This is true in throwing darts, in shot putting, and in a lunge in fencing (Figure 11.4). Because of the angular motions of the forearm and upper arm, the hand travels linearly and thus is able to impart linear force to the dart, to the shot prior to the release, and to the foil.

Kinds of Motion Experienced by the Body

The human body experiences all kinds of motion. Because most of the joints are axial, the body segments must undergo primarily angular motion (Figure 11.5). A slight amount of translatory motion is seen in the gliding movements of the plane or irregular joints, but these movements are negligible in themselves. They occur chiefly in the carpal and tarsal joint and in the joints of the vertebral arches in conjunction with angular movements in neighboring axial joints.

The body as a whole experiences rectilinear movement when it is acted on by the force of gravity, as in coasting down a hill (Figure 11.1) or in a free fall (Figure 11.6), and likewise when acted on by an external force, as in water skiing (Figure 11.7). It experiences general motion in forward and backward rolls on the ground and in somersaults in the air, and rotary motion in twirling on ice skates. It experiences curvilinear translatory motion in diving and jumping, and it experiences reciprocating motion when swinging back and forth on a swing or a bar.

Factors That Determine the Kind of Motion

Thus far we have considered the cause of motion and the various kinds of motion on the basis of movement patterns or paths. Now we must turn to another question. What determines the kind of motion that will result when an object is made to move? The best way for the student to discover the answer is to produce each kind of motion and then analyze what was done to obtain the desired motion.

To make an object move linearly, we discover that it must be free to move and that either we must apply force uniformly against one entire side of the object or we must apply it directly in line

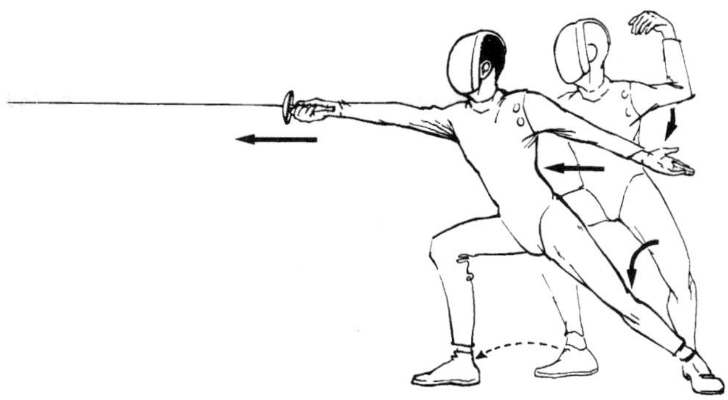

Figure 11.4 General motion: linear motion of one part of the body (the hand) resulting from angular motion of several segments of the body. (a) Just before lunge (thrust). (b) At completion of lunge.

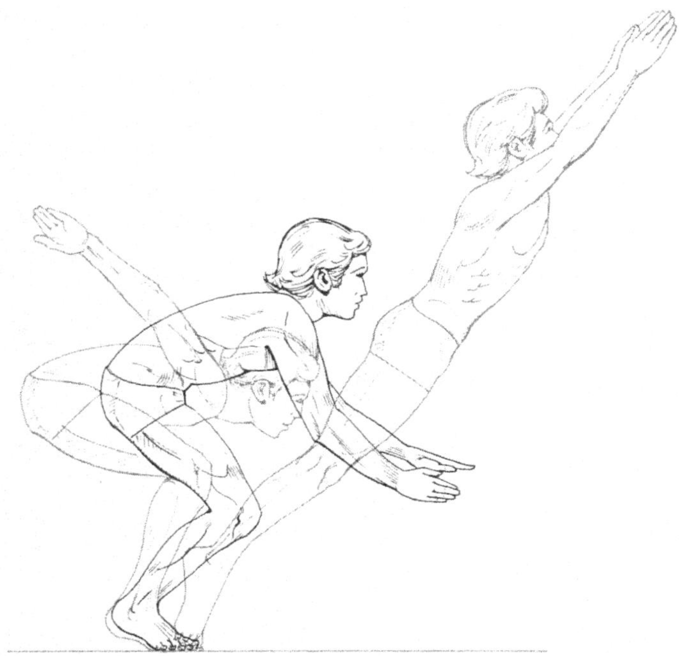

Figure 11.5 An example of movement of the body caused by the body's own muscular activity. Movements of individual body segments are primarily angular.

with the object's center of gravity. The object will move in a straight line, provided it does not meet an obstacle or resistance of some sort. If its edge hits against another object or encounters a rough spot, the moving object will turn about its point of contact with the interfering obstacle. If we attempt to push a tall cabinet across a supporting surface that provides excessive friction, such as a cement floor, the cabinet will tip, even though we place our hands exactly in line with the cabinet's center of gravity and push in a horizontal direction. To move it linearly, it is necessary to apply the push

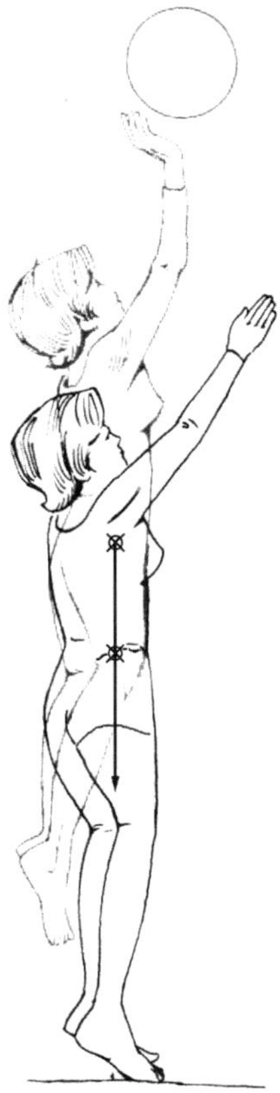

Figure 11.6 Descent from a vertical jump. An example of linear movement of the body caused by the force of gravity.

lower than the cabinet's center of gravity to compensate for the friction.

If one part of an object is "fixed," rotary motion will occur when sufficient force is applied on any portion of the object that is free to move. A lever undergoes rotary motion because, by definition, some portion of it remains in place. To move an object in the manner of a lever, it is necessary to provide a "fulcrum" or an axis and to apply force to the object at some point other than at the fulcrum. Thus, if rotary motion of a freely movable object is desired, it is necessary to apply force to it "off center" or to provide an "off center" resistance that will interfere with the motion of part of the object.

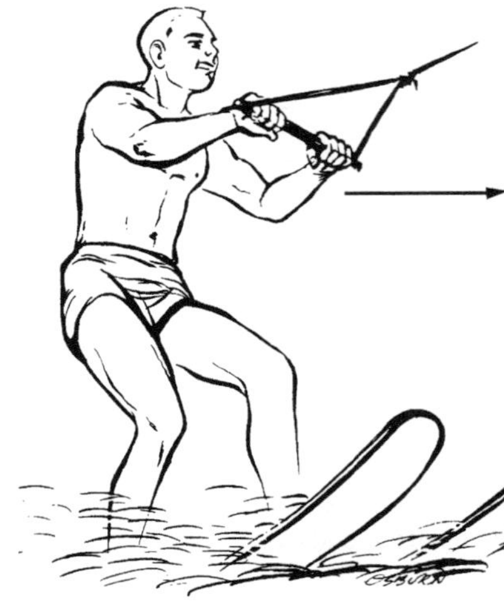

Figure 11.7 An example of movement of the body caused by an external force.

Reciprocating motion is caused by a uniform repetition of opposing force applications, and the oscillation of a pendulum is produced by repeated applications of gravitational force to a suspended object that is free to move back and forth and that is in any position other than its resting position.

In summary, the kind of motion that will be displayed by a moving object depends primarily on the kind of motion permitted in that particular kind of object. If it is a lever, it is permitted only angular motion; if it is a pendulum, oscillatory motion; and so on. If it is a freely movable object, it is permitted either translatory or rotary motion, depending on the circumstances. These circumstances include the point at which force is applied with reference to the object's center of gravity, the environmental pathways of movement available to the object, and the presence or absence of additional external factors that modify the motion.

Factors Modifying Motion

Motion is usually modified by a number of external factors, such as friction, air resistance, and water resistance. Whether these factors are a help or a hindrance depends on the circumstances and the nature of the motion. The same factor may facilitate one form of motion, yet hinder another. For instance, friction is a great help to the runner because maximum effort may be exerted without danger of slipping; on the other hand, friction hinders the rolling of a ball, as in field hockey, golf, and croquet. Again, wind or air resistance is indispensable to the sailboat's motion, but unless it is a tailwind, it impedes the runner. Likewise, water resistance is essential for propulsion of the body by means of swimming strokes and of boats through the use of oars and paddles, yet at the same time it hinders the progress of both the swimmer and the boat, especially if these present a broad surface to the water. For this reason, swimmers keep the body level, and designers plan streamlined boats. One of the major problems in movement is to learn how to take advantage of these modifying factors when they contribute to the movement in question and how to minimize them when they are detrimental to the movement. A more detailed discussion of forces influencing motion is presented in Chapters 12 and 13.

The motion of the segments of the body is also modified by anatomical factors. These include friction in the joints (minimized by synovial fluid), tension of antagonistic muscles, tension of ligaments and fasciae, anomalies of bone and joint structure, atmospheric pressure within the joint capsule, and the presence of interfering soft tissues. Except for the limitations because of fat or muscle bulk, these modifying factors are classified as internal resistance.

KINEMATIC DESCRIPTION OF MOTION

Motion has been defined as the act or process of changing place or position with respect to some reference point. Thus, to talk about motion, a starting point must be identified. Once this is done, the resultant motion, regardless of whether it is translatory or rotary, may be characterized according to the distance and direction away from the starting point, the speed of the movement, and any change in speed that may occur. This kind of motion study is called kinematics. Motion is described in terms of displacement, velocity, and acceleration with no consideration of or reference to the forces that cause or modify the motion. Linear kinematics is concerned with translatory motion and angular kinematics with rotary motion.

Linear Kinematics

Distance and Displacement

The distance an object is removed from a reference point is called its displacement. Displacement does not indicate how far the object travels in going from point A to point C. It only indicates the final change of position. A person who walks north for 3 kilometers to point B and then east for 4 kilometers to point C has walked a distance of 7 kilometers, but the displacement with respect to the starting point is only 5 kilometers (Figure 11.8). Similarly, a basketball player who

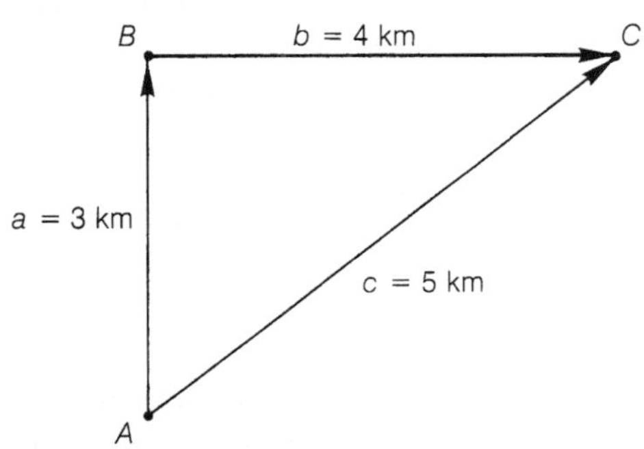

Displacement, c = 5 km

Solution:
$$c^2 = a^2 + b^2$$
$$c^2 = 3^2 + 4^2$$
$$c = \sqrt{9 + 16} = \sqrt{25}$$
$$c = 5 \text{ km}$$

Figure 11.8 Displacement is the resultant distance an object is removed from its starting point.

runs up and down the court several times has traveled a considerable distance, but the displacement with respect to one of the end lines may be zero. Or consider the poor golfer who, blinded by the late afternoon sun, hits the ball so erratically and frequently that the route to the green, 450 yards away, crosses and recrosses the fairway many times. Regardless of the zigzag path to the green and the many changes of direction needed to get there, the ball's displacement is the straight-line distance from the tee to the green.

Displacement is a vector quantity having both magnitude and direction. It is not enough to indicate only the amount of positional change. That alone would be *distance,* a scalar quantity. The direction of the vector must also be defined. When the golfer finally reaches the green, the displacement from the hole to the green is 450 yards west. And the walker's displacement in Figure 11.8 is 5 km, in a northeast direction.

Speed and Velocity

Speed and *velocity* are frequently used to describe how fast an object is moving. These terms are often used interchangeably, but in fact there is a significant difference. Speed is related to distance and velocity to displacement. Speed tells how fast an object is moving—that is, the distance an object will travel in a given time—but it tells nothing about the direction of movement.

$$\text{Average speed} = \frac{\text{distance traveled}}{\text{time}} \text{ or } = \frac{\mathbf{d}}{\mathbf{t}}$$

Examples of speed measurements are a car traveling at 7 km/hr, the wind blowing at 60 mph, a ball thrown with a speed of 30 m/sec, or a sprinter running at 10 m/sec.

Velocity, on the other hand, involves direction as well as speed. Speed is a scalar quantity, whereas velocity is a vector quantity. In many activities this difference is of no concern, but in others it is of extreme importance. The speed of a football player carrying the ball may be impressive, but if the speed is not directed toward the opponent's goal, it is not providing yardage for a first down. Although the speed may be great, the velocity in the desired direction may indeed be zero. Velocity is speed in a given direction. It is the amount of displacement per given unit of time. This is the same as saying that velocity is the rate of displacement, or

$$\text{Average velocity} = \frac{\text{displacement}}{\text{time}} \text{ or } = \frac{\mathbf{s}}{\mathbf{t}}$$

In the diagrams in Figure 11.9, displacement values (s) are represented on the y-axis and the time values (t) are on the x-axis. If displacement values are plotted to correspond with their time values, the line formed by connecting these plotted values represents the rate of displacement or velocity (v). When the rate of displacement does not change—that is, when the distance and direction traveled is the same for each equal time period—the velocity is constant, and the velocity line on the diagram is a straight line. In Figures 11.9a, b, and c, the velocity is constant; but in Figure 11.9d the curved line indicates that the rate of displacement changes, and therefore the velocity is not constant. When there is greater displacement per unit of time, the velocity increases, as does the slope of the velocity line in the diagram. Figure 11.9b shows the fastest velocity and c the slowest. In d, the displacement starts at a slow rate and then increases. If a, b, c, and d represent runners on a straight track, a, b, and c would each be running at a constant but different velocity, with b's velocity the fastest and c's the slowest. Runner d starts out at a slow velocity but increases the rate of displacement until the resultant velocity is the fastest of all four.

Where velocity is constant, as in Figure 11.9a, b, and c, the motion is said to be uniform. When the amount of displacement per unit of time varies, nonuniform motion occurs. Uniform motion is not a common characteristic of human motion, because most human movements are likely to have many variations in the rate of displacement. When the velocity of human motion is given, it is usually an average velocity that tells only the total displacement occurring in a stated period of time. Although a long-distance runner who ran the Boston Marathon (a distance of 26 miles, 385 yards), in 2.5 hours had an average velocity of 10.4 mph, it is doubtful that the velocity was uniformly 10.4 mph throughout the run. If one

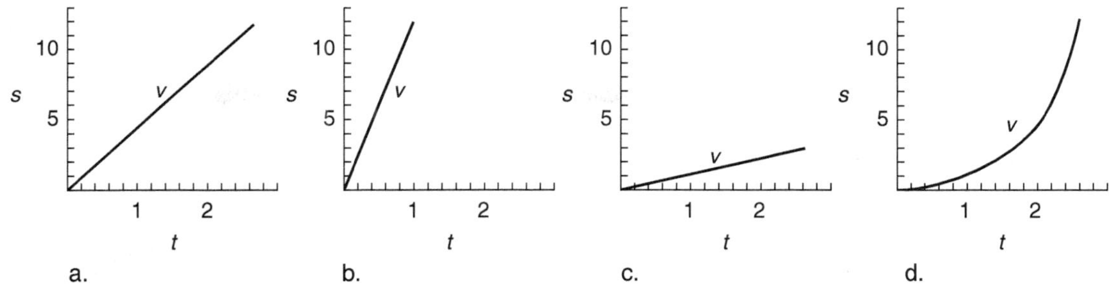

Figure 11.9 Examples of displacement–time graphs for uniform and nonuniform motion. The velocity in (a), (b), and (c) is constant.

were to record the time at which the runner passed frequent and equally spaced distance points along the route, a displacement–time graph could be prepared to show the variations in the runner's speed at various points in the course of the race. This kind of information can be quite useful in helping a coach or participant analyze the performance and strategy of the race and plan changes where needed. The narrower the distance intervals used, the greater is the possibility that critical variations in speed will become apparent. The use of motion analysis systems permits a similar analysis of brief and fast events. The distance and time data necessary for graphing and analyzing the motion patterns are obtained indirectly from the video or digital record.

In equation form, average velocity is

$$\bar{v} = \frac{s}{t}$$

The symbol s represents displacement, and t represents time. The average velocity of a tennis ball served 19 meters in 0.35 second is 19 divided by 0.35, or 54.3 m/sec in the direction of the service court.

Acceleration

When velocity changes, its rate of change is called *acceleration*. A sprint runner has an initial velocity of 0 m/sec. When the gun signals the beginning of a race, the sprinter's velocity begins to change by increasing. The rate of change in velocity is acceleration. Acceleration may be positive or negative. An increase is considered positive, and a decrease such as slowing down at the end of the race is negative. Negative acceleration is also called deceleration.

In equation form, acceleration is expressed as

$$\bar{a} = \frac{v_f - v_i}{t}$$

where $\bar{a}$ represents average acceleration, v_f is the final velocity and v_i is the initial velocity. In other words, acceleration is any change in velocity divided by the time interval over which that change occurred.

In the example of the sprint runner, a graph of the sprinter's velocity throughout the race can be used to illustrate acceleration (Figure 11.10). As the sprinter is waiting in the starting blocks, the velocity is zero. In section a of the race, the sprinter changes from a velocity of 0 to a velocity of 9 m/sec after the first 5.6 seconds. Because this is an increase in velocity, this is positive acceleration. The acceleration for this phase of the race, the rate of change in velocity, equals the difference between the final velocity (9 m/sec) and the initial velocity (0 m/sec) divided by the time interval (5.6 sec), or 1.8 m/sec^2. In section b of the race, the velocity does not change but remains at a constant 9 m/sec. Because there is no change in velocity, the acceleration for this phase would be zero. To prove this, we use the equation

$$\bar{a} = \frac{v_f - v_i}{t} = \frac{9^m/_s - 9^m/_s}{9 - 5s} = \frac{0^m/_s}{4s} = 0^m/_{s^2}$$

In section c, the sprinter increases velocity again just before the finish. In this phase the acceleration

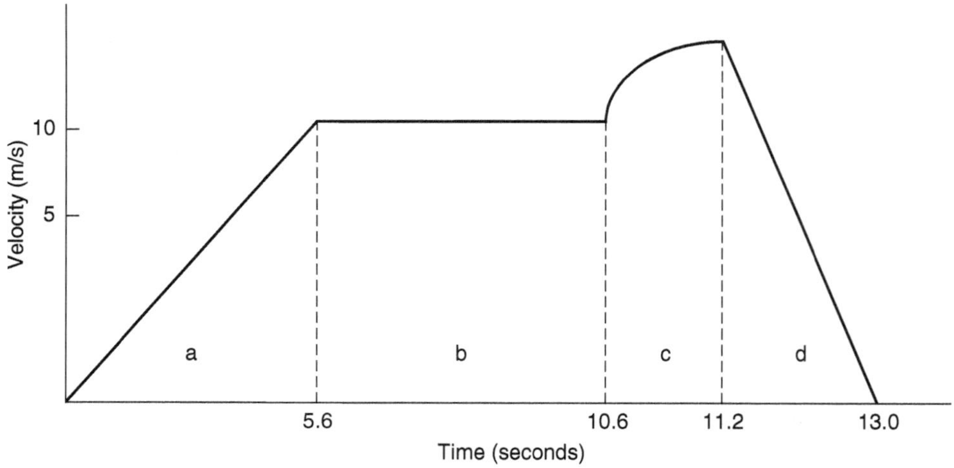

Figure 11.10 An acceleration curve showing a constant acceleration (uniform change in velocity) in (a), zero acceleration (no change in velocity) in (b), varying acceleration in (c), and constant deceleration (uniform slowing) in (d).

is not constant, so calculating an average velocity would not produce a true representation of the changes in velocity that are occurring. It is more accurate to calculate several instantaneous accelerations to plot a curve. By visually examining the curve, it can be seen that the acceleration at the beginning of this short phase is greater than the acceleration at the end of the phase. Section d of the race starts as the sprinter crosses the finish line. At this point the velocity is 10 m/sec. The sprinter now decreases velocity to come to a stop (0 m/sec) after the race. This slowing down represents negative acceleration, or deceleration.

Because velocity is always displacement divided by time and acceleration is velocity divided by time, acceleration is really displacement divided by time divided by time, and the units for measurement must reflect this. The time unit must appear twice in acceleration units. The logic for this is apparent when the units of m/sec are used for velocity in the equation for average acceleration:

$$\bar{a} = \frac{\left(\frac{\text{final m}}{\text{sec}} - \frac{\text{initial m}}{\text{sec}}\right)}{\text{sec}}$$

After the subtraction is completed, this equation becomes

$$\bar{a} = \frac{\frac{\text{m}}{\text{sec}}}{\text{sec}}$$

or, as commonly written, m/sec/sec or m/sec^2. Thus, the average acceleration of the runner in the example is 1.6 m/sec^2.

One usually thinks of acceleration in terms of a change in the amount of distance covered in equal units of time. Acceleration also occurs when, although the speed remains constant, there is a change in direction. The example given for Figure 11.10b is that of a runner keeping a steady pace on a straight track with no acceleration. If the runner, still running at the same speed, shifts to a circular track, acceleration occurs because of the change in direction, and the velocity–time graph would look more like Figure 11.10c.

Uniformly Accelerated Motion

When the acceleration rate is constant, the velocity change is the same during equal time periods. Under these conditions, motion is said to be uniformly accelerated. This type of acceleration does not occur with great frequency, because the change in velocity of bodies in motion is usually irregular and complicated. However, one common type of uniform acceleration is important in sport and physical education—the acceleration of freely falling bodies.

Neglecting air resistance, objects allowed to fall freely will speed up or accelerate at a uniform rate owing to the acceleration of gravity. Conversely, objects projected upward will be slowed at a uniform rate that is also due to the acceleration of gravity. The value for the acceleration of gravity changes with different locations on the earth's surface, but for most of the United States this value can be considered to be 32 ft/sec^2 or 9.80 m/sec^2. Regardless of its size or density, a falling object will be acted on by gravity so that its velocity will increase 9.8 m/sec each second it is in the air. A dropped ball starting out with a velocity of 0 m/sec will have a velocity of 9.8 m/sec at the end of 1 second, 19.6 m/sec at the end of 2 seconds, 29.4 m/sec at the end of 3 seconds, and so on. A second ball weighing twice as much will fall with exactly the same acceleration. It too will have a velocity of 29.4 m/sec at the end of 3 seconds. Of course, this example does not consider the resistance or friction of air, which can be appreciable. The lighter the object, the more it is affected. After an initial acceleration, light objects such as feathers or snowflakes may stop accelerating entirely and fall at a constant rate. Consider, for instance, the difference between the behavior of a badminton shuttle and a golf ball when dropped from a height.

The denser and heavier the free-falling object, the less air friction affects it, especially if the distance of the fall is not too great. Even heavy objects, such as sky divers falling from great distances, eventually reach a downward speed large enough to create an opposing air resistance equal to the accelerating force of gravity. When this happens, the diver no longer speeds up but continues to fall at a steady speed. This speed is called terminal velocity and amounts to approximately 120 mph (53 m/sec) for a falling sky diver. With the parachute open, the diver's velocity decreases to 12 mph steady velocity.

Laws of uniformly accelerated motion In spite of the reality of air resistance, much can be learned about the nature of free-falling bodies and uniform acceleration through a knowledge of the laws of uniformly accelerated motion. Because the acceleration of gravity is constant, the distance traveled by a freely falling body, as well as its downward velocity, can be determined for any point in time by application of these laws. Expressed in equation form, they are

$$v_f = v_i + at$$
$$s = v_i t + \tfrac{1}{2}at^2$$
$$v_f^2 = v_i^2 + 2as$$

Galileo's experiments with inclined planes enabled him to work out these equations. They apply to any type of linear motion in which acceleration is uniform. Their specific application to the effect of gravity on freely falling objects is presented in Table 11.1. If the initial velocity (v_i) is zero, as it is when an object is allowed to fall freely from a stationary position, the equations may be simplified:

$$v_f = at$$
$$s = \tfrac{1}{2}at^2$$
$$v_f^2 = 2as$$

The student may also discover that some authors, when applying these equations specifically to gravity, replace a, the symbol for acceleration, with g, the symbol for gravity.

The time an object takes to rise to the highest point of its trajectory is equal to the time an object takes to fall to its starting point. Similarly, the release speed and landing speed are the same. Other than the fact that the directions are reversed, the upward flight is a mirror image of the downward flight. Proof that the release velocity and landing velocity are equal in amount but opposite in direction can be shown mathematically by substitution of values in the motion equations. Following vector conventions, velocities upward are positive and those downward are negative. Thus the acceleration of gravity is treated as a negative value.

TABLE 11.1 Effect of Gravity on a Freely Falling Object

	Time	Distance Traveled $s = v_i t + \frac{1}{2} at^2$	Final Velocity $v_f = v_i + at$	Average Velocity $\bar{v} = \frac{v_i - v_f}{2}$
U.S.	1 sec	16 ft	32 ft/sec	16 ft/sec
$a = 32$ ft/sec^2	2 sec	64 ft	64 ft/sec	32 ft/sec
	3 sec	144 ft	96 ft/sec	48 ft/sec
	4 sec	256 ft	128 ft/sec	64 ft/sec
	5 sec	400 ft	160 ft/sec	80 ft/sec
Metric	1 sec	4.9 m	9.8 m/sec	4.9 m/sec
$a = 9.81$ m/sec^2	2 sec	19.6 m	19.6 m/sec	9.8 m/sec
	3 sec	44.1 m	29.4 m/sec	14.7 m/sec
	4 sec	78.4 m	39.2 m/sec	19.6 m/sec
	5 sec	122.5 m	49 m/sec	24.5 m/sec

Example Assuming that a ball is thrown upward so that it reaches a height of 5 meters before starting to fall, what is its initial velocity as it leaves the hand? What is its final velocity as it lands in the hand?

Upward Thrown Velocity

Given: $v = 0$

$a = -9.80\ \text{m/s}^2$

$s = 5\ \text{m}$

Find: $v_i = ?$

Downward Landing Velocity

Given: $v_i = 0$

$a = -9.80\ \text{m/s}^2$

$s = 5\ \text{m}$

Find: $v_f = ?$

Solution: Using eq. (11.3) $v_f^2 = v_i^2 + 2as$

$$v_f^2 = v_i^2 + 2as$$
$$v_i^2 = v_f^2 - 2as$$
$$v_i^2 = 0 + (2 \times 9.81\,{}^{m}/_{s^2} \times 5\ \text{m})$$
$$v_i^2 = 98\,{}^{m^2}/_{s^2}$$
$$v_i = \sqrt{98\,{}^{m^2}/_{s^2}}$$
$$v_i = -9.90\,{}^{m}/_{s}$$

$$v_f^2 = v_i^2 + 2as$$
$$v_i^2 = 0 - (2 \times 9.81\,{}^{m}/_{s^2} \times 5\ \text{m})$$
$$v_i^2 = -98\,{}^{m^2}/_{s^2}$$
$$v_i = -\sqrt{98\,{}^{m^2}/_{s^2}}$$
$$v_i = -9.90\,{}^{m}/_{s}$$

Projectiles

An object that has been given an initial velocity and then allowed to move in free fall under the influence of gravity is a projectile. Balls that are thrown, kicked, or hit; javelins; bullets or missiles; and jumpers, divers, and gymnasts while in the air are all examples of projectiles.

An object or a body is projected into the air for any of several reasons. In the case of the diver or the gymnast, the purpose of the projection is to gain maximum time in the air, or time of flight. The longer the *time of flight* the athlete can produce, the greater the number of acrobatic moves that can be performed. In other activities, a decreased time of flight may serve to deceive or avoid an opponent, as in the volleyball spike, or a smash in tennis, or an onside kick in football. Projectiles may also be released for the purpose of producing *maximum horizontal displacement.* The long jumper, the discus thrower, the shot-putter, and the batter in baseball are all examples of projection of an object for distance. Maximum displacement may also be in the vertical direction. Projections for maximum vertical displacement include such activities as the high jump and the pole vault. Projection of a body or an object for *maximum accuracy* is the purpose of actions such as shooting in basketball or soccer, passing, archery, or golf. When accuracy is the primary concern, a compromise often must be made between horizontal displacement and time in the air.

Once released, projectiles follow a predictable path. If air resistance is ignored because it is considered negligible, this path will be a parabola. The characteristic parabolic path of a projectile is the result of the constant downward force of gravity. This means that gravity will decelerate any upward motion at a rate of 9.8 m/sec^2 or will accelerate any downward motion at the same rate (Figure 11.11). All objects in free fall have the same downward acceleration whether they start from a resting position with a drop or fall or have been given some initial velocity.

Two forces, then, are acting on a projectile: the projecting force and gravity. The projecting force is a vector quantity that may act at any desired angle, depending on the purpose of the projection. The application of the projecting force produces an initial velocity in the object at some angle of projection. Because this initial release velocity is a vector quantity, it can be resolved into two component velocities, one vertical and one horizontal. The vertical component of velocity, being a vector parallel to gravity, will be directly affected by gravity. The horizontal component will not. Gravity is also a vector force that always acts in a vertical, downward direction. This downward force of gravity acts completely independently of any horizontal component of the projecting force (Figure 11.12).

If an object or a body is projected with only a horizontal velocity, then gravity, as the second force, will still act to cause that object to fall. If one object falls freely from rest at the same time that another is projected horizontally from the same height, both objects will hit the ground at the same time. However, they will hit in different places. The dropped object will land immediately below the point of release, whereas the projected object will land some distance away. Gravity has acted on both objects equally, giving them equal vertical velocities in the downward direction, so they will fall at the same rate and land at the same time. The difference in landing points is the result of the horizontal velocity possessed by the projected object. In the time it took both objects to fall, the horizontal velocity of the projected object carried that object some distance from the point of release. This distance can be calculated using the velocity equation

$$v = s/t \qquad \text{or} \qquad s = v \times t$$

If, for instance, these two objects were balls released at a height of 2 meters, they would take 0.64 second to fall to the ground. If one was projected horizontally with a velocity of 20 m/sec, it would strike the ground at a distance of 12.8 meters from the release point (s = 20 m/sec × 0.64 sec; Figure 11.13).

To change the time an object is in the air, the velocity produced by projection must have some vertical component. This may be an upward component, opposing gravity, or a downward component being added to gravity. The time an object is in the air may also be varied by altering the height of release. If the balls in the previous examples were released from a height of 3 meters, both balls would be in the air for 0.78 seconds. Using the velocity equation again, it can be determined that the horizontally projected ball would now travel 15.6 meters from the point of release (s = 20 m/sec × 0.78 sec = 15.6 meters).

An object that is projected with only upward velocity will be decelerated by gravity until it reaches a velocity of zero. At this point, it will start to drop back toward the release point, accelerating as it falls. When the object reaches the release point, it will possess the same velocity it was given at release. The time required to reach the

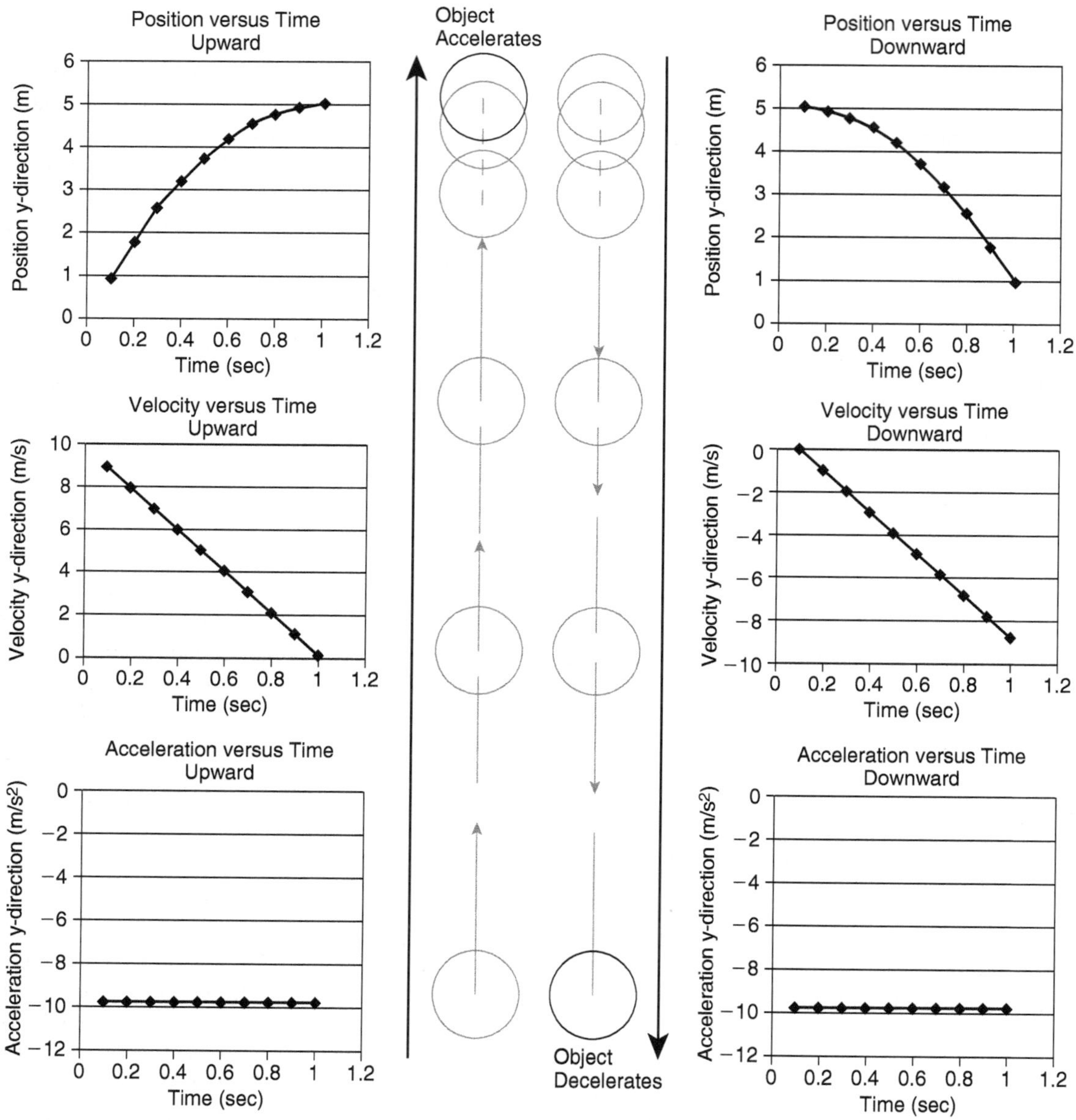

Figure 11.11 Objects projected upward are decelerated by the downward force of gravity at the same rate as those allowed to fall downward are accelerated. Both objects will cover the same distance in the same time.

highest point will be equal to the time it takes to fall back to the height from which it was released.

More often than not, objects put into flight will be projected in some direction other than exactly vertical or horizontal. A projectile of this type has both horizontal and vertical components of the initial velocity vector. Again, these two component velocities are considered independently. The horizontal component of velocity remains constant following release (if air resistance is neglected), as no force is available to change this velocity. The vertical component

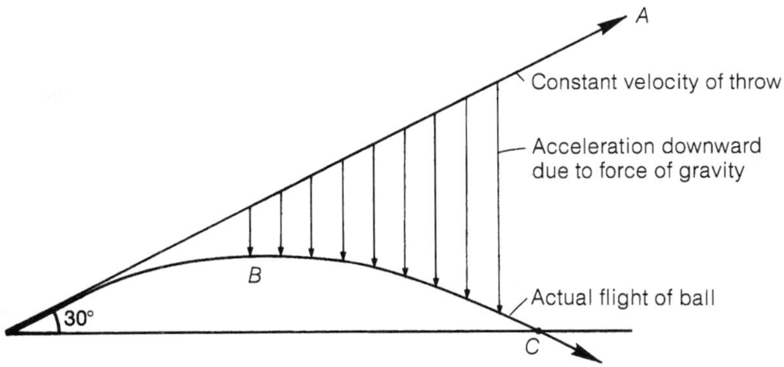

Figure 11.12 Effect of gravity on the flight of a projectile.

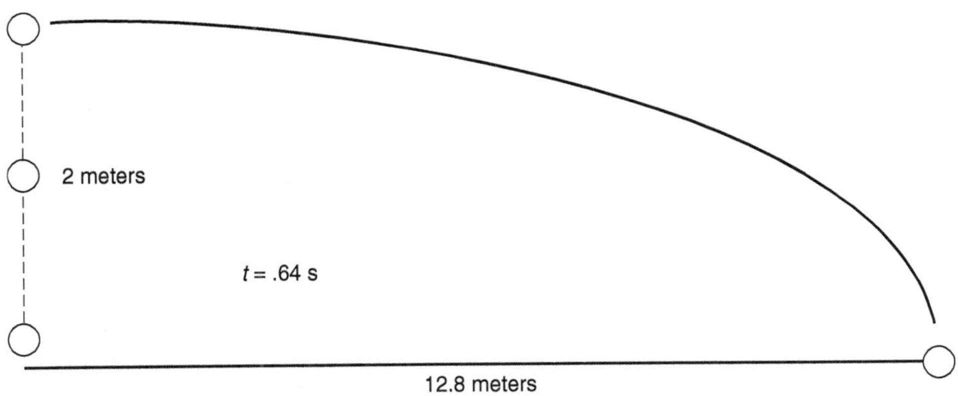

Figure 11.13 A horizontally projected object and a free-falling object released from the same height will land at the same time but in different places.

of velocity will be subject to the uniform acceleration of gravity. When the object is projected with some upward angle, gravity will act to decelerate the object to zero vertical velocity and then accelerate the object again as it falls downward. During this period of vertical deceleration and acceleration, the object is also undergoing constant horizontal motion. This combination of these two independent factors produces the parabolic flight path of the projectile as portrayed in Figure 11.14.

The horizontal distance an object will travel in space depends on both its horizontal velocity and the length of time the object is in the air, or time of flight. The time of flight depends on the maximum height reached by the object, and that, in turn, is governed by the vertical velocity imparted to the object at release. Thus the horizontal distance an object will travel depends on both the horizontal and vertical components of velocity. As will be remembered from the earlier discussion of vectors, the magnitudes of these two components will be determined by the magnitude of the initial projection velocity vector and by the angle that indicates the direction of this vector, referred to as the angle of projection. With this in mind, it can be seen that a projectile with a low angle of projection will have a relatively high horizontal velocity in relation to the vertical velocity. The low vertical velocity does little to resist the pull of

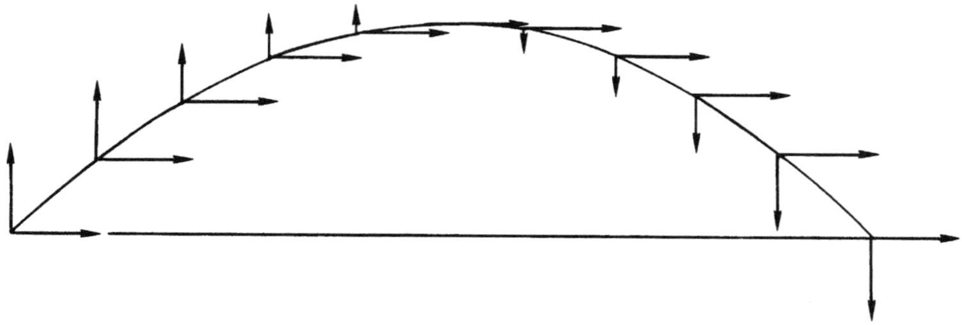

Figure 11.14 Magnitude of horizontal and vertical velocities during projectile flight.

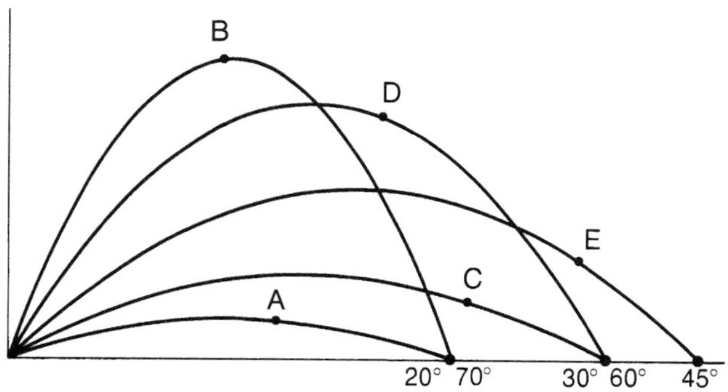

Figure 11.15 The angle of projection influences the horizontal and vertical distance covered by a projectile. Complementary angles of projection produce the same horizontal displacement.

gravity, which therefore requires very little time to decelerate the object to a vertical velocity of zero and start the drop back down. In this instance, vertical distance is low, and therefore time of flight is short, allowing little time for horizontal travel. On the other hand, if the angle of projection is large, it takes longer for the object to decelerate to zero velocity, allowing a much longer time of flight. In this instance, however, there is little horizontal velocity, so little distance can be covered in the time available. Thus it would seem that the optimum angle of projection would be a 45-degree angle, with equal magnitudes for the horizontal and vertical components. In fact, the actual optimal angle of projection depends on several factors, including purpose of the projection. A 45-degree angle of projection will maximize horizontal distance only if release height and landing height are the same. In this case, the object will approach the landing at approximately the same angle as that at which it was projected (Figure 11.15).

If an object is projected from above the ground, as in many throwing events, a lower angle of projection may produce optimum results. This is because the object thrown will have a somewhat increased time of flight as it covers the extra distance between the height of release and the ground as it falls. With this increased time of flight, a slightly reduced vertical velocity and a slightly increased horizontal velocity will usually be optimal. The greater the difference between release height and landing height, the lower the angle of projection needs to be. If initial velocity can be increased, the optimum angle can also be increased back toward a 45-degree angle. From this discussion, then, it can be concluded that *speed of release, angle of projection,* and *height of release* are the three factors that control the range of a projectile.

Angular Kinematics

Angular kinematics is very similar to linear kinematics because it is also concerned with displacement, velocity, and acceleration. The important difference is that the displacement, velocity, and acceleration are related to rotary rather than to linear motion, and although the equations used to show the relationships among these quantities are quite similar to those used in linear motion, the units used to describe them are different (Table 11.2).

Angular Displacement

The human skeleton is made up of a system of levers that by definition are rigid bars that rotate about fixed points when force is applied. When any object acting as a rigid bar moves in an arc about an axis, the movement is called rotary, or angular, motion. An attempt to describe angular motion in linear units presents real problems. As an object moves in an arc, the linear displacement of particles spaced along that lever varies. Particles near the axis have a displacement in inches, meters, feet, or centimeters that is less than those farther away. For example, in the underarm throw pattern, the hand moves through a greater distance than the wrist and the wrist a greater distance than the elbow. Rotary motion needs rotary units to describe it. As might be expected, these units relate to the units of a circle and the fact that the circumference of a circle C is equal to $2\pi r$, where r is the radius and π is a constant value of 3.1416.

There are three interchangeable rotary, or angular, units of displacement: degrees, revolutions, and radians. One radian is the same as 57.3 degrees, and one full revolution is the same as 360 degrees or 2π radians of displacement. The word *revolution* is not stated, but it is understood when we say that a diver executed a 1 1/2

TABLE 11.2 Quantities in Linear and Angular Motion

	Linear	Angular
SYMBOLS		
Displacement	s	θ
Velocity	v_f, v_i, v	$\omega_f, \omega_i, \omega$
Acceleration	a, a	α, α
Time	t	t
EQUATIONS		
Velocity	$v = s/t$	$\omega = \theta/t$
Acceleration	$a = \frac{v_f - v_i}{t}$	$\alpha = \frac{\omega_f - \omega_i}{t}$
LINEAR AND ANGULAR CONVERSIONS		
Displacement	$s = \theta r$	$\theta = s/r$
Velocity	$v = \omega r$	$\omega = v/r$
Acceleration	$a = \alpha r$	$\alpha = a/r$

somersault tuck. The dive could also be described as a tuck somersault of 540 (360 + 180) degrees or 3π radians. Degrees are used most frequently in the measurement of angles; but radians, the term favored by engineers and physicists, are the units most often required in equations of angular motion. The advantage of using radians is that they have no units and, therefore, may be used in equations with linear kinematic terms, as we will see. A radian is the angle at which the subtended arc of a circle is equal to the radius. The result of having 2π radians in a circle is that there are 6.28 radians in 360 degrees. If the circle is divided by the 6.28 radians it contains, it can be seen that each radian is 57.3 degrees. The symbol for angular displacement is the Greek letter θ (theta).*

Angular Velocity

The rate of rotary displacement is called angular velocity, symbolized as ω (omega). Angular velocity is equal to the angle through which the radius turns divided by the time it takes for the displacement:

$$\overline{\omega} = \frac{\theta}{t}$$

It is expressed as degrees/second, radians/second, or revolutions/second. A softball pitcher who moves the arm through an arc of 140 degrees in 0.1 second has an average angular velocity of 1,400 degrees per second. This could also be expressed as 3.88 revolutions per second or 24.43 radians per second. This velocity is called average velocity because film studies of pitchers show that the angular displacement during the execution of the skill is not uniform, and a velocity such as this represents the average velocity over the time span through which the displacement is measured. As with linear movements, most angular human movements are likely to be variable and not uniform. The longer the time span through which the displacement is measured, the more variability is averaged. Thus, if one is interested in the velocity at a specific instant in a skill, the displacement must be measured over an extremely small time span.

Figure 11.16 shows the variations in displacement during the execution of a golf drive. Each displacement between images occurs over the same time period (approximately 0.0067 seconds), so greater spacing between images indicates greater angular displacement over the same time or greater velocity. When the total angular displacement of the golf club was measured from the beginning of the downswing to the point of contact with the ball and divided by the time it took for the swing, the average velocity of the club was 2,148 degrees/second (37.5 rad/sec). The "instant" velocity at a, however, was 1,432 degrees/sec, and at b it was 2,864 degrees/sec. Illustrations such as this, which show a motion as it occurs over very small spans of time, are produced with high-speed film or video. This golfer was filmed at a rate of approximately 150 frames per second, or 0.0067 seconds per picture.

Angular Acceleration

In the discussion of linear velocity, a change in velocity was called acceleration. The same is true for changes in angular velocity. Angular acceleration α (alpha) is the rate of change of angular velocity and is expressed in equation form as

$$\alpha = \frac{\omega_f - \omega_i}{t}$$

where ω_f is final angular velocity, ω_i is initial velocity, and t is time. If, in Figure 11.16, the angular velocity is 25 rad/sec at a and 50 rad/sec at b and the time lapse between a and b is 0.11 seconds, the angular acceleration between a and b is 241 rad/sec/sec. This value for α, indicating that the velocity increased 241 radians per second each second, would be true, of course, only if the velocity increased at a uniform rate. Otherwise this value has to be considered as an average of accelerations that may have been higher or lower during the time period studied.

*For a review of the geometry of circles and an additional explanation of degrees, radians, and revolution, see Appendix D, Part 5.

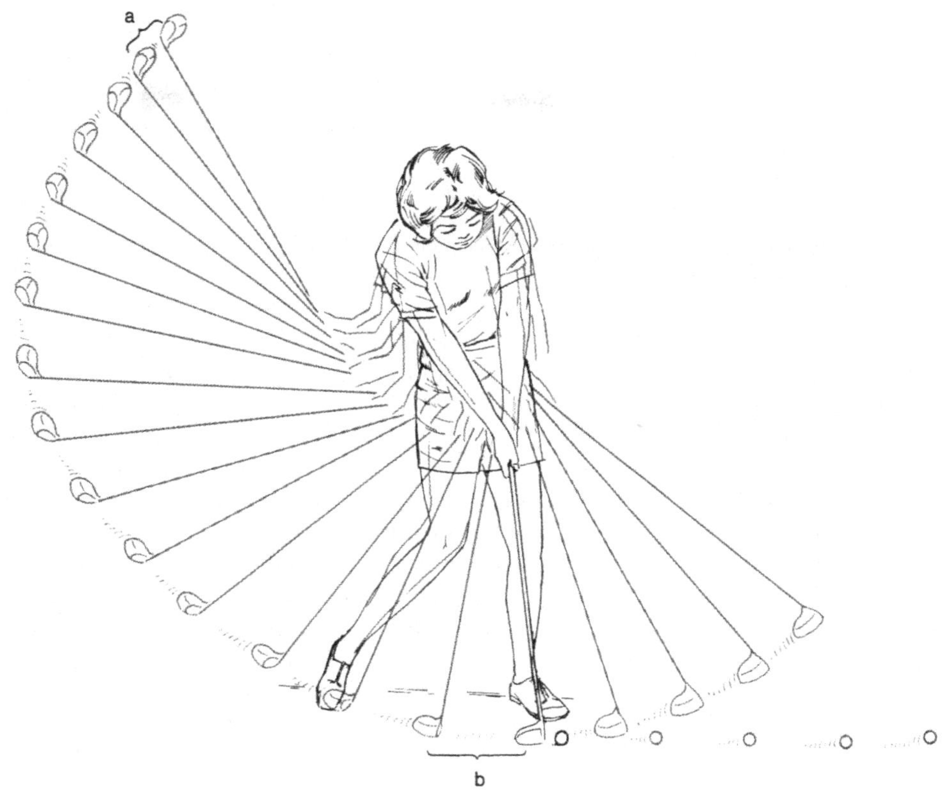

Figure 11.16 Variations in the angular displacement of a golf club over equal time intervals during the execution of a golf drive.

Relationship Between Linear and Angular Motion

The description of angular motion in terms of displacement, velocity, and acceleration can tell us a great deal about human movements, but nothing in such a description accounts for or shows the effect of the length of the radius on the outcomes of the movements. We know that, all other things being equal, a baseball hit in the middle of a bat will not go as far as one hit at the end, that a ball hit by a tennis racket will travel farther than a ball hit with the hand, and that a golf driver will cause a struck ball to travel farther than a nine iron. In each instance, greater force is imparted to the struck object because the radius of the striking implement (distance between axis and point of contact) is longer, and greater linear velocity is generated at its end.

As can be seen in Figure 11.17, lever *PA* is shorter than lever *PB*, and lever *PB* is shorter than lever *PC*. If all three levers move through the same angular distance in the same amount of time, it is apparent that point *C* traveled farther in a curvilinear manner than either point *A* or point *B*. This curvilinear distance is difficult to measure but may be easily calculated if the angular displacement (θ) and the length of the radius (r) are known. The equation that expresses the relationship between angular and linear displacement is $s = \theta r$. Because the linear displacement of point *C* took the same amount of time as the displacements of points *A* and *B*, point *C* moved with a

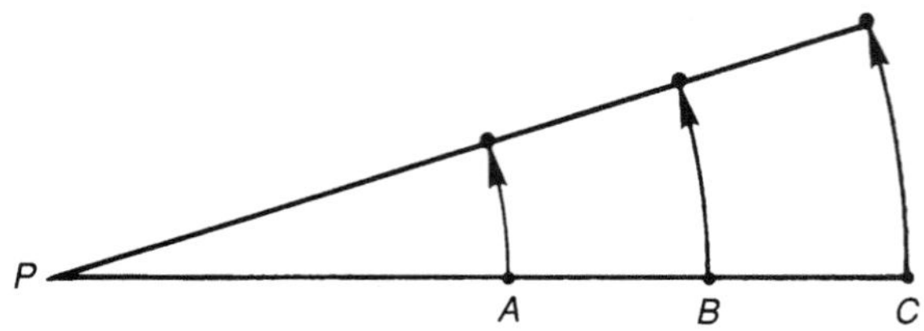

Figure 11.17 Lever $PA < PB < PC$. Although the angular displacement for all three levers is the same, the linear displacement at the end of the longer levers is greater than that at the end of the shorter levers.

greater linear velocity than either of the other two points. Point *B* had a smaller linear velocity than point *C* but a larger linear velocity than point *A*. All three levers have the same *angular velocity,* but linear velocity of the circular motion at the end of each lever is proportional to the length of the lever. An object moved at the end of a long radius will have a greater linear velocity than one moved at the end of a short radius, *if the angular velocity is kept constant. The longer the radius, the greater is the linear velocity of a point at the end of that radius.* Thus it is to the advantage of a performer to use as long a lever as possible to impart linear velocity to an object if the long lever length does not cause too great a sacrifice in angular velocity. The longer the lever, the more effort it takes to swing it. Therefore, the optimum length of the lever for a person depends on the individual's ability to maintain angular velocity. A child who cannot handle the weight of a long radius is better off with a shortened implement that can be controlled and swung rapidly, whereas a strong adult profits by using a longer radius.

If the reverse occurs—that is, if the linear velocity is kept constant—an increase in radius will result in a decrease in angular velocity. Once an object is engaged in rotary motion, the linear velocity at the end of the radius stays the same because of the conservation of momentum. The radius of rotation for a pike somersault dive is longer than that for a tuck somersault, and the radius for a layout somersault is longer than that for a pike somersault. If one starts a dive in an open position and then tucks tightly, the radius of rotation decreases but, because the linear velocity does not change, the angular velocity increases. The same situation occurs when a figure skater rotates slowly about a vertical axis with arms and one leg out to the side and brings the arms and leg close to the axis. The radius decreases and the angular velocity increases. To slow down, the skater again reaches out with arms and leg. Figure 11.18 shows the effect of shortening the radius while maintaining a constant linear velocity at the end of the radius. *Shortening the radius will increase the angular velocity, and lengthening it will decrease the angular velocity.* Points *a* and *b* on radii *A* and *B* have moved through the same linear distance, but the angular displacement for *A* is greater than that for *B*. If the displacements of *a* and *b* each take place in the same amount of time, the linear velocities will be equal, but the angular velocity for *A* will be greater than that for *B*.

The relationship that exists between the angular velocity of an object moving in a rotary fashion and the linear velocity at the end of its radius is expressed by the equation

$$\bar{v} = \omega r$$

To use any of the equations relating linear and angular motion, the angular measures must be

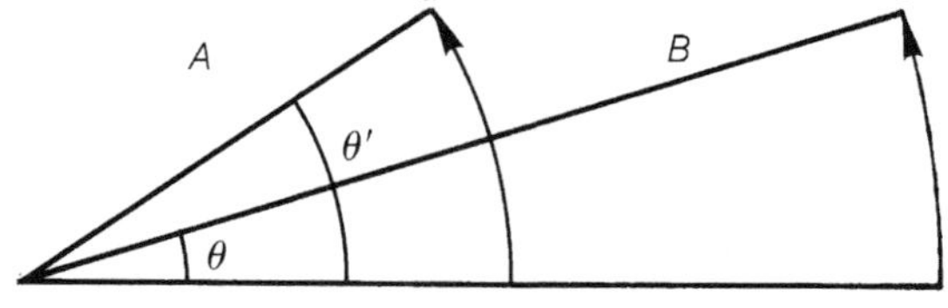

Figure 11.18 Increasing the length of the radius decreases the angular velocity when the linear velocity remains constant.

expressed in radians. If the angle is expressed in degrees, it can be converted to radians simply by dividing by 57.3.

Either form of the equation shows the direct proportionality that exists between linear velocity and the radius. For any given angular velocity, the linear velocity is proportional to the radius. If the radius doubles, the linear velocity does likewise. And for any given linear velocity, the angular velocity is inversely proportional to the radius. If the radius doubles, the angular velocity decreases by half. To achieve higher linear velocities at the end of levers, the motions must be done with longer levers or higher angular velocities (Figure 11.19).

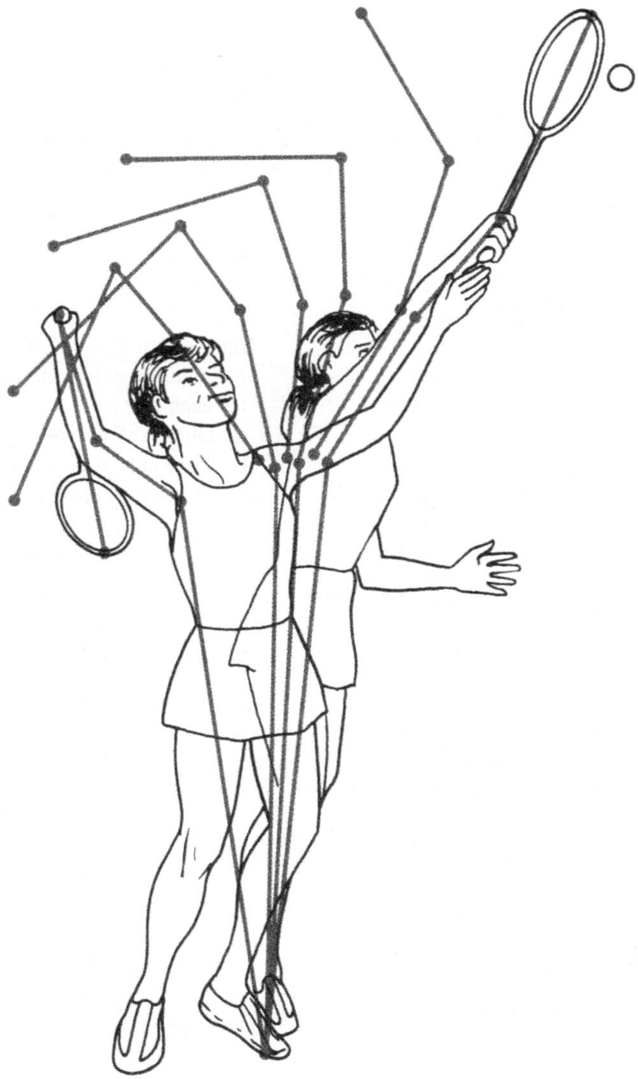

Figure 11.19 Long levers and high angular velocities result in high linear velocities at the ends of the levers. Thus the tennis racket, an extension of a long body lever, is able to impart high linear velocity to the ball.

References and Selected Readings

Bartlett, A. A. (2005). Television, football, and physics: Experiments in kinematics. *The Physics Teacher,* 43, 393.

Dapena J., Gutierrez-Davila, M., Soto, V. M., & Rojas, F. J. (2003). Prediction of distance in hammer throwing. *Journal of Sports Sciences,* 21(1), 21–28.

Ozkaya, N., Nordin, M., & Frankel, V. H. (1999). *Fundamentals of biomechanics: Equilibrium, motion, and deformation* (2nd ed.). New York: Springer.

Trizeren, A. (2000). *Human body dynamics: Classical mechanics and human movement.* New York: Springer.

Zatsiorsky, V. M. (1998). *Kinematics of human motion.* Champaign, IL.: Human Kinetics.

Laboratory Experiences

1. Define the following key terms:

Linear motion	Velocity
Angular or rotary motion	Acceleration
Distance	Gravity
Speed	Projectile
Displacement	

2. Choose one of the following activities:
   Running long jump
   Basketball jump shot
   Softball pitching
   Identify the critical linear and angular kinematic elements of the selected skill. Explain how each of these elements contributes to successful performance.
3. An Olympic skater who participated in the men's speed-skating events had the following times: 1,500 m in 2 min 2.96 sec; 5,000 m in 7 min 23.61 sec; and 10,000 m in 15 min 1.35 sec. What was his average speed for each of these events?
4. Using the concept of acceleration, explain how a swimmer can have a better time for a 100-m race in a 25-m pool than in a 100-m pool.
5. How much time will a batter have to decide to swing at a pitch and still hit it under these circumstances?
   a. The pitcher throws the ball at 80 mph.
   b. The distance from the ball release to the plate is 56 ft.
   c. It takes the batter 0.30 sec to get the bat to the desired contact point.
6. With the help of several classmates, prepare a displacement–time graph and a velocity–time graph for your performance on two 50-m dash efforts: one in which you run through the end, and one in which you stop right at 50 m. Class members should be spaced at 5-m intervals along your running path, each with a stopwatch. On the signal for you to go, each timer will start the watch and stop it when you pass that timer's position. Prepare a table with the following data for each run:
   a. Distance intervals
   b. Times recorded at each interval
   c. Times over each 5-m interval (subtract adjacent times)
   d. Average velocity over each 5-m interval
   For each set of data, prepare a displacement–time graph and a velocity–time graph for the whole run. Describe your run in terms of displacement, velocity, and acceleration. Compare your graphs to those of other groups and note any differences.
7. An arrow shot straight up into the air reached a height of 75 m. With what velocity did it leave the bow? How long was the arrow in the air?
8. Place one coin near the edge of a table and another on the end of a ruler (as shown in Figure 11.20). While pressing the center of the ruler to the table with an index finger, strike one end of it in the direction indicated so that both coins land on the ground. Diagram the path of each. Which hits the floor first? Explain.
9. Throw a ball so that it is projected vertically upward. Catch it at the same height it was released. Have a partner measure the time the ball is in the air—that is, from the time of release to the time the ball lands in your hand.

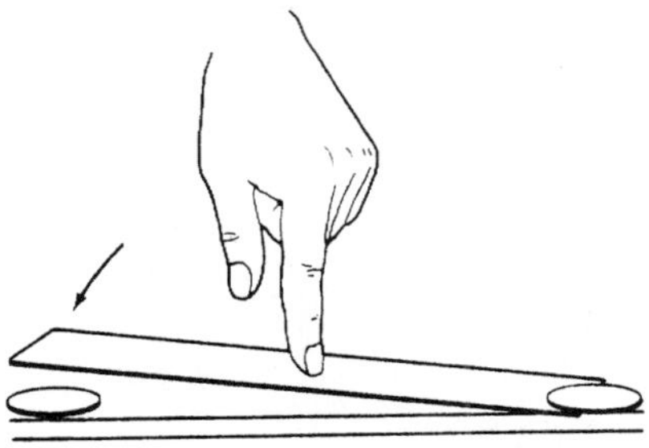

Figure 11.20

Determine the velocity of the ball at the moment of release and the distance the ball traveled before it started its descent. Graph the flight of the ball on a piece of graph paper. Break the flight of the ball into five sections: (1) from initiation of upward motion of the hand to just prior to release, (2) from moment of release to just before maximum height, (3) at maximum height, (4) from maximum height to just before you catch the ball, (5) from the ball contact to the ball being brought to rest. For each section, describe the displacement, velocity, and acceleration.

10. While walking along at a constant speed, project a ball vertically into the air. If you continue to walk without changing your speed or direction, where will the ball land? Explain. Draw a diagram of the ball's flight, indicating the forces acting on it.
11. Assume that you are able to throw a ball with a velocity of 24 m/sec and at an angle of 45 degrees with the horizontal. If it is caught at the same height from the ground at which it was released, neglecting air resistance, how far will it go? How long will it be in flight? Repeat with a 30-degree angle of release. How would these values change if the landing height were lowered?
12. Using Figure 11.3, determine the angular velocity of the lower leg at the knee joint at the beginning of the force phase and at the moment of foot contact with the ball. The time between each stick-figure tracing is 0.0156 sec. What is the linear velocity at the ankle at the moment of contact if the lower leg is 35 cm (knee joint to ankle joint)?

CHAPTER

12

THE CONDITIONS OF LINEAR MOTION

OUTLINE

- ***The Nature of Force***
  - Aspects of Force
  - Resolution of Forces
  - Composite Effects of Two or More Forces
- ***Newton's Laws of Motion***
  - Law of Inertia
  - Law of Acceleration
  - Law of Reaction
- ***Forces that Modify Motion***
  - Weight
  - Contact Forces
  - Elasticity and Rebound
  - Fluid Forces
- ***Free-Body Diagrams***
- ***Work, Power, and Energy***
  - Work
  - Energy
- ***The Analysis of Linear Motion***
- ***Laboratory Experiences***

OBJECTIVES

At the conclusion of this chapter, the student should be able to:

1. Name, define, and use the following terms properly as they apply to linear motion: *force, inertia, mass, weight, momentum,* and *impulse.*
2. Explain what is meant by the terms *magnitude, direction,* and *point of application of force,* and use these terms properly as they apply to internal and external forces.
3. Explain the effect of specified changes in the magnitude, direction, and point of application of force on the motion state of a body.
4. Define and give examples of the terms *linear forces, concurrent forces,* and *parallel forces.*
5. Determine the magnitude, direction, and point of application of muscle forces in hypothetical situations in which specific muscles are considered in isolation.
6. State Newton's laws as they apply to linear motion.
7. Explain the cause-and-effect relationship between the forces responsible for linear motion and the objects experiencing the motion.
8. Name and define the basic external forces responsible for modifying motion: weight, normal reaction, friction, elasticity, buoyancy, drag, and lift.
9. Draw and analyze simple two-dimensional free-body diagrams in which all applicable external forces are properly accounted for.
10. Explain the work–energy relationship as it applies to a body experiencing linear motion.
11. Define and use properly the terms *work, power, kinetic energy,* and *potential energy.*
12. Using the concepts that govern linear motion, perform a mechanical analysis of a selected motor skill.

THE NATURE OF FORCE

Objects start moving when they are pushed or pulled, that is, when some type of force acts on them. Forces produce motion, stop motion, and prevent motion. They may increase speed, decrease speed, or cause objects to change direction. They may push or pull to cause motion or produce a net effect so that bodies remain stationary. *Force is defined as that which pushes or pulls through direct mechanical contact or through the force of gravity to alter the motion of an object.* It is the effect that one body has on another. The identification of forces that act to produce motion of the body or of an object is an important element of a kinesiological analysis.

The action of a force may be internal or external. Internal forces are defined as forces exerted by bodies on other bodies within a defined system, whereas external forces are those exerted by bodies within an arbitrarily specified system on bodies outside the specified system. Internal forces cause differences in body shape, and external forces cause displacement of the body. In kinesiology, the system under consideration is the human body. Internal forces are therefore usually classified as muscle forces that act on the various structures of the body, and external forces are those outside the body. The best-known external force is weight, or gravitational force. Wind or water resistance forces, friction, or forces due to other objects acting on the body are also external forces.

Aspects of Force

Force is a vector quantity. Force possesses both magnitude and direction, as do all vector quantities. Force also has an exact point of application on the object. To describe a force fully, all three of these characteristics must be identified and taken into account. A change in any one of them alters the nature of the motion. Applying a force of insufficient magnitude, for instance, might produce no motion. A weight lifter trying to lift a 250-N barbell with 150 N of force would be unsuccessful. If the force applied by the weight lifter were increased to 260 N, the barbell would move if the force were applied in the proper direction and at the proper point of application. If the direction of the force is downward, the barbell will not be lifted upward. If the force is applied to only one end of the barbell, the bar will rotate rather than move upward in a linear manner. To successfully lift the 250-N barbell, the lifter must apply a force greater than 250 N in an *upward direction,* through the center of gravity of the barbell.

Magnitude, direction, and point of application as they relate to both external and internal forces are explained in the following sections.

Magnitude

The amount or size of the force that is being applied makes up the magnitude of the force vector. The basic unit of force in the U.S. system is the pound, and in the metric system it is the newton. In the weight-lifting example just used, the magnitude of the muscle force used in the first unsuccessful attempt was 150 N. The force being exerted by the barbell had a magnitude of 250 N. This 250-N force was the result of the pull of gravity acting on the mass of the barbell. This force is commonly referred to as weight. Weight can be expressed as mass times the acceleration due to gravity, or

$$w = mg$$

When one holds a ball in the hand, the pull of gravity is felt as the weight of the ball. The ball stays in the hand as long as an equal and opposite force acting between the hand and the ball balances the downward gravitational force. In this example, the equal and opposite force is muscular. When the opposing force is removed, the ball drops and gravity's pull is apparent in the downward motion of the ball. The weight of the ball is the magnitude of the force of gravity acting on the ball.

The magnitude of muscular force is in direct proportion to the number and size of the fibers in the muscle that is contracting. If muscles contracted individually, it would be a relatively easy matter to measure the force exerted by each one in a given movement. Because they normally act in groups, however, their force or strength is measured collectively. It is customary to measure maximum muscular strength by performing a simple movement against the resistance of a dynamometer or similar instrument. The instrument thus serves as the resistance to an anatomical lever whose force is provided by a group of muscles that act as a functional team to produce the movement of the lever. Among the muscle groups that are frequently measured by this method are the finger flexors (grip strength), elbow flexors, and knee extensors.

The magnitudes of external forces other than gravity depend on other factors. Most of these external forces will be discussed in more detail later in this text.

Point of Application

The point of application of a force is that point at which the force is applied to an object. Where gravity is concerned, this point is always through the center of gravity of an object. For practical purposes, it may be assumed that the point of application of muscular force is the center of the muscle's attachment to the bony lever. This usually corresponds to the muscle's insertion or distal attachment. Technically, however, it is the point of intersection between the line of force and the mechanical axis of the bone or segment serving as the anatomical lever. This axis does not necessarily pass lengthwise through the shaft of the bony lever. If the bone bends or if the articulating process projects at an angle from the shaft, the greater part of the axis may lie completely outside the shaft, as in the case of the femur (see Figure 2.3). *The mechanical axis of a bone or segment is a straight line that connects the midpoint of the joint at one end with the midpoint of the joint at the other end or, in the case of a terminal segment, with its distal end.*

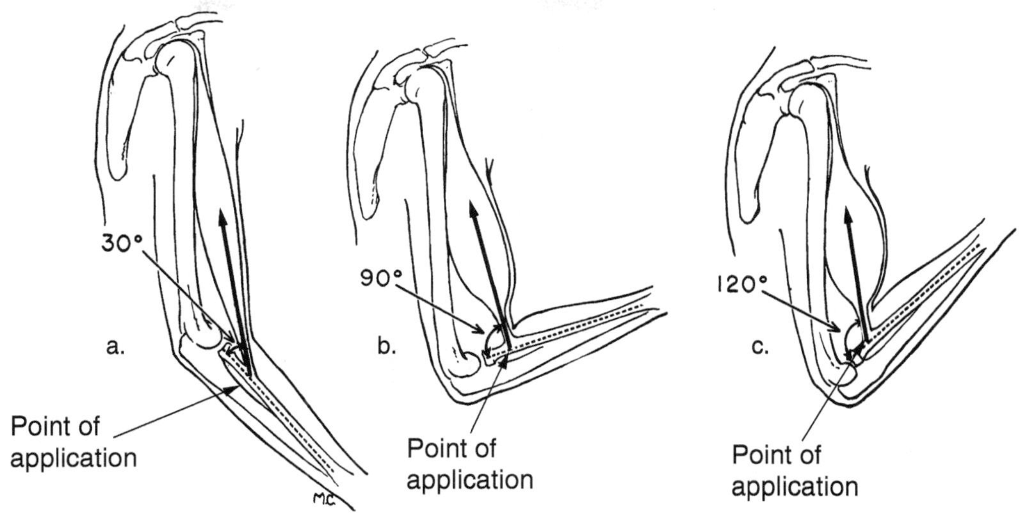

Figure 12.1 Angles of muscle pull: (a) an angle less than 45 degrees; (b) an angle of 90 degrees; (c) an angle greater than 90 degrees.

Direction

The direction of a force is along its action line. Because the force of gravity pulls all objects toward the earth's center, the direction of gravitational forces is vertically downward. The force of gravity acting on an object would be represented as a downward-directed vector starting at the center of gravity of the object.

The direction of a muscular force vector is in the direction of the muscle line of pull. This direction is identified by the muscle angle of pull, which is defined as the angle between the line of pull and that portion of the mechanical axis of bone that lies between the point of application of the muscle force and the joint, which acts as the fulcrum (Figure 12.1).

Resolution of Forces

Because force has the qualities of both magnitude and direction, it is a vector quantity. Graphically, the magnitude of the force is represented by the length of the vector line. The point of application of the force is the point where the force vector starts. The vector line represents the line of force, and the arrowhead indicates the direction of the force application (Figure 12.2).

Angle of Pull

As with any vector, a force may be resolved into a vertical and a horizontal component, and the relative size of these component vectors depends on the angle at which the force is applied. Where muscles are involved, the size of a muscle's angle of pull changes with every degree of joint motion, and consequently so do the sizes of the x and y components. The x- and y-axes refer to a local reference frame, in which the x-axis is always the mechanical axis of the bone. These changes have a direct bearing on the effectiveness of the muscle's pulling force in moving the bony lever. The larger the angle between 0 degrees and 90 degrees, the greater the y component and the less the x component (see Figure 12.1).

The component along the y-axis of the muscle is always perpendicular to the lever and is called the rotary component. It is that part of the force that moves the lever. The component along the x-axis is parallel to the lever and is the nonrotary (stabilizing) component. It does not contribute to the lever's movement. The angle of pull of most muscles in the resting position is less than a right angle, and it usually remains so throughout the movement (see Figure 12.1a). This means that the

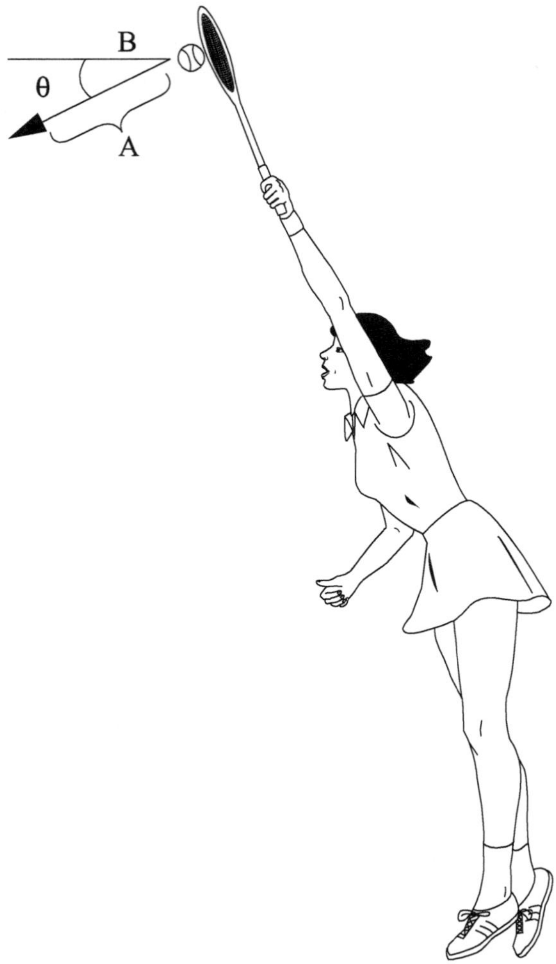

Figure 12.2 Graphic representation of a force vector. The magnitude of the force is the vector line, A; the point of application is the beginning of the vector, B; and the direction of the vector is represented by the arrowhead and the angle θ.

nonrotary component of force is directed toward the fulcrum, which gives it a stabilizing effect. By pulling the bone lengthwise toward the joint, it helps maintain the integrity of the joint. Under most circumstances, therefore, muscular force has two simultaneous functions—movement and stabilization. In the latter capacity it supplements the ligaments, an excellent example of the body's efficiency because muscles perform this stabilizing function only during the period when the segment is moving, at which time the integrity of the joint may be threatened.

Occasionally the angle of pull becomes greater than a right angle, which means that the nonrotary component of force is directed away from the fulcrum and is therefore a dislocating component. This does not happen in many instances, however, when it does, the muscle is close to the limit of its shortening range and is therefore not exerting much force (see Figure 12.1c).

When the angle of pull is 90 degrees, the force is completely rotary. When it is 45 degrees the rotary and stabilizing (nonrotary) components are equal. Because the angle of pull usually remains less than 45 degrees, more of the muscle's force serves to stabilize the joint than to move the lever. In fact, there are some muscles whose angles of pull are always so small that their contributions to motion would seem to be negligible. This appears to be true of the coracobrachialis and the subclavius muscles. It is interesting to note that the upper extremity is frequently called upon to perform violent, powerful movements, as well as to support the body weight in suspension. The joints that bear the brunt of this violence and strain are the shoulder and sternoclavicular joints. They might well become dislocated more easily than they do, were it not for the coracobrachialis and the subclavius muscles, which pull the bones lengthwise toward their proximal joints and thus serve to stabilize these joints.

The effect the angle of pull has upon the rotary force of a muscle for a given angle is demonstrated in the following problem. The solution clearly shows an increase in rotary force with each increase in angle size.

Example

Muscle *M* exerts a force of 100 N at insertion and is pulling at an angle of 30 degrees. How much of its force is rotary? Stabilizing? How do these values change when the angle of pull is 10 degrees? 75 degrees? (See Figure 12.3.)

Solution

Angle of pull of 30°:

Construct a right triangle where $\sin 30° = \frac{A}{100}$.

Rotary component equals $100 \times \sin 30° = 50$ N.
Stabilizing component equals $100 \times \cos 30° = 86.6$ N.

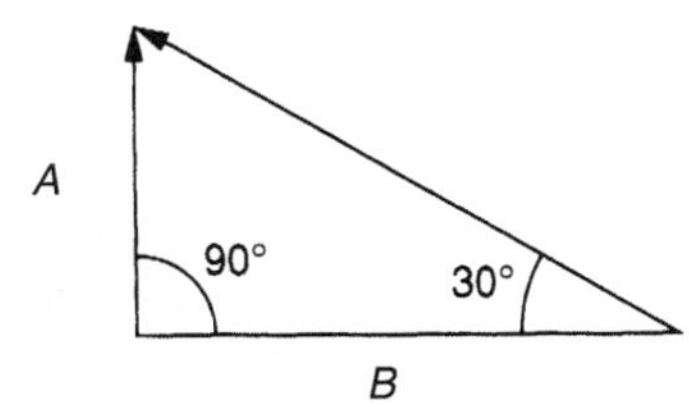

Angle of pull of 10°:

Construct a right triangle where $\sin 10° = \frac{A}{100}$.

Rotary component *A* equals $100 \times \sin 10° = 17.36$ N.
Stabilizing component *B* equals $100 \times \cos 10° = 98.48$ N.

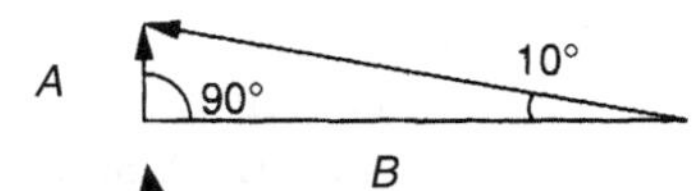

Angle of pull of 75°:

Construct a right triangle where $\sin 75° = \frac{A}{100}$.

Rotary component equals $100 \times \sin 75° = 96.59$ N.
Stabilizing component equals $100 \times \cos 75° = 25.88$ N.

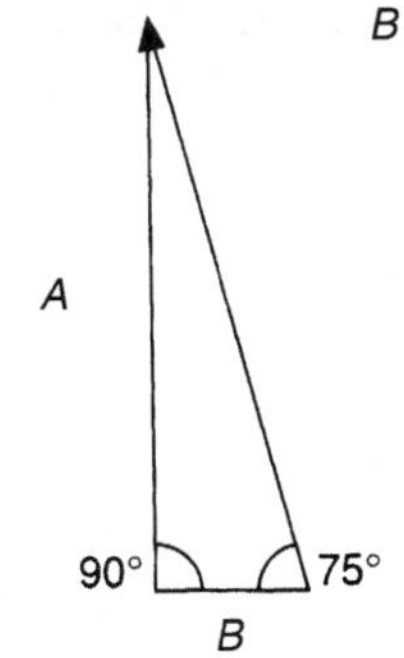

Anatomical Pulley

The small angle of pull that most muscles have when in their normal resting position has already been noted. Were it not for anatomical devices that serve as fixed single pulleys, some muscles would probably be unable to effect any movement whatsoever. The anatomical pulley serves the same purpose as the mechanical fixed single pulley, that of changing the direction of force by changing the angle of pull of the muscle providing the force.

An anatomical pulley can alter the way a muscle acts on a joint in a number of ways. First,

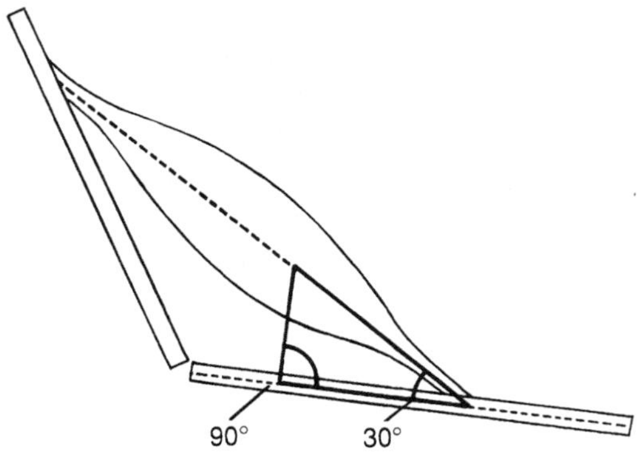

Figure 12.3 Method of constructing a right triangle for the purpose of determining the components of muscular force by the trigonometric method. Note that the hypotenuse coincides with a portion of the muscle's line of pull, and the side adjacent coincides with the mechanical axis of the bone into which the muscle is inserted.

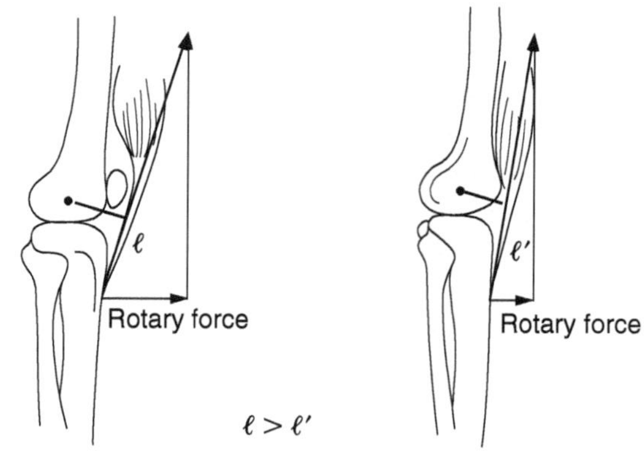

Figure 12.4 By increasing the angle of pull, the patella increases the rotary force component of the quadriceps femoris. *Source:* From *Biomechanics of Human Motion,* by M. Williams & H. R. Lissner. Copyright © 1962, W. B. Saunders, Orlando, FL. Reprinted by permission.

a pulley may act to improve the muscle angle of pull and increase the rotary component, such as the way in which the patella moves the quadriceps tendon away from the knee joint (Figure 12.4). Another example of this might be the condyles of the femur and tibia, effectively pushing the gracilis away from the joint (Figure 12.5). Second, a pulley may change the direction of the muscle action. A good example would be the peroneus longus, passing behind the lateral malleolus before it turns under the foot (Figure 12.6). If the peroneus longus did not do this, it would produce dorsiflexion. Another configuration with a pulley action is the pronator teres, which rotates the radius over the ulna. Tendons and ligaments may also act as pulleys. A good example of this is the pulley action of the finger and thumb flexor sheaths.

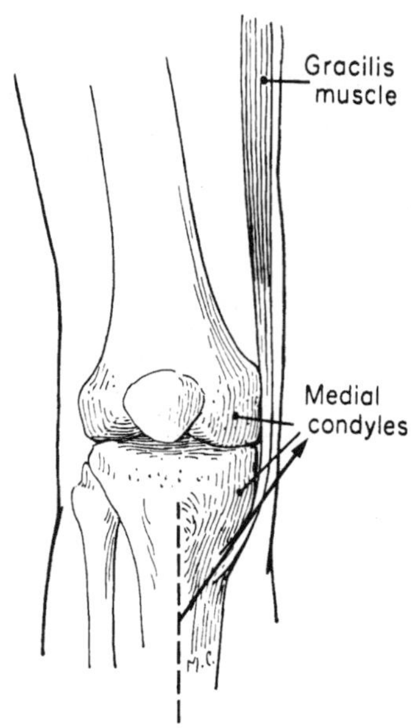

Figure 12.5 The medial condyles at the knee joint serving as a pulley to increase the angle of pull of the gracilis tendon.

Resolution of External Force

The resolution of a single external force vector into component force vectors acting at right angles to each other is accomplished in the same manner as that explained for muscular forces and would be used when the force is applied at an oblique angle. If, instead of giving a piece of furniture a horizontal push, one pushes it by standing close to it with the arms held at a forward-downward slant, only part of the force will push the table forward (Figure 12.7). The force is applied to the

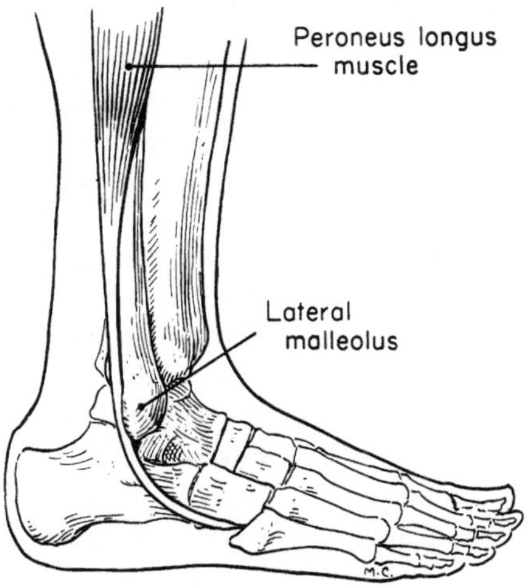

Figure 12.6 The lateral malleolus serving as a pulley for the peroneus longus tendon.

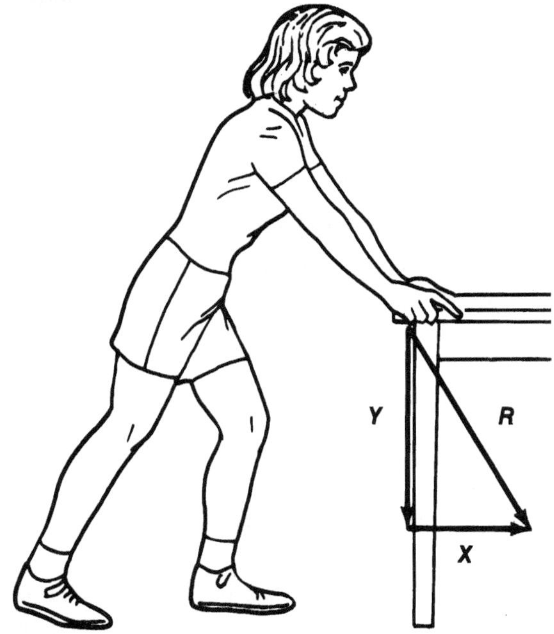

Figure 12.7 The diagonal pushing force (*R*) consists of a horizontal and a vertical component. Only the horizontal component (*X*) serves to overcome the table's resistance to being moved. The vertical component (*Y*) adds to the resistance.

table at an oblique angle and thus has both a vertical and a horizontal component. Whether or not the table moves forward depends on the amount of the total force applied in the horizontal direction. If sufficient, only the horizontal component of force will overcome the table's resistance to move. The downward component merely pushes the table against the floor and increases the friction between the floor and the table. The closer one can come to applying all the available force in the desired direction of movement, the more efficient will be the action. Another example of this principle is demonstrated in pulling actions. If a child's sled or wagon is drawn by too short a rope, there will be a relatively large lifting component and a small forward pulling component. Because the purpose is to pull the wagon horizontally, it is more efficient to use a long rope because this gives a relatively greater horizontal or pulling component.

Composite Effects of Two or More Forces

Frequently, two or more forces are applied to the same object. A canoe may be acted on by both the wind and the paddler. One force tends to send the canoe north and the other east. While in flight a punted ball's path is the result of the force imparted to it by the kicker, the downward force of gravity, and the force of the wind, if any. In the body it is rarely, if ever, the case that an individual muscle acts by itself. For example, at least four muscles may act in flexion of the forearm, and more than five contribute to flexion of the leg at the knee joint. The effect that composite forces have on the human body to cause or modify motion may be classified according to their direction and application as linear, concurrent, or parallel.

Linear Forces

Forces applied in the same direction along the same action line are called linear forces. If a horizontal push is applied to a piece of furniture and the push is applied in line with the object's center of gravity, the object will move forward in a horizontal direction, if, of course, there is no additional conflicting force or resistance. If another force is applied to the furniture in line with and in the same direction as the first force, the resultant of the two forces has a value equal to the sum of the two forces ($a + b = c$).

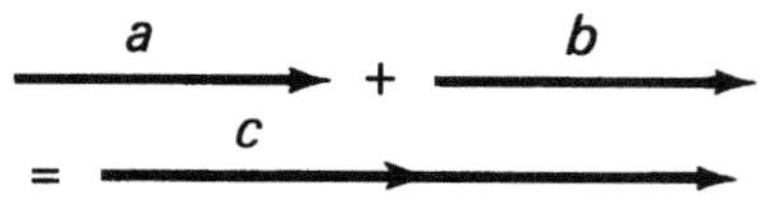

Similarly, if the forces act in opposite directions, the resultant still equals the algebraic sum of the two forces ($a + (-b) = c$). This might be the case in a tug-of-war.

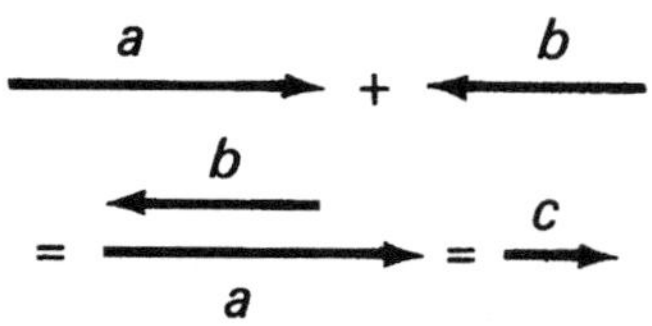

Examples of more than one force applied at the same point and acting in identical directions in the body are rare. Possibly there are two such examples: the gastrocnemius and the soleus acting at the ankle joint, and the psoas and the iliacus acting at the hip joint. In each of these examples, the two muscles have a common tendon for their distal attachments.

Concurrent Forces

Forces acting at the same point of application but at different angles are called concurrent forces. Several football players opposing each other in a blocking situation furnish opposing forces that may be considered as acting at one point (Figure 12.8). The resultant outcome of the blocking is found using the method known as the combination of vectors described in Chapter 10. This method assumes a common point of application. Although this situation is common externally, it is not true of the majority of muscles that act on the same bone. Very few muscles have a common point of attachment. Nevertheless, the principle of finding the composite effect of two or more forces, with respect to magnitude and direction, is as true for forces acting on body segments as for forces acting on external objects. The important thing to remember is that the resultant magnitude of two or more concurrent forces is not their arithmetic sum, and the resultant direction of two concurrent forces is not halfway between them unless the two forces are of equal magnitude. The *resultant of two or more concurrent forces depends on both the magnitude of each force and the angle of application*—that is, the direction of each force.

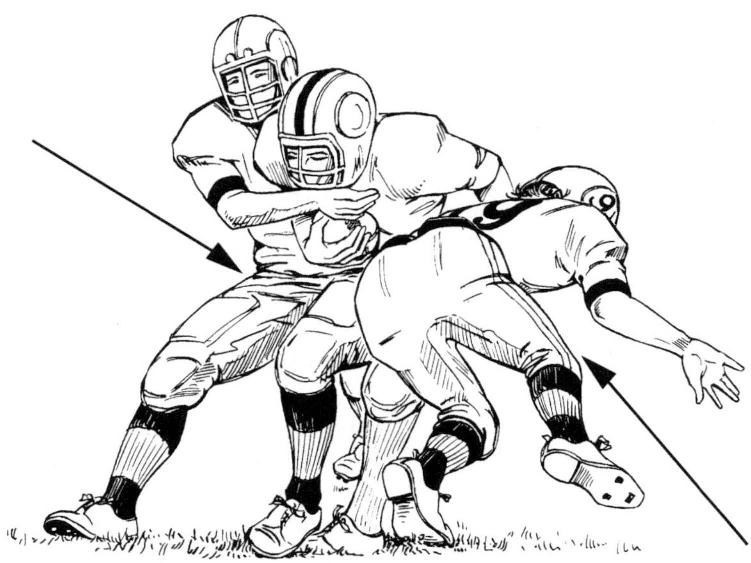

Figure 12.8 Opposing forces acting at one point but at different angles are called concurrent forces.

The techniques of vector resolution and combination must be used when doing force calculations.

Parallel Forces

In addition to linear forces, in which all forces occur along the same action line, and concurrent forces, in which forces acting at different angles are applied at the same point, another situation exists in which forces not in the same action line but *parallel* to each other act at different points on a body. An example of this is holding a 10-N weight in the hand when the forearm is flexed so that the angle of pull of the biceps is 90 degrees. The force of gravity may be represented as acting at two different points to push the forearm and the weight down while the force of the biceps acting in the opposite direction at another point pulls the forearm up (Figure 12.9).

The effect parallel forces have on the object they act on depends on the magnitude, direction, and application point of each force.

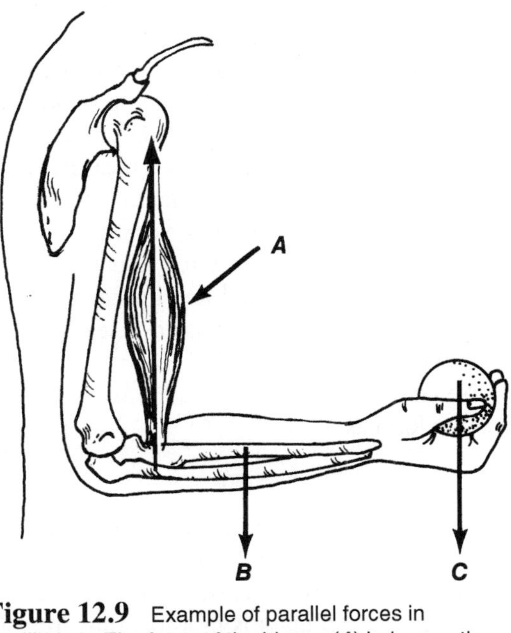

Figure 12.9 Example of parallel forces in equilibrium. The force of the biceps (*A*) balances the opposite force of gravity acting on the forearm at its center of gravity (*B*) and on the weight held in the hand?(*C*).

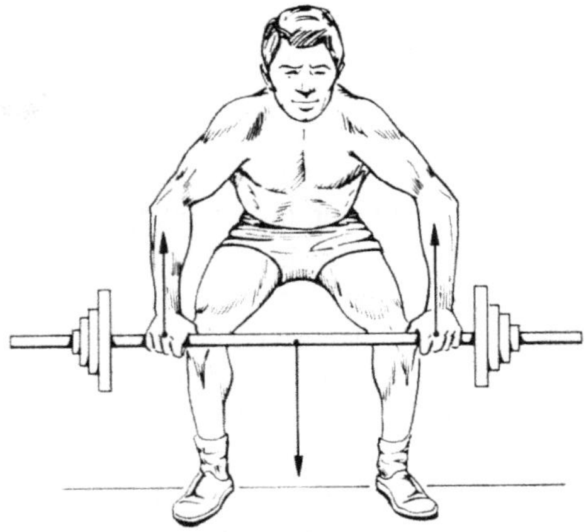

Figure 12.10 Example of parallel forces producing linear motion.

Parallel forces may act in the same or opposite directions. They may be balanced and cause no motion, or they may cause linear or rotary motion. When parallel forces act on an object, their relationship to the object's fixed axis or to its center of gravity, if it can move freely, determines the resultant action. Another example of parallel forces is shown in Figure 12.10.

NEWTON'S LAWS OF MOTION

The fact that motion is related to force in a precise manner was observed by Sir Isaac Newton in the seventeenth century. He formulated three laws of motion that explain why objects move as they do. Although all of these laws cannot be proved on earth, even in ideal experimental situations, they are accepted as universal truths to explain the effects of force.

Law of Inertia

Newton's first law of motion states that **a body continues in its state of rest or of uniform motion unless an unbalanced force acts on it**. This Law of Inertia means that an object at rest remains at rest, and one in motion will continue at a constant speed in a straight line unless acted on by a force. In effect, the law identifies the conditions under which there is no external force. The fact that objects at rest need a force to move them seems obvious, but the need for force to slow or stop an object in motion is not always as apparent. We have all seen moving objects come to rest of their own accord, or what seems to be their own accord, but, in fact, other forces in the form of friction or air resistance caused the change in velocity. The tendency for a body to stay in motion for long periods of time is possible to observe more clearly in laboratory conditions where the effects of friction and air resistance can be minimized. Nevertheless, numerous examples of Newton's first law can still be observed in sport and everyday experiences. Base runners in baseball know that it takes force to change velocity suddenly to avoid overrunning a base. Skiers continue into space if they traverse a hill or mogul at high speed (Figure 12.11). And nearly everyone at some time or another has experienced the frightening situation of continuing to move forward when the vehicle in which one is riding stops suddenly.

The property of an object that causes it to remain in its state of either rest or motion is called *inertia*. Because of inertia, force is needed to change the velocity of an object. The amount of force needed to alter the object's velocity is directly related to the amount of inertia it has. The measure of inertia in a body is its mass, that is, the quantity of matter it possesses. The greater the mass of an object, the greater its inertia. A bowling ball obviously has greater inertia than does a volleyball. A tennis racquet has greater inertia than a badminton racquet, and a textbook more than a magazine.

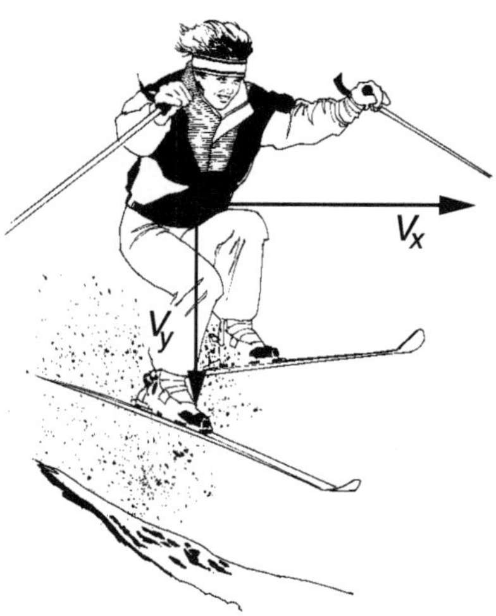

Figure 12.11 An example of Newton's first law of motion.

Law of Acceleration

Newton's second law of motion, the Law of Acceleration, concerns acceleration and momentum, and it tells how the quantities of force, mass, and acceleration are related and how to measure force when it exists. The law states that **the acceleration of an object is directly proportional to the force causing it, is in the same direction as the force, and is inversely proportional to the mass of the object.** It is quite easy to show that change in velocity (acceleration) of an object is proportional to the force and in the direction of the force. The velocity of a pitched ball reflects the force with which it is thrown, and it moves in the direction of the line of force at the moment of release. Similarly, it takes less braking force to stop a baseball moving at 5 meters per second than it does to stop a pitch of 50 meters per second. In both instances, the change in velocity is directly proportional to the amount of force and is in the direction of the force. The mass of the ball is a measure of its inertia, and the greater the inertia, the more force it takes to change the object's velocity. Thus, a bowling ball requires more force to put it in motion than a playground ball, and the same is true for stopping it. Acceleration is inversely proportional to mass.

Newton's second law may be expressed in equation form as

$$F = ma$$

For this to be possible, the force unit is the pound when acceleration is in feet/second/second and mass is in slugs. When acceleration is in meters/second/second and mass is in kilograms, force is expressed in newtons.

With this equation it is possible to determine the force needed to produce a given linear acceleration of a body if the weight of the body is known. Because we know that $m = \frac{w}{g}$ the equation for force, $F = ma$, can be written as $F = \frac{w}{g} \times a$, the force needed to accelerate a 300-N object 2 m/sec² is 61 N, or

$$\left(\frac{300}{9.8 \text{ m/sec}^2} \times 2 \text{ m/sec}^2\right)$$

Impulse

The Law of Acceleration dictates that when sufficient force is applied to a mass, an acceleration will occur according to the equation

$$F = ma$$

Because acceleration is the rate of change in velocity, this equation can be rewritten as

$$F = \frac{m(v_f - v_i)}{t}$$

substituting for $\frac{v_f}{t} - \frac{v_i}{t}$ for a. Multiplying both sides by time produces a new equation:

$$Ft = m(v_f - v_i)$$

In other words, the product of a force and the time over which this force acts will produce a change in the velocity of the mass. This product of force and time is called *impulse*. From the impulse equation, $Ft = m(v_f - v_i)$, it should be apparent that the force required to produce a given change of velocity in a given time period is proportional to the mass. It is also easy to see that as any change in velocity of an object of a given mass increases, so must the impulse increase proportionately. Conversely, if either force or time is increased, the velocity of the mass must also increase. Doubling either the force or the time over which a force is applied will double the velocity change.

The importance of creating as large an impulse as possible is evident in the skillful execution of many sports techniques. A baseball pitcher uses a form that allows the longest time over which to apply the force to the ball before releasing it. This same long windup is seen in the technique used by hammer throwers, discus throwers, and shot-putters. In each instance, the performer accelerates the object to be thrown as much as possible by generating as much force as strength permits and by using body segment adjustments that increase the time over which the force can be applied (Figure 12.12).

Consider a pitcher throwing a 5-oz (0.142-kg), 90-mph baseball (40 m/s). If we know that the

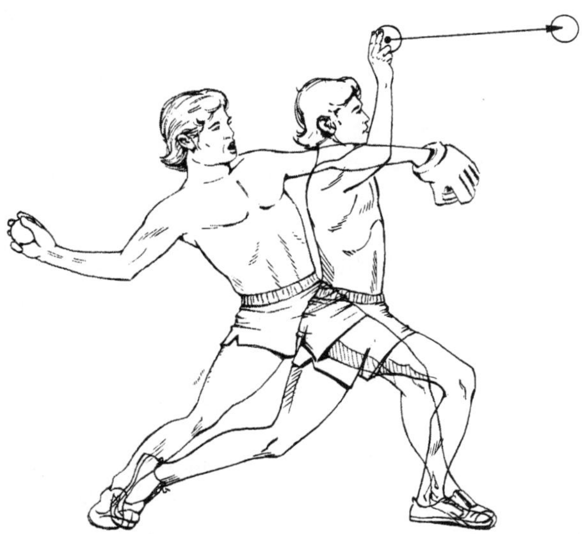

Figure 12.12 Example of impulse generation.

time of the forward motion of a throw is approximately 0.03 seconds, then using the impulse momentum relationship, the force required to bring about the change in velocity from 0 m/s (at the beginning of the forward motion) to 40 m/s at ball release can be determined.

$$Ft = m(v_f - v_i)$$

$$F(0.03s) = (0.142kg)(40^m/_s - 0^m/_s)$$

$$F = \frac{(0.1442kg)(40)^m/_s}{0.03s}$$

$$F = 192.26 \text{ N}$$

To change the velocity of a baseball from rest to 40 m/s takes a force of 192.26 N (44.12 lbs).

Next, consider taking part in an egg-toss game. When watching this activity, it is easy to see how the catchers are using the impulse momentum relationship to catch the egg without breaking it. In this situation, the catcher wants to increase the time over which the force is being exerted to diminish the amount of force being applied. To increase the amount of time over which the force is being exerted, the catcher will "give" with egg.

$$Ft = m(v_f - v_i)$$

The right side of the equation will remain the same, and the velocity of the egg will be reduced to zero. The catcher can control only the left side of the equation. The egg can be brought to rest quickly (a small time and a large force), or it can be brought to rest over a longer time period (longer time and smaller force).

The impulse relationship also shows that force cannot be generated to cause a change in velocity unless time is available over which the force is applied. This helps explain the value of the follow-through in throwing, kicking, and striking movements. Although the follow-through does not affect the flight of the object once the object has left the throwing or striking implement, it does help ensure that the missile will stay in contact with the implement that is imparting force to it for as long as possible. The ball is actually carried along by the foot, golf club, or tennis racquet, and the longer the time the force of the implement can be applied to the ball, the greater will be the change in velocity in the ball.

Momentum

The impulse equation is also written as

$$Ft = mv_f - mv_i$$

The product of mass and velocity (mv_i or mv_f) is *momentum,* and any change in momentum is equal to the impulse that produces it. Momentum is a quantity of motion that may be increased or decreased by increasing or decreasing either the mass or the velocity. The shot-putter who is able to push the shot with a greater speed than the opponent will cause the shot to have greater momentum at the moment of release. And, even though the mass is less, a small child may topple an adult if the child's faster speed is sufficient to produce a larger momentum than the person the child collides with. Similarly, heavier bowling balls released with the same speed as lighter balls have greater momentum, and a heavier tennis racquet will strike a tennis ball with greater momentum and cause a greater change in momentum in the tennis ball than will a lighter racquet.

An increase in momentum occurs when the force is applied in the direction of the motion. Force applied in the opposite direction produces a slowing down or decrease in momentum. This is what happens when one catches a fast ball or lands from a jump or a fall. In both instances relatively large momentums are reduced to zero, and large impulses occur. The momentum of the ball is large because of its large velocity, and the momentum of the person falling is great because of a large mass. Looking again at the impulse equation, $Ft = mv_f - mv_i$, it can be seen that a short stopping time will require a larger stopping force and that an increase in stopping time will reduce the amount of stopping force needed to change the momentum of the object to zero. This is why it is necessary to increase the stopping time by "giving" when catching the ball or when landing from a jump or fall. Without the "give" the impulse will not be enough, the momentum will not decrease to zero, and the ball will not be caught, or the momentum will reach zero but the force will be so great that injury in the form of damaged bones, joints, and soft tissue may result. A 20-N force falling for 5 seconds has the same impulse as a 100-N force falling for 1 second.

Law of Reaction

Newton's third law of motion considers the way forces act against each other. A book lying on a table (Figure 12.13) exerts a downward force on the table, and because the book is stationary, another equal and opposite force must be acting on the book. Newton's first law states that unbalanced forces produce motion. Because we have no motion here, we must have a balanced force system. The downward force of the book on the table is balanced by an upward force of the table on the book. The same is true when a person walks across a floor. The feet push back against the floor with the same magnitude as the floor pushes forward against the feet. Without the forward push of the floor against the feet, forward progress would not be possible. Notice how the front part of the foot in the footprint in Figure 12.14 makes a deeper impression than the heel. To accelerate forward, the walker has to push backward. For this reason, runners push against starting blocks at the beginning of a race so that a strong forward reaction push can be received from the blocks. In each of these instances, forces of equal magnitude are exerted in opposite directions. One force is called the action force and the other is the reaction force.

Newton's Law of Reaction states that **for every action, there is an equal and opposite reaction.** Whenever one body exerts a force on a second body, the second body exerts an equal and opposite force on the first.

In locomotion on the surface of the earth (ground or floor), this reaction force is referred to as *ground reaction force*. The ground reaction force vector is equal in magnitude and opposite in direction to the force vector that is being applied to the ground. In walking, as the foot pushes down and back against the ground, the ground pushes up and forward against the foot. Again, notice how the front part of the footprint in Figure 12.14 makes a deeper impression in the front than the heel does in the back. Notice also

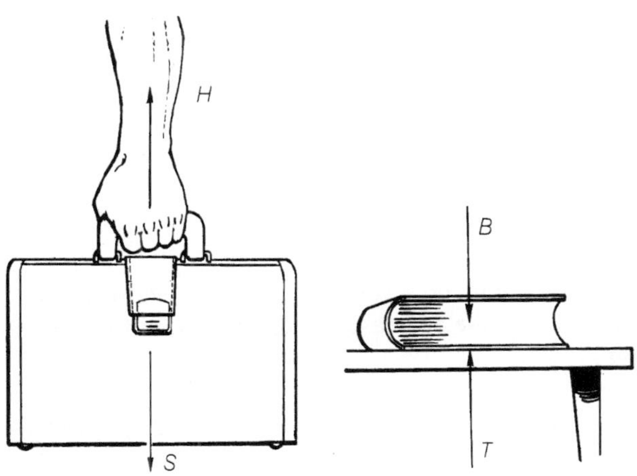

Figure 12.13 Equal and opposite reactions: $H = S$ (forces of hand and bag) and $B = T$ (book and table).
Source: From *Biomechanics of Human Motion,* by M. Williams & H. R. Lissner. Copyright © 1962, W. B. Saunders, Orlando, FL. Reprinted by permission.

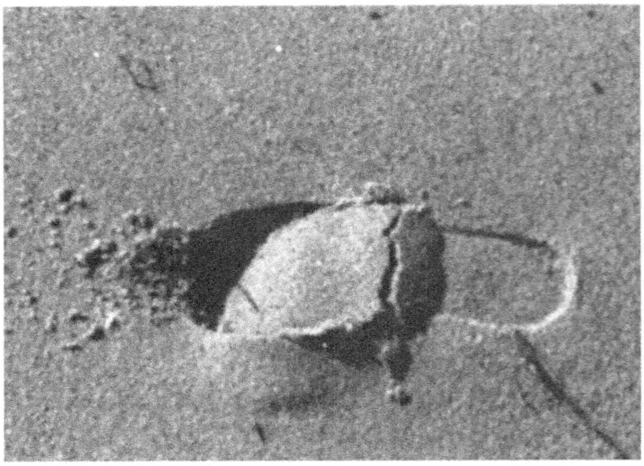

Figure 12.14 To accelerate forward, a walker must push backward. Notice how the front part of the footprint in the sand is more deeply depressed than the rear.

how the sand had to be compressed by the walker before it was solid enough to produce an equal and opposite reaction. This is one reason that walking on soft sand or snow is more difficult than walking on a firm surface.

Although ground reaction force is necessary for locomotion, such forces do place stress on the body. It sometimes becomes necessary to minimize ground reaction force to prevent injury. A pole vaulter, for example, uses ground reaction force in the run and the takeoff but needs to minimize the ground reaction force at landing. The use of a landing pit or crash pad allows the vaulter to alter momentum by increasing the time over which velocity is reduced. In the impulse equation, $Ft = m(v_f - v_i)$, if time (t) is increased, force (F) must decrease. A decrease in the force component of impulse is a decrease in the action force. With the Law of Reaction, a decrease in the action force will produce an equal and opposite decrease in the ground reaction force.

Action and reaction show up in countless other ways when objects are in motion. When a boat is rowed, the oars exert a force against the water and the water pushes against the oars with an equal and opposite reaction, causing the boat to be pushed forward as the force is transferred from the oar to the boat through the oarlock. The force of a volleyball can be felt pushing back against the hand as it is served with a forward force. A similar force is observed when a gun is shot or an arrow is released from a bow. The recoil of the gun or bow is due to the reaction force of the bullet or arrow to the action force of the gun or bow.

Conservation of Momentum

When an object is set in motion by a force, the momentum (mv) of the object is changed. Because the force that causes this change in momentum must have an equal and opposite force, another equal and opposite momentum change must occur in the object producing the reactive force. The time the objects are in contact with each other would also be equal, and therefore the impulses (Ft) would be equal. This means that $m_1v_{1f} - m_1v_{1i} = m_2v_{2f} - m_2v_{2i}$. This principle is summarized in the Law of Conservation of Momentum, which states that **in any system where forces act on each other, the momentum is constant.** Thus, if an impact or action between objects occurs, the momentums before impact must equal the momentums after the impact—provided, of course, that no momentum is lost through friction or other forces. The momentum of a golf ball changes from zero to a larger quantity after it is struck by a club (Figure 12.15). Neglecting air resistance and friction, the momentum of the club will also change so that the momentum of ball and club after impact will equal the momentum of ball and club before impact.

This is proved by using the impulse equation

$$m_bv_{bf} - m_bv_{bi} = m_cv_{cf} - m_cv_{ci}$$

where the subscript b refers to the ball and the subscript c to the club. Rearranged, this equation becomes

$$m_bv_{bi} - m_cv_{ci} = m_bv_{bf} - m_cv_{cf}$$

That is, the combined momentums before impact equal the combined momentums after impact. Momentum is conserved; none is lost.

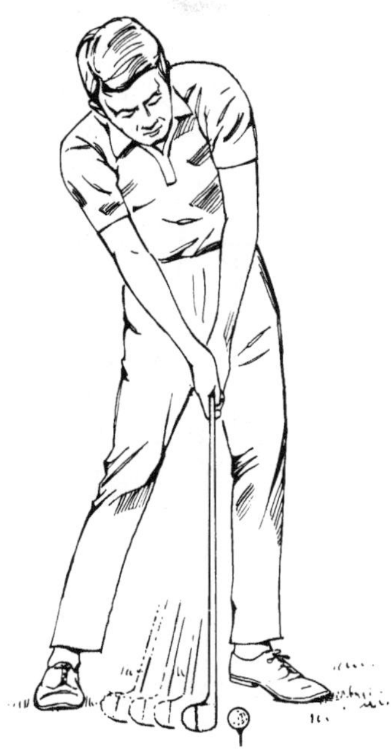

Figure 12.15 Momentum of club and ball before impact equals momentum of club and ball after impact.

The conservation of momentum may be easily apparent in some instances, whereas in others it is harder to visualize. When one steps out of a canoe onto a dock, the canoe is pushed back by the passenger as the passenger is pushed forward by the canoe. The change in momentum of the canoe backward ($m_1v_{1f} - m_1v_{1i}$) will equal the change in momentum of the passenger forward ($m_2v_{2f} - m_2v_{2i}$). Here the action–reaction relationship is evident in the movements of both the canoe and the person. But if the same person steps off an ocean liner, the change in momentum of the ship is imperceptible, yet it will still equal the change in momentum of the passenger. Because the mass of the ship is so great, its velocity is not apparent. In both instances, the change in the mass–velocity product of the passenger equals the change in the mass–velocity product of the boat (canoe or ship), and momentum is conserved. Incidentally, if the passenger disembarking from the canoe does not account for the backward acceleration of the canoe, the step toward the dock may be a wet one.

Summation of Forces

The forces generated by the muscle structure of the body may be summated from one segment to another. In generating momentum, these forces, applied over a period of time, are used to build momentum, which is then transferred from segment to segment. In a typical throwing pattern, for instance, force is first generated in the muscles of the lower extremity as the legs extend to push against the ground. The momentum generated is transferred to the trunk, where the application of further muscular force acts to increase momentum, primarily through an increase in velocity. This momentum is then transferred to the upper arm. The great decrease in mass when moving from trunk to upper arm produces an increase in velocity, in accord with the momentum equation (*mv*) and the fact that momentum within a system must be conserved. If the muscles of the shoulder contract to provide further impulse, velocity will increase further. This sequential transfer of momentum continues with mass decreasing and velocity increasing until momentum is finally transferred to the thrown ball.

Forces that Modify Motion

In addition to the forces that produce motion, a number of forces act to modify motion in some manner. These modifying forces must be considered when studying the kinetics of linear motion. When the kinesiological analysis model presented in Chapter 1 is applied to a motor skill, the forces that modify motion must be included in any discussion of the nature of the forces involved. Six of these forces are commonly categorized as follows:

1. **Weight**
2. **Contact forces**
   a. Ground reaction force
   b. Friction

3. **Fluid forces**
   a. Buoyancy
   b. Drag
   c. Lift

For purposes of discussion in this chapter, an additional category of elasticity and rebound has been added.

Weight

In what came to be known as the Law of Gravitation, Newton (remember the apple) was the first to point out that all bodies are attracted to each other in direct proportion to their masses and in inverse proportion to the square of the distance between them. The amount of this attraction between bodies on earth is negligible except for the attraction between the earth itself and the bodies on it. Because of the earth's huge mass, this attraction is quite noticeable. The force is called gravity, and it is measured as the weight of the body applied through the center of gravity of the body and directed toward the earth's axis (Figure 12.16). The closer a body is to the earth's center, the greater is the gravitational pull and, therefore, the more it weighs. When the body moves far enough away from the earth's center, such as to the moon, the decrease in the gravitational pull is apparent, as in the ease of giant leaps made by astronauts. The mass of the body is the same as on earth, but the weight has decreased in proportion to the gravitational pull. The relation between weight, mass, and gravity is represented in equation form as $w = mg$. The force of weight must be considered in all motion analyses.

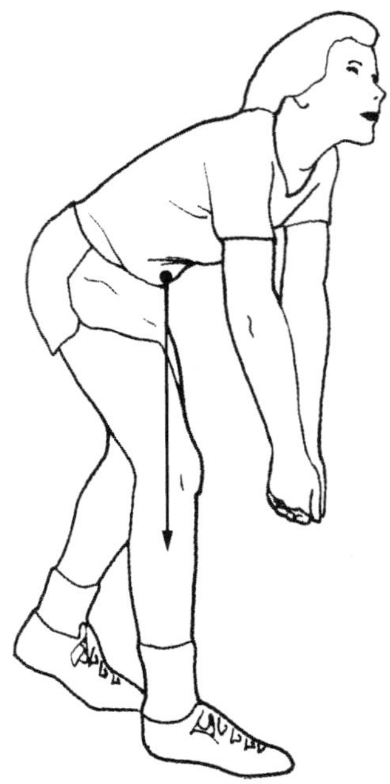

Figure 12.16 Gravitational force is measured as the weight of the body applied through the center of gravity of the body and directed toward the center of the earth.

Contact Forces

Ground Reaction Force

As Newton's third law states, for every action there is an equal and opposite reaction. Anytime a force is exerted on an object, that object will exert a force back. As you sit and read this section, you are exerting a force on a chair and the chair is exerting an equal and opposite force on you. If the chair did not exert an equal and opposite force, you would be falling toward the floor. If you are sitting still, the ground reaction force is equal to your body weight. Likewise, when you walk, run, or jump, the ground pushes back on you with the same force that you exert on the floor. In Figure 12.17, the high jumper exerts a force on the ground (action), and the ground exerts a force on the jumper's foot (reaction force).

Without the reactive force, there would be no motion. You cannot walk without the ground reaction force. When the heel strikes the ground, the ground brings the foot to rest so the body can pass over the planted foot. Then the ground reaction force pushes back against the toe at push-off. Ground reaction force is usually measured with a force platform and during jogging can be as high as two to three times body weight. If a book (4.45 N) is sitting on the floor, the ground reaction force is equal to the weight of the book (4.45 N). If you were to push directly down on the

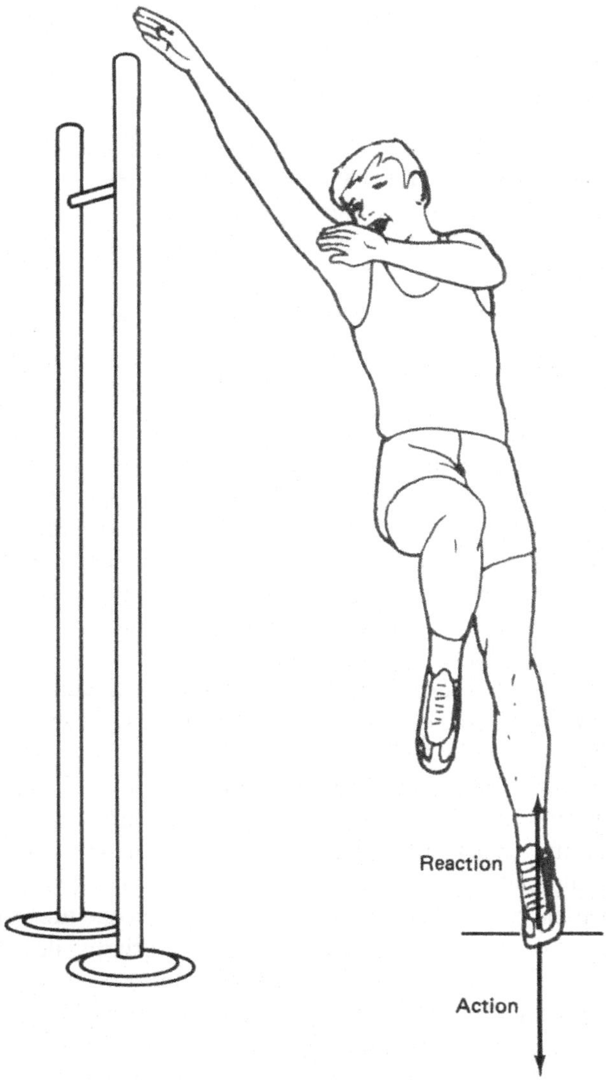

Figure 12.17 Example of normal reactive force. As the jumper pushes down on the ground, the ground pushes back.

book, the ground reaction force would be the sum of the weight of the book plus the pushing-down force. If the force that you exerted on the book was not directly down, but at an angle, the ground reaction force would be the sum of only that part of the force acting downward plus the weight of the book.

Friction

Friction is the force that opposes efforts to slide or roll one body over another. Without friction it would be impossible to walk or run or do much of any kind of moving. On the other hand, friction increases the difficulty of moving objects about with its deterrent effect. There are numerous examples in which we attempt to *increase* friction for more effective performance. The use of rubber-soled shoes on hardwood floors or wet decks, spikes on golf shoes, and rubber knobs on hiking boots improves friction with the supporting surface. To decrease slippage, gymnasts chalk their hands, people wear work gloves, and tennis racquets have cloth grips. Even the surfaces of balls are designed to increase friction through irregularities such as the fuzz on the tennis ball or the dimples on a golf ball. Attempts to decrease friction are also evident in physical activity. The sole of one of a bowler's shoes is made to have little friction so that it can slide more easily in the approach. Sharp ice skates apply pressure on the ice and cause slight melting, thus making it easier for the skates to move across the ice. Ice covered with a slight film of water is more slippery than colder, drier ice. Skis are waxed, bicycles are greased, and in-line skates have ball bearings, each for the purpose of minimizing the retardant effect of friction.

The amount of friction between one surface and another depends on the nature of the surfaces and the forces pressing them together. Generally speaking, smooth surfaces have less friction than rough surfaces. The area of surfaces in contact with each other does not affect friction. A footlocker pulled along on one end would take as much force to pull as one on its side. An empty footlocker, however, would take less force than one full of books. **Friction is proportional to the force pressing two surfaces together.**

In Figure 12.18, the book is pressing down on the table with a force (W) equal to its weight. The reactive force of the table pushing up against the book is called the normal force (N). The normal force acts perpendicular to the support surface and in this case is equal and opposite to the weight of the book. The maximum force that can be applied to the book *before* it begins to slide is called the force of static friction (F_{max}). The ratio of the force of static friction to the normal force is a quantity called the coefficient of static friction (μ_s).

$$\mu_s = \frac{F_{max}}{N}$$

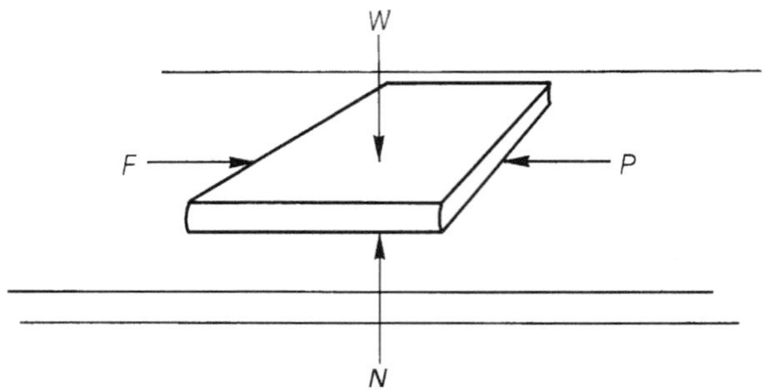

Figure 12.18 The coefficient of friction is the ratio between the force needed to overcome the friction P to the force holding the surfaces together W.

The symbol μ_s (mu) represents the coefficient of static friction and is an experimentally determined quantity that is a constant for any two surfaces. The larger the coefficient, the more the surfaces cling together, and the more difficult it is for the two surfaces to slide over each other. Police officers use this information every day in investigating automobile accidents. To determine how fast a car was going, they look to the length of the skid marks and determine how much friction (the coefficient of friction) was between the tires and the road. This is achieved experimentally through use of a drag sled. A portion of a tire filled with concrete to approximate the weight on one tire of a car is pulled along the road by a spring scale. The reading of the spring scale just before the sled moves is recorded as F_{max}. The total weight of the car divided by four is the N, and the coefficient of friction is F_{max}/N. From this information, the police officers can tell how fast the car was going and if it was traveling over the posted speed limit.

From an exercise science perspective, friction is a very important concept and is taken into consideration when looking at shoe-to-floor interface. It is used to answer such questions as which court shoes give better traction on hardwood floors or clay tennis courts.

Up to this point the discussion has centered on static friction, which is the amount of attraction between two surfaces that must be overcome for one of those surfaces to begin to move along the other. Once motion has been achieved, other types of friction take over, such as sliding friction and rolling friction. Static friction will always be greater than sliding friction or rolling friction for a given set of surface conditions. It is easier to keep something moving than to get it moving in the first place. As the name implies, *sliding friction* is a measure of the resistance of one surface to continue to slide along another and can be used to explain how far from a base a player needs to begin a slide. *Rolling friction* considers how easily one surface can continue to roll over, another surface. Rolling friction helps soccer players and golfers determine how a ball will react on short grass versus high, thick grass, and helps people determine which surface is better for in-line skating. The smaller the coefficient, the easier it is for the two surfaces to begin sliding or rolling over each other. A coefficient of 0.0 would indicate completely frictionless surfaces. The equation also shows that the coefficient of friction is totally dependent on the force holding the surfaces together (N) and the force needed to slide one surface over the (F_{max}). The coefficient will decrease as F_{max} decreases.

The coefficient of friction between two objects may also be found by placing one object on the second and tilting the second until the first starts to slide. The tangent of the angle of the second object with the horizontal is the coefficient of friction (Figure 12.19). An interesting application of the use of μ can be seen with respect to the gripping power of basketball shoes. The amount of lean a player may safely take is equal to the angle θ that the player makes with the vertical,

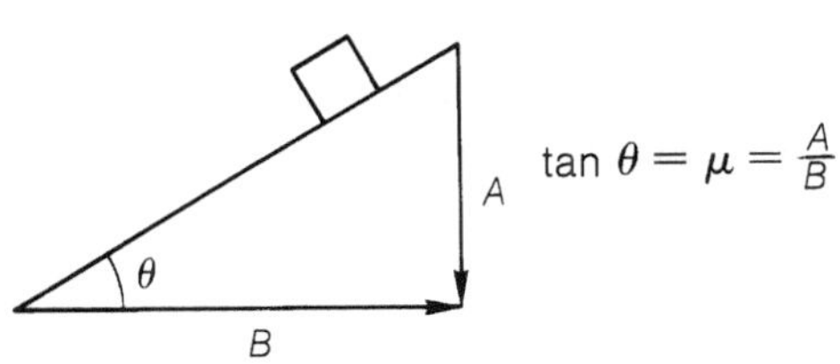

Figure 12.19 An inclined plane may be used to determine the coefficient of friction μ between two surfaces.

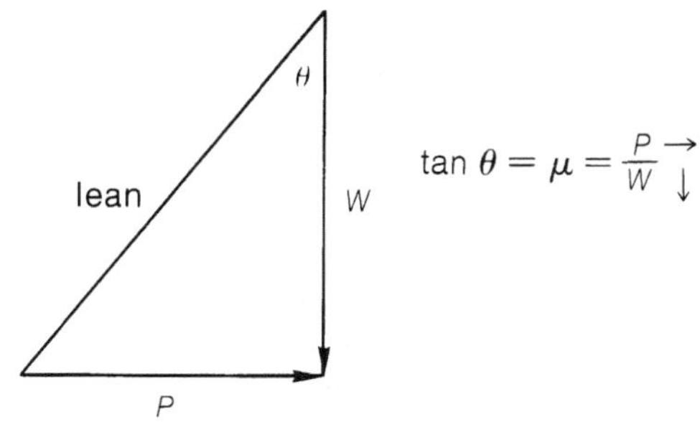

Figure 12.20 The amount of lean a basketball player can safely assume depends on the friction between the floor and his or her shoes.

whose tangent $= \frac{P}{W}$, P is the amount of horizontal force needed to cause the feet to start sliding horizontally, and W is the weight of the player (Figure 12.20). Shoes allowing a greater lean would certainly afford their wearers an advantage in the game. For this information to be of use to shoe manufacturers, however, a standard type of floor surface would have to be determined.

Elasticity and Rebound

Objects that rebound from each other do so in a fairly predictable manner. The nature of a rebound is governed by the elasticity, mass, and velocity of the rebounding surfaces, the friction between the surfaces, and the angle with which one object contacts the second.

Anytime two or more objects come into contact with each other, some distortion or deformation occurs. Whether or not the distortion is permanent depends on the elasticity of the interacting objects. Elasticity is the ability of an object to resist distorting influences and to return to its original size and shape when the distorting forces are removed. The force that acts on an object to distort it is called *stress*. The distortion that occurs is called *strain* and is proportional to the stress causing it. Stress may take the form of tension, as in the stretching of a spring; compression, as in the squeezing of a tennis ball (Figure 12.21); bending, such as the bending of a

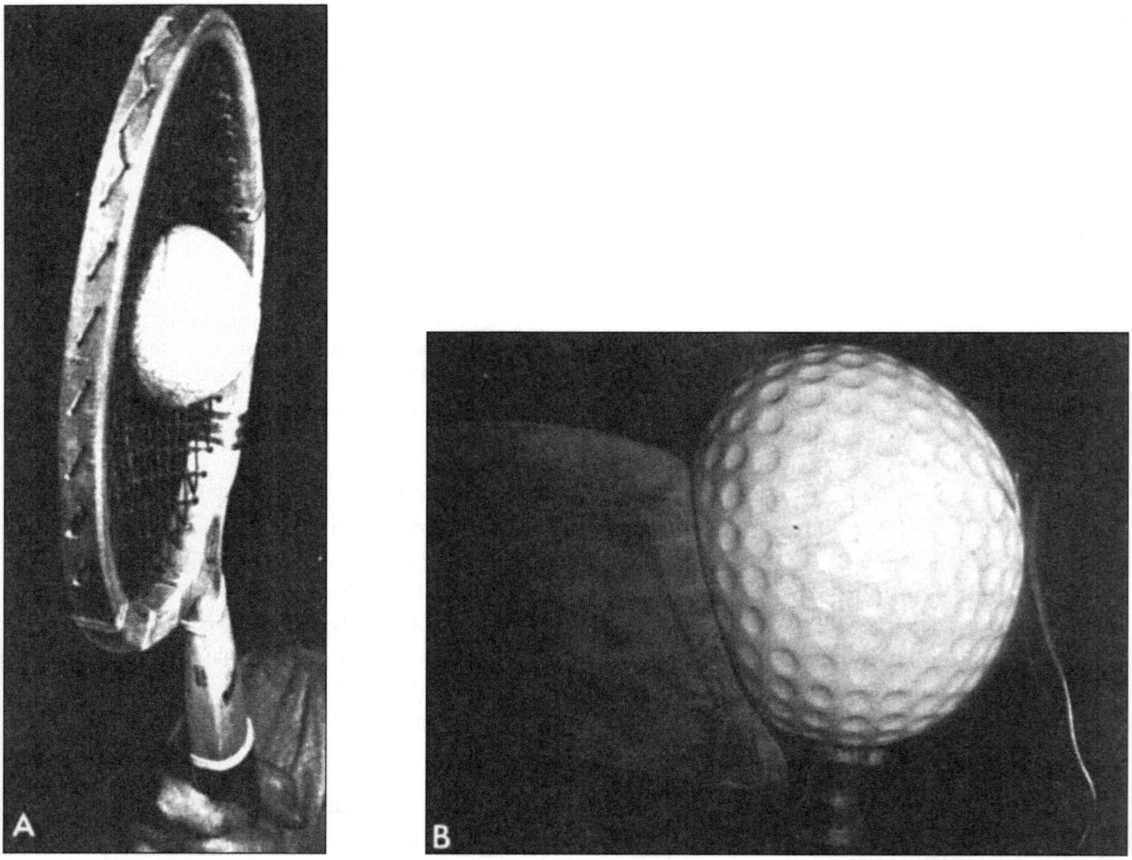

Figure 12.21 Compression of tennis ball (a) and golf ball (b) at moment of impact. Courtesy of H. E. Edgerton.

fencing foil; or torsion, as in the twisting of the spring. In all cases the object tends to resume its original shape when the stress is removed. If the stress is too large, the elastic limit of the object is exceeded and permanent distortion occurs.

Coefficient of Elasticity

Substances vary in their resistance to distorting forces and in their ability to regain their original shapes after being deformed. One usually thinks of a material such as rubber as being highly elastic because it yields easily to a distorting force and returns to its original shape. Actually, substances that are hard to distort and return perfectly to their original shapes are more elastic. Gases, liquids, highly tempered steel, and brass are examples. In comparing the elasticity of different substances, coefficients of elasticity are used. A coefficient of elasticity or restitution is defined as the stress divided by the strain.

The coefficient of elasticity most commonly determined in sports activities is that caused in the compression of balls. If one drops a ball onto a hard surface like a floor, the coefficient of restitution may be determined by comparing the drop height with the bounce height in the equation

$$e = \sqrt{\frac{\textbf{bounce height}}{\textbf{drop height}}}$$

where e = coefficient of restitution or elasticity. The closer the coefficient approaches 1.0, the more perfect the elasticity. Rules require that a basketball should be inflated to rebound to a height of 49 to 54 inches at its top when its bottom is dropped from a height of 72 inches. For the maximum bounce height, this is a coefficient of ·781. In comparison, a volleyball dropped from the same height and inflated to 6 psi (pounds per square inch) rebounds to 51 inches and has a coefficient of .84. A tennis ball has a coefficient of ·73, and a leather-covered softball one of ·46.

The coefficient of elasticity may also be found in another way. Because the Law of Conservation of Momentum states that the total momentum in any impact between two objects must remain the same, the momentum of one object may be reduced, so long as the momentum of the other object increases proportionately. If the objects are numbered 1 and 2 and it is assumed that mass of the objects remains constant, it is possible to find the coefficient of elasticity by using the change in velocity of the two objects:

$$e = \frac{v_{f1} - v_{f2}}{v_{i1} - v_{i2}}$$

where v_{f2} and v_{f1} are the velocities after impact, and v_{i1} and v_{i2} are the velocities before impact.

Angle of Rebound

An elastic object dropped vertically onto a rebounding surface will compress uniformly on its underside and rebound vertically upward. An elastic object that strikes a rebounding surface obliquely will compress unevenly on the bottom and rebound at an oblique angle. The size of the rebound angle compared with that of the striking angle depends on the elasticity of the striking object and the friction between the two surfaces. The rebound of a perfectly elastic object is similar to the reflection of light: *The angle of incidence (striking) is equal to the angle of reflection (rebound)* (Figure 12.22). Variations from this ideal are to be expected as the coefficient of restitution varies. Low coefficients will generally produce angles of reflection greater than angles of incidence.

For example, an underinflated volleyball will not have a great coefficient of restitution. It will therefore rebound at an angle much less, or much closer to the floor, than the striking angle. The coefficient of restitution acts to affect the vertical component of rebound. In rebound at an oblique angle, friction affects the horizontal component of the rebound. An increase in friction will produce a decrease in the angle of rebound. It is possible to produce an angle of rebound equal to the angle of incidence by decreasing both the horizontal component (increased friction) and the vertical component (elasticity) proportionately. If the proportions between the two components are constant, the angle of rebound will equal the angle of incidence, but the resultant velocity of the object after impact will be decreased.

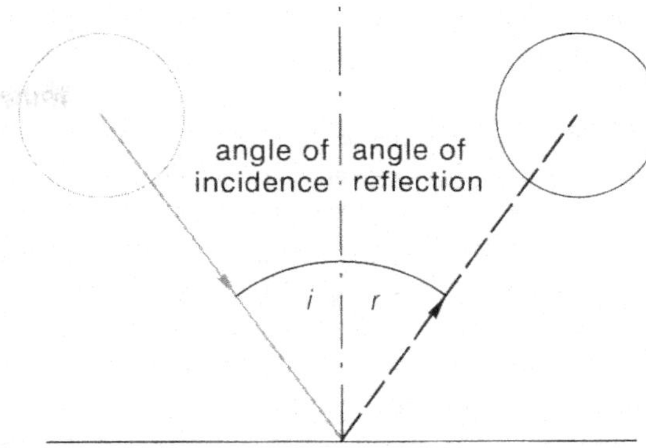

Figure 12.22 The angle of incidence and the angle of reflection in oblique rebounds.

Effects of Spin on Bounce

Spin also influences rebounding angles. Balls thrown with topspin will rebound from horizontal surfaces lower and with more horizontal velocity than that with which they struck the surface. They will tend to roll farther also, an action often desirable on long golf drives. Balls hitting a horizontal surface with backspin rebound at a higher bounce and are slower. Balls with backspin also roll for shorter distances than those with topspin or no spin. Because of the compression of the ball and the friction between it and the surface, a ball with no spin hitting the surface at an angle will develop some topspin on the rebound, and a ball hitting with topspin will develop greater topspin upon rebounding. With backspin, however, the spin may be completely stopped or reversed. A ball with sidespin will rebound in the direction of the spin. A ball spinning or curving to the right will "kick" to the right upon rebounding, and a left-spinning ball will do the reverse.

When spinning balls hit vertical surfaces, such as a basketball backboard or a racquetball court wall, they respond in relation to the surface in the same manner as with horizontal surfaces. When the vertical surface is struck from below, a ball with no spin or topspin will have added spin on rebound, and the angle of reflection will be greater than the angle of incidence. With backspin the spin will stop or reverse, and the angle of reflection will be less than the incidence angle. For this to be true, a backspinning ball approaching a vertical wall from above must be regarded as moving with topspin in relation to the rebounding surface. Similarly, a topspinning ball hitting the vertical surface from above is in actuality spinning backward with respect to the rebounding surface.

When a spinning ball meets a forward-moving object, as in tennis or table tennis, the ball will rebound in a direction that results from the forces acting on it at impact. For example, a ball with topspin striking a stationary vertical surface head-on will rebound upward. That same ball (with topspin) striking a moving vertical surface, like a tennis racquet, will also rebound upward; but not as much, because the resultant rebound has a horizontal force component from the forward-moving tennis racquet. Nevertheless, the upward direction may be sufficient to send the ball out of bounds. To counteract the upward direction, the racquet face can be turned obliquely downward, thus adding a downward-compensating force component as well as changing the spin of the ball.

The resultant force path of a rebounding ball is controlled by several factors. When one attempts to predict the direction of the rebound, the momentums of both the ball and the striking implement must be considered as well as the elasticity of the two objects, the spin of the ball, and the angle of impact. Awareness of these factors and the ways in which they affect play have numerous and valuable applications in sports such as handball, squash, racquetball, table tennis, paddleball, and tennis.

Fluid Forces

Water and air are both fluids and as such are subject to many of the same laws and principles. The fluid forces of buoyancy, drag, and lift apply in both mediums and have considerable effect on the movements of the human body in many circumstances. A discus sails, a baseball curves, a volleyball "wobbles," and a shuttlecock drops because of contact with air currents. Sky divers and hang gliders control their flight paths by interacting with the air currents, whereas downhill racers, swimmers, and underwater divers streamline their bodies to minimize the effect of fluid resistance.

Buoyancy

If an adult female stands in shoulder-deep water and abducts her arms as she lays her head back on the water's surface, most likely her feet will leave the bottom as her legs begin to rise. At some point between the vertical and horizontal, the swimmer will come to rest, and she will be in a motionless back float. For this to occur, an upward force must counterbalance the weight (force) of her body, acting vertically downward at her center of gravity. This upward force is called *buoyancy* and, according to **Archimedes' Principle,** the magnitude of this force is equal to the weight of water displaced by the floating body. Specifically, Archimedes' Principle states that **a solid body immersed in a liquid is buoyed up by a force equal to the weight of the liquid displaced.** This principle explains why some objects float and others do not, why some individuals float motionless like bobbing corks, and why others struggle to keep their noses above water while attempting a back float. When a body is immersed in water, it will sink until the weight of the water it displaces equals the weight of the body. Sinking objects never do displace enough water to equal their body weight and eventually settle to the bottom. If such objects are weighed underwater, they will be found to weigh less than when weighed in air. That difference in weight equals the weight of the water displaced and is the buoyant force acting on the immersed objects. Even a body that floats has some part of its volume beneath the surface and thus displaces a volume of water. The weight of the water it displaces equals the *total* weight of the floating object. Any object stops sinking when the weight of the water it displaces equals its weight.

The ratio between the weight of an object and its volume is referred to as density. The more weight per volume, the greater the density. An inflated volleyball, for example, has a slightly greater volume than a bowling ball. The bowling ball, however, weighs much more. Because the bowling ball has more weight for its volume than does the volleyball, it is said to have greater density.

The ratio between the density of any given object and that of water is called specific gravity. If an object or a body has the same density as water, or the same weight and volume ratio, it possesses a specific gravity of 1.0. Those objects with greater density will have a specific gravity greater than 1.0 and will sink. The bowling ball, being very dense, will sink very quickly. Objects with a density less than that of water will have a specific gravity less than 1.0 and will float with some part of the object or body exposed. An example is the inflated volleyball, which is composed primarily of air.

Human beings differ in specific gravity depending on individual body composition. Human bone and muscle tissue both have a specific gravity greater than water and as a result tend to sink. Fat and air, on the other hand, have specific gravities much less than that of water and will float. The ease with which one floats and the floating position assumed are therefore determined by the distribution of muscle, bone, fat, and air within the body. The specific gravity of the various body parts differs accordingly.

Usually the legs have a high specific gravity and consequently are the part of the body that most often sinks during the back float. The thoracic region is the most buoyant part, having the lowest weight for its volume. A person can increase the buoyancy of this region by keeping the lungs inflated with air, thus increasing the ease of floating. Some individuals have overall specific gravities greater than 1.0. It is impossible for these people to do a motionless float because they are "sinkers." A practical way to determine whether a person is a floater or a sinker is to have the person assume the tucked jellyfish float position with lungs inflated. If any portion of the individual's back is on or above the surface, the individual can learn to maintain a motionless floating position that, even though it may be more nearly vertical than supine, is still called a back float.

A floater has to be concerned with two forces, the downward force of the body's weight and the upward buoyancy of the water. When these forces act on the body so that their resultant is zero, the forces will be in equilibrium and the body will be in a motionless float. The downward force acts at the center of gravity of the body, a point somewhere in the pelvis. The buoyant force acts at the center of buoyancy of the body, a point that varies with individuals but is usually closer to the head than the center of gravity. If the body were of uniform density, the center of gravity and the center of buoyancy would coincide, but because the body has less mass toward the head, the center of buoyancy is usually higher in the body than the center of gravity. The center of buoyancy is the point where the center of gravity of the volume of displaced water would be if the water were placed in a vessel the shape and size of the floater's body. Because the water is of uniform density, its center of gravity will be in the direction of the greater volume, that is, near the chest region. If the center of gravity and center of buoyancy are not in the same force line with each other, as shown in Figure 12.23a, the body will rotate in the direction of the forces until the forces are equal and opposite in line, direction, and magnitude. At this point the floater will be in a balanced float (Figure 12.23b). Individuals who float horizontally have the center of gravity and

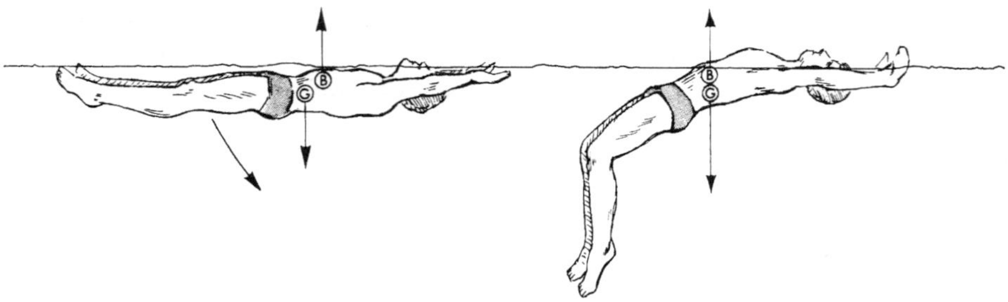

a. b.

Figure 12.23 A balanced float occurs when the gravity and the center of buoyancy are in the same force line. *G* = downward force of body weight; *B* = upward force (buoyancy) of water.

center of buoyancy in the same vertical line while in the horizontal position. These are usually individuals whose bodies contain a high percentage of fat. Those floaters whose legs tend to drop when attempting the back float will have a balanced position somewhere between the horizontal and vertical at that point where the center of gravity and center of buoyancy are in the same vertical line.

The angle of the floating position with the horizontal may be decreased by making adjustments in the position of the body segments that move the center of gravity in closer alignment with the center of buoyancy. Raising the arms over the head, bending the knees, and flexing the wrists to bring the hands out of the water all contribute to moving the center of gravity closer to the head and thus closer to the center of buoyancy (Figure 12.23b).

Lift and Drag

The fluid resistance to movement through air or water consists of two forces: *drag* and *lift*. The fluid flow that produces these two resistance forces is the result of either fluid or object velocity, which acts to produce pressure. Putting one's hand into a calm swimming pool will produce no fluid flow and no feeling of pressure because there is no velocity. Moving the hand back and forth in the pool (object velocity) or placing the hand in a fast-running stream (fluid velocity) produces definite pressure sensations because of fluid flow. Similarly, a softball thrown at 30 mph on a calm day will produce an airflow around the ball in the opposite direction of 30 mph. If the ball were thrown into a 5-mph headwind, the airflow velocity around the ball would be 35 mph. The magnitude of the fluid flow is directly proportional to the fluid and object velocities.

The resistance to forward motion experienced by objects moving through a fluid is called drag. Drag force is the result of fluid pressure on the leading edge of the object and the amount of backward pull produced by turbulence on the trailing edge. In fluid flow, the layer of fluid next to the object is called the *boundary layer.* There will usually be some amount of friction between the boundary layer and the object, which will cause resistance to forward motion. This friction is referred to as *surface drag.* If the flow of fluid around an object is smooth and unbroken, it is referred to as *laminar flow.* Laminar flow usually occurs in fluids passing around a smooth surface at relatively slow speeds. In laminar flow, the boundary layer is slowed down slightly by surface drag but continues in a smooth, unbroken flow around the object (Figure 12.24a). A smooth surface will produce much less surface drag than a rough surface. New, smoother swimsuit fabrics and the practice of shaving body hair before competition are both examples of attempts to reduce surface drag in competitive swimming.

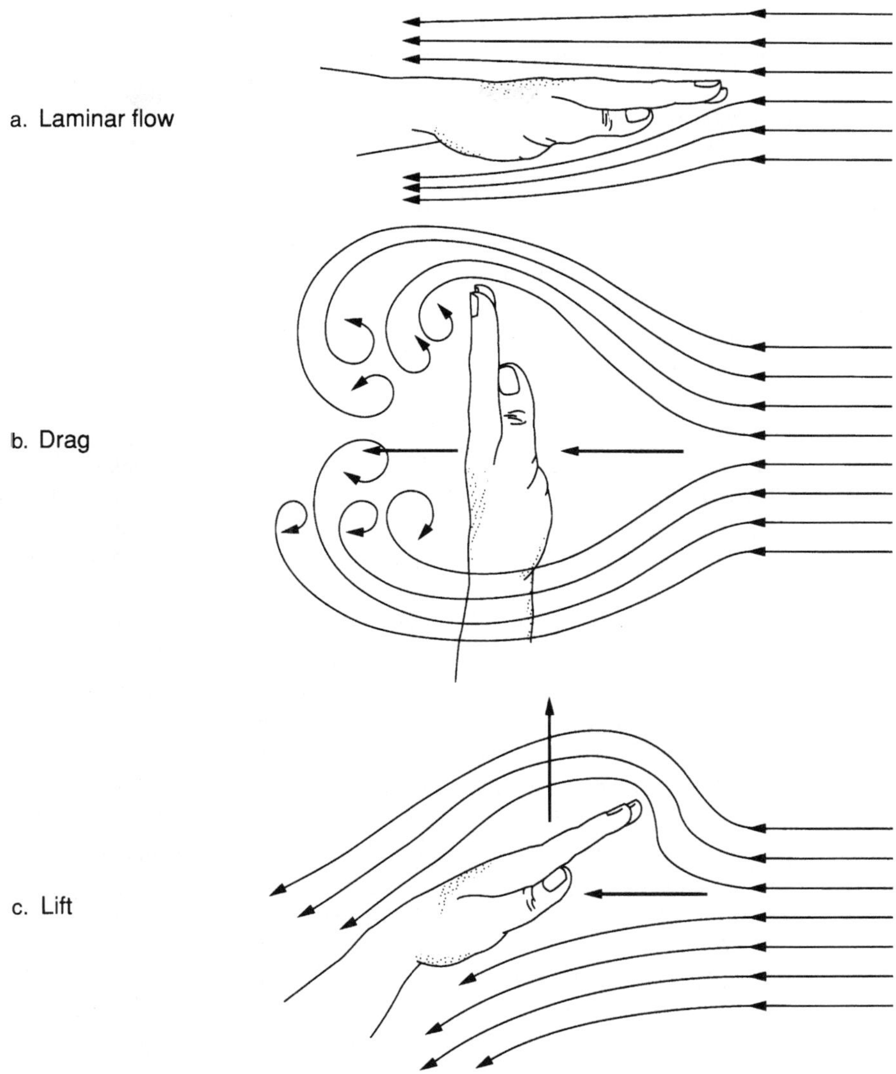

Figure 12.24 Patterns of flow around an object vary with the shape of the frontal surface. (a) Smooth, unbroken flow is laminar flow. (b) Flow that is disrupted and creates turbulence on the trailing edge creates drag. (c) Lift is produced when flow over one side of the object is faster than flow over the other side.

If the surface area presented by the object is great or if the flow velocity is high, there will be greater flow pressure on the leading edge of the object than on the trailing edge. In this situation, the boundary layer does not flow completely around the object. The boundary layer separates, creating a vacuum behind the trailing edge. Fluid rushes in to fill this vacuum, causing a backflow of fluid that is called *turbulence*. Turbulence produces a suction force backward, against the direction of motion. This turbulence is the result of *form drag*. In form drag the shape of the object is such that the fluid, moving at a given velocity, cannot follow the contours of the object (Figure 12.24b). Drivers on interstate highways often experience turbulence caused by form drag. When approaching a large truck from behind, the driver of a small car may experience an agitated airflow that tends to make the car harder to control. The driver may also feel a pull toward the truck. Both of these are the effects of turbulence. This turbulence might also increase as the velocity of the truck increases.

Form drag often can be reduced by streamlining. Examples of streamlining are common any time one desires to move easily and quickly through air or water. The crouch position on a racing bicycle, the shape of a race car, and the sharp bow of a boat are all examples of streamlining. The shape of a discus is also meant to take advantage of the effects of streamlining. The discus is tapered at both leading and trailing edges, so the airflow does not have to make any abrupt changes in direction. This streamlining principle will work only if the discus is thrown so that air flows past the tapered edges. If the discus is thrown with the flat side leading, air must make a very abrupt change of direction. There will be increased pressure on the leading edge and turbulence on the trailing edge, creating a large form drag. For this reason, streamlining makes the angle between the long axis of the object and the direction of fluid flow very important. This angle is often referred to as the *angle of attack*.

The angle of attack is also critical in producing and utilizing the fluid force known as *lift*. Lift is the result of changes in fluid pressure as the result of differences in airflow velocities. An extremely important principle in understanding the mechanism of lift is **Bernoulli's Principle.** Simply stated, Bernoulli determined that **the pressure in a moving fluid decreases as the speed increases.** The design of an airplane wing is based on Bernoulli's Principle of lift. The top side of an airplane wing has a higher curve than the bottom. To avoid creating a vacuum, airflow over the top will be at a higher velocity than the flow across the bottom. Pressure will therefore be lower on top of the wing. Lift will act upward, from the area of high pressure toward the area of low pressure, causing the wing to move upward. The swimmer uses lift in much the same way. Creating lift toward the forward surface of the hand is one force that aids in propelling the body forward. Lift, therefore, is the result of fluid on one side of an object having to travel farther in the same amount of time to avoid creating a vacuum. Lift always acts perpendicular to the fluid flow and therefore to the drag force (Figure 12.24c).

Ball Spin

Bernoulli's Principle applies for moving objects passing through a stationary fluid as well as for fluids passing stationary objects and, in addition to explaining why airplanes can fly, it also explains why balls with spin follow a curved path. This latter application of Bernoulli's Principle is called the Magnus effect after the German physicist who first explained the phenomenon. A ball moving through the air will also move in the direction of least air pressure. As shown in Figure 12.25a, the ball spinning in a clockwise direction drags around a boundary layer of air. At the bottom of the ball, this air current is moving in the same direction as the oncoming air. At the top, the boundary air is moving in the opposite direction. The air at the bottom is moving faster, and therefore the pressure is reduced. The air at the top moves more slowly and the pressure is increased. Thus the ball will move in a downward curve in the direction of least pressure. Viewed from the side, this would be the behavior of a ball with topspin imparted to it. Balls with topspin drop sooner than balls with no spin. A ball with a counterclockwise or backspin will move in an upward curve and thus stay aloft longer than a ball with no spin (Figure 12.25b). Balls spinning about a vertical axis have sidespin. Right spin causes the ball to curve to the right and occurs when the forward edge of the ball moves to the right. Left spin is the opposite.

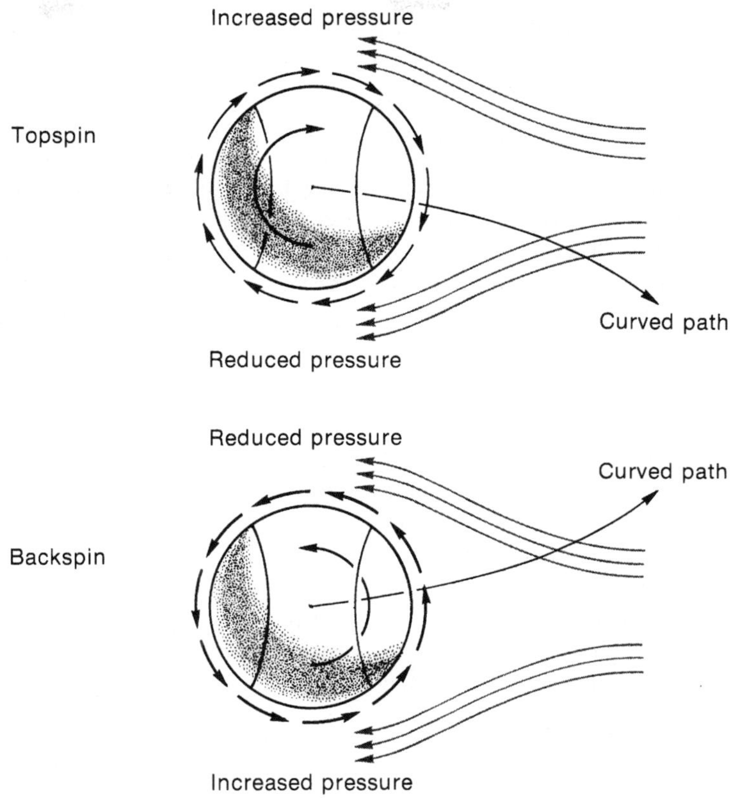

Figure 12.25 A spinning ball follows a curved path moving in the direction of least pressure. (The curve is exaggerated for clarity.)

The amount of air a ball drags around with it when spinning depends on the surface of the ball and the speed of the spin. Rough or large surfaces, small mass, and a fast spin speed all produce a more noticeable spin and curve deflection. The small mass of a table tennis ball, the fuzz on a tennis ball, and the seams on a baseball all enhance spin, an important element in each game's strategy. The deflection will also be more pronounced if the forward velocity is slow. This may occur because of little force imparted to the ball or a strong headwind. Spin on a ball may also smooth its flight by acting as a stabilizer. Like a gyroscope, a football or discus spinning around one axis resists spinning about another axis and therefore is less likely to tumble through the air.

FREE-BODY DIAGRAMS

In analyzing any technique, the student should consider all the external forces by methodically accounting for the effect of each one on the body. To do this, it is helpful to look at the body as if it were isolated from its surroundings. The isolated body is then considered to be a separate mechanical system whose boundaries have been defined. The isolation makes it easier to identify the forces and to represent them as vectors in a diagram of the body. This type of representation is called a *free-body diagram* and can help settle any doubts about the application and direction of the various forces acting on the body in any given time frame. The direction of each of the external forces and the point through which each acts are summarized in Table 12.1.

TABLE 12.1 Direction and Point of Application of External Forces

Force	Direction of Force	Point of Application
Weight (*W*)	Downward (toward center of earth)	Center of gravity of body
Ground reaction force (*R*)	Perpendicular to contact surface	Point of contact
Friction (*F*)	Along contact surface (perpendicular to normal reaction)	Point of contact
Buoyancy (*B*)	Upward	Center of buoyancy of body
Drag (*D*)	Opposite the direction of oncoming fluid flow	Center of gravity of body
Lift (*L*)	Perpendicular to drag	Center of gravity of body

In Figure 12.26, the magnitude of each external force acting on the body is represented by the arrow length. The direction of the force is represented by the arrowhead, and the point of application is located at the arrow tail. The body is acted on by its weight (*W*) applied through the center of gravity, the reactive force (*R*) and the friction force (*F*), both applied at the point of contact with the vault, and the horizontal force (*H*) directed through the center of gravity.

Free-body diagrams are also used to show the forces acting on an isolated body segment. In Figure 12.27, the thigh has been isolated from the rest of the lower limb, and the forces acting on it are shown. The forces acting on the limb include the weight of the thigh (*W*), the resultant muscle force acting across the hip joint (M_h), the resultant muscle force acting across the knee joint (M_k), and the reactive force components acting across the hip joint (H_x and H_y) and knee joint (K_x and K_y).

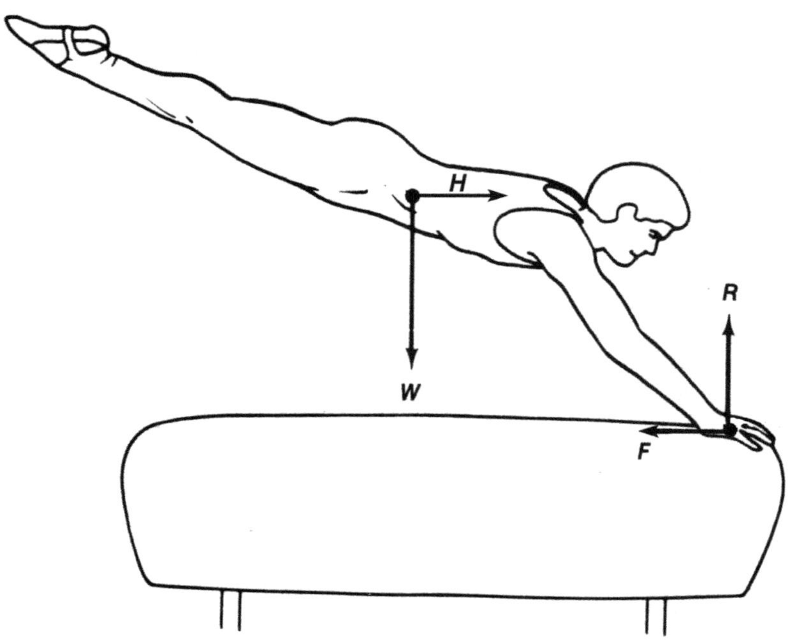

Figure 12.26 A free-body diagram showing the application and direction of the external forces acting on the vaulter: weight (*W*), horizontal force (*H*), normal reaction (*R*), and friction (*F*).

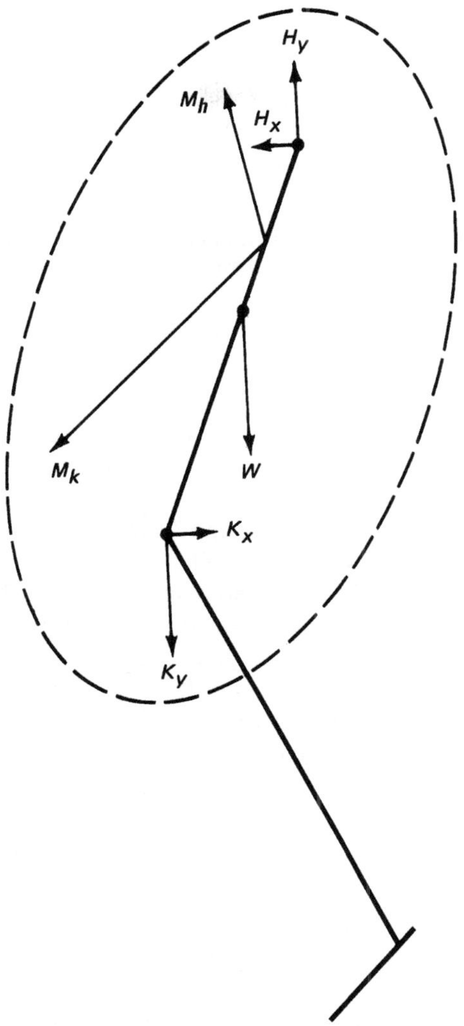

Figure 12.27 Free-body diagram of forces acting on a stationary thigh. Isolation of the limb is shown by the dotted line. Composite muscle forces are M_h and M_k. Reactive forces at the hip are H_y and H_x and at the knee are K_y and K_x. The weight force is W. *Source:* Adapted from *Biomechanics of Sports,* by D. I. Miller & R. C. Nelson. Copyright © 1973, Lea & Febiger, Malvern, PA. Reprinted by permission.

WORK, POWER, AND ENERGY

Work

Simple machines such as the lever are devices designed to do work. In each instance the machine aids in the use of a force to overcome a resistance. When the resistance is overcome for a given distance, *work* is done. Mechanically speaking, **work is the product of the amount of force expended and the distance through which the force succeeds in overcoming a resistance it acts upon.** For work done in making a body move in a linear fashion, this may be expressed as

$$W = Fs$$

where W stands for work, F for force, and s for the distance along which the force is applied. Units for expressing work are numerous because any force unit may be combined with any distance unit to form a work unit. In the U.S. system the foot-pound is the most common work unit; the joule is the most frequently used unit in the metric system. A joule is equivalent to $10^7 \times 1$ gram of force exerted through 1 centimeter.

In computing work, the distance s must always be measured in the direction in which the force acts, even though the object whose resistance is overcome may not be moving in the same direction. If one lifts a 20-N suitcase from the floor to place it on a shelf 2 meters above the floor, the work accomplished is 40 newton-meters (Nm). If, on the other hand, that same weight is lifted an equal distance upward but along a 4-meter inclined plane, the amount of work done is still 40 N·m (Figure 12.28). The work done along the incline is the same as the work done to lift the weight to the height of the incline. The horizontal distance the suitcase moves is not included.

Work done in the same direction that the body moves is called *positive* work, whereas work done in the opposite direction is called *negative* work. When an individual does a deep knee bend, the extensor muscles of the leg contract eccentrically to resist the effect of gravity on the body. The body moves in a direction opposite to the upward force of the muscles, and thus negative or resistive work is performed by the muscles. In the return to standing from the knee-bend position, the body moves in the same direction as the concentrically contracting extensors, and the work of the muscles is positive. The net work accomplished during the

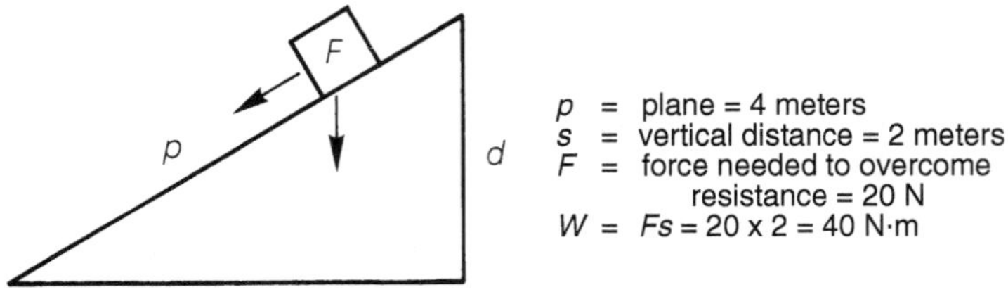

Figure 12.28 Work is the product of force needed to overcome a resistance and the direction over which the force is applied. The force lifting the 20-N weight 2 vertical meters does 40 N·m of work even though the 20 N are moved 4 meters along the plane.

down and up movement of the knee bend is the sum of the positive and negative work.

Consider the mechanical work done during a 444-N (50 lbs) bench press cycle. If the weight is moved through a distance of 0.33 m (13 in.), then the work done would be

Downward Phase	Upward Phase
$W = Fs$	$W = Fs$
$W = (444 \text{ Nm})(0.33 \text{ m})$	$W = (444 \text{ Nm})(0.33 \text{ m})$
$W = -146.52 \text{ Nm}$	$W = 146.52 \text{ Nm}$
The downward phase would be considered negative work because the force and the motion are in opposite directions.	The upward phase would be considered positive work because the force and the motion are in the same direction.

If the question was, "How much mechanical work is done in one complete bench press cycle?" the answer would be zero. Because the weight started and ended at the same point, no net motion occurred and, as such, no mechanical work was done.

When the exertion of effort produces no motion, such as might happen during a tug-of-war, no work is accomplished. Static contraction of muscles may be evident and considerable physiological effort may be expended but, in the strict mechanical sense, no work is being done. The physiological measure of such efforts is determined by obtaining the energy costs, which in turn are usually measured by computing the amount of oxygen consumed during the effort and converting it to calories per minute.

Theoretically, the mechanical work performed by an individual muscle can also be determined using the equation $W = Fs$. Suppose, for instance, that there is a rectangular muscle, 10 centimeters long and 3 centimeters wide, that exerts 240 newtons of force as it turns a bony lever. Because the average muscle fiber shortens to one-half its resting length and the fibers of a small rectangular muscle run the full length of the muscle, the force of the muscle in question is exerted over a distance of 5 cm (the amount of shortening equal to one-half the resting length). Therefore, $F = 240$ N and $s = 5$ cm, the muscle is performing 1200 newton-centimeters, or 120 newton-meters, of work. In brief: $W = F\ (240 \text{ N}) \times s\ (5/100 \text{ meters})$.

If the force of the muscle is not known, it is computed from the muscle's cross section. Assuming the muscle in question to be 1 cm thick and the force per square inch of cross section to be 360 N, the following steps are taken:

1. Find the muscle's cross section:
   Cross section = width × thickness.
   3 cm × 1 cm = 3 sq cm (cross section).
2. Find the amount of force exerted by the muscle:
   Average force = 360 N per sq cm.
   Cross section = 3 sq cm.
   $F = 360 \times 3 = 1{,}080$ N.
3. Find the amount of work performed by this muscle, first in N·cm, then in N·m:
   $W = Fs$.
   $W = 1{,}080 \text{ N} \times 5 \text{ cm} = 5{,}400$ N·cm.
   $5{,}400/100 = 540$ N·m.

For purposes of simplification, the internal structure of the hypothetical muscle used in these examples was rectangular. This means that a simple geometric cross-sectional measure could be used. For penniform and bipenniform muscles, however, it would be essential to determine the physiological cross section. It must also be remembered that *s* in the work equation represents one-half the length of the average fiber in the muscle and that this may or may not coincide with the total length of the fleshy part of the muscle, depending on its internal structure. The number of pounds of force per square inch exerted by the average human muscle must be selected arbitrarily, depending on whose research the student accepts.

A single equation for computing the work performed by a muscle whose average fiber length is known and whose physiological cross section (PCS) has been determined is as follows:

$$W = 360 \times \text{PCS (in square centimeters)} \times 1/2 \text{ the length of the fibers (in centimeters)}$$

This gives work in terms of newton-centimeters. Because it is customary to measure work in terms of newton-meters, the result should be divided by 100. The following equation includes this step:

$$W = \frac{360\ (\text{PCS in square cm})(1/2 \text{ the fiber length in cm})}{100}$$

Any measure of work does not account for the time involved in performing the work. When one lifts 200 N a distance of 2 meters, 400 N·m of work is done, regardless of the time it takes to do it. Work per unit time or the rate at which work is done is called power.

$$\boldsymbol{Power = \frac{Work}{Time} = \frac{W}{t}}$$

Recall that $W = Fs$ and that by substituting Fs for work, a different version of the power equation can be written:

$$Power = \frac{Fs}{t} \quad \text{or} \quad Power = F\frac{s}{t}$$

Recall that $\frac{s}{t}$ is the equation for velocity, so a different version of the power equation can be written:

$$\boldsymbol{Power = Fv}$$

Any form of the equation clearly points out that the machine or person who can perform more work in a given unit of time or who takes less time to do a specified amount of work is more powerful.

In the U.S. system, power is expressed as ft.lb/sec or as horsepower (550 ft.lb/sec = 1 horsepower). The metric system unit is the watt, which is equivalent to 1 joule/second.

Energy

Energy is defined as the capacity to do work. A body is said to possess energy when it can perform work, and the energy that the body possesses is measured as the work accomplished. Energy may take numerous forms, and it is common for it to be converted from one form to another, although according to the Law of Conservation of Energy it can be neither created nor destroyed. Some forms that energy may take are heat, sound, light, electric, chemical, nuclear, and mechanical. When a ball is hit with a bat, some of the mechanical energy is converted to sound and heat energy, but none of the energy is lost. **The total amount of energy possessed by a body or an isolated system remains constant.**

Potential energy and kinetic energy are two classifications of mechanical energy that have important implications in biomechanics. Potential energy is the capacity for doing work that a body has because of its position or configuration. A raised weight such as a diver standing on a platform, a bent bow, or a compressed spring all have potential energy. Measured in work units, potential energy is the product of the force an object has and the distance over which it can act. The potential energy of a 150-pound diver whose center of gravity is 20 feet above the water surface is 3,000 foot-pounds. In this instance the appropriate form for the potential energy equation is

$$\boldsymbol{PE = mgh}$$

where m is the mass of the body, g is the acceleration of gravity, and h is the height between the diver's center of gravity and the water surface. The product of m and g (mg) is the same as the diver's weight.

The distance selected for h in the potential energy equation is established by choosing an arbitrary zero level. The potential energy of someone standing on a table 1 meter from the floor can be increased by boring a large hole in the floor directly in front of the table. The individual's potential for dropping farther is now greater because h is greater.

The kinetic energy of a body is the energy due to its motion. The faster a body moves, the more kinetic energy it possesses. When a body stops moving, the kinetic energy is dissipated. This is readily seen in the equation for kinetic energy

$$KE = 1/2\, mv^2$$

where m is the mass of the object and v is its velocity. If v is zero, then KE is also zero.

Energy has been defined as the capacity to do work, and because energy can neither be created nor destroyed, the work done is equal to the kinetic energy acquired, or

$$Fs = 1/2\, mv^2$$

This relationship is extremely helpful in explaining the value of "giving" when receiving the impetus of any moving object. In attempting to catch a fast-moving ball, one's chances of success are improved by increasing the distance used for stopping the ball's motion. The work of the kinetic energy against the hands depends on the kinetic energy the ball possesses when it hits the hand. Whether that work consists of a large F and a small s or a small F and a large s depends on the technique used by the catcher. As s increases in $Fs = 1/2\, mv^2$, the force of the impact F must decrease. The skillful performer knows this and will decrease the possibility of injury and increase the chances of holding onto the ball with the choice of a small F and a large s. Achieving a gradual loss of kinetic energy is likewise advantageous when landing from a jump or a fall (Figure 12.29).

Energy is frequently transformed from kinetic into potential energy or conversely from potential to kinetic energy. The diver who jumps from a platform above the water begins immediately to lose potential energy in proportion to the gain in kinetic energy. At platform height all of the diver's energy is potential. At zero elevation all of the potential energy has been converted into an equivalent amount of kinetic energy. Barring no conversion of energy to other forms (heat, sound, and so forth) the potential energy at the top equals exactly the kinetic energy at the bottom.

The transformation from one energy state to another is interesting to note in a gymnast swinging on the flying rings. Like a pendulum, the

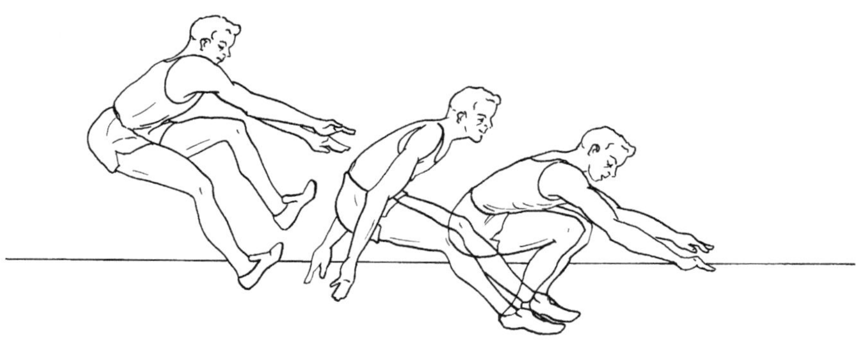

Figure 12.29 Effecting a gradual loss of kinetic energy by bending the knees upon landing from a jump.

swinger's energy is transformed from kinetic to potential on every swing. As the suspended body moves upward, the kinetic energy is continuously changed to potential energy, and the higher the swinger goes, the greater the potential becomes for doing work on the downswing. At the top of the swing, the conversion to potential energy is complete. Once more as the gymnast begins to fall, kinetic energy again develops and becomes greatest at the bottom of the swing, when the speed is greatest and potential energy is zero. Theoretically the swinging should continue uninterrupted, but because of friction some energy is converted to heat and eventually the "pendulum" will come to rest.

The Analysis of Linear Motion

Establishing the mechanical principles that are used in the analysis of linear motion involves first identifying the nature of the forces involved in the motion of interest. As discussed in this chapter, several forces must be considered.

1. Weight—applied downward through the center of gravity.
2. Propulsive forces—forces generated by muscles, which, in turn, move segments to produce contact forces.
3. Ground reaction—applied equal and opposite to contact forces, perpendicular to contact surfaces.
4. Friction—applied perpendicular to normal reaction forces along contact surfaces opposite the direction of the propulsive force.
5. Buoyancy—acting in opposition to gravity to support the body in a fluid.
6. Drag—resistance to motion caused by fluid pressure and turbulence, acting in the direction of fluid flow.
7. Lift—acting perpendicular to the direction of fluid flow.

In the long jump example used throughout this text, weight is the resistance force that must be overcome in order for the jumper to leave the ground. The propulsive force is muscle force acting to produce forceful extension of the lower extremities and flexion of the upper extremities. The flexion of the upper extremities produces a downward reaction force. This, along with the downward-directed force produced by lower extremity extension, generates a downward-directed normal force and a backward-directed tangential force. It is the equal and opposite ground reaction force and the friction force that propel the body into the air as a projectile.

The principles that govern the mechanical aspects of a movement performance can be summarized by examining some of the basic concepts involved in the kinetics of linear motion. Some general movement principles based on these concepts might be as follows:

Inertia An object will resist any change in motion state, based on mass or momentum (mass × velocity).

Impulse Any change in the motion state depends on the applied force and the time over which it is applied. An impulse is required for any change in momentum.

Work The amount of work done by the movement system is equal to the amount of force applied and the distance over which it is applied.

Kinetic energy The amount of work done on a body or object is equal to the kinetic energy produced. Energy can be imparted to move objects or be dissipated to cause objects to stop motion.

To return to the long jump example, the inertia that must be overcome is the mass of the jumper's body. The impulse generated in the propulsion phase must be one that will give maximum linear velocity to the body for its projectile flight. When this impulse is applied, work is done on the body. The result of this work is the production of the kinetic energy necessary to carry the body forward in flight. The amount of kinetic energy generated will be directly dependent on the impulse applied.

The student must understand that the linear forces that produce motion in the human body are often the result of the rotary motion of the body segments occurring at the joints. For this reason, an analysis of linear mechanics alone cannot fully describe the mechanical attributes of performance. Chapter 13 provides the student with the knowledge to analyze the rotary components of human motion.

REFERENCES AND SELECTED READINGS

Burnfield, J. M., Tsai, Y. J., & Powers, C. M. (2005). Comparison of utilized coefficient of friction during different walking tasks in persons with and without a disability. *Gait and Posture,* 22(1), 82–88.

Giatsis, G., Kollias, I., Panoutsakopoulos, V., & Papaiakovou, G. (2004). Biomechanical differences in elite beach-volleyball players in vertical squat jump on rigid and sand surface. *Sports Biomechanics,* 23(1), 145–158.

Grezios, A. K., Gissis, I. T., Sotiropoulos, A. A., Nikolaidis, D. V., & Souglis, A. G. (2006). Muscle-contraction properties in overarm throwing movements. *Journal of Strength and Conditioning Research,* 20(1), 117–123.

Havriluk, R. (2005). Performance level differences in swimming: A meta-analysis of passive drag force. *Research Quarterly for Exercise and Sport,* 76(2), 112–118.

Ireson, G. (2001). Beckham as physicist? *Physics Education,* 36, 10–13.

Kjendlie, P. L., Stallman, R. K., & Stray-Gundersen, J. (2004). Passive and active floating torque during swimming. *European Journal of Applied Physiology,* 93(1–2), 75–81.

Lees, A., Vanrenterghem, J., & De Clercq, D. (2006). The energetics and benefit of an arm swing in submaximal and maximal vertical jump performance. *Journal of Sports Sciences,* 24(1), 51–57.

Lees, A., Vanrenterghem, J., & De Clercq, D. (2006). Understanding how an arm swing enhances performance in the vertical jump. *Journal of Biomechanics,* 37(12), 1929–1940.

Minetti, A. E., & Ardigo, L. P. (2002). Halteres used in ancient Olympic long jump. *Nature,* 420(6912), 141–142.

Mollendorf, J. C., Termin, A. C., Oppenheim, E., & Pendergast, D. R. (2004). Effect of swim suit design on passive drag. *Medicine and Science in Sports and Exercise,* 36(6), 1029–1035.

Ozkaya, N., Nordin, M., & Frankel, V. H. (1999). *Fundamentals of biomechanics: Equilibrium, motion, and deformation* (2nd ed.). New York: Springer.

Pain, M. T., Mills, C. L., & Yeadon, M. R. (2005). Video analysis of the deformation and effective mass of gymnastics landing mats. *Medicine and Science in Sports and Exercise,* 37(10), 1754–1760.

Parker, K. (2001). Use of force platforms in physics and sport. *Physics Education,* 36, 18–22.

Pendrill, A. M., & G. Williams. (2005). Swings and slides. *Physics Education,* 40, 527–533.

Powers, C. M., Burnfield, J. M., Lim, P., Brault, J. M., & Flynn, J. E. (2002). Utilized coefficient of friction during walking: Static estimates exceed measured values. *Journal of Forensic Science,* 47(6), 1303–1308.

Schade, F., Arampatzis, A., Brüggemann, G. P., & Komi, P. V. (2004). Comparison of the men's and women's pole vault at the 2000 Sydney Olympic Games. *Journal of Sports Sciences,* 22, 835–842.

Souza, A. L., Shimada, S. D., & Koontz, A. (2002). Ground reaction forces during the power clean. *Journal of Strength and Conditioning Research,* 16(3), 423–427.

Tcizeren, A. (2000). *Human body dynamics: Classical mechanics and human movement.* New York: Springer.

Vennell, R., Pease, D., & Wilson, B. (2006). Wave drag on human swimmers. *Journal of Biomechanics,* 39(4), 664–671.

Zhang, S., Clowers, K., Kohstall, C., & Yu, Y. J. (2005). Effects of various midsole densities of basketball shoes on impact attenuation during landing activities. *Journal of Applied Biomechanics,* 21(1), 3–17.

LABORATORY EXPERIENCES

1. Define the following key terms and give an example of each that is not used in the text:
   Force
   Inertia
   Mass
   Weight
   Momentum
   Impulse
2. In the diagram of the biceps muscle in Figure 12.30, find the size of the angle of pull.
3. Place a book on a table and stand a small bottle on top of it. Pull the book toward you with a quick jerk. Note the action of the bottle. Stand the bottle on the book again and pull the book across the table with a steady pull. How does the bottle move? Now pull the book and stop it suddenly. Explain the action of the bottle in all three instances.
4. Hit a softball with a bat from a tee, from a self-toss, and from a pitch. Which hit goes the farthest? Explain.
5. Lie on your back in the water with your arms over your head. Raise your legs by flexing your hips. What happens to your arms and trunk? Explain. Devise another experiment that demonstrates the same principle.
6. While both of you have on ice skates or roller skates, stand facing someone whose weight is the same as yours. Push against each other. Observe and compare the distance and velocity each of you moves. Repeat the procedure with someone who weighs considerably more or less than you do. Explain the difference between the two performances.
7. Place a long, wide board on some rollers (pencils, dowels, or pipes) so that there is very little friction between the board and the floor. Carefully step on the board and attempt to walk normally along it. What happens to you? To the board? Take the board off the rollers and place it on the floor. Walk along it. Explain the reason for the differences in the behavior of the board and your ability to walk along it. The use of spotters is advised for this exercise.
8. Determine the coefficient of restitution for each of the following objects dropped from a height of 2 meters onto a wooden floor:
   a. Tennis ball
   b. Racquetball

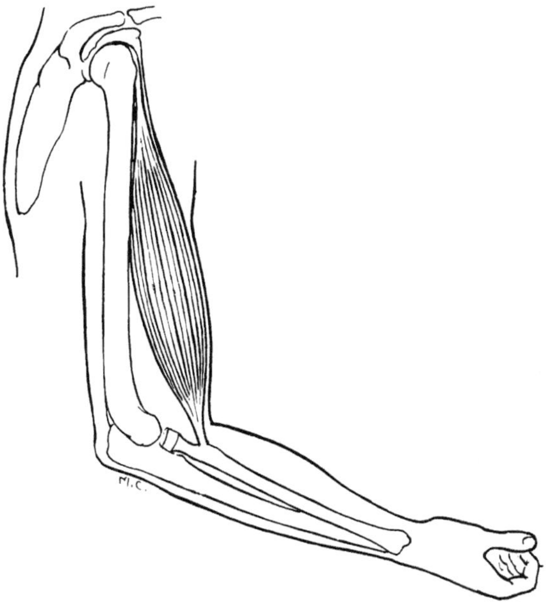

Figure 12.30 The forearm as a lever with the biceps providing the force.

c. Golf ball
d. Soccer ball
e. Baseball
Repeat the calculations for the same objects rebounding from concrete, from asphalt tile, from artificial turf, and from a tumbling mat.

9. Using a tennis racquet or a paddle, impart topspin, backspin, no spin, and sidespin to a ball. Note the effect on the velocity and angle of reflection when the ball rebounds from a horizontal surface, from a vertical surface when struck from above, and from a vertical surface when struck from below.
10. Assume a back-lying position in the water with your arms at your sides. Note and explain any shift in body position. Slide your arms from your sides to a side horizontal position, keeping them close to and parallel to the surface of the water. What effect does this have on body position? Continue moving your arms until they are overhead. Next, flex the wrists so the hands are out of the water. Finally, flex the legs at the knees. Explain the effect of these last three moves on your position in the water.
11. Record the body weight for each of five subjects. Using a stopwatch, record the time necessary for each subject to run up two flights of stairs. Determine the vertical distance from the bottom of the first flight to the top of the second flight. Calculate the work done by each subject and the power of each. Complete the chart below.
    a. Which subjects did the most work? Why?
    b. Did those who did the most work have the most power? Explain.
    c. If power is an important part of an event, how should an athlete train for it?
12. Estimate the cross section of your own biceps muscle. Approximately how much force should it be able to exert?
13. Approximately how much force should your triceps be able to exert?
14. In each of the following movement patterns, identify the nature of the motion for each phase. State the underlying mechanical objectives and describe what must occur to achieve optimum results. Consider carefully the application of linear mechanical principles.
    Front crawl stroke
    Bench press
    High jump

Subject	Weight	Time	Work	Power
1.				
2.				
3.				
4.				
5.				

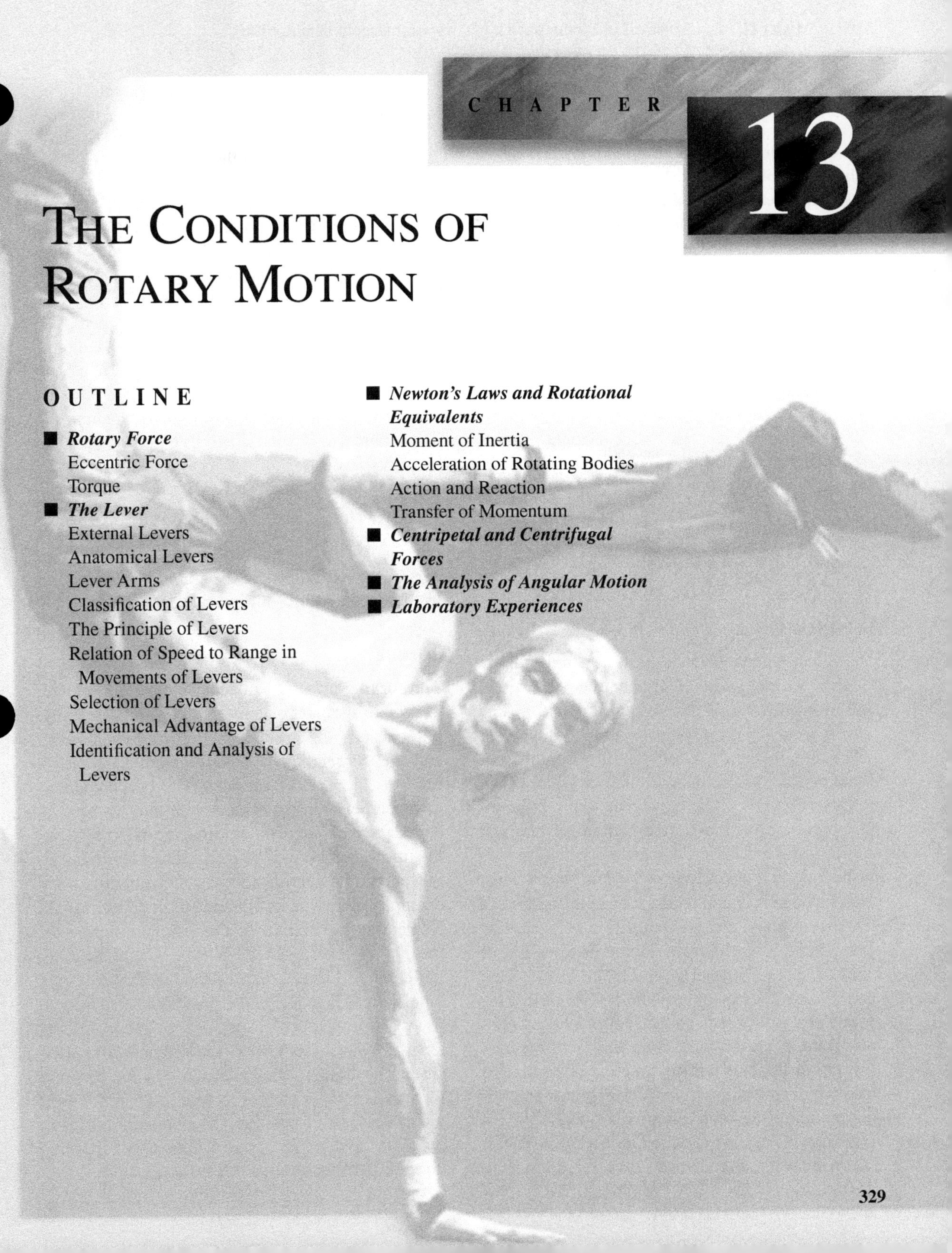

CHAPTER 13

THE CONDITIONS OF ROTARY MOTION

OUTLINE

- ***Rotary Force***
  - Eccentric Force
  - Torque
- ***The Lever***
  - External Levers
  - Anatomical Levers
  - Lever Arms
  - Classification of Levers
  - The Principle of Levers
  - Relation of Speed to Range in Movements of Levers
  - Selection of Levers
  - Mechanical Advantage of Levers
  - Identification and Analysis of Levers
- ***Newton's Laws and Rotational Equivalents***
  - Moment of Inertia
  - Acceleration of Rotating Bodies
  - Action and Reaction
  - Transfer of Momentum
- ***Centripetal and Centrifugal Forces***
- ***The Analysis of Angular Motion***
- ***Laboratory Experiences***

OBJECTIVES

At the conclusion of this chapter, the student should be able to:

1. Name, define, and use the following terms properly as they relate to rotary motion: *eccentric force, torque, couple, lever, moment of inertia,* and *angular momentum.*
2. Solve simple lever and torque problems involving the human body and the implements it uses.
3. Demonstrate an understanding of the effective selection of levers by relating speed, range of motion, and mechanical advantage to the properties of given lever systems.
4. Explain the analogous kinetic relationships that exist between linear and rotary motion.
5. State Newton's laws of motion as they apply to rotary motion.
6. Explain the cause-and-effect relationship between the forces responsible for rotary motion and the objects experiencing the motion.
7. Define centripetal and centrifugal force, and explain the relationships that exist between these forces and the factors influencing them.
8. Identify the concepts of rotary motion that are critical elements in the successful performance of a selected motor skill.
9. Using the concepts that govern rotary motion, perform a mechanical analysis of a selected motor skill.

ROTARY FORCE

Eccentric Force

The effect forces have on an object depends on the magnitude, point of application, and direction of each force. When force is applied in line with a freely moving object's center of gravity, linear motion occurs. When the direction of force is not in line, a combination of rotary and translatory motion is likely to occur. This relationship between force application and direction and the resulting motion are apparent when a book is pushed along a table. Linear motion occurs when sufficient force is applied in line with the book's center of gravity, and a combination of linear and rotary motion results from a force directed left or right of center. Similarly, an object with a fixed axis, like a door or one of the body's limbs, rotates when the force is applied off center but does not rotate when the force is in line with the axis of rotation. A force whose direction is not in line with the center of gravity of a freely moving object or the center of rotation of an object with a fixed axis of rotation is called an **eccentric force.** There must be an eccentric force for rotation to occur. Some examples of the application of eccentric force are shown in Figure 13.1.

Torque

The turning effect of an eccentric force is called *torque,* or moment of force. The torque about any point equals the product of the force magnitude and the perpendicular distance from the line of force to the axis of rotation. The perpendicular distance between the force vector and the axis is called the *moment arm,* or torque arm. In this text, the turning effect will be referred to as torque and the perpendicular distance as moment arm. An example of torque is illustrated in Figure 13.2. Neglecting the weight of the arm, the torque or turning effect caused by a 9-N weight held in the hand with the forearm flexed at the elbow to a horizontal position is the product of the weight times its perpendicular distance, or moment arm length, from the elbow. If the moment arm d is 0.3 m, the amount of torque or downward-turning force is 3 newton-meters (N·m). To keep the arm motionless in this position, the elbow flexors must exert an equal and opposite torque or upward-directed turning force of 3 N·m.

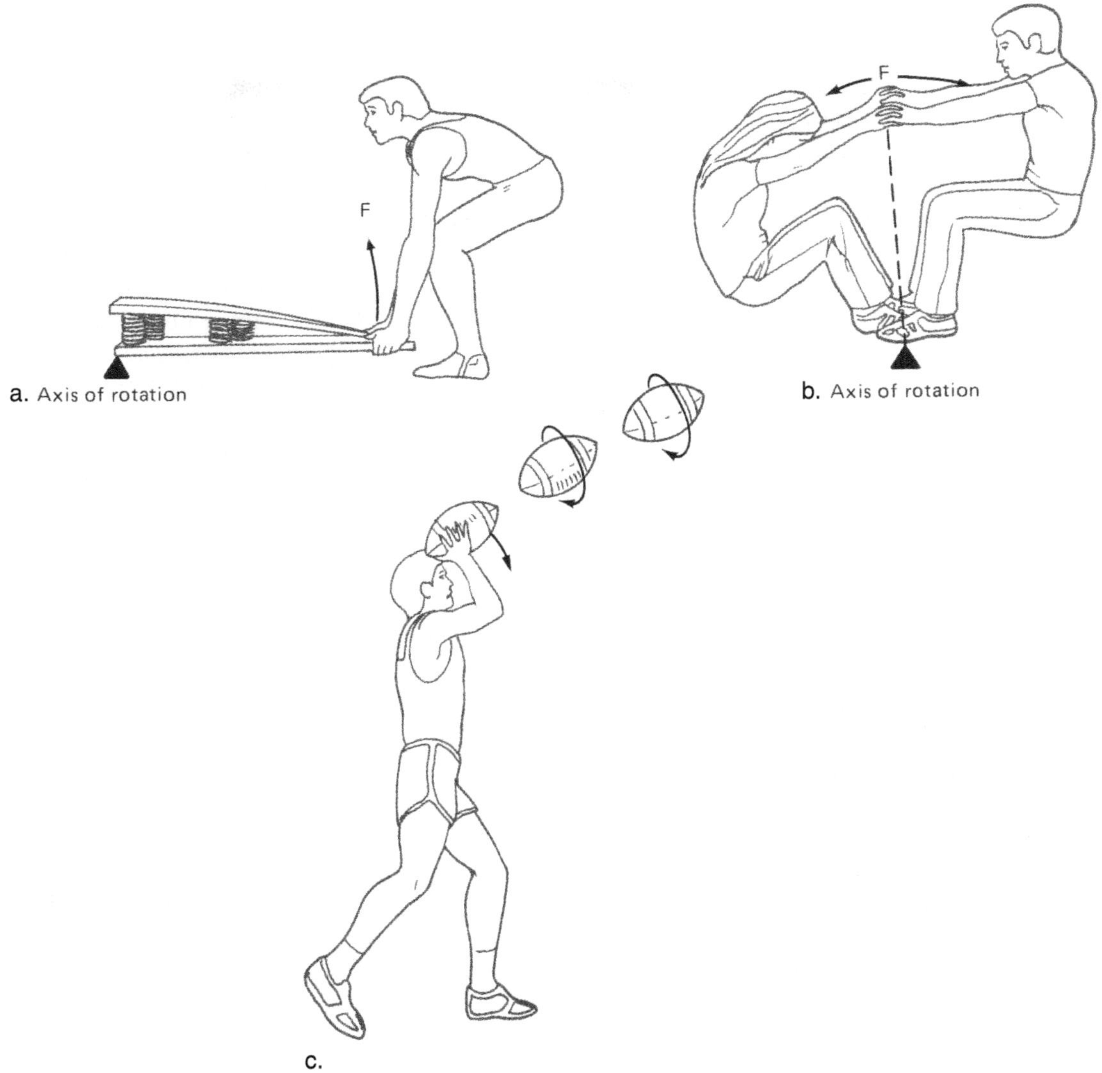

Figure 13.1 Examples of the application of eccentric force.

Because torque is the product of force and the length of the moment arm, it may be modified by changing either the force or the moment arm. Torque may be increased by increasing the magnitude of the force or by increasing the length of the moment arm. Decreasing either of these factors will produce a decrease in torque. In the preceding example, for instance, if the magnitude of the weight held in the hand were decreased to 6 N, the torque would also decrease, in this case to 2 N·m. Conversely, increasing the weight would increase the torque. If, however, the weight is increased but is moved closer to the axis (the elbow), the torque produced by the heavier weight would be reduced through reducing the length of the moment arm.

It is important to emphasize that the moment arm is the *perpendicular* distance from the direction of force to the axis of rotation. In the example just given, the moment arm length was the same as the length of the forearm because the horizontal forearm was perpendicular to the vertical direction of the force, and therefore the forearm length was equal to the perpendicular distance from the force direction to the axis. If the arm were in some position other than the horizontal, its length would no longer be equal to the moment arm distance between the force direction and axis. Suppose the forearm's position is shifted from the horizontal to one of 45 degrees of flexion with the horizontal. Now the force line of the weight is not at right angles to the forearm (Figure 13.3). This means that the length of the moment arm is no longer the length of the forearm because, by definition, the moment arm is the perpendicular distance from the direction or line of force to the axis of motion. The moment arm now is considerably shorter. Using trigonometric relations (see Chapter 10), we find that the moment arm length is 0.2 m. Consequently, the torque decreases from 3 N·m to 1.9 N·m, and the amount of muscular effort needed to counteract this downward force decreases proportionately.

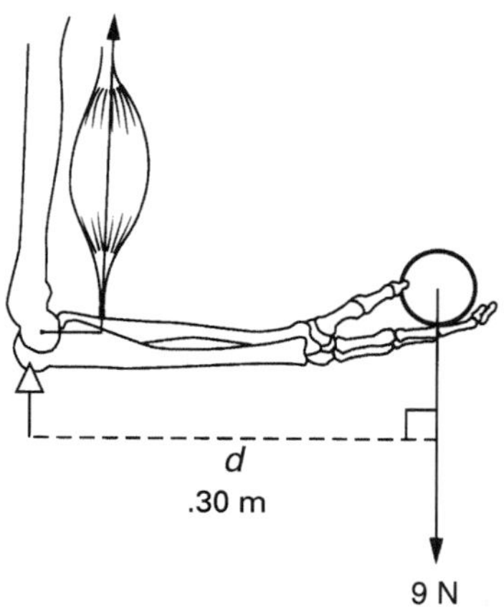

Figure 13.2 A weight applied at some distance (d) from the axis (elbow) produces torque.

In the human body, the mass or weight of a segment cannot be altered instantaneously. Therefore, the torque of a segment that is due to gravitational force can be changed only by changing the length of the moment arm in relation to the axis. This is done by moving a body segment so that the force line of the weight is closer to or farther from

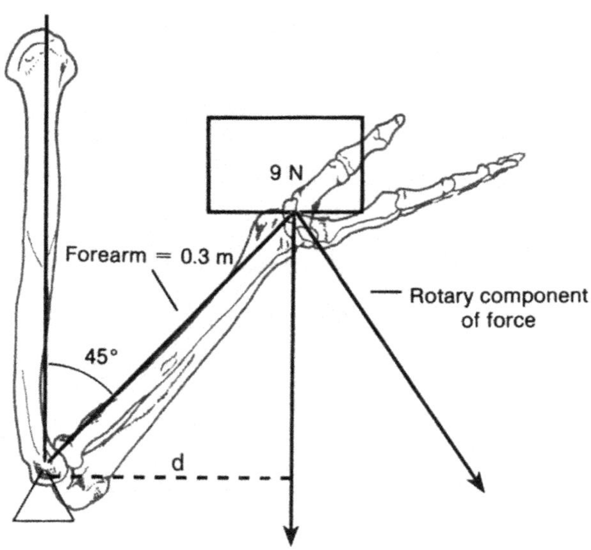

Figure 13.3 The torque of the 9-N weight about the elbow joint is the product of the rotary component of the weight and the distance from the rotary component to the axis of rotation.

the axis. The effect of doing this is quite apparent in the stages of the sit-up. Compare the gravitational torque on the trunk when the trunk is just leaving the floor with the torque when the trunk is at a 30-degree angle from the floor (Figure 13.4).

Muscle forces also exert torque on rotating segments. The amount of torque depends on both the magnitude of the muscle force and the moment arm length. Unlike gravitational torque, each of these factors can be altered. The moment arm length depends on the point of insertion of the muscle and the position of the body segment at any point in a given motion. Figure 13.5 shows how the moment arm of the biceps changes for every change of arm position during elbow flexion. The magnitude of the force of the muscle contributing to the torque changes also as its length, tension, and angle of pull change.

With changes in muscle angle of pull, the magnitude of the force effectively producing torque also changes. When muscle force vectors are resolved into their two components, it can be seen that only the rotary component—that which is perpendicular to the mechanical axis of bone—is actually a factor in torque production. The stabilizing component of the muscle force acts along the mechanical axis of the bone through the axis of rotation; thus this component is not an eccentric, or off-center, force and cannot contribute to torque. It has a moment arm length equal to zero. Once a muscle force is resolved into a rotary and a stabilizing component, the moment arm is the distance between the axis of rotation and the point of application of the rotary component of the muscle force. Because the rotary component of any known force can be calculated trigonometrically,

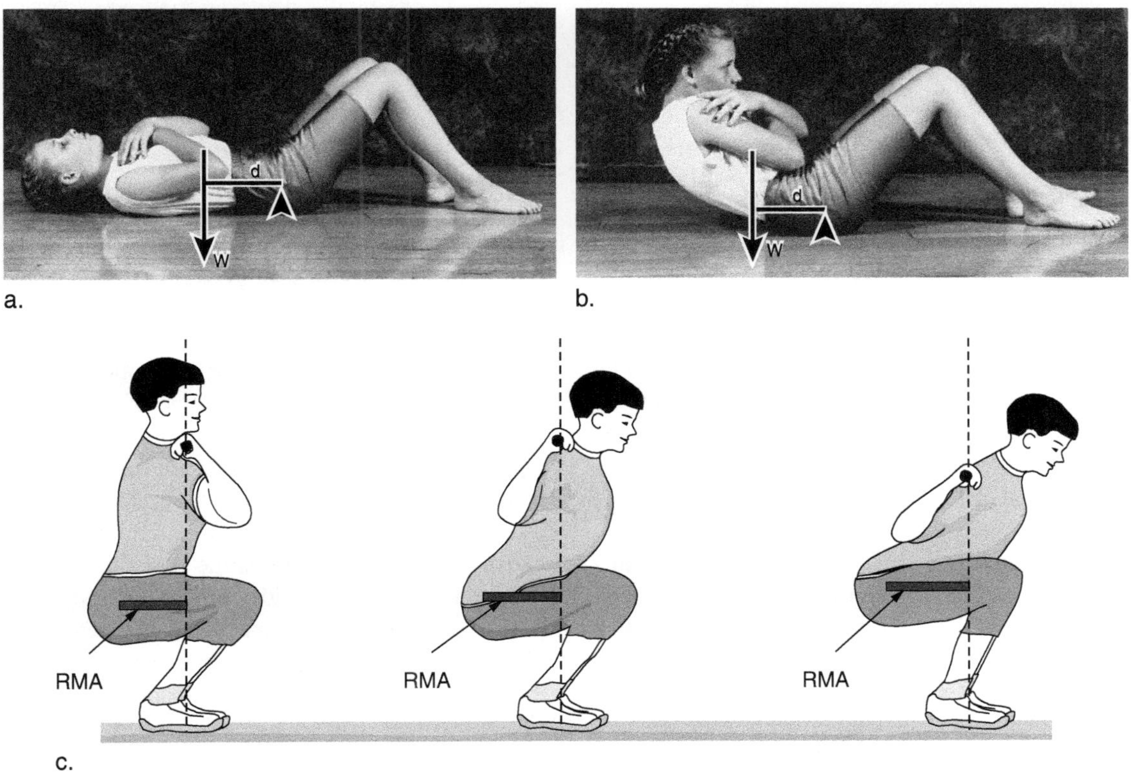

Figure 13.4 Gravitational torque *d* decreases in going from (a) to (b) as the force line moves closer to the axis. The torque is 0 at 90 degrees. In figure c, the resistance moment arms (RMA) from the bar to the lower back are indicated. Notice that the moment arm for the third position is the longest.

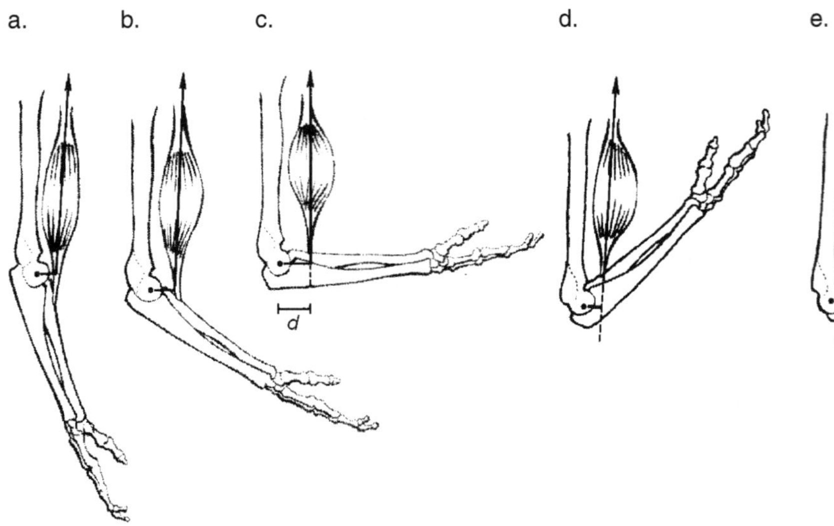

Figure 13.5 The biceps at various points of elbow flexion, showing variations in the moment arm. *Source:* From *Williams and Lissner: Biomechanics of Human Motion* (2nd ed.), by B. F. Leveau. Copyright © 1977, W. B. Saunders, Orlando, FL. Reprinted by permission.

given the angle between the line of force and the mechanical axis, torque can be calculated as the product of the rotary component of the force (Fy) times the moment arm along the lever (d; see Figure 13.9). In the example used earlier, the angle between the line of force for the weight and the mechanical axis of the bone is 45 degrees. Using the angle and the 9-N magnitude of the force, the rotary component of the force is calculated to be 6.4 N. When multiplied by the 0.3-m length of the moment arm, the torque is 1.9 N·m, the same value found when calculating the length of the true moment arm in Figure 13.3. Either method of finding torque is satisfactory.

The important thing to remember from this discussion is that the turning effect, or torque, produced on objects free to rotate depends on two factors: the magnitude of the applied force and the perpendicular distance from the force vector to the axis. Change in turning effect occurs when either of these factors is altered. Shortening the moment arm distance or decreasing the force magnitude will decrease the torque. Lengthening the moment arm or increasing the force magnitude will increase the turning effect and consequently the necessary effort to resist it.

Summation of Torques

The sum of two or more torques may result in no motion, linear motion, or rotary motion. When equal parallel eccentric forces are applied in the same direction on opposite sides of the center of rotation of an object, either no motion or linear motion will occur. An example of no motion is two children balanced on a seesaw. When the equal parallel forces are adequate to overcome the resistance of the object, linear motion will occur. This could be the situation with paddlers in a canoe, with one paddling on the port side and the other on the starboard side. When equal and opposite parallel forces are exerted on opposite sides of the axis of rotation, rotary motion will occur. The effect of equal parallel forces acting in opposite directions is called a *couple,* or *force couple.* An example of this type of movement is steering a car when both hands are used on opposite sides of the wheel (Figure 13.6). Another example is that of turning in a rowboat by simultaneously pulling

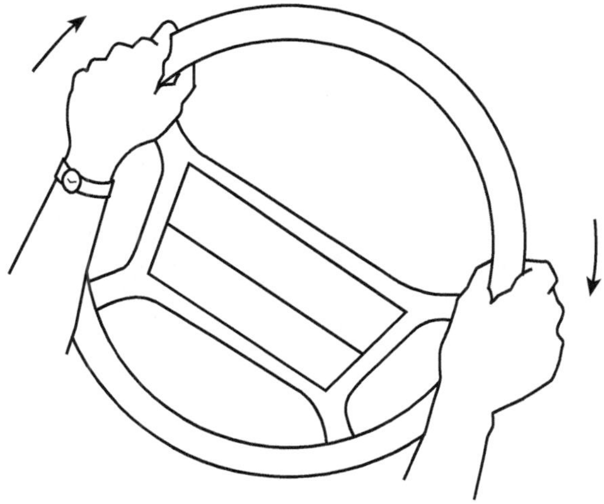

Figure 13.6 When one steers with two hands, the hands act as a force couple.

on the handle of one oar while pushing on the handle of the other.

There are many examples in the human body in which two muscles rotate a bone by acting cooperatively as a force couple; for instance, trapezius II and the lower portion of serratus anterior are a force couple, rotating the scapula upward. Trapezius II and IV, acting on the two extremities of the spine of the scapula, similarly serve as a force couple to help rotate the scapula upward, as do the oblique abdominals in acting to rotate the trunk (Figure 13.7).

Principle of Torques

It is common for more than one torque to act on a body at any given time. The resultant effect of these torques is expressed in the principle of the summation of torques, which states that the **resultant torques of a force system must be equal to the sum of the torques of the individual forces of the system about the same point.** Because torques are vector quantities, the summation must consider both magnitude and direction. The direction of rotation is expressed as either clockwise or counterclockwise direction. Clockwise torques are usually labeled as negative, and counterclockwise torques as positive. Their signs must be accounted for when they are summed.

When the sum of counterclockwise torques equals the sum of clockwise torques, no turning will occur. This idea may also be expressed by stating that rotation will be absent when the sum of the torques of all forces about any point or axis equals zero. When the sum of clockwise torques does not equal the sum of the counterclockwise torques, the resultant turning effect (torque) will be the difference between the two opposing forces and in the direction of the larger.

In Figure 13.8 all the forces are applied perpendicular to the lever. Force A is 1.5 m from the axis, and B is 3 m away. Both A and B are clockwise forces. Force C is a counterclockwise force that also is 3 m away from the axis. The sum of these torques produces a resultant torque of 22.5 N·m in a clockwise direction about the center of rotation.

When an eccentric force is applied at an angle to the lever other than 90 degrees, the moment arm is not along the lever line. Before the torque can be found, the length of the moment arm must be determined. This can be done using trigonometric functions. An example of this procedure is shown in the following problem:

> What muscular force F pulling at an angle of 25 degrees would be required to keep the abducted arm in a position of 20 degrees with the

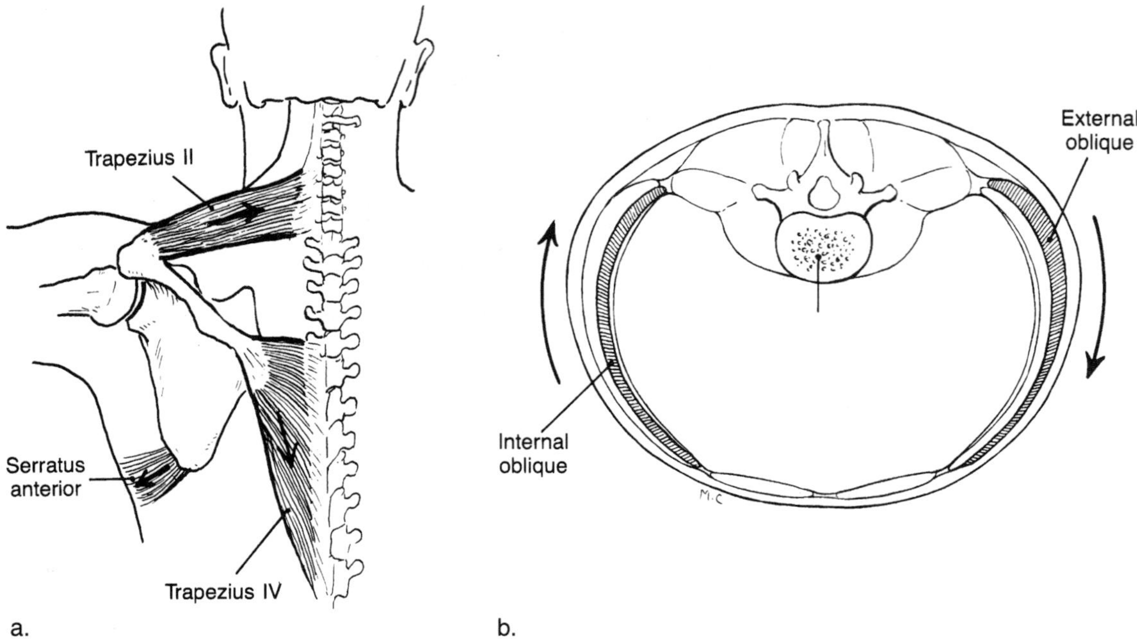

Figure 13.7 (a) Two force couples acting on the scapula to rotate it upward. Trapezius II and lower serratus anterior are an excellent example. Trapezius II and the lower fibers of IV also tend to act as a torce couple although their pulls are not in opposite directions. (b) A cross section of the trunk in which the oblique abdominal muscles act as a force couple to rotate the trunk.

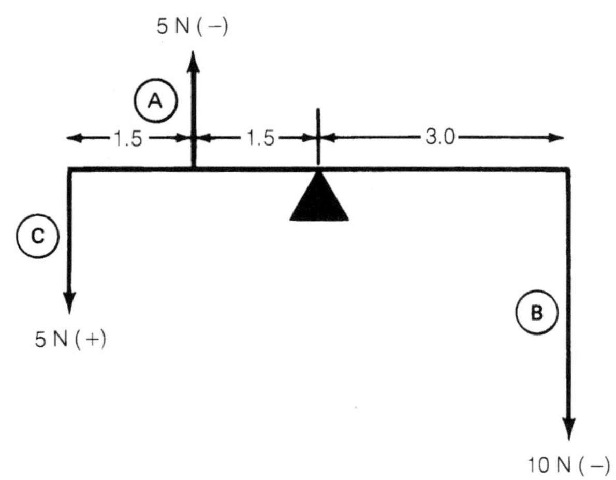

Figure 13.8 Summation of moments. The resultant moment about a point is equal to the sum of the moments of the individual forces about the same point. Clockwise moments are negative, and counterclockwise moments are positive. The sum of the moments about the fulcrum on this diagram is 22.5 newton-meters in a clockwise direction.

horizontal? The muscle inserts 10 cm from the shoulder joint. The arm weighs 50 N and its center of gravity is located 30 cm from the shoulder. A 45-N weight is held in the hand 60 cm from the shoulder joint. *Note:* For the arm to be held stationary, the sum of the counterclockwise torques must equal the clockwise torques ($\Sigma CCW = \Sigma CW$). (See Figure 13.9 for solution.)

THE LEVER

A simple machine that operates according to the principle of torques is the **lever.** A lever is a rigid bar that can rotate about a fixed point when a force is applied to overcome a resistance. When they move, levers serve two important functions. They are used either to overcome a resistance larger than the magnitude of the effort applied or to increase the speed and range of motion through which a resistance can be moved. When there is no motion, the torque produced by the effort and the torque produced by the resistance are equal and the lever system is said to be balanced.

External Levers

We use levers every day of our lives. In the workshop or around the house, pry bar, wrench, and wheelbarrow are levers. What do these implements have in common? Even though their shapes vary and their structures differ in complexity, each of these is a rigid bar. When a force is applied to one of them, it turns about a fixed point known as a **fulcrum,** and it overcomes a resistance that may, in some cases, be no more than its own weight. All the levers mentioned are designed to enable use of a relatively small force to overcome a relatively large resistance. In levers such as these, the range of movement of the resistance is relatively slight, whereas the range of movement of the effort is large. The crowbar, for instance, lifts a rock only a few centimeters, whereas the handle moves through a much larger distance. In other words, the force to overcome a considerable resistance is gained at the expense of range of motion.

The striking implements used in sports are levers that do the opposite of this. The golf club, for instance, is used to gain range of motion at the expense of force. The length of the shaft enables the club head to travel through a large arc of motion, but it is used to overcome the relatively slight resistance of the weight of the club itself. Tennis and squash rackets, baseball bats, hockey sticks, and fencing foils are other examples of levers used to gain distance at the expense of force. These levers do not save the strength of the user, as do the household levers mentioned, but they increase the user's range and speed of movement. By striking a ball with a racket, for instance, the striker can impart more speed to it and send it a greater distance than could be done by striking it with the hand. This is because the head of the racket travels a greater distance, and therefore at a greater speed, than the hand alone is able to do.

A still different kind of lever is seen in the seesaw on the playground, the scales in the laboratory, and the mobile hanging in the art gallery. These levers gain neither force nor distance but provide for a balancing of weights. If the loads are equal, they will balance each other when they are equidistant from the fulcrum. If they are unequal, they will balance only if the heavier load is placed closer to the fulcrum. There is an exact relationship between the magnitude of the weights and their respective distances from the fulcrum, so that when the torques are summed, the resultant is zero.

This kind of lever may also be used to balance a force and a load. The skier carrying skis over one shoulder, balanced by a hand holding the other end, is an example. The amount of effort exerted by the hand depends on what portion of the ski is in contact with the shoulder. If the weight of the skis is evenly distributed on each side of the shoulder, the hand needs to exert little or no effort.

Anatomical Levers

But where in the human body do we have anything even faintly resembling a punch can opener, hockey stick, or seesaw? When we recognize each of these levers as a rigid bar that turns about a

How much muscle force is needed to hold the arm and the 45-N weight in this position?

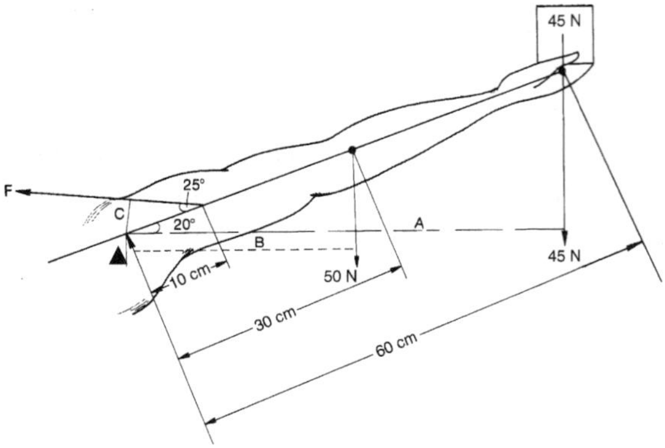

Solution Finding Moment Arm

▲ = axis
F = force of muscle
A = moment arm for 45 = N weight
B = moment arm for 50 = N weight
C = moment arm for F
To balance, clockwise torques must equal counterclockwise torques.

1. Clockwise torques
   a. 45 N × A = 45 N × (60 cm × cos 20)
      45 N × (60 cm × .940) = 2538 N·cm
   b. 50 N × B = 50 N × (30 cm × cos 20)
      50 N × (30 cm × .940) = 1410 N·cm
2. Counterclockwise torques
   a. F × C = F × (10 cm × sin 25)
      F × (10 cm × .423) = F × 4.23 cm
3. CCW = CW
   a. F × 4.23 cm = 2538 N·cm + 1410 N·cm
   b. F × 4.23 cm = 3948 N·cm
   c. $F = \dfrac{3948 \text{ N·cm}}{4.23 \text{ cm}}$
   d. F = 933.3 N

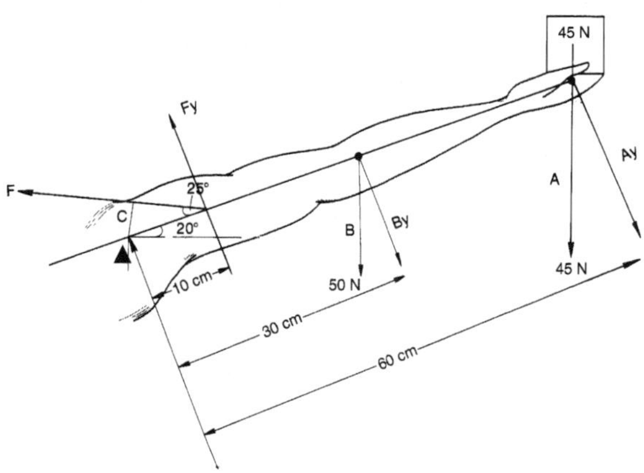

Solution Finding Rotary Components

A = 45 N force B = 50 N force

1. Clockwise torques
   a. A_y = 45 N × cos 20
      A_y = 45 N × .940
      A_y = 42.3 N
   b. B_y = 50 N × cos 20
      B_y = 50 N × .940
      B_y = 47 N
2. CCW = CW
   a. F_y × 10 cm = (A_y × 60 cm) + (B_y × 30 cm)
   b. F_y × 10 cm = (42.3 N × 60 cm) + (47 N × 30 cm)
   c. F_y × 10 cm = 3948 N·cm
   d. F_y = 3948 N·cm/10 cm = 394.8 N
   e. F = Fy/sin 25 = 394.8 N·m/.423
   f. F = 933.3 N

Figure 13.9 Summation of torques using trigonometric functions. The amount of muscle force needed to counteract the force of gravity in this example is 933.3 N.

fulcrum when force is applied to it, it is then apparent that nearly *every bone* in the skeleton can be looked upon as a lever. The bone itself serves as the rigid bar, the joint as the fulcrum, and the contracting muscles as the force. A large segment of the body, such as the trunk, the upper extremity, or the lower extremity, can likewise act as a single lever if it is used as a rigid unit. When the entire arm is raised sideward, for instance, it is acting as a simple lever. The center of motion in the shoulder joint serves as the fulcrum. The effort is supplied mainly by the deltoid muscle, and the resistance in this instance is the weight of the arm itself. The point at which the effort is applied to the lever is approximately the point at which the deltoid inserts into the humerus, and the point at which the resistance is applied is the center of gravity of the extended arm. If a weight is held in the hand, the resistance point is then the center of gravity of the arm plus its load and is located closer to the hand than before. If a relatively heavy weight is lifted, for practical purposes the weight of the arm may be disregarded and the resistance point may be assumed to be the center of the object's point of contact with the hand.

Anatomical levers do not necessarily resemble bars. The skull, shoulder blade, and vertebrae are notable exceptions to the definition. The resistance point, also, may be difficult to identify, especially in the seesaw type of lever. It is not always easy to tell whether the resistance is the weight of the lever itself or is the resistance afforded by antagonistic muscles and fasciae that are put on a steadily increasing stretch as the movement progresses. For instance, when the head is turned easily to the left, the resistance point may be regarded as the center of gravity of the head. We can only guess at the approximate location of this. If the turning of the head is resisted by the pressure of someone's hand against the left side of the chin, the resistance point is the midpoint of the contact area. If the head is turned without external resistance but is forced to the limit of motion, resistance to the movement is afforded by the antagonistic rotators, and possibly by the ligaments and fasciae. The resistance point in such a case is the midpoint of the area over which these resisting forces act on the head. As in the first example, the location of this point can only be estimated.

Lever Arms

Lever arms are commonly defined as the portion of the lever between the fulcrum and the force points. The effort arm is the distance between the fulcrum and the effort point, and the resistance arm is the distance between the fulcrum and the resistance point. These definitions are valid, however, only when the effort and resistance are applied at right angles to the lever. When the effort and resistance are applied at some angle other than 90 degrees to the lever, these definitions are inaccurate. A better definition of a lever arm that applies regardless of the angle of force application is one synonymous to that of a moment arm. Indeed, a lever arm is a moment arm. In a lever the perpendicular distance between the fulcrum and line of force of the effort is the *effort arm (EA)*. Similarly, the perpendicular distance between the fulcrum and the line of resistance force is the *resistance arm (RA)*. In Figure 13.16, *EA* is the effort arm and *RA* is the resistance arm.

Classification of Levers

Three points on the lever have been identified: the point about which it turns, the point at which effort is applied to it, and the point at which the resistance to its movement is applied or concentrated. Because there are three points, there are three possible arrangements of these points. Any one of the three may be situated between the other two. The arrangement of these three points provides the basis for the classification of levers.

First-Class Levers

In a first-class lever, the axis lies between the effort and the resistance (Figure 13.10a). The mechanical advantage of the first-class lever is balance. The first-class lever also can be used to magnify the effects of the effort or to increase the speed and range of motion on the basis of the relative lengths of the

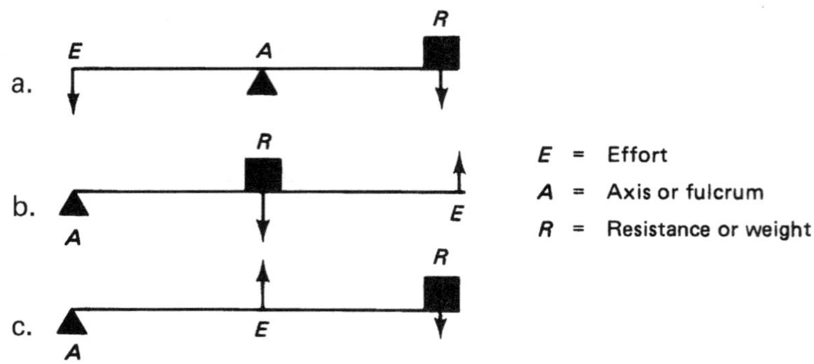

Figure 13.10 Levers: (a) a lever of the first class; (b) a lever of the second class; (c) a lever of the third class.

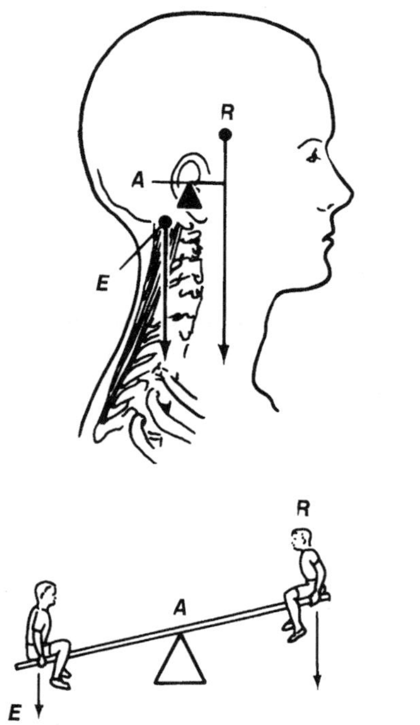

Figure 13.11 The head acting as a first-class lever like the seesaw. *A* = the approximate position of the axis or fulcrum; *E* = the point where the force is applied; *R* = the approximate point where the resistance is concentrated.

effort moment arm (*EA*) and the resistance moment arm (*RA*). Examples of external first-class levers are the seesaw, balance scale, crowbar, scissors, and automobile jack (Figure 13.11).

The head, tipping forward and backward, is a good example of a first-class lever in the body (Figure 13.11). The effort is supplied by the extensors of the head, notably the splenius and upper portions of the semispinalis, and is applied to the head at the base of the skull. The resistance to the movement is furnished by the weight of the head itself, together with the tension of the antagonistic muscles and fasciae, as the limit of motion is approached.

Another first-class lever is seen in the foot when it is not being used for weight bearing, as when the knees are crossed in the sitting position. As the soleus pulls upward on the heel, the foot plantar flexes at the ankle joint where the fulcrum is situated. The resistance seems to be provided by the tonus of the dorsiflexor muscles.

The forearm is another example of a first-class lever *when it is being extended by the triceps muscle against a resistance* (Figure 13.12). The fulcrum is situated at the elbow joint, the effort is applied at the olecranon process, and the resistance point is located at the forearm's center of gravity when no external resistance is present, and at the hand when the latter is pushing against an external resistance. Internal resistance does not appear to be a factor in this movement.

Second-Class Levers

In a second-class lever, the resistance lies between the axis and the effort (Figure 13.10b). In this lever, the *EA* is always longer than the *RA*. This arrangement has the advantage of magnifying the

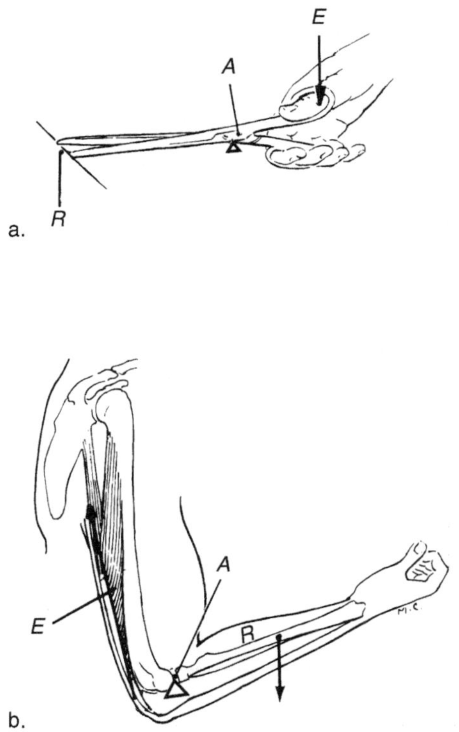

Figure 13.12 The forearm acting as a first-class lever, similar to a pair of paper shears.

effects of the effort so that it takes less force to move the resistance. Its disadvantage is that range of motion is sacrificed. Examples of external second-class levers are the wheelbarrow, door (effort applied at the knob), and nutcracker. Whether or not there are any second-class levers in the body seems to be a controversial matter among anatomists and kinesiologists. Some claim that when the foot is being plantar flexed in a weight-bearing position, as when rising on the toes, it is a second-class lever. The fulcrum is said to be at the point of contact with the ground, the effort point at the heel where the tendon of Achilles attaches, and the resistance at the ankle joint where the weight of the body is transferred to the foot.

There are numerous second-class levers involving body segments if those actions where gravity supplies the effort for the movement and muscles control or resist the movement through eccentric contraction are included. The forearm in slow downward extension is an example. The fulcrum is at the elbow joint, the effort may be considered to be applied at the center of gravity of the forearm, and the resistance at the insertion of the elbow flexor, which for this example is considered to be the brachialis. The brachialis through eccentric contraction resists the downward-directed weight of the arm (Figure 13.13). Another example is the slow lowering of the leg at the knee from an extended to a flexed position. The fulcrum is at the knee joint, the effort is the lower leg applied at its center of gravity, and the resistance is the eccentric contraction of the quadriceps at its point of insertion on the tibial tuberosity.

Third-Class Levers

In a third-class lever, the effort lies between the axis and the resistance (see Figure 13.10c). In this lever, *RA* is always the longer of the two moment arms. This means that it will take greater effort to overcome a given resistance. However, a very small motion by the effort will produce a large motion in the resistance. The advantage of the third-class lever is speed and range of motion at the expense of force.

There are not many examples of external third-class levers. One example is a screen door with a spring closing. There are, however, many examples of anatomical third-class levers. Most body segments that are moved by muscular effort fall into this class. The forearm is a good example of a third-class lever when it is being flexed by the biceps and the brachialis (Figure 13.14). Another third-class lever is seen in the example cited earlier—namely, the arm as it is abducted by the deltoid muscle (Figure 13.15).

The Principle of Levers

A lever of any class will balance when the product of the effort and the effort arm equals the product of the resistance and the resistance arm. This is known as the **principle of levers.** It enables us to calculate the amount of effort needed to balance a known resistance by means of a known lever or to

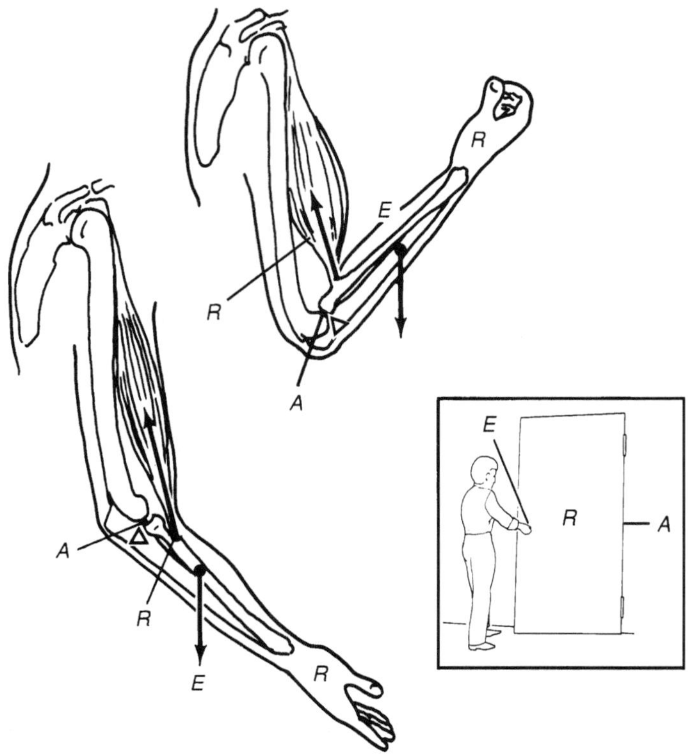

Figure 13.13 The forearm acting as a second-class lever, similar to pushing open a door.

calculate the point at which to place the fulcrum to balance a known resistance with a given effort. If any three of the four values are known, the remaining one can be calculated by using the following equation:

$$E \times EA = R \times RA$$

(effort times effort arm equals resistance times resistance arm)

This equation restates a principle already studied under the summation of torques. When the torques in one direction equal the torques in the opposite direction, equilibrium exists. $E \times EA$ is a torque, as is $R \times RA$. When applied to Figure 13.16, this means that it will be possible to balance the weight in the hand when the product of the weight and the perpendicular distance from its vector line of action to the fulcrum ($R \times RA$) equals the product of the muscle effort and the perpendicular distance from its vector line of action to the fulcrum ($E \times EA$).

The lever equation also shows the importance of lever arm lengths in determining the amount of effort needed to balance a given resistance. If *EA* is lengthened while $R \times RA$ remains constant, the amount of effort needed to balance the lever must decrease. If, on the other hand, *RA* is increased, the amount of effort must increase. For this reason, second-class levers require less effort to balance or move heavier resistances, whereas third-class levers require more effort than the resistance they must balance or move (see Figures 13.14 and 13.15). The first-class lever may have either a longer *EA* or *RA*, depending on the placement of the fulcrum (see Figures 13.11 and 13.12).

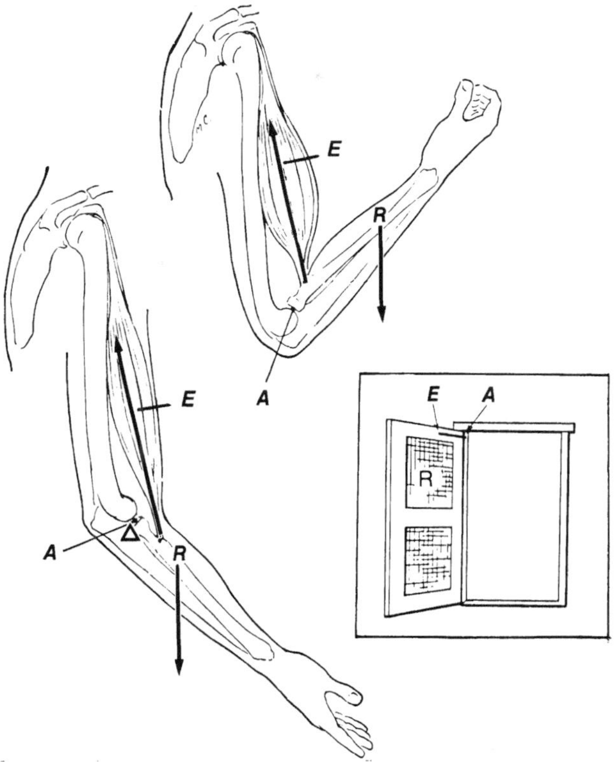

Figure 13.14 The forearm acting as a third-class lever, similar to a screen door.

A lever whose effort arm is the longer of the two moment arms, whether it be a first- or second-class lever, is said to favor force. Less effort is required to overcome a resistance with this kind of lever than it would take to overcome the same resistance without the aid of the lever. This advantage is gained at the expense of speed and range of movement. The heavier resistance will always move through a smaller distance than the effort (Figure 13.17). Conversely, a lever whose resistance arm is longer, whether it be a first- or third-class lever, is said to favor speed and distance. However, more effort is required to move it than would be the case if the relative lengths of the effort and resistance arms were reversed. Furthermore, an object of negligible weight can be moved a greater distance and more rapidly by this kind of lever than it could without the aid of the lever.

Relation of Speed to Range in Movements of Levers

The reader will have noticed that in the foregoing discussion of levers, the terms *speed* and *range* were usually linked together. There is a reason for this. In angular movements, speed and range are interdependent. For instance, if two third-class levers of different lengths each move through a 40-degree angle at the same angular velocity, the tip of the longer lever will be traveling a greater distance or range than the tip of the shorter lever. Because it covers this distance in the same amount of time it takes the tip of the shorter lever to travel the shorter distance, the former must be moving faster than the latter. This is easily seen if the shorter lever is superimposed on the longer, as in Figure 13.18. Here the shorter lever *AB* has been

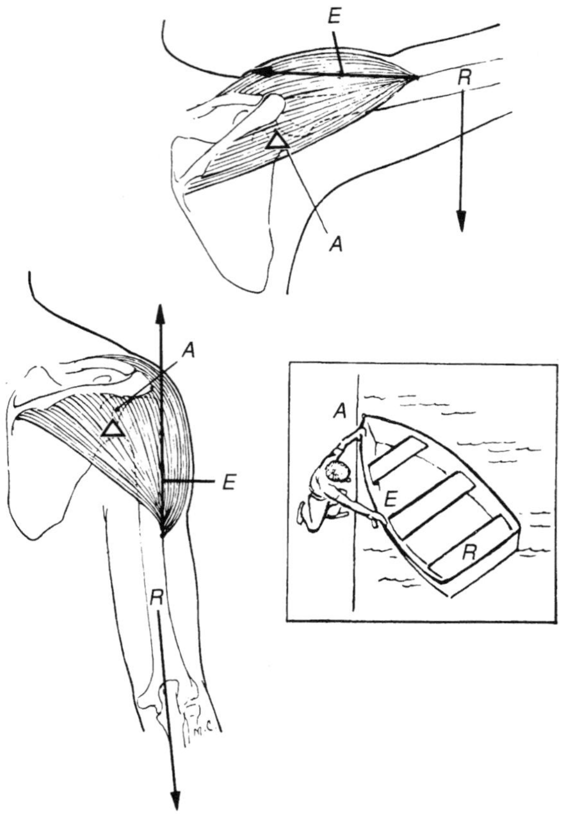

Figure 13.15 The humerus acting as a third-class lever, somewhat like a boat being pulled alongside the dock.

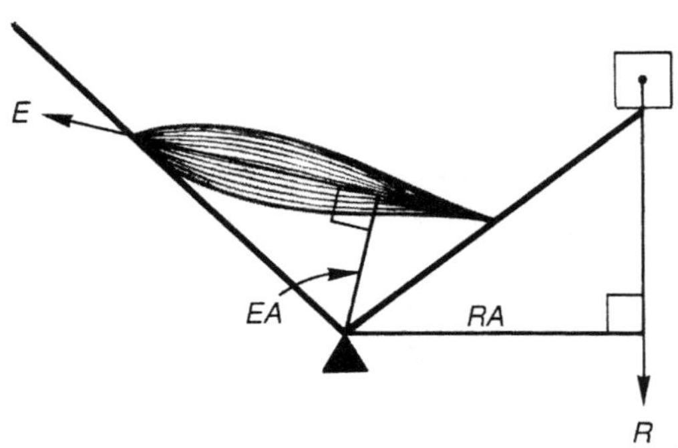

Figure 13.16 Lever arms, like moment arms, are the perpendicular distance between the fulcrum and the force line.

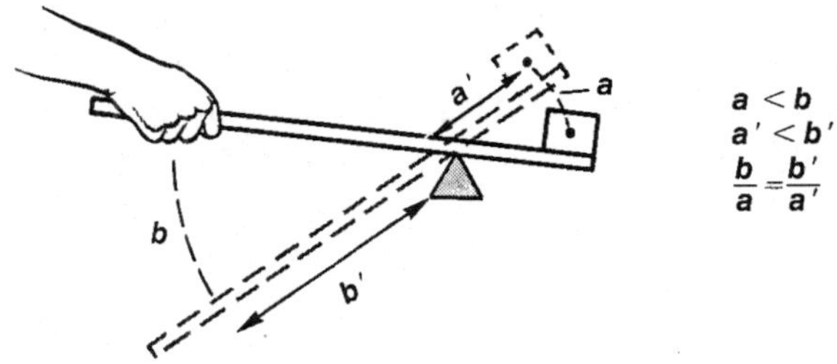

Figure 13.17 The range of motion increases as the lever arm length increases.

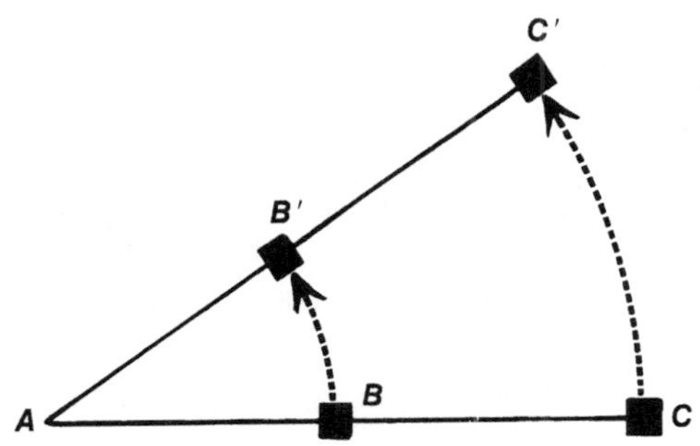

Figure 13.18 Comparison of a long and a short lever turning the same number of degrees. It takes B the same amount of time to reach B' that it takes C to reach C'.

superimposed on the longer lever AC. The levers are moving from the horizontal position to the diagonal one. Because point C travels to its new position C' in the same time it takes B to travel to B', point C must obviously be moving farther and faster than point B. This is the same relationship that was discussed in Chapter 11. The linear kinematics at the end of a lever vary with the length of the radius. Thus, the greater the length of the lever, the greater the linear displacement, velocity, and acceleration that occur at the distal end point of the lever.

The effort arms in the skeletal lever systems of the human body are determined by the point of muscle attachment, usually close to the proximal end of the lever, and the muscle angle of pull. Because of these two factors, with few exceptions the effort arm in skeletal levers is shorter than the resistance arm. Thus anatomical levers tend to favor speed and range of movement at the expense of effort. Examples of this preference are the throwing of a baseball or the kicking of a soccer ball. The hand in the one case and the foot in the other travel through a relatively long distance at considerable speed. Both movements require strong muscular action, even though the balls are relatively light in weight. This type of leverage is the reverse of the kind usually seen in mechanical implements such as the crowbar and the automobile jack, both of which are used to move heavy weights a relatively short distance. Sports implements that may serve as levers in themselves or as artificial extensions of the human arm also favor speed and range of movement. Frequently the sport implement, arm, and a large part of the rest of the body act together as a system of levers. In hitting a baseball, for instance, the trunk forms one lever, the upper arms another, the forearms another, and the hands and bat still another. This use of multiple leverage builds up speed at the tip of the bat because the greater this speed, the greater the force that can be imparted to the ball.

Selection of Levers

Skill in motor performance depends on the effective selection and use of levers, both internal and external. Long golf clubs are selected for distance, and shorter clubs for accuracy at close range. Heavy baseball bats are chosen by those with the strength to swing them, whereas children are often taught tennis with short-handled rackets. In most instances external levers are designed for a specific purpose and are selected accordingly. The levers of the human body, on the other hand, are not designed for one action or purpose. Body parts or segments may be held in numerous positions for any given joint action and thus provide a great variety of lever arrangements. Consequently, skill depends on the right choice of joint axis, joint action, and moment arm length. In all three instances in Figure 13.19, the ball in the hand is carried forward by virtue of the counterclockwise (as seen from above) rotation of the pelvis that takes place at the left hip joint. The pelvis carries the trunk with it, but no movement occurs in any joint other than the left hip. In all three positions the resistance moment arm for the action is the perpendicular distance between the hip axis and the line of action of the resistance (the weight of the ball). However, the resistance moment arm is a different length in each situation. It is smallest in (a) and largest in (c). Consequently, when the angular velocity is the same in each instance, the linear velocity of the ball is largest in (c) and smallest in (a; see Figure 13.19). Similarly, if flexion of the shoulder is the joint action, the position of the arm that will provide the greatest linear velocity to the object in the hand at the moment of release is one in which the elbow is extended and the arm is perpendicular to the desired direction of flight (Figure 13.20).

It is not always desirable to choose the longest lever, however. The positioning of body parts to form short levers enhances the angular velocity of the levers while sacrificing linear speed and range of motion at the end of the lever. And although forming the longest possible lever can increase speed and range of motion at the end of the lever, the strength needed to maintain the desired angular velocity increases as the lever lengthens. This

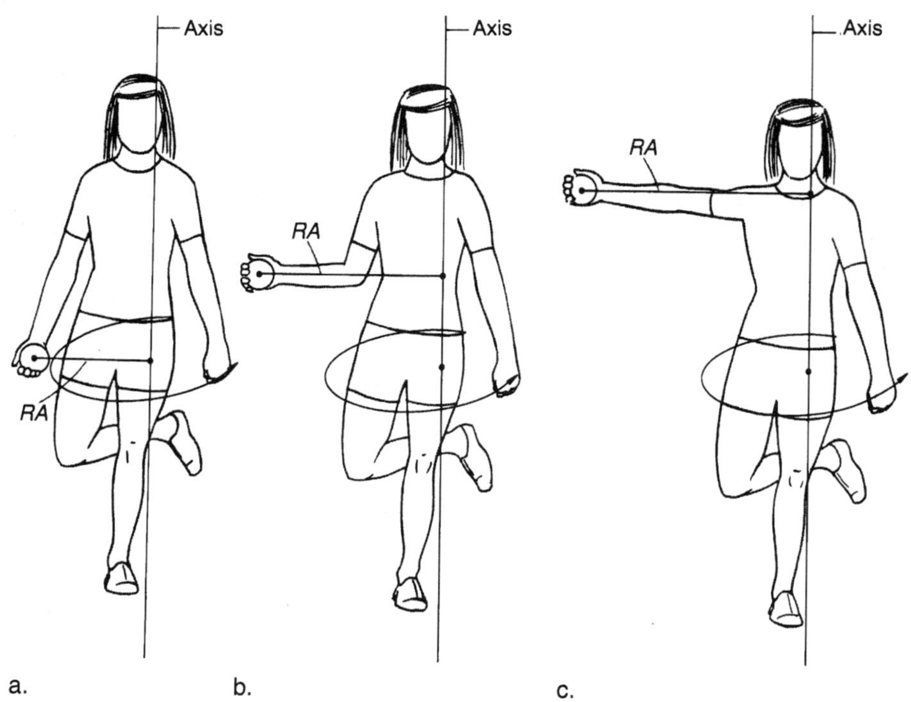

Figure 13.19 The length of the *RA* determines the linear velocity at the end of the lever. In the positions pictured, when the pelvis rotates to the left, the linear velocity of the ball is least in (a) and greatest in (c). The movement occurs at the left hip and results in the lower extremity being medially rotated, relative to the pelvis.

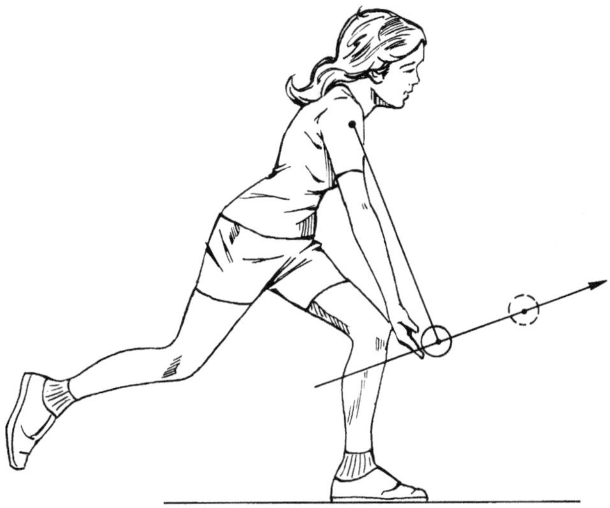

Figure 13.20 A straight arm perpendicular to the desired line of flight provides the greatest linear velocity to the ball when the joint action is shoulder flexion.

is why the tennis player may flex the elbow in the forehand drive or the batter may "choke up" when swinging a heavy bat. As the magnitude of the resistance to be moved increases, the more the performer may want to shorten the lever. Moving very large weights produces very high levels of external torque. This torque can be reduced by decreasing the *RA*. One should not attempt to move heavy loads by using a long lever and high movement speeds.

Mechanical Advantage of Levers

Machines are judged good if they are efficient, poor if they are inefficient. How is the efficiency of a machine measured? Because the machines used in industry and in the workshop are usually for the purpose of magnifying force, it is customary to measure their efficiency in terms of their *mechanical advantage*—in other words, their ability to magnify force. Another way to express this ability is to state the "output" of the machine relative to its "input." In levers this is the ratio between the effort applied to the lever and the resistance overcome by the lever. It may be expressed in terms of the following equation: Mechanical advantage equals the ratio of the resistance overcome to the effort applied, or, simply,

$$MA = \frac{R}{E}$$

Because the balanced lever equation may also be expressed as

$$\frac{R}{E} = \frac{EA}{RA}$$

the mechanical advantage may be expressed in terms of the ratio of the effort arm to the resistance arm. Hence, if

$$MA = \frac{R}{E}$$

it also holds that

$$MA = \frac{EA}{RA}$$

When a muscle is said to have poor leverage, it means that it has poor mechanical advantage. In other words, the effort arm of the lever on which it is acting is short compared with the resistance arm.

There are four functions of a simple machine:

Balance two or more forces
Favor force production
Favor speed and range of motion
Change the direction of the applied force

Depending on the relative lengths of *EA* and *RA*, a lever can achieve one or more of these functions.

Identification and Analysis of Levers

Figures 13.11 to 13.15 depict certain anatomical levers and their mechanical counterparts. These should enable the student to understand the principle of leverage as it applies in the human body and to see how the anatomical levers compare with the levers of everyday life. For each of these levers and for every lever that the student observes, these questions should be answered: (1) What are the locations of the fulcrum, effort point, and resistance point? (2) At what angle is the effort applied to the lever? (3) At what angle is the resistance applied to the lever? (4) What is the effort arm of the lever? (5) What is the resistance arm of the lever? (6) What are the relative lengths of the effort and resistance arms? (7) What kind of movement does this lever favor? (8) What is the mechanical advantage? (9) What class of lever is this?

NEWTON'S LAWS AND ROTATIONAL EQUIVALENTS

When applied to angular motion, Newton's laws of motion may be stated as follows:

1. A body continues in a state of rest or uniform rotation about its axis unless acted upon by an external torque.
2. The acceleration of a rotating body is directly proportional to the torque causing it, is in the same direction as the torque, and is inversely proportional to the moment of inertia of the body.
3. When a torque is applied by one body to another, the second body will exert an equal and opposite torque on the first.

TABLE 13.1 Analogous Quantities in Linear and Rotary Motion

Unit	Linear Motion	Angular Motion
Distance	s	θ (theta)
Velocity	v	ω (omega)
Acceleration	a	α (alpha)
Mass	m	I (moment of inertia)
Force	F	T (torque)
Force equation	$F = ma$	$T = I\alpha$
Momentum	mv	$I\omega$
Impulse	Ft	Tt
Work	Fs	$T\theta$
Power	Fv	$T\omega$
Kinetic energy	$\frac{1}{2}mv^2$	$\frac{1}{2}I\omega^2$

The laws themselves are analogous to those stated for linear motion. To comprehend their application to angular motion, however, an understanding of the rotary equivalents of linear mass, momentum, and force is necessary. These parallel relationships between linear motion and angular motion quantities become quite apparent when presented side by side, as in Table 13.1.

Moment of Inertia

In the preceding discussion of Newton's laws, the ability of a body to resist change in its state of motion was identified as inertia. The inertia of a body with respect to linear motion was shown to be directly proportional to the mass of the object. The heavier an object is, the greater the force that is required to start it moving and to stop it. This is also true in angular motion. Once they are set in motion, spinning bodies tend to keep spinning. As with linear motion, the amount of force needed to start or stop a spinning object is related to its mass: the heavier the object, the greater the effort that is required to start or stop its rotation. However, an additional factor needs to be considered. As an example, the hammer thrower knows that it takes more effort to start the weight moving in a circular fashion at the end of the wire than it does to start it moving in a linear fashion. It is also true that once the hammer is moving in a circular fashion, it is more difficult to slow it down than if it were moving in a straight line. Therefore, it seems that the hammer's inertia is greater when moving in an angular pattern than when moving in a linear path. Because the mass of the hammer does not change, this increase in inertia must be due to some other element. In the same way that the torque causing rotation depends on the magnitude of force and the distance from the line of action of the force to the the axis, the inertia of a rotary body is affected by both the mass and the distance between the mass and the axis of rotation. A ball rotating on the end of a long string is harder to stop and start than one on a short string. As the distance between the axis and the mass increase, the inertia increases. Thus the size of the angular inertia, called the *moment of inertia, I,* depends on both the quantity of the rotating mass and its distribution around the axis of rotation. The exact nature of this relationship is shown in the equation for the moment of inertia:

$$I = \Sigma mr^2$$

where m is the mass of a particle in the rotating body and r is the perpendicular distance between the mass particle and the axis of rotation. Thus the moment of inertia of an object is the sum of the mass of each of the particles multiplied by the square of the distance to the axis (Figure 13.21). If the mass of an object is concentrated close to the axis of rotation, the object is easier to turn because the radius for each particle is less, thus making I less. Conversely, if the mass is concentrated farther away from the axis, I becomes greater and the rotating body will require more force to start or stop it.

In the human body the mass distribution may be altered by changing the body position, thereby changing the moment of inertia. A runner is able to move the recovery leg forward more rapidly when it is in a flexed position than when it is extended. The mass of the leg is the same in both instances, but it is closer to the axis when the leg is flexed and the moment of inertia is less.

Using a method similar to finding the center of gravity of the body by the segmental method (see Chapter 14, pp. 381–386), Hay (1993) reported the moment of inertia of the human body in some common rotating positions. In the tuck position, I about the body's center of gravity was 3.5 kg·m^2; in the pike position it was 6.5 kg·m^2 and in the layout, 15.0 kg·m^2. The moment of inertia about the hands of the giant swing position was 83.0 kg·m^2. These figures verify that inertia to rotation increases as the mass is distributed farther away from the axis.

When one is interested in the moment of inertia of a specific body segment, it is usually taken

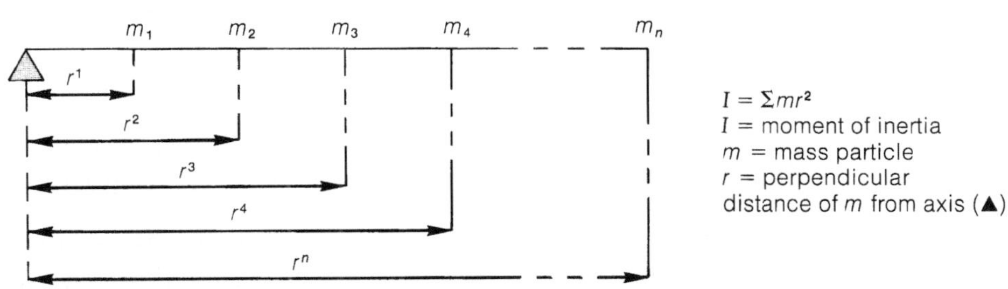

Figure 13.21 The moment of inertia about an axis is the sum of the mass particles multiplied by the square of the distance of each particle from the axis: ($I = \Sigma mr^2$).

about the center of the joint serving as the axis, although other axes may be chosen. If another axis is selected, such as the center of gravity of the segment, I will change accordingly because values of r will be different in the equation $I = \Sigma mr^2$.

Acceleration of Rotating Bodies

The equation for Newton's second law of motion when applied to linear motion was shown to be $F = ma$. The rotational equivalent is $\boldsymbol{T = I\alpha}$—that is, rotary force, or torque (T), is equal to the product of the moment of inertia (I) of the rotating object and the angular acceleration (α). The angular equivalent of linear force is torque, the angular equivalent of mass is the moment of inertia, and the angular equivalent of linear acceleration is angular acceleration. With a little transposing of the equation, it becomes apparent how the rotary equivalent of Newton's second law of motion states that the change in angular velocity (α) is directly proportional to the torque (T) and inversely proportional to the moment of inertia (I)—that is, $\alpha = T/I$.

When a net unbalanced torque is applied to a mass, this mass will begin to accelerate angularly according to the equation

$$T = I\alpha$$

Where T is torque, I is the mass moment of inertia, and α is the angular acceleration. Because angular acceleration is the time rate of change of angular velocity (rad/sec), this equation can be rewritten as

$$T = \frac{I(\omega_f - \omega_i)}{t}$$

$$Tt = I(\omega_f - \omega_i)$$

In other words, the product of a torque and the time over which this torque acts will produce a change in angular velocity of the mass, provided that the distribution of the mass is constant. Called angular impulse, it is the effect of a torque, applied over a given time, on the change of angular velocity of an object with a certain mass and mass distribution. Consider the exercise where you lie on your back and your partner stands above you. You bring your feet upward, and your partner throws your feet downward. During this downward motion, your abdominals are resisting the anterior pelvic girdle rotation. If your partner throws your legs at the same rate each time, then we know the change in angular momentum, specifically, from that initial angular velocity to 0 rad/sec. To stop the downward rotation of your legs quickly will take a relatively large torque (very strong abdominals). However, if you use the whole range of motion to stop the legs before they hit the floor, less torque is required.

Angular Momentum

Momentum is a measure of the force needed to start or stop motion. Objects undergoing angular motion have momentum in the same fashion as objects engaged in linear motion. Linear momentum is the product of mass and velocity. Angular momentum is the product of the angular equivalents of mass and velocity—that is, the moment of inertia I and angular velocity ω.

$$\text{Linear momentum} = mv$$

$$\text{Angular momentum} = I\omega$$

The momentum of a skater skating in a straight line is mv. The momentum of the skater spinning is $I\omega$.

Angular momentum can be increased or decreased by increasing or decreasing either the angular velocity or the moment of inertia. A heavy bat swung with the same velocity as a light bat has greater angular momentum. However, increasing the velocity of the lighter bat could produce an angular momentum equal to or greater than that of the heavier bat. Similarly, the angular momentum of a kicking leg can be increased by increasing its angular velocity. Conversely, it will decrease if the leg is flexed at the knee (thus decreasing this moment of inertia) while keeping the velocity constant.

Conservation of Angular Momentum

Newton's first law as applied to rotary motion can also be stated in terms related to momentum. Worded thus, it states that the total angular momentum of a rotating body will remain constant unless acted upon by external torques. This is why the law is also known as the *law of conservation of angular momentum.* Like linear momentum, angular momentum is conserved. Once a spinning body is in motion, its angular momentum will not change, provided, of course, that no outside forces are introduced. Divers, gymnasts, dancers, and other rotating performers all make use of the conservation of angular momentum to control the speed of bodily spin. A skater starts to spin with the arms outstretched. After spinning slowly in this position, the skater brings the arms in close to the body and immediately begins to spin rapidly. The increase in angular velocity occurs with no effort on the skater's part. By bringing the arms in closer to the axis of rotation, the moment of inertia is decreased about that axis. Because the angular momentum must remain constant, a decrease in I produces an increase in ω. Increasing I by stretching the arms and perhaps a leg out to the side will again slow down the skater. A diver performing a tuck somersault can control the speed of rotation by changing the tightness of the tuck, thus changing the moment of inertia. If the diver thinks the entry into the water will be spoiled because of too rapid a rotation, the I can be increased and the angular velocity decreased proportionately by "opening up" or loosening the tuck (Figure 13.22).

Action and Reaction

As previously explained, the force for angular motion is torque. For every torque exerted by one body on a second body, there is another torque equal in magnitude and opposite in direction exerted by the second body on the first. This is Newton's third law of motion as applied to angular movement. A force that causes a change in angular momentum must have an equal and opposite force creating an equal and opposite momentum change. In other words, angular momentum is conserved. When one jumps straight up from a trampoline bed with arms stretched upward and then swings the legs forward and up, the body will jackknife at the hips. The torque acting on the legs results in an equal and opposite torque acting on the rest of the body. A change in angular velocity is observed in both body segments, although that in the trunk segment is less because I is greater. Another jump upward followed by a sharp flexion of the wrists only will also produce an equal and opposite torque on the rest of the body. However,

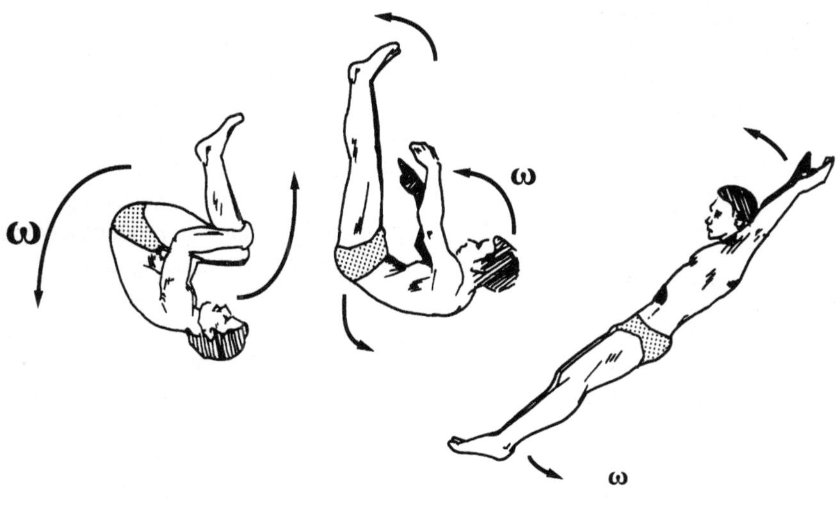

Figure 13.22 Lengthening the radius of rotation increases the moment of inertia and decreases the angular velocity. The angular momentum of the rotating diver is conserved.

in this case the change in angular velocity of the arms and trunk resulting in forward-upward motion will be barely visible. *I* for the arms and trunk is so large compared with *I* for the hands that the opposite rotation will be very slight. The angular velocity of the two moving parts is inversely proportional to their moments of inertia about the axis of motion (the wrist joint in the example just given). Axes for such actions may be in any plane, but the reactions must be in the same or parallel planes. The arms swinging horizontally across in front of the trunk will produce an opposite action of the rest of the body in the transverse plane (Figure 13.23). Movement of one arm downward in the frontal plane produces an equal and opposite action of the rest of the body in the frontal plane. This is the movement that may be used to regain balance on a beam or tightrope. If one falls to the left, a downward movement of the left arm produces a reaction of the rest of the body to the right and hopefully prevents a fall.

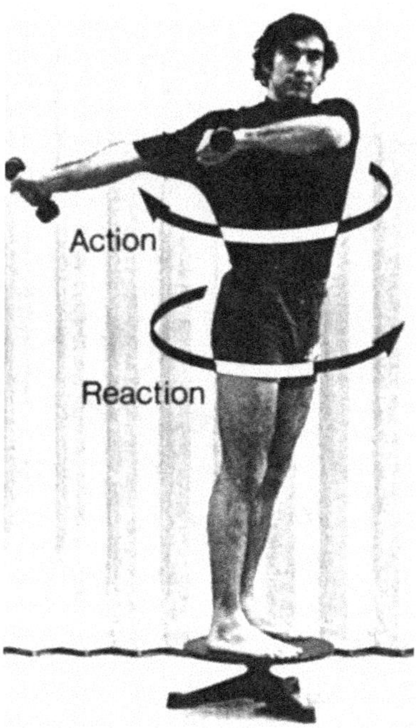

Figure 13.23 Angular action and reaction. As the arms swing across the body in one direclion, an equal and opposite reaction occurs in the rest of the body.

The equation describing this action–reaction relationship may be written as

$$I(\omega_{1f} - \omega_{1i}) = I(\omega_{2f} - \omega_{2i})$$

Any changes in the moments of inertia of the two bodies (I_1 and I_2) or of their respective angular velocities (ω_1 and ω_2) will produce equal and opposite momentum changes so that $I_1(\omega_{1f} - \omega_{1i})$ and $I_2(\omega_{2f} - \omega_{2i})$ continue to be equal and opposite.

Sometimes action and reaction in specific body parts is not desired and should be controlled. This can be done by substitution or absorption of the undesired action. In walking and running, the rotation of the pelvis and legs about a vertical axis produces an undesired reaction of the upper trunk in the opposite direction if it is not compensated in some fashion. To prevent this, the arms move in opposition to the legs to "absorb" the reaction by producing a countertwist that cancels out the reaction of the body to the leg action. The faster one moves or the more massive the legs, the more vigorous must be the arm action. The arms are used in the same fashion to prevent undesired trunk reaction to leg action in hurdling, diving, and jumping.

Transfer of Momentum

Because of the law of conservation of momentum, angular momentum may be transferred from one body or body part to another as the total angular momentum remains unaltered. In the suspended balls shown in Figure 13.24, the sudden checking of motion in ball *A* produces a comparable action in ball *E*. Similarly, checking the simultaneous motion in *A* and *B* produces equal momentum in *D* and *E*. Examples of transfer of angular momentum in movement patterns are numerous. As a back diver leaves the board, the arms are swung upward until the motion is checked by the limitation of range of motion in the shoulder joint. The checked momentum transfers to the body and increases its angular momentum, thus helping turn the body in the air. In the racing dive, the angular momentum of the diver's arms is also transferred to the body as the diver stops the upward movement of the arms in the forward reach, and in a jump twist, the dancer transfers twisting momentum from the upper arms and trunk to the legs as the feet leave the ground. In each of these instances the body is in contact with the ground while the momentum is developing. Otherwise, an equal and opposite reaction, rather than a transfer, would occur. The effect that the transfer of angular momentum has on unsupported bodies is discussed in Chapter 20.

A very common example of the transfer of angular momentum is the series of sequential segmental rotation that occurs in throwing, kicking, and striking actions. In an efficient performer, a throwing motion involves a series of rotations of progressively smaller body segments. The initial angular momentum generated by the application of torque to the fairly massive leg and trunk segments is transferred to the much lighter upper arm. The decrease in moment of inertia between the trunk and the arm produces an increase in the angular velocity of the upper arm. By the time this angular momentum has been transferred to the hand, angular velocity will be at a maximum.

Angular momentum also can be transferred or converted into linear momentum, or the reverse can occur. The angular momentum of the hammer becomes linear momentum when it is released. Conversely, a ball that hits the ground with no spin but rebounds spinning has had some of its linear momentum converted to angular momentum. Similarly, a long jumper's linear momentum most often is partially converted to angular momentum at the takeoff. Those who advanced the somersault technique for long jumping thought that as long as the angular momentum existed, it should be used to advantage. Unfortunately there were too many disadvantages, and the style is no longer legal. The hitch kick technique that most good jumpers currently use provides the necessary "opposite"

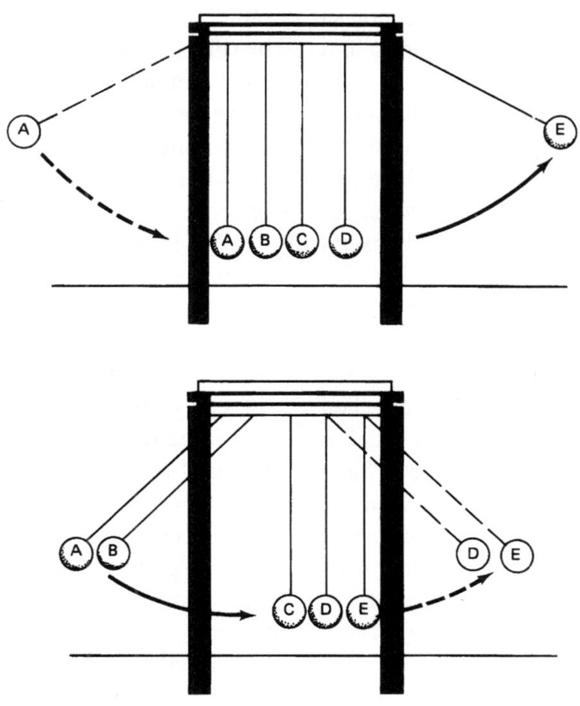

Figure 13.24 Example of conservation of angular momentum resulting in transfer of angular momentum from one body to another.

reaction to minimize the undesired forward rotation "action" of the trunk while putting the feet in an optimum landing position.

CENTRIPETAL AND CENTRIFUGAL FORCES

A weight whirling around on the end of a string is engaged in linear motion of the circular type (see pp. 270–271), while the string itself is undergoing rotary motion about an axis. If one lets go of the string, both the string and weight fly off and experience linear motion. This is expected because, according to Newton's first law, a moving body left alone travels uniformly in a straight line. To make that body leave the straight path requires application of an additional force. In the case of the weight on the string, the force has to be applied in a manner that will cause the weight to change direction and move in a circular path about the axis. This force is called *centripetal force.* It is a constant center-seeking force that acts to move an object tangent (at right angles) to the direction in which it is moving at any instant, thus causing it to move in a circular path.

The centripetal force acting on the weight is an external force that is applied by the finger through the string to the weight. The finger, in turn, must have a force pulling on it because, according to Newton's third law, if one body exerts a force on the second body, that body will reciprocate with an equal and opposite force on the first body. This outward-pulling force is called *centrifugal* (center-fleeing) *force* and is felt in the tension exerted on the finger by the string attached to the circling object. Centrifugal force is equal in magnitude to centripetal force. If centripetal force ceases, there is no longer an inward pull on the object and the latter then flies off at a tangent to the direction in which it was moving at the instant the force stopped. Without centripetal force, there will be no centrifugal reaction, and the object will once more travel uniformly in a straight line.

Even though the speed of a whirling object is constant, its direction changes continually—that is, there is a constant change in velocity. This, in effect, is the same as saying that the weight is uniformly accelerating because, by definition, acceleration is the rate of change of velocity. The amount of acceleration that a whirling object possesses increases with the speed with which it is orbiting and decreases with the distance from the axis to the object. This relationship is represented in equation form as $a = v^2/r$. The substitution of this value for acceleration in the equation obtained from Newton's second law of motion, $F = ma$, results in the equation for centripetal force:

$$F_c = mv^2/r$$

The equation for centrifugal force is the same, because it is equal in magnitude and opposite in direction to centripetal force.

From the equation it can be seen that the amount of centripetal force necessary to keep an object moving in a circular path is proportional to its mass and the square of its velocity and inversely proportional to its radius. Doubling the mass doubles the centripetal force, whereas doubling the radius decreases it by half. Changes in velocity have an even greater impact and are more dramatic. Doubling the velocity along the curve increases the centripetal force fourfold, and decreasing the velocity by one-half decreases to one-fourth the force needed to keep the object in orbit.

When runners or bicyclists negotiate corners with any appreciable speed, they lean into the curve. If they did not, they would tend to topple outward. In the same manner that centripetal force was exerted by the finger on the weight at the end of the string, the ground exerts centripetal force on the body of the runner through the feet and on the body of the cyclist through the bicycle wheel.

Centrifugal force, acting equal and opposite, tends to pull the body outward, back into a linear path. This centrifugal force produces a torque on the body in an outward direction, with the foot or the bicycle wheel acting as the axis. To maintain equilibrium against this torque, the runner or the bicyclist must lean inward, using the body weight to produce an equal and opposite inward torque. In

Figure 13.25a, this outward-rotating torque $F_c y$ is shown as the product of the centripetal–centrifugal force and the distance between the center of gravity of the runner and the axis of rotation about the foot. When one leans in, an opposite reacting torque is created, also about the feet, and is equal to the product of the weight and the perpendicular distance from the direction of weight to the axis. In Figure 13.25b, the torque that is due to the lean (Wx) balances the opposite acting torque that is due to centripetal force, so $F_c y = Wx$. This relationship demonstrates that as F_c increases, the amount of lean will also have to increase. As this occurs, x increases, y decreases, and W, of course, remains the same. It also shows that the lower the center of gravity of a body negotiating a curve, the smaller will be the outward-rotating force because the moment arm y will be less.

Where speeds are too great or radii too small for participants to negotiate curves successfully, the track may be banked. The amount of banking is determined for the particular radius and the average expected velocity so that the performer may remain perpendicular to the surface while rounding the curve. As might be expected, the greater the anticipated velocity for negotiating the curve, or the smaller the radius of the turn, the more the track must be banked.

Centripetal–centrifugal forces are evident in many instances in which the body imparts force

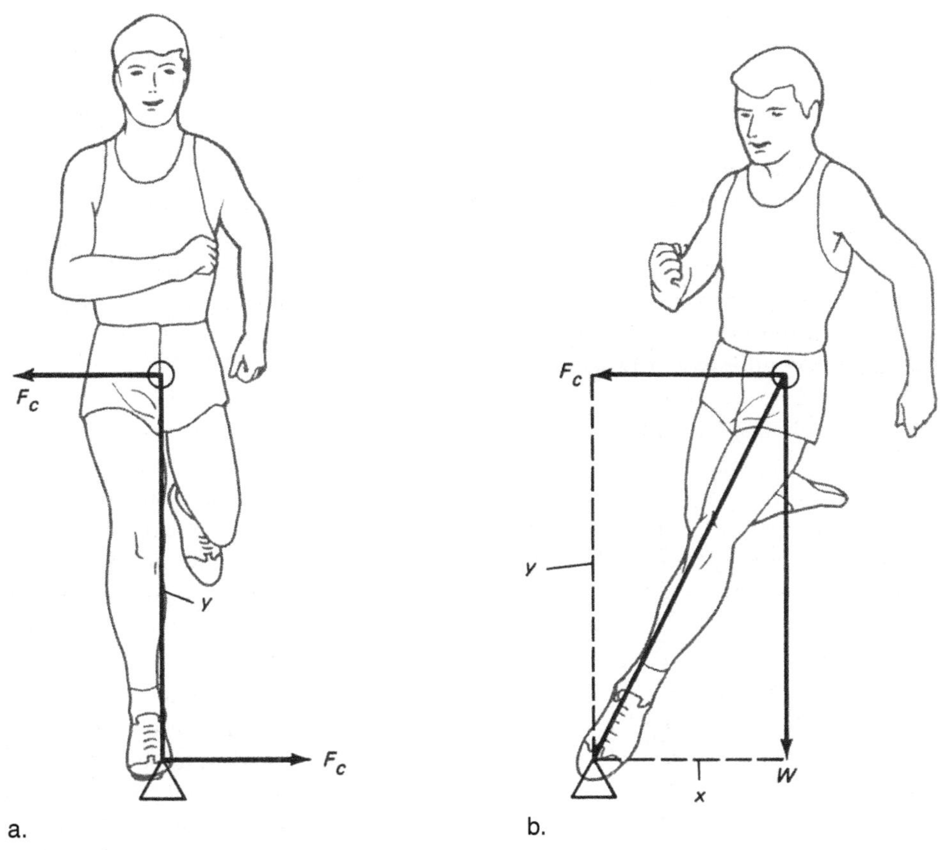

Figure 13.25 A runner must lean in when going around a corner to balance an outward-pulling torque ($F_c y$). The outward-pulling torque ($F_c y$) will topple the runner unless it is counterbalanced by an opposite torque (Wx) so that $F_c y = Wx$.

to an external object. Overarm, sidearm, or underarm throwing patterns all involve the application of force to the object to be thrown in order to keep it moving in a circular path for all or part of the time before it is released. As soon as the object is released, its inertia causes it to move in a straight line. In the hammer throw (Figure 13.26), the thrower transmits force to the head of the hammer along the flexible wire. This is centripetal force directed inward toward the axis of rotation. As the performer increases the speed of rotation, the velocity of the hammer increases, and the increased centripetal force the thrower must exert is proportional to the square of the velocity. The outward-pulling centrifugal force increases accordingly on the thrower, who must adjust by leaning back or be pulled off balance. A hammer thrower needs considerable strength to resist centrifugal force.

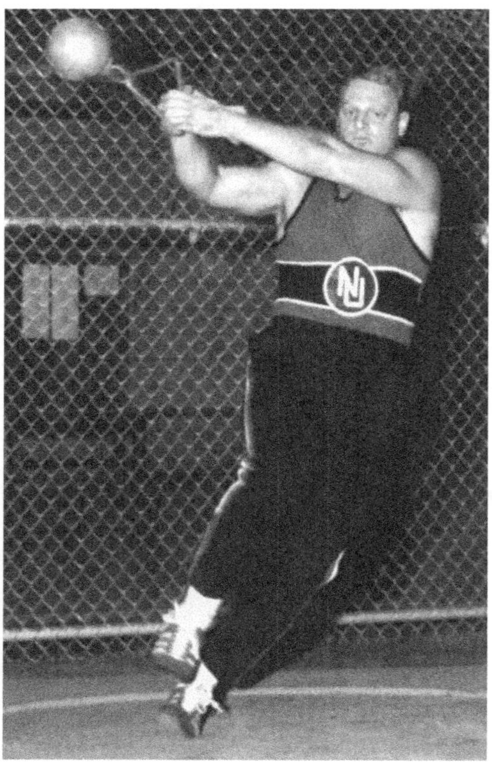

Figure 13.26 Centripetal–centrifugal forces operating in weight event. Photograph courtesy of Northeastern University.

This is also true with discus throwers who generate considerable centripetal force during the turn prior to delivery, or baseball pitchers whose elbows are subject to great forces because of the tremendous speed with which the forearm is whipped forward in the pitch. Another instance in which centripetal force is an important factor is in all swinging activities in gymnastics.

The Analysis of Angular Motion

As most motions of the human body involve rotation of a segment about a joint, any mechanical analysis of movement requires an analysis of the nature of the rotary forces, or torques, involved. In examining and evaluating performance of any movement skill, both internal and external torques must be considered. Internal torques will be generated by applied muscle forces as identified in the anatomical portion of the skill analysis. External torques now must be identified as they are produced by the external forces identified in the analysis of linear motion.

The principles that govern angular motion are based primarily on the production of torque and the results of torque production. Some general principles of angular motion might be stated as follows:

Torque The torque about any point equals the product of the force magnitude and its perpendicular distance from the line of action. The force rotating the body segments depends on the related joint torques, which are governed by the muscle forces and the locations of their attachments.

Summation of Torques The resultant torque of a force system equals the sum of the individual torques. Therefore, if a maximum resultant is desired, all body segments that have the capability must contribute to their maximum. Torques may be summed either simultaneously or sequentially.

Conservation of Angular Momentum In the absence of any outside torque, an object undergoing rotary motion will continue to rotate. Because angular momentum is conserved, alterations in the moment of inertia will produce changes in the angular velocity and vice versa. In other words, a decrease in the moment of inertia will produce an increase in angular velocity, with the opposite also being true.

Principle of Levers Any lever will balance when the torque of the effort equals the torque produced by the resistance. The amount of effort required may be calculated using this principle if the resistance torque and the length of the effort arm are known.

Transfer of Angular Momentum Angular momentum may be transferred from one body part to another when total angular momentum remains unchanged. In many motions, this transfer of momentum moves from more massive segments to less massive segments. When this occurs, the velocity of rotation increases with each transfer based on the conservation of angular momentum.

In the continuing example of the long jump, for instance, the force applied to generate the propulsive impulse will be the result of the joint torques generated. To be most effective, these joint torques must be summed, meaning that each body segment that has the capability must contribute to its maximum. Maximum thrust of the body in the jump depends on maximum resultant torques developed at the individual joints.

References and Selected Readings

Bahamonde, R. E. (2000). Changes in angular momentum during the tennis serve. *Journal of Sports Sciences,* 18(8), 579–592.

Cross, R., & Bower, T. (2006). Effects of swing-weight on swing speed and racket power. *Journal of Sports Sciences,* 24(1), 23–30.

Hay, J. G. (1993). *The biomechanics of sports techniques.* Englewood Cliffs, NJ: Prentice Hall.

Hiley, M. J., & Yeadon, M. R. (2001). Swinging around the high bar. *Physics Education,* 36, 14–17.

King. D., Smith, S., Higginson, B., Muncasy, B., & Scheirman, G. (2004). Characteristics of triple and quadruple toe-loops performed during the Salt Lake City 2002 Winter Olympics. *Sports Biomechanics,* 3(1), 109–123.

King, M. A., & Yeadon, M. R. (2004). Maximising somersault rotation in tumbling. *Journal of Biomechanics,* 37(4), 47 1–477.

Koh, M., Jennings, L., & Elliott, B. (2003). Role of joint torques generated in an optimized Yurchenko layout vault. *Sports Biomechanics,* 2(2), 177–190.

Leardini, A., & O'Connor, J. J. (2002). A model for lever-arm length calculation of the flexor and extensor muscles at the ankle. *Gait and Posture,* 15(3), 220–229.

Özkaya, N., Nordin, M., & Frankel, V. H. (1999). *Fundamentals of biomechanics: Equilibrium, motion, and deformation* (2nd ed.). New York: Springer.

Royer, T. D., & Martin, P. E. (2005). Manipulations of leg mass and moment of inertia: Effects on energy cost of walking. *Medicine and Science in Sports and Exercise,* 37(4), 649–656.

Southard, D., & Groomer, L. (2003). Warm-up with baseball bats of varying moments of inertia: Effect on bat velocity and swing pattern. *Research Quarterly for Exercise and Sport,* 74(3), 270–276.

Tözeren, A. (2000). *Human body dynamics: Classical mechanics and human movement.* New York: Springer.

Laboratory Experiences

1. Define the following key terms and give an example of each that is not used in the text.

Torque	Moment of inertia
Moment arm	Angular momentum
Lever	Centripetal force
Mechanical advantage	Centrifugal force

2. For each of the following anatomical levers, estimate the approximate length of the effort arm, that is, the perpendicular distance. Refer to anatomical illustrations or to a muscle mannequin to help you estimate the angle of pull of the muscles. Unless otherwise stated, assume that the segments are in their normal resting position. (*Hint:* Use the mechanical axis of the segment for the lever.)
   a. The forearm lever with the biceps providing the effort.
   b. The upper arm lever with the middle deltoid providing the effort.
   c. The upper arm lever in the side-horizontal position with the entire pectoralis major providing the effort. (*Hint:* Which view would show you the angle of pull for this movement, facing the subject or looking down from above?)
   d. Same lever as in c, with the anterior deltoid providing the effort.
3. Referring to the diagrams in Figure 13.5, assume that a weight is suspended from the wrist. Find the resistance arm of the forearm lever in positions b, d, and e. Consider that the scale for these diagrams is 2 cm = 25 cm.
4. Assume that a muscle having a force of 300 N is pulling at an angle of 75 degrees. Find the components of the force by the trigonometric method.
5. Assuming that the weight used in Experience 3 is 8 kg, determine the rotary and nonrotary components of the weight by the trigonometric method.
6. Referring to Figure 7.21, make a tracing of the femur and the adductor longus muscle. Draw a straight line to represent the mechanical axis of the femur and another to represent the muscle's line of pull (connecting the midpoints of the proximal and distal attachments).
   a. Using a protractor, measure the angle of pull (i.e., the angle facing the hip joint) formed by the intersection of the muscle's line of pull with the bone's mechanical axis.
   b. Measure the effort moment arm of the lever (i.e., the perpendicular distance from the fulcrum [center of hip joint] to the muscle's line of pull). To convert this to a realistic figure, use the scale 1 cm = 0.25 m.
   c. Assuming the muscle's total force to be 900 N, calculate the moment of force (i.e., the torque) of the lever.
   d. Calculate the rotary and the stabilizing components of force.
7. Place a pole across the back of a chair, hang a pail or basket containing a 3-kg weight on one end, and hold the other end of the pole. Now adjust the pole so that it becomes increasingly difficult to balance the weight of the pail with one hand. Stop when you reach the point where you are barely able to lift the pail by pushing down on the opposite end of the pole. Have an assistant measure the effort arm and the resistance arm of the lever. Without shifting the position of your hand, draw the pole toward you until you can easily lift the pail by pushing down on the opposite end of the pole with one finger. Again, have an assistant measure the effort and resistance arms of the lever. What do you conclude concerning the relative length of the two arms? In which case does the pail move through the greater distance? What do you conclude about the relationship between the effort required to move an object by leverage and the distance that the object is moved?
8. Balance a pole across the back of a chair, hanging a 3-kg weight at each end. Let one of these represent the effort and the other the resistance. The effort arm and the resistance arm should be exactly equal if the pole is symmetrical. Now add 3 more kilograms at another point on the resistance end and adjust the pole until it balances. Measure the effort and resistance moment arms. What do you conclude about:
   a. The relationship between the resistance and the resistance arm? Between the effort and the effort arm?
   b. The relationship between the resistance and the resistance arm, given a changing resistance and a constant effort?
9. Compute the amount of effort necessary to lift a resistance of 20 N with a 2-m, first-class lever

whose fulcrum is located 0.5 m from the point at which the weight is attached and 1.5 m from the point at which the effort is applied. Assume that both the effort and the resistance are applied at right angles to the lever.

10. Where would the fulcrum have to be located in the above-mentioned 2-m, first-class lever if only 5 N of effort were available to balance the 20-N weight? Determine this by experiment. Check your answer by the algebraic method.
11. For each of the anatomical levers listed, identify the class of lever represented; identify the fulcrum, effort point, and resistance point; and name the kind of movement favored by this type of lever.
    a. Leg being flexed at knee by hamstrings
    b. Leg being extended at knee by quadriceps femoris
    c. Pelvis being tilted to right by left quadriceps lumborum
    d. Clavicle being elevated by trapezius I
    e. Lower extremity being abducted by gluteus medius
    f. From supine lying position, lower extremities being raised by hip flexors
    g. From supine lying position, trunk being raised by hip flexors
12. Perform the following paired movements, noting the difference in the effort needed. Diagram and explain the reasons for the difference.
    a. A push-up from the toes and a push-up from the knees
    b. A sit-up with hands on the thighs and a sit-up with a 3-kg weight held behind the head
    c. A 3-kg weight held in the hand with the arm outstretched horizontally sideward and a 3-kg weight suspended from the elbow crotch when the arm is outstretched sideward
13. Explain the difference in effort needed to hold the body levers in Experience 12a, b, c, at a 10-degree angle with the horizontal compared with holding them at a 30-degree angle and a 45-degree angle.
14. What muscular effort *E*, pulling at an angle of 80 degrees, would be required to keep the lower leg in a position of 10 degrees with the horizontal? The muscle inserts 8 cm from the knee joint. The lower leg and foot weigh 35 N and the center of gravity is located 18 cm from the knee joint. A 50-N weight is hung from the ankle 33 cm from the knee joint.
15. A gymnast weighing 56 kg attempts a handstand on the balance beam. Her center of gravity is 1 m above the beam. What is the moment of force tending to pull her over if her center of gravity moves 3 cm ahead of the center of her support? 15 cm ahead?
16. Perform a vertical jump with and without the use of your arms. Have someone compare the height of the two jumps by noting the level of the top of your head. A chart with numbered horizontal lines on the wall behind you will help in scoring. The observer's eyes should be at the level of the top of your head at the peak of the jump. Repeat several times and compare your results with those of others doing the same experiment. Explain the results.
17. Stand on a frictionless turntable or sit on a swivel stool. Hold a 3-kg weight in each hand and hold your arms out to the side. Have a partner spin you around. Alternately bring your hands in to your shoulders and move them out to the side. Explain the changes in your angular velocity.
18. Stand on a frictionless turntable or sit on a swivel stool. Determine how you can rotate yourself moving just your arms. Explain why your arm motions make the rotation possible.
19. Firmly tape equal-length chains of small rubber bands to a golf ball and a table tennis ball.
    a. Holding the end of the elastic, swing the golf ball around in a circle. Repeat with the lighter ball, swinging it at the same speed as the heavier ball.
    b. Swing the table tennis ball at different speeds.
    c. Swing the table tennis ball with one-half the radius length; one-fourth the radius length. What does this experiment tell about the relationship of mass, velocity, and radius to centripetal force? How can you tell whether the centripetal force is increasing or decreasing?
20. In each of the following movement patterns, identify the nature of the motion for each phase. State the underlying mechanical objectives and describe what must occur to achieve optimum results. Consider carefully the application of rotary mechanical principles.
    Fencing lunge
    Bowling delivery
    Shot put
    Tennis lob

CHAPTER

14

THE CENTER OF GRAVITY AND STABILITY

OUTLINE

- ***Center of Gravity***
  - Definition of Center of Gravity
  - Placement of Center of Gravity in Humans
- ***Stability and Equilibrium***
  - Factors Affecting Stability
  - Principles of Stability
  - Mobility
- ***Center of Gravity and Posture***
  - Postural Adaptation
  - Dynamic Posture
  - Principles Applied to Posture
- ***Finding the Center of Gravity in the Human Body***
  - Reaction Board Method
  - Segmental Method
- ***Laboratory Experiences***

OBJECTIVES

At the conclusion of this chapter, the student should be able to:

1. Define the term *center of gravity,* and explain the basis for its location in the human body.
2. Estimate the location of the center of gravity of individuals in any position.
3. State the principles of equilibrium, and explain and demonstrate applications of each.
4. Discuss the factors that affect the stability and energy cost of the erect posture.
5. Explain the effects that the postural adaptations have on static and dynamic postures.
6. Explain the value of both anticipatory and compensatory postural adjustments.
7. Locate the center of gravity of an individual using either the reaction board or the segmental method.

CENTER OF GRAVITY

Definition of Center of Gravity

The **center of gravity** of a body is sometimes described as its balance point or that point about which a body would balance without a tendency to rotate. For this reason, the center of gravity is often identified as the point where all the weight of the body or object is concentrated. More accurately, it is the point where the weight of the body may be said to act.

The ability to locate the center of gravity of a body is based on the knowledge of what it takes for a system to be balanced, or in equilibrium. Two conditions must be met:

1. All the linear forces acting on the body must be balanced.
2. All the rotary forces (torques) must be balanced.

Another way of expressing these necessary conditions for equilibrium is to say that the sum of all the forces acting on the body must equal zero. If there is a downward-directed linear force, there must be an equal upward force so that the vector sum of these forces equals zero. If there is a negative clockwise torque, it must be canceled out by a positive counterclockwise torque of equal magnitude (Figure 14.1).

In this illustration it is represented as the intersection of the *x*-, *y*-, and *z*-axes. It may be located by application of the principle of torques.

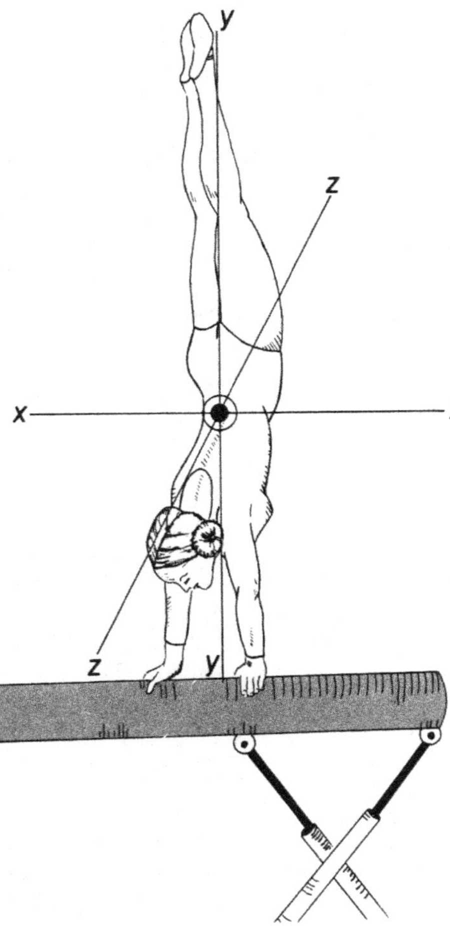

Figure 14.1 The center of gravity of a body is the point where all forces acting on the body equal zero.

A simple experiment to locate the center of gravity, or balance point, consists of suspending an irregularly shaped object by a string and letting it hang until it ceases to move (Figure 14.2). A vertical line is drawn on the object from the point of suspension in a line that is a continuation of the string. The object is then suspended from another point, and the vertical string continuation line is drawn again. This procedure is repeated one more time. The point at which the three drawn lines intersect is the center of gravity. If the object is suspended from this point, it will hang in whatever position it is placed because the weight of the object is equally distributed about this point and no unbalanced forces (torques) exist.

The location of the center of gravity of any object remains fixed as long as the body does not change shape. In rigid bodies of homogeneous mass, the center of gravity is at the geometric center. Where the density of a rigid body varies, the center of gravity is not at the geometric center but is shifted toward the more weighted section. If an object's shape or position changes, the location of the center of gravity will also change. This happens in the human body (Figure 14.3). It is a segmented structure, capable of numerous positions, and the location of its center of gravity changes accordingly. This is an important consideration in the execution of sports skills. The evolution of the technique for the high jump shows how the change of placement of the center of gravity in the body increased the height of the bar over which the jumper could project himself (Figure 14.4). As one changes the relationship of the body segments to each other, the center of gravity may even be located completely outside the body itself.

Placement of Center of Gravity in Humans

The location of the center of gravity of a human being in the normal standing position varies with body build, age, and sex. It is generally accepted that in the transverse plane the center of gravity in females is located at approximately 55% of the standing height, whereas in males the center of gravity is at approximately 57% of standing height. The center of gravity will be higher in infants, whose head size is still quite large in relation to the rest of the body. As the infant body grows and changes, the center of gravity descends to the adult position, a point level with the first sacral segment, which is approximately behind the navel and about 6 inches above the crotch.

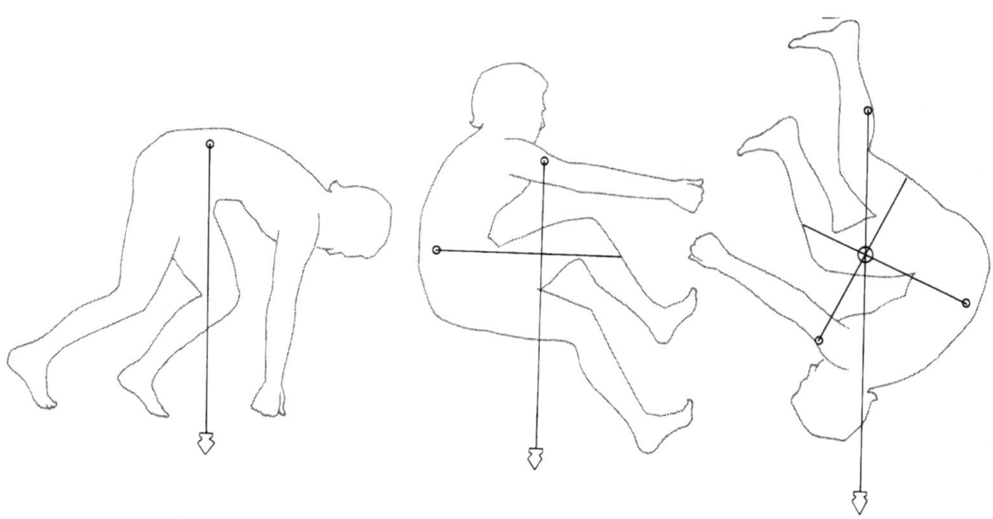

Figure 14.2 Location of the center of gravity in an irregularly shaped object.

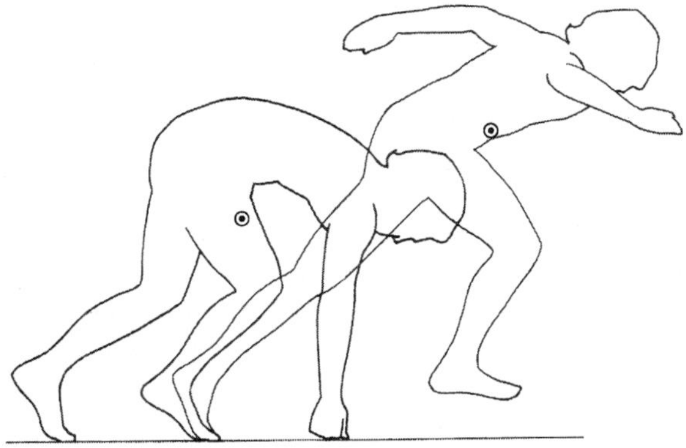

Figure 14.3 A shift in segment configuration results in a relocation of the body's center of gravity.

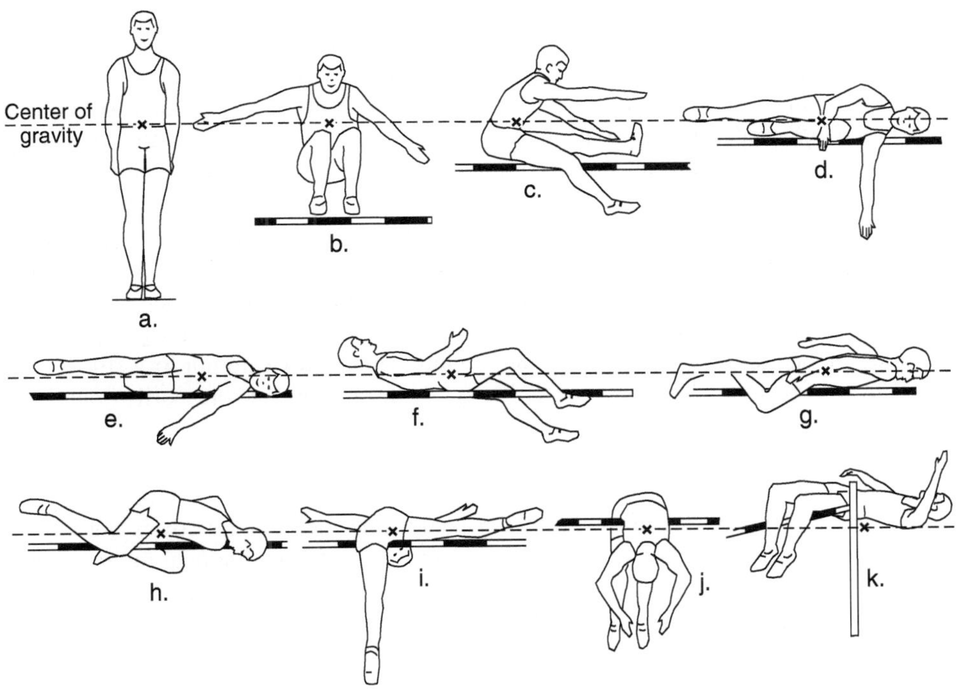

Figure 14.4 Effect of shift in center of gravity on high jump performance. *Source:* From *The Mechanics of Athletics*, by G. H. G. Dyson. Copyright © 1970, University of London Press, London. Reproduced by permission of Hodder & Stoughton, Ltd./New English Library, Ltd.

In quiet standing, the center of gravity of the body can be considered to be held almost directly over the *center of pressure.* The center of pressure is that point at which the force vector for ground reaction force can be said to be applied. During normal standing, there will be some motion in the head region, which will in turn produce a pendulum-like motion in the center of gravity. As the center of gravity shifts slightly, the center of pressure will also shift slightly in the foot–ground interface. This slight motion is referred to as postural sway. Postural sway is normally measured in both the sagittal plane (anteroposterior or AP sway) and the frontal plane (mediolateral or ML sway). AP sway has been found to average 2 to 3 cm, whereas ML sway averages 1 to 2 cm (Raymakers et al., 2005).

Postural sway magnitude and velocity can be affected by a number of factors. Age, fatigue, injury, bracing, obesity, and the stability of the external environment have all been found to influence postural sway. Increased postural sway has been found to be related to falling in the elderly and in some pathological conditions. The presence of excessive postural sway should be viewed as an indication that there may be problems with stability.

Stability and Equilibrium

All objects at rest are in equilibrium. All the forces acting on them are balanced; the sum of all linear forces equals zero, and the sum of all torques equals zero. However, all objects at rest are not equally stable. If the position of an object is slightly altered and the object tends to return to its original position, the object is in stable equilibrium. *Stable equilibrium* occurs when an object is placed in such a fashion that an effort to disturb it would require its center of gravity to be raised. Thus it would tend to fall back into place (Figure 14.5a). The more its center of gravity has to be raised to upend it, the more stable it is. A brick on its side is more stable than one on end because its center of gravity needs to be raised higher to upend it. The wrestler and defensive lineman both know the value of shifting body position to increase stability by lowering the center of gravity. In fact, if for any reason the equilibrium is too precarious, assuming a crouching, kneeling, or sitting position will lower the center of gravity and increase stability.

Unstable equilibrium exists when it takes only a slight push to destroy it. This is the situation when the center of gravity of the object drops to a lower point when the object is tilted (Figure 14.5b). A pencil on end or a tightrope walker displays unstable equilibrium because the center of gravity is bound to be lowered if either loses its balance. Swimmers standing on the starting block poised for the start of a race or sprint runners at the start of their race are in unstable equilibrium, as are toe dancers on point or balance beam performers. In each instance, the center of gravity will be lowered if the individual is perturbed so that rotation occurs around the point of support.

The third classification of equilibrium is called *neutral equilibrium* and exists when an object's center of gravity is neither raised nor lowered when it is disturbed (Figure 14.5c). A ball lying on a table is in neutral equilibrium. Objects in neutral equilibrium will come to rest in any position without a change in level of the center of gravity. Upon receiving a slight push, such objects fall neither backward nor forward.

Because people ordinarily hold themselves in an upright position and because the effect of gravity is always in operation on this earth, the problems of stability are ever present. Probably the only time the human body is not adjusting itself in response to gravitational force is when it is in a position of complete repose. Either consciously or unconsciously, human beings spend most of their

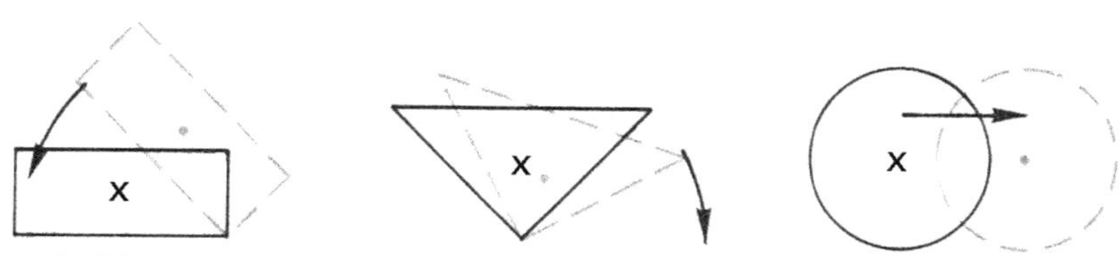

a. Stable b. Unstable c. Neutral

Figure 14.5 Types of equilibrium.

waking hours adjusting their positions to the type of equilibrium best suited to the task.

Factors Affecting Stability

The ability to maintain one's balance under unfavorable circumstances is recognized as one of the basic motor skills. Standing on tiptoe or on one foot without losing one's balance or maintaining a headstand or a handstand for an appreciable length of time is such a skill. These particular feats are examples of static balance, and the mark of skill is to accomplish them with a minimum of motion. Familiarity with the following factors affecting the stability of a performer's equilibrium state should make the analysis of balance easier and may suggest means for improvement of the skill with which the technique is executed.

The three most critical factors affecting stability are the size of the base of support, the relation of the line of gravity to the base of support, and the height of the center of gravity. Other factors such as mass of the body, friction, segmental alignment, visual and psychological factors, and physiological factors may also play a role in stability.

Size and Shape of the Base of Support

The size of the base of support is a primary factor in the stability of an object. Much of the difficulty experienced in balancing on one leg on a balance beam, a tightrope, or another small surface is due to the narrow base of support. The problem is to keep the center of gravity over the base of support, a requisite for maintaining equilibrium. The wider the base, the easier this is.

The base of support includes the part of a body in contact with the supporting surface and the intervening area (Figure 14.6). In a person whose weight is supported entirely by the feet, the base of support includes the two feet and the space between. If the feet are separated, the base is widened and the equilibrium improved. The person supported by crutches in Figure 14.7 has a base of support that encompasses the area bounded by the feet and crutches. He will be more stable if he places the crutches forward, making a triangular base instead of a linear one. There is another factor, however, that must not be overlooked. If one takes a stride position that is wider than the breadth of the pelvis, the legs will assume a slanting position. This introduces a horizontal component of force that, if accompanied by insufficient friction between the feet and the supporting surface, as when standing on ice, does not make for greater stability. In fact, the wider the stance, the less one can control the sliding of the feet. From this we see that we must observe all the principles that apply to a situation. Observance of only one may not bring the results expected.

In addition to the size of the base of support, the shape is also a factor in stability. To resist lateral external forces, the base should be widened in the direction of the oncoming force. In Figure 14.7c, the position provides great stability for lateral forces from the side but very little from the front or back. Where the forces are known to be coming from a forward-backward direction, as when catching a swift ball or spotting a performer in gymnastics, a forward-backward stance is recommended. A similar adjustment is made when one stands in a bus or a subway train. The tendency to be thrown backward when the vehicle starts up is resisted either by standing sideways with the feet in a moderately wide stance, or by facing forward and leaning forward with one foot placed forward. These automatic reactions to external forces are for one purpose only—namely, to enable one to keep the center of gravity over the base of support in spite of the perturbing external forces. When the direction of oncoming force cannot be predicted, a slight oblique stance is probably best.

Height of the Center of Gravity

Ordinarily, the center of gravity in an adult human being is located approximately at the level of the upper third of the sacrum, but *only* during the normal standing position. If the arms are raised or if a weight is carried above waist level, the center of gravity shifts to a higher position, and it becomes more difficult to maintain one's equilibrium. Activities and stunts such as walking on stilts, canoeing, and balancing a weight on the head are difficult or dangerous

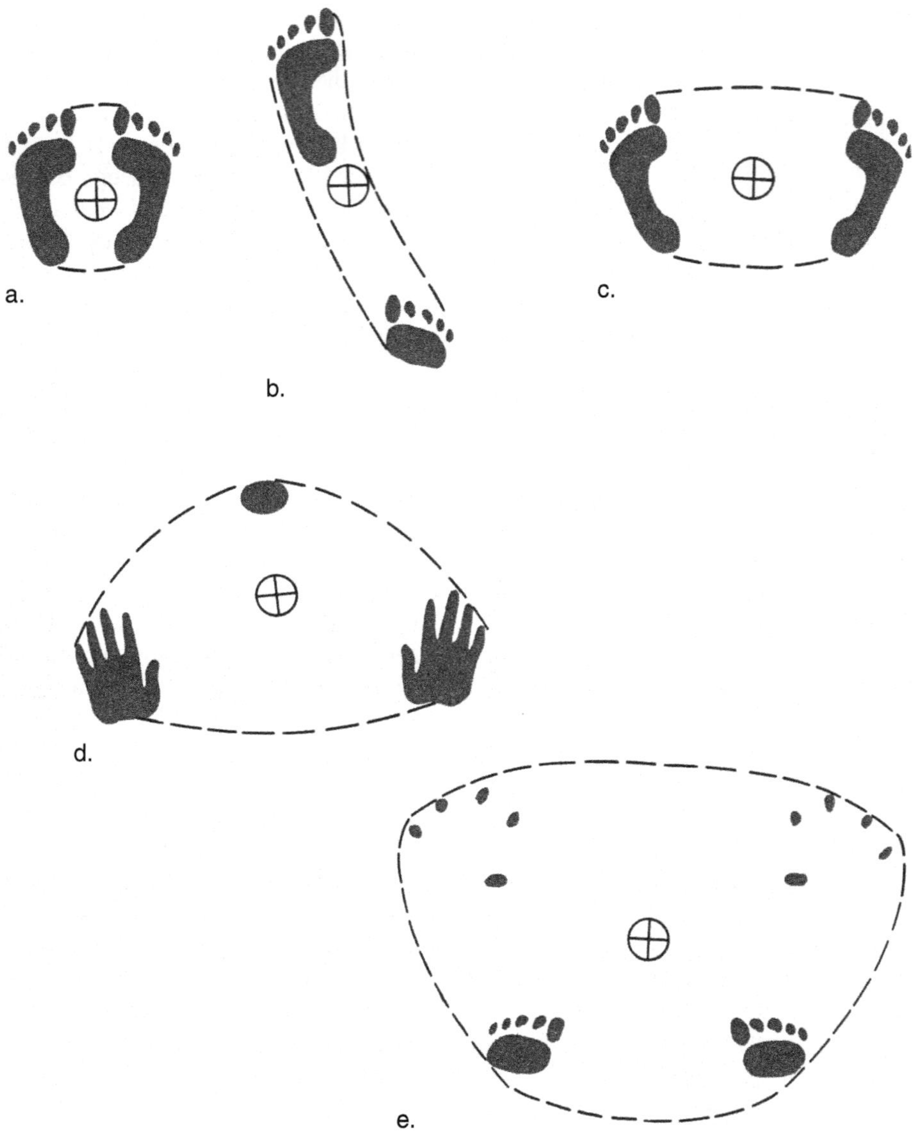

Figure 14.6 The base of support includes the part(s) of the body in contact with the supporting surface and the intervening area. What can you conclude about the stability of the base of support in these illustrations? In (a), (b), and (c) the weight is supported by the feet; in (d) it is supported by the forehead and hands during a headstand; in (e) the weight is supported by the hands and feet while the body is in a squat position. Circled crosses indicate point of intersection of line of gravity with base of support.

because of the relatively high center of gravity. Lowering the center of gravity will increase the stability of the body because it allows greater angular displacement of the center of gravity within the bounds of the base of support (Figure 14.8).

Relation of the Line of Gravity to the Base of Support

An object retains its equilibrium only so long as its line of gravity falls within its base of support. When the force that the body is resisting is the

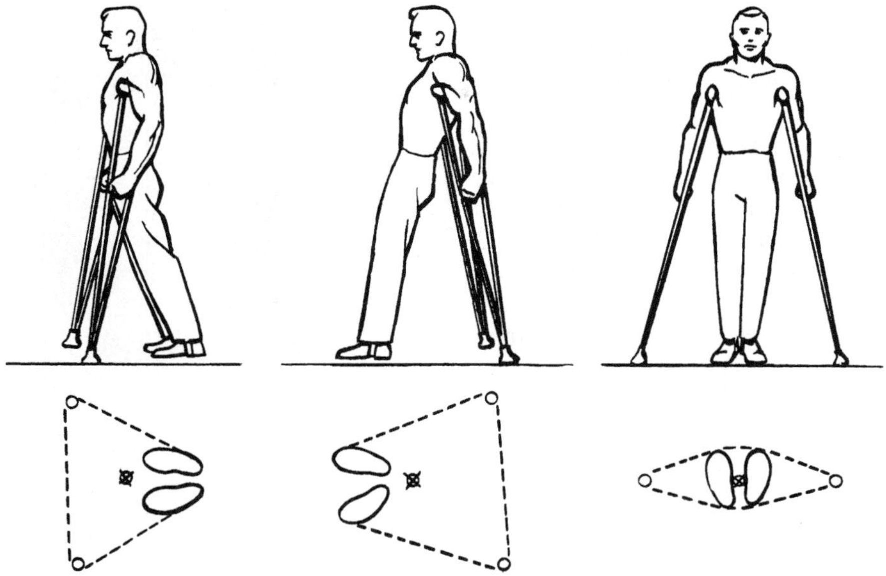

a. b. c.

Figure 14.7 Bases of support with varying degrees of stability. Can you rank these from most stable to least stable? The subject in (a) and (b) is secure primarily in the anteroposterior direction; the position in (c) provides greater stability in the frontal plane than in the sagittal plane. *Source:* From *Williams and Lissner: Biomechanics of Human Motion* (2nd ed.), by B. Leveau. Copyright © 1977, W. B. Saunders, Orlando, FL. Reprinted by permission.

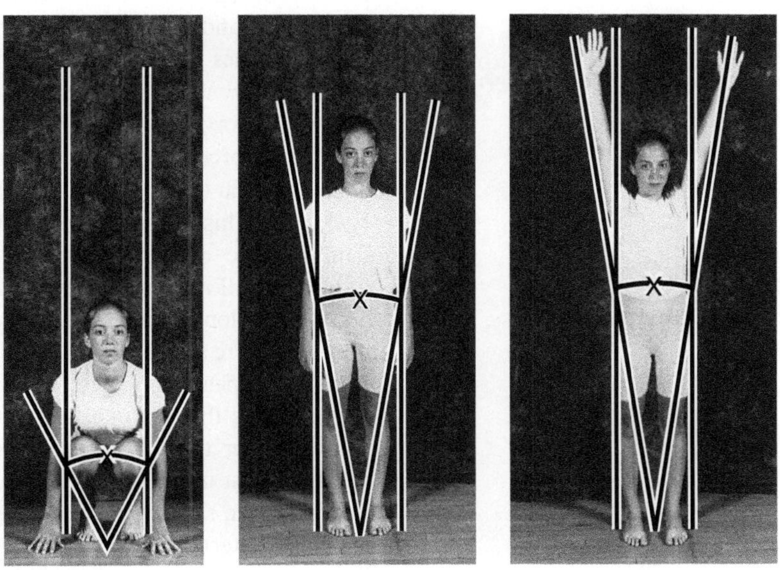

a. b. c.

Figure 14.8 The height of the center of gravity changes with a change in body position. *X* = center of gravity. As the center of gravity moves closer to the base of support, more angular displacement of the center of gravity can occur before it goes beyond the vertical line marking the edge of the base of support. The angle in (a) is greater than that in (b), and the angle in (b) is greater than that in (c). Thus, a > b > c with respect to lateral stability.

downward force of gravity, the nearer the line of gravity to the *center* of the base of support, the greater the stability (Figure 14.9); and, conversely, the nearer the line of gravity to the *edge* of the base of support, the more precarious the equilibrium (Figure 14.10). Positions of instability occur when gravity can "pull us over." This occurs when the force of gravity changes from a linear force to a rotational force, or torque. Consider a brick standing on its end. If this brick is tilted and balanced on one of the edges, the line of force from the center of gravity acts through the base of support, or in this case, the axis of rotation. The brick is stable, and the lever arm of the force of gravity is zero. However, any shift in the location of the center of gravity of the brick will produce a lever arm, and the brick will rotate and fall. This is what happens to humans. When the center of gravity gets outside the base of support, the force of gravity immediately has a lever arm, and the human begins to rotate about the axis of rotation (the feet). For example, consider someone performing a trust fall (in which you close your eyes and someone stands behind you and promises to catch you). As you lean back, you feel yourself getting less and less stable as your center of gravity approaches the edge of your base of support. Once your center of gravity passes outside your base of support, a lever arm is established through which the force of gravity can produce a torque and cause you to rotate about your feet as you fall backward. This factor constitutes the major problem in some dance techniques, balance stunts, tightrope walking, and pyramid building.

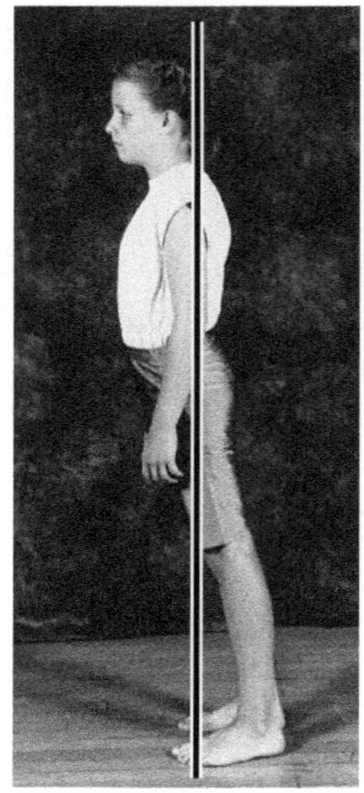

Figure 14.10 Position of the body in which the line of gravity falls near the anterior edge of the base of support. This position is less stable than the one shown in Figure 14.9.

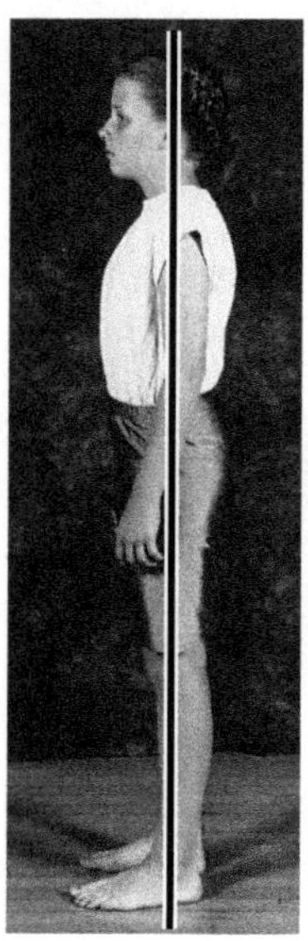

Figure 14.9 Position of the body in which the line of gravity falls approximately through the center of the base of support. This is a stable position.

To develop the neuromuscular control necessary to acquire such skills as these, there is no substitute for repeated practice. There are, however, a few methods that help keep the center of gravity centered over the base of support. One of these we do almost unconsciously. If we carry a heavy weight at one side of the body (e.g., a suitcase or a pail of water), *this constitutes a unilateral load* that, if uncompensated, would shift the center of gravity to that side, bringing it dangerously close to the edge of the base of support. By raising the opposite arm sideways, by bending or leaning to

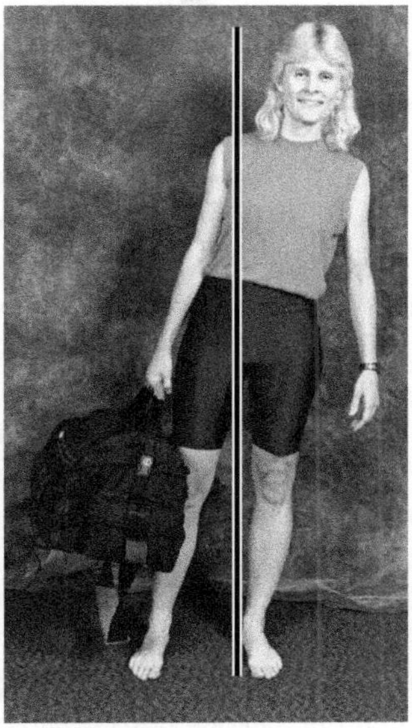

Figure 14.11 Compensating for a unilateral load by inclining the entire body to the opposite side.

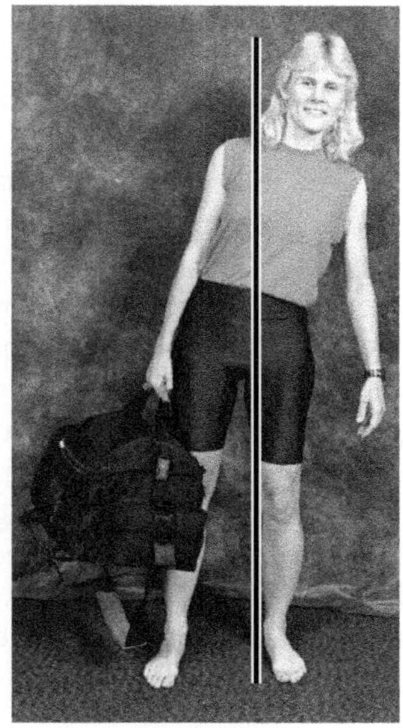

Figure 14.12 Compensating for a unilateral load by bending to the opposite side.

the opposite side, or by a combination of these, we counterbalance the external load and keep the line of gravity close to the center of the base of support (Figures 14.11 and 14.12). Another application of the principle of keeping the line of gravity over the center of the base of support is seen in the tightrope walker who carries a balancing pole or, to a lesser degree, in the gymnast walking on a balance beam with arms extended sideward.

When the external force acting on a body is a lateral one, stability is increased if the line of gravity is placed so that it will continue to remain over the base even when forced to move by the external force. Leaning into the wind (Figure 14.13) or pushing a heavy chest are examples of when the line of gravity should be close to the edge of the base of support nearest the oncoming force. Pulling in a tug-of-war is an example of having the gravity line near the edge of the base of support farthest away from the external force. When one is not certain from which direction an external force may be applied, equilibrium is most stable when the line of gravity is in the center of the base of support.

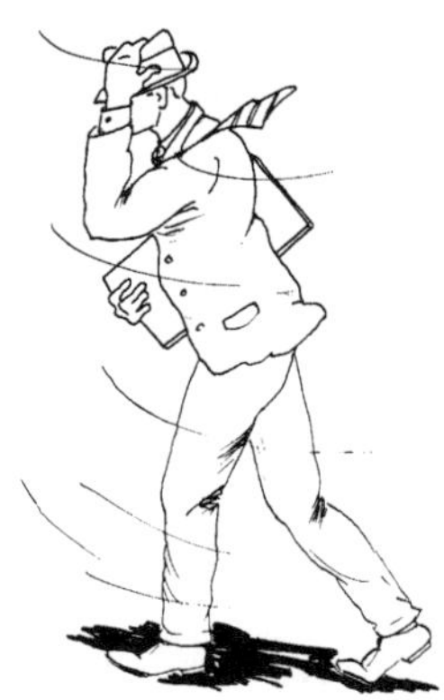

Figure 14.13 Leaning into the wind to balance the effect of its force on the body.

Mass of the Body

The mass or weight of an object is a factor in equilibrium only when motion or an external force is involved. Then, as Newton's second law states, $F = ma$. The amount of force needed to effect a change in motion (acceleration) is proportional to the mass being moved. The greater the mass (inertia), the greater the stability. It is a matter of common observation that an empty cardboard carton is more likely to blow down the street than one filled with canned goods. Likewise, a lineman weighing 120 kg is less likely to be brushed aside than one weighing 60 kg. In all sports involving physical contact, the heavy, solid individual stands a better chance of keeping his or her footing than does the lighter one. Recall that mass is a measure of an object's inertia, and inertia is a measure of resistance to change in motion state (Newton's first law). Therefore, the greater the mass, the greater the resistance to change in position or motion. When all factors are considered, however, mass is less a factor in stability than are the location of the line of gravity and the height of the center of gravity.

Friction

Friction as a factor in stability has already been suggested in relation to the size of the base of support. It has even greater influence when the body is in motion or is being acted on by an external force. Inadequate friction is what makes it difficult to keep one's equilibrium when walking on icy pavement, particularly if an active dog tugs unexpectedly on its leash. When the supporting surface presents insufficient friction, the footgear can make up for it. The person who must walk on icy pavement can wear "creepers" on the shoes, the golfer and the soccer player can wear cleats, and the basketball player can wear rubber-soled shoes.

Segmental Alignment

If, instead of being in one solid piece, an object consists of a series of segments placed one above the other, the problem of retaining its equilibrium is a multiple one. Maximum stability of a segmented body is ensured when the centers of gravity of all the weight-bearing segments lie in a vertical line that is centered over the base of support. In a column of blocks, this means that each block must be centered over the block beneath. In a jointed column, as in the human body, one segment cannot slide off another, but it is quite possible for the segments to be united in a zigzag alignment. Such is all too often the case in human standing posture. In fact, the alignment of the body segments is a widely used criterion for judging standing posture. When the segments are aligned in a single vertical line, the posture is not only more pleasing in appearance to most of us, but there is less likelihood of strain to the joints and muscles. When one segment gets out of line, there is usually a compensatory misalignment of another segment in order to maintain a balanced position of the body as a whole. (For every "zig" there is a "zag.") At every point of angulation between segments, there is uneven tension thrown on the ligaments and uneven tension in opposing muscle groups. This causes fatigue, if not actual strain.

The addition of an external weight to the body, as when one carries books, babies, or suitcases, may be thought of as the addition of a segment. The additional segment will add mass to the body and change its stability somewhat. More important, though, is the effect on the height of the center of gravity and the location of the line of gravity. The center of gravity will be displaced in the direction of the added weight, and the line of gravity will shift accordingly. Its new location will be governed by the nature of compensation made to accommodate the additional weight (see Figures 14.11 and 14.12).

Visual and Psychological Factors

Factors that belong in this category are less easily explained than the others but are familiar to everyone. Consider how difficult it is to stand on one foot with eyes closed versus eyes open. The giddiness that many experience when walking close to an unprotected edge high above the ground or when crossing a swirling river on a footbridge is a real detriment to one's equilibrium. Even if the supporting surface is entirely adequate, the sense of balance may be disturbed. A common means of preserving the balance, both in this type of situation and when walking on a narrow rail, is to fix the eyes on a stationary spot above or beyond the "danger area." This seems to facilitate neuromuscular control by reducing the disturbing stimuli.

Physiological Factors

In addition to the visual and psychological factors, there are also physiological factors related to the physical mechanism for equilibrium—namely, the semicircular canals. In addition to actual lesions of this mechanism, any disturbance of the general physical condition is likely to affect the sense of balance. Feelings of dizziness accompanying nausea or any form of debility reduce one's ability to resist other factors that threaten the equilibrium. Colds, viruses, and other problems that affect the inner ear may also interfere with balance. These physiological factors are largely beyond our control. One principle that can be derived from them, however, is that it is better to avoid situations likely to threaten the equilibrium when there is a temporary physiological disturbance. The same would be true of any decrease in proprioception, as often occurs with injury.

Principles of Stability

The principles of stability are stated here as simply and concisely as possible, and several examples are suggested in each case.

1. Other things being equal, the lower the center of gravity, the greater will be the body's stability.

Examples *a.* When landing from a jump, one usually flexes at the knees, both to absorb force and to lower the center of gravity in order to regain one's balance.

b. In canoeing, the kneeling position represents a compromise position that combines the advantages of stability and ease of using the arms for paddling. Kneeling is preferable to sitting on the seat because the lowering of the center of gravity makes the position a more stable one. Although it is less stable than sitting on the floor of the canoe, it is a more convenient position for paddling. A position frequently recommended is kneeling and sitting against a thwart or the edge of a seat.

c. A performer on a balance beam quickly squats when he or she feels as if balance is being lost.

d. A wrestler tries to remain as stable as possible by lowering the center of gravity.

2. Greater stability is obtained if the base of support is widened in the direction of the line of force.

Examples *a.* This helps an individual keep from being thrown off balance when punching with force, pushing a heavy object, or throwing a fastball. It also enables the puncher to "put the full body weight behind the punch" because, with a relatively wide forward-backward stance, the weight can be shifted from the rear foot to the forward foot as the force is delivered.

b. In pushing and pulling heavy furniture, the whole body can be put into the act without loss of balance.

c. When catching a fast-moving object such as a baseball, or a heavy one such as a medicine ball, widening the base in line with the direction of the force enables the catcher to "give" with the catch and, in this way, to provide a greater distance in which to reduce or stop the motion of the object. It also ensures greater accuracy by reducing the likelihood of rebound.

d. The military "at ease" is more stable than the position of "attention."

e. Keeping one's balance when standing on a bus or train that is accelerating or decelerating is facilitated by widening the stance in the direction that the vehicle is moving, that is, in a forward-backward direction in relation to the vehicle.

3. For maximum stability, the line of gravity should intersect the base of support at a point that will allow the greatest range of movement within the area of the base in the direction of forces causing motion.

Examples *a.* A football player knowing he will be pushed from in front should lean forward so that he can "give" in a backward direction without losing his balance.

b. A person in a tug-of-war line leans backward in preparation for absorbing a strong forward pull from the opponent.

c. A tennis player anticipating the opponent's return will keep the line of gravity centered so that the center of gravity can be shifted quickly in any direction without loss of balance.

d. Dragging a heavy box forward on a high shelf and then lifting it down is an activity in the home to which this principle applies. Assuming a forward-backward stance and leaning forward for this act gives the individual a wider distance to receive the weight of this forward-moving object. This decreases the likelihood of being thrown off balance when the box suddenly comes free of the shelf. It also enables one to take a step backward, which makes it easier to lower the box in front and to keep control of it. With a sideward stance, one would be more likely to be thrown off balance as the box comes free. There is also the danger of exerting so much horizontal force that, instead of lowering the box in front, the individual swings back overhead, hyperextending the spine and running the risk of straining the back.

e. Basketball and other team games involving running often require sudden reversals of direction. If the player tries to turn while the feet are close together, the momentum is likely to throw the runner off balance. This can be prevented by spreading the feet to check the forward motion and leaning back so that the line of gravity will be toward the rear. The runner can then quickly pivot to reverse direction.

4. Other things being equal, the greater the mass of a body, the greater will be its stability.

Example *a.* In sports in which resistance to impact is a factor, heavy, solid individuals are more likely to maintain their equilibrium than lighter ones. This provides one basis for selecting linemen in football.

5. Other things being equal, the most stable position of a vertical segmented body (such as a column of blocks or the erect human body) is one in which the center of gravity of each weight-bearing segment lies in a vertical line centered over the base of support or in which deviations in one direction produce torques that must be balanced by deviations producing torque in the opposite direction.

Examples *a.* This principle applies to postural adjustments for achieving a well-balanced alignment of the body segments, both with and without external loads.

b. In balance stunts in which one person (or group of persons) supports the weight of another person or persons, the chief problem is one of either aligning or balancing the several centers of gravity over the center of the base of support.

6. Other things being equal, the greater the friction between the supporting surface and the parts of the body in contact with it, the more stable the body will be.

Example Wearing cleats and rubber-soled shoes for sport activities not only aids in locomotion but also serves to increase one's stability in positions held momentarily between quick or forceful movements, as in basketball, fencing, football, field hockey, lacrosse, and other sports.

7. Other things being equal, a person has better balance in locomotion under difficult circumstances when the vision is focused on stationary objects rather than on disturbing stimuli.

Example Beginners learning to walk on a balance beam or to perform balance stunts, and others who for any reason have difficulty in keeping their balance, can minimize disturbing visual stimuli by fixing their eyes on a stationary spot in front of them, either at eye level or somewhat above eye level.

8. There is a positive relationship between one's physical and emotional state and the ability to maintain balance under difficult circumstances.

Example Persons should not be permitted to attempt dangerous balance stunts or activities requiring expert balance ability when their physical or emotional health is impaired.

9. Regaining equilibrium is based on the same principles as maintaining it.

Examples *a.* After an unexpected loss of balance, such as when starting to fall or after receiving impetus when off balance, equilibrium may be more quickly regained if a wide base of support is established and the center of gravity is lowered.

b. Upon landing from a downward jump, stability may be more readily regained if the weight is kept evenly distributed over both feet or over the hands and feet, and if a sufficiently wide base of support is provided.

c. Upon landing from a forward jump, the balance may be more readily regained if one lands with the weight forward and uses the hands, if necessary, to provide support in the direction of motion.

From this emphasis on stability, it might seem that one should seek maximum stability in all situations. This is not true regarding certain stunts and gymnastic activities that are designed for the purpose of testing and developing body control under difficult circumstances. In many gymnastic vaults, for instance, "good form" stipulates that the performer land with the heels close, the knees separated, the arms extended sideward, and the trunk as erect as possible while the knees bend slightly to ensure a light landing. In teaching beginners, it seems wiser to postpone emphasis on form from the point of view of appearance and to stress good mechanics and safety.

Mobility

There is an inverse relationship between stability and mobility. The greater the stability of a given body, the more difficult it will be to start the body moving. Conversely, the greater the mobility of the body, the less stability it possesses. A critical point in this relationship is the change from a position of stability to a state of mobility and eventually back to a position of stability. An example of this transition is seen in walking. The stationary standing position is a stable position with the line of gravity centered over the base of support. To initiate the step, a force is exerted downward and backward against the ground. The ground reaction force acts to move the center of gravity slightly up and to shift the line of gravity forward of the base of support, initiating the forward step. The swing leg then moves forward to reestablish a base of support either to regain stability or to initiate the next step.

Often in sport and physical activity, it is necessary to alter stability intentionally to become mobile. To initiate forward motion, swimmers and runners waiting for the start of a race assume a position in which they may lose balance rapidly (Figure 14.14a). A football lineman in a three-point stance is also in a position to lose balance and apply forward force quickly. In many instances the ability to start, stop, or change direction quickly depends on manipulating the stability of the body.

Both the speed and the direction of the desired mobility are used to determine the nature of the change in stability required to initiate the motion. To enhance the speed of a start in a given direction, the line of gravity should be as close as possible to the edge of the base of support in the direction of the desired motion. The opposite is true if a performer is attempting to stop quickly. A quick stop requires that stability be established quickly. To accomplish this, the performer must enlarge the base of support, lower the center of gravity, and move the line of gravity away from the leading edge of the base of support (Figure 14.14b).

CENTER OF GRAVITY AND POSTURE

When we speak of posture, we are speaking of the shape or configuration of the body. Of primary concern is the way in which the parts of the body relate to each other and to the external environment. For all practical purposes, no individual's posture can be described completely. Posture means position, and a multisegmented organism such as the human body cannot be said to have a single posture. It assumes many postures and seldom holds any of them for an appreciable time. We look at posture as being either static or dynamic. In reality, all postures are dynamic, involving muscle activity for the maintenance of position.

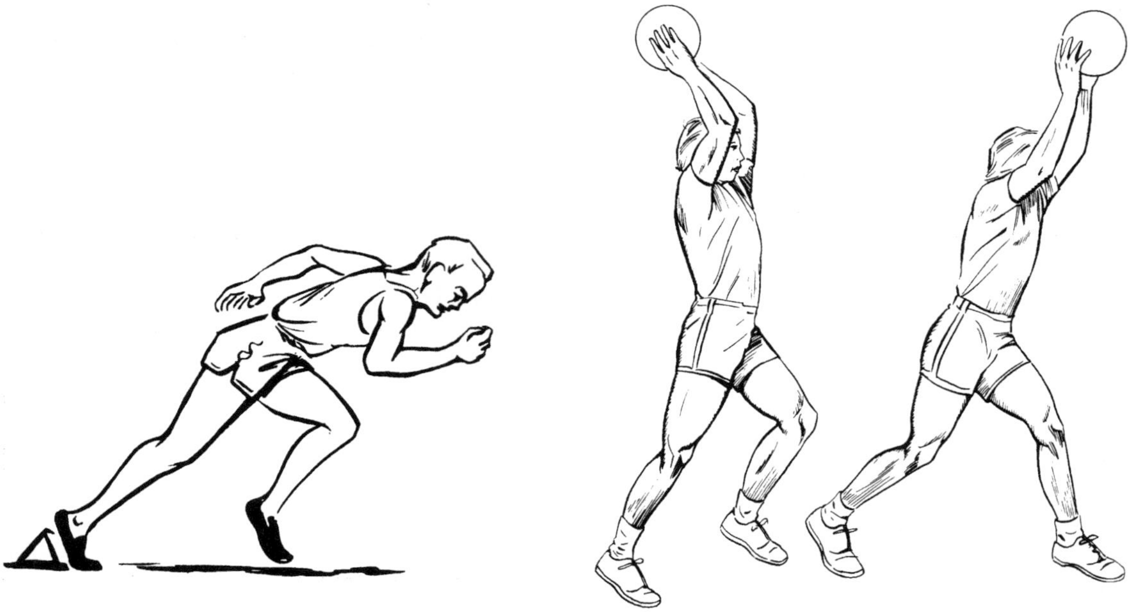

a. b.

Figure 14.14 (a) Becoming unstable in order to move quickly. (b) Reestablishing stability to stop motion.

Because dynamic postures should be of greater concern than static postures to those who specialize in human movement, it may be well to say a word in defense of the practice of examining static posture. It is admitted that the posture in a static position is of little importance in itself, unless this posture must be maintained for long periods of time. In reality, all posture is somewhat dynamic. Even when standing still, the body is in motion, undergoing postural sway. The motion of the center of gravity—and the center of pressure—is used as a measure of postural stability. The alignment of the body when maintaining the erect standing posture becomes important in controlling and maintaining the appropriate level of postural sway. It also becomes significant when taken as the point of departure for the many postural patterns assumed by the individual, both at rest and in motion. Because there is an almost endless variety of active postures and because these are extremely difficult to judge, a convenient custom is to accept the standing posture as the individual's basic posture from which all other postures stem. Hence, as a reflection of the individual's characteristic postural patterns, the standing posture takes on an importance it would not otherwise have.

Static posture by definition implies a state of equilibrium. In quiet standing, for example, one assumes that the body is balanced within itself. In reality, this is not completely true. To maintain a static posture such as standing, each segment of the body must be balanced with respect to the inferior, supporting segments. Given the irregular, nonrigid shapes of the body and the segments, this is not feasible. For this reason, even in quiet standing, there must be muscular activity in order to maintain segmental balance. Evidence of this can be seen in the postural sway described earlier. In postural sway, projection of the center of gravity (line of gravity) moves slightly within the base of support. The magnitude of this motion reflects to a large extent the stability of the body. The larger the magnitude of the postural sway, the less stable the static posture. A less stable posture requires a greater level of muscular activity, although there is no clear-cut point at which postural sway becomes detrimental. The reasons why the body produces this sway are unclear. Postural sway may have its origins in the postural reflexes that aid in the maintenance of upright posture (Visser et al., 2008). Measures of sway have been used to quantify static balance and to distinguish the existence of neurological disorders, load-carrying demands, aging, or attentional demands. Postural sway is measured in many ways, the most popular being computerized dynamic posturography. More recently, several researchers (Forth et al., 2007; Haddad et al., 2006) have demonstrated that the "time to contact" (TtC) method appears to provide greater clinical sensitivity. This measure includes the velocity as well as location of the center of mass.

Slight perturbations in static postures will produce changes in the pattern of postural sway. For example, lifting the arm forward (shoulder flexion) will produce a torque in the forward and/or downward direction. This will necessitate that an equal and opposite torque be produced in order to maintain equilibrium. To accomplish this, the body weight (center of gravity) will be shifted slightly backward. This will increase the magnitude of the postural sway in the AP plane somewhat. An example of this can be seen in the center of pressure traces presented in Figure 14.15. Any variation in the standing posture will affect sway in some manner.

Postural Adaptation

A number of conditions necessitate postural adjustment if one is to maintain a reasonably balanced standing position. These include standing on either an uphill or a downhill slope; standing on the level but wearing high heels; standing on a moving surface, such as a bus, streetcar, subway, or train; holding a heavy bundle against the front of the body; pregnancy; and standing on one foot.

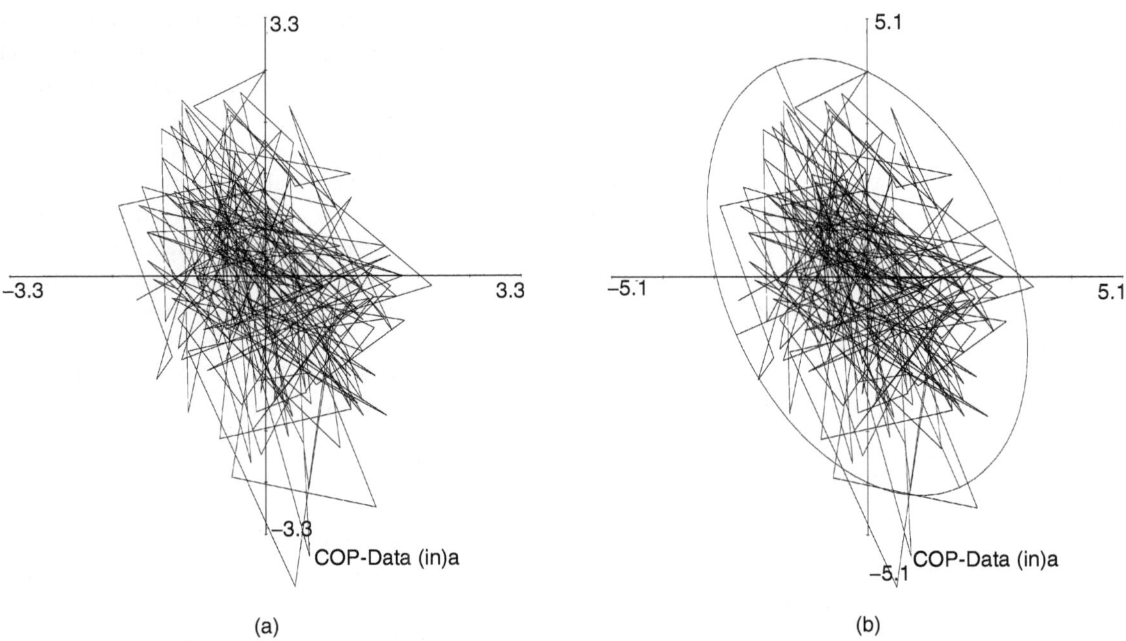

Figure 14.15 (a) Center of pressure during quiet standing. (b) Center of pressure as arms are raised.

In all of these conditions, the body can be relied upon to adjust automatically through the function of proprioceptors and the feedback mechanism.

Maintaining postural control in various environments and under varying surface conditions requires adaptations by the body. Researchers have identified two main strategies that help negotiate specific threats to balance. The hip strategy is used to navigate slippery surfaces, and the ankle strategy is used to navigate uneven surfaces. It is probable that these strategies exist on a continuum with the hip strategy on one end and the ankle strategy on the other. The different challenges to balance lie along this continuum and usually require a combination of responses to maintain upright posture (Bardy et al., 2002).

The hip strategy is easily observable when someone is walking across a slippery surface. Adjustments made to maintain the center of gravity over the base of support are achieved through trunk flexion–extension and hip flexion–extension. Based on a review of previous literature, Blackburn et al. (2003) concluded that the hip plays a substantial role for balance in the sagittal plane.

The ankle strategy is more subtle and is observable as a person walks over gravel or moves the head suddenly. While navigating these surfaces, the ankle/foot adopts a position that allows the person walking to maintain a level gaze. The knee may bend slightly; however, the hip and knee joint angles remain relatively static when the ankle strategy is employed.

The ability to remain upright, in quiet stance, is a complicated process that requires integration of the information from the visual, vestibular, and proprioceptive systems.

Consider trying to get a skeleton to remain upright just by balancing the bones one on top of another. Next, think about how the skeleton would lean if the left arm were raised and how the muscular system would have to respond to this shift. Now, think about how unstable the skeleton would become if it were standing on one leg, which happens with each step we take. The human body must interpret threats to remaining upright, devise a plan to counteract these threats, and implement that plan in time to prevent a fall.

When standing in a moving bus, streetcar, or train, one should be prepared to make three adjustments: acceleration, deceleration, and side-to-side sway. The same principle applies to all three—namely, establishing a comfortably wide stance in the direction of motion (forward-backward for acceleration and deceleration, and sideward for a steady speed, especially if there is a pronounced sway). During sudden acceleration, especially, the person tends to be thrown toward the back of the vehicle, in keeping with Newton's first law of motion.

The foot toward the rear, therefore, should be well braced, and more weight should be borne by the forward foot in anticipation of the jerk. The reverse is true during deceleration and stopping. In both acceleration and deceleration, the body is less likely to be thrown off balance if the knees are slightly flexed; doing so shortens the lever upon which the vehicle's motion acts and also lowers the center of gravity of the body.

The adjustment to standing on one foot is a delicate one but is usually managed automatically by the muscle, joint, and labyrinthine proprioceptors, and by the reflex response. The adjustment consists of a shift in the body weight to the single supporting limb and in the support of the pelvis on the side of the free limb. The latter adjustment requires additional effort by the quadratus lumborum and the abductors (gluteus medius and minimis, tensor fasciae latae, and oblique abdominal muscles on the support side). The iliopsoas, which is continuously active during all standing, increases its activity in steadying the lumbar spine (Basmajian & DeLuca, 1985). In addition, there is probably a continuous interplay of the deep muscles of the lumbar spine and possibly of many of the lower extremity muscles. The alternating action of the foot and ankle muscles, especially the tarsal pronators and supinators, is quite pronounced in their effort to keep the center of gravity over the narrow base of support. This problem can be helped somewhat by turning the toes slightly outward (i.e., rotating the thigh slightly outward) before assuming the one-legged stance.

Dynamic Posture

Movements of the body will cause a disruption, or perturbation, to the static posture. As illustrated earlier with the raising of the arm, any motion perturbs the static posture. When this perturbation occurs, the posture becomes dynamic. In dynamic postures, we must remember Newton's law of action and reaction. Every motion of a body segment produces an instantaneous reaction throughout the kinetic chain. These reactions also are transmitted to the supporting surface. This implies that there must be some muscular activity to counteract these reaction forces and torques. As more segments are added to the motion, the perturbations become greater. When the point is reached where the body moves from a state of stability to one of mobility, the posture is completely dynamic, or constantly changing. In this dynamic state, postural stability depends on the motion of both the center of pressure and the center of gravity. If both are aligned in relation to one another, static postural stability might be attained at the conclusion of the motion. If these two constructs are not aligned, balance may be lost. The more critical factor, however, is the relationship between center of pressure, center of mass, and momentum. If the motion vectors of the center of pressure and the center of gravity are not in the same direction as the momentum vector of the system (body), the regaining of static balance may be difficult if not impossible.

Postural Adjustments

During movement activities, postural adjustments take place almost continuously. Some of these adjustments are in response to proprioceptive feedback and help to maintain posture during the motion. Other postural adjustments are anticipatory in nature. These adjustments take place before the motion occurs. The purpose of these anticipatory postural adjustments is to prepare the body to maintain a dynamic equilibrium when the motion starts. A good example of an anticipatory postural adjustment might be the slight backward lean that occurs in preparation for lifting a weight in front of the body. Postural adjustments occur throughout the course of the movement. These adjustments, both feedback and feedforward in nature, rely on information from the neuromuscular system, as discussed in Chapter 4.

Postural adjustments, therefore, occur before, during, and after movement. Anticipatory postural adjustments prepare the body to move while maintaining dynamic balance. Postural adjustments during the motion (compensatory adjustments) act to keep the body in a state where stability is possible at the conclusion of the voluntary movement.

Principles Applied to Posture

By this time, the reader should understand that posture influences all we do and that it is not a static but a dynamic configuration. It should also be understood that no single ideal postural model is appropriate for all individuals. Instead, there must be an understanding of the principles that govern efficient posture. These principles must then be applied to each individual.

1. The weight-bearing segments of the body are so aligned in good standing posture that angles of inclination in the trunk and in the pelvic girdle are within "normal" limits. These limits are based on an erect posture of the pelvic girdle (lack of either posterior or anterior tilt) and the maintenance of normal spinal curves.
2. To be stable, the intersection of the line of gravity with the base of support will be close to the geometric center of the base. Maximum postural stability usually occurs when the line of gravity is over the center of pressure.
3. Standing posture is a position of extension of the weight-bearing joints. This should be an easy, balanced extension and should not be accompanied by strain or tension (Figure 14.16).

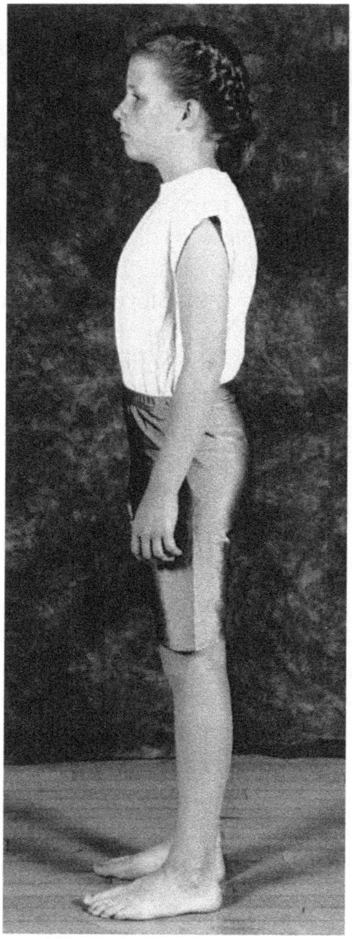

Figure 14.16 Except for a slightly forward head, the subject shows good alignment and extension without strain.

4. From the viewpoint of energy expenditure, efficient posture would seem to be a position that requires a minimum expenditure of energy *for the maintenance of good alignment.* Excess energy expenditure indicates hypertonicity, poor neuromuscular coordination, or both.
5. Efficient posture, both static and dynamic, requires a minimum of muscle force. This implies adequate development of the antigravity muscles to resist the pull of gravity successfully and to maintain alignment without excessive effort or tension. It also implies a balance between antagonistic muscle groups. There is no indication, however, that "the stronger the muscles, the better the posture."
6. Posture, both static and dynamic, requires sufficient flexibility in the structures of the weight-bearing joints to permit good alignment without interference or strain. Poor flexibility may be caused by tight ligaments or fasciae, short muscles, or hypertrophied muscles. The flexibility should not be so great, however, that excessive muscular effort is needed to keep the weight-bearing joints in alignment.
7. Posture requires coordination. This implies neuromuscular control and well-developed postural reflexes.
8. Adjustments in posture can be made more readily by individuals who have a good kinesthetic awareness of the postures they assume and of the degree of tension in their muscles.
9. The characteristics of normal posture change with age. Young children typically have a protruding abdomen and hollow lower back. Loss of muscle strength, inactivity, and balance problems in older persons show up in a wider stance, forward head, and rounded upper back, and limited flexibility in the trunk, hips, and knees.

Finding the Center of Gravity in the Human Body

The location of the center of gravity in human beings is of interest to scientists in many areas. Anatomists, kinesiologists, orthopedists, physical therapists, space engineers, and equipment design engineers have all shown interest in methods of determining the location of the center of gravity. Early experiments located the center of gravity by balancing the body over a wedge. Various other methods have since been developed to estimate the location of the center of gravity, either at rest or in motion. Two of these procedures, easily replicated with a minimum of equipment, are described here.

Reaction Board Method

It is a fairly simple matter to find an estimate of the center of gravity of a motionless body by using the *reaction board method.* Making use of the principle of moments, this procedure relies on the fact that the sum of the moments acting on a body in equilibrium is zero. Using this information, the location of the gravitational line is found for each plane. The center of gravity of the body becomes the intersection of the values for each of these three planes. Directions for locating the center of gravity in three planes follow.

Apparatus (Figure 14.17)

1. Scales: preferably either the Toledo or the spring balance type.
2. A stool or block the same height as the platform of the scales.
3. A board about 40 cm wide and 200 cm long. A knife edge should be attached to the underside of each end so that when the board is placed in a horizontal position, it rests on the knife edges. To simplify the calculations, the distance from knife edge to knife edge should measure exactly 200 cm. The front edge of the board should be marked in centimeters. The board should be tested with a level to make certain it is horizontal.

Directions (Refer to Figure 14.17)

1. Find the subject's total weight, ***W.***
2. Put one knife edge of board on the scale platform and the other edge on the box platform. Use a spirit level to make sure the board is horizontal. Note the reading on the scales. This is the partial weight of the board, ***B.***
3. Have the subject lie supine on the board with the heels against the footrest at the end of the board away from the scales. The position the subject assumes should be as similar to the standing position as possible. Record the reading on the scales. This is the partial weight of the subject and board, ***S.***
4. For equilibrium to exist about the pivot point ***P,*** the counterclockwise torques must equal the clockwise torques. If ***W*** is the total weight of the subject; ***B,*** the partial weight of the board; ***S,*** the partial weight of the subject and board; ***L,*** the length of the

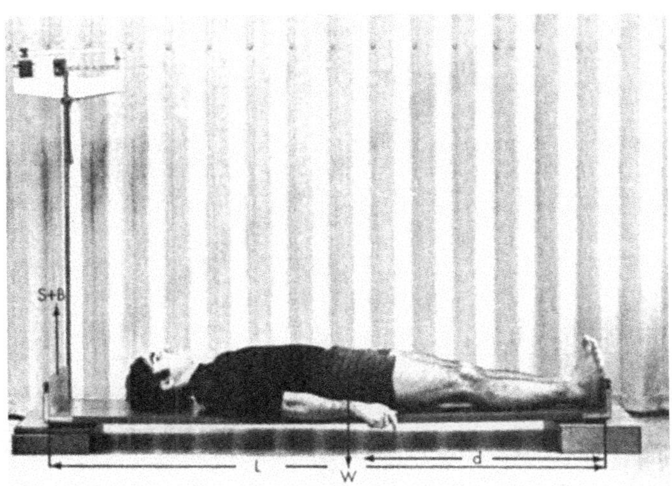

Figure 14.17 Reaction board method for locating the height of the center of gravity.

board; and ***d,*** the perpendicular distance from ***P*** to ***W;*** then

$$d \times W = (S - B)L$$

(clockwise torques = counterclockwise torques)

$$d = \frac{(S - B)L}{W}$$

Rearranged, the distance between the subject's feet and center of gravity is ***d.*** This is comparable to the distance between the ground and the center of gravity when the subject is standing but must be viewed as an estimate because of shifts in body organs and tissues when lying down.

5. The percentage height of the center of gravity with respect to the subject's total height is found by dividing the value of ***d*** in the transverse plane (supine lying position) by the subject's total height and multiplying by 100.

$$\text{Percent} = \frac{d \text{ in transverse place}}{\text{subject's height}} \times 100$$

6. To locate the center of gravity in the frontal or sagittal planes, the procedure must be repeated with the subject standing on the board (preferably near the middle). For the sagittal plane, the subject stands with the side to the scales (Figure 14.16) and for the frontal plane location, the subject stands facing the scales. Use the same formula

$$d = \frac{(S - B)L}{W}$$

to solve for ***d.*** The value of ***d*** represents the distance from the knife edge ***P*** to the plane in which the subject's center of gravity is located.

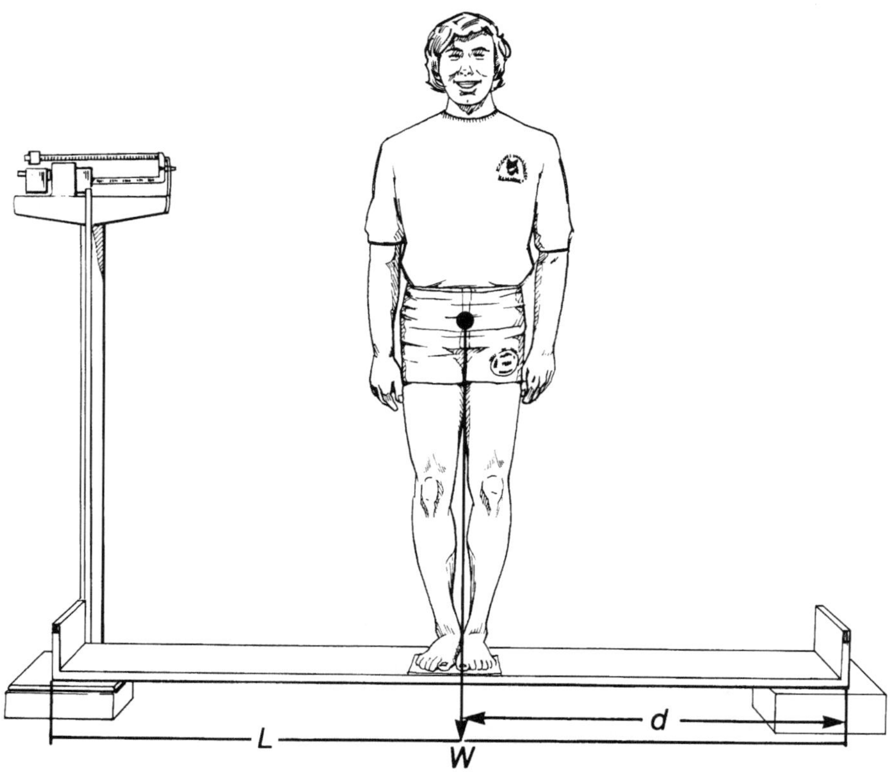

Figure 14.18 Reaction board method for locating the line of gravity in the sagittal plane.

7. To find the single point representing the spot where the line of gravity intersects the base of support, a piece of paper should be placed under the subject's feet for the side-view measurement. The outline of the feet is traced on the paper. When the first ***d*** is found, the distance is measured and marked on both the left and right sides of the paper. The paper should then be removed and the points connected by a straight line. When the subject faces forward for the second measurement, the paper should be placed on the board so that the subject's feet will fit in the footprints. When the second *d* is found, the distance should be measured and marked on both edges of the paper, and the place where two lines intersect represents the approximate position of the point where the line of gravity strikes the base of support. This is a crude method of locating this point and is not strictly accurate, because the subject may not be standing in exactly the same posture for both measurements. Furthermore, the element of swaying always introduces a source of error.

A modification of the reaction board method involves the use of a large triangular board supported by scales on two corners and a platform of equal height under the third corner (Waterland & Shambes, 1970). Each corner makes contact with its support through a pointed bolt. Again, it is important that the board be horizontal. If this triangle is equilateral, the moments are taken about lines forming two sides of the triangle, and the perpendicular distance from each line to the center of gravity is determined as follows:

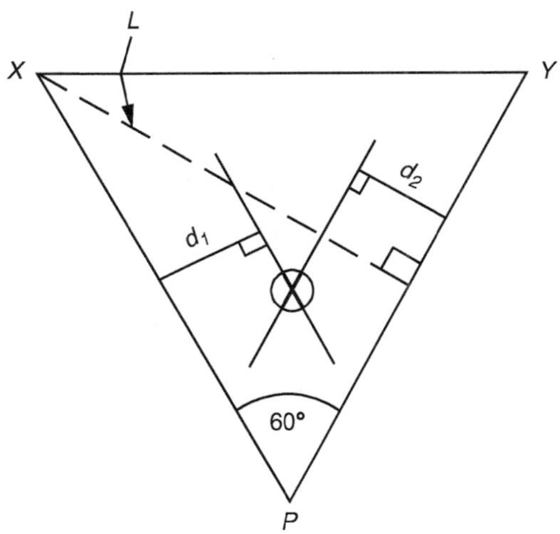

$$d_1 = \frac{(S_Y - B_Y)L}{W}$$

$$d_2 = \frac{(S_X - B_X)L}{W}$$

where

d_1 = distance between *XP* and center of gravity
d_2 = distance between *YP* and center of gravity
S_X = partial weight of subject and board on scale *X*
S_Y = partial weight of subject and board on scale *Y*
B_X = partial weight of board recorded on scale *X*
B_Y = partial weight of board recorded on scale *Y*
W = weight of subject
L = altitude of triangle (perpendicular distance from scale to line about which moment is being taken)

Segmental Method

Experiments using the reaction board are convincing in showing how the body automatically compensates for external loads and segmental adjustments. It is revealing also to see how the body adjusts for the sideward raising of an arm, the forward bending of the trunk, a briefcase carried in one hand, or a load of books carried on the hip. Such analysis, however, is limited to the body in a stationary position. The location of the center of gravity of someone in action requires the use of another method. A highly useful procedure is one called the *segmental method.* This technique makes use of a photograph of the subject and involves finding the location of the center of gravity of each of the body segments, the position of these individual gravity points with respect to arbitrarily placed x- and y-axes, and knowledge of the ratio between the individual segment weights and the total body weight.

Considerable research has been done to determine values for the proportionate weights of body segments and the locations of the segmental centers of gravity. These data have been obtained through the weighing and suspension of cadaver segments, determination of the weight of segments of living subjects through the amount of water displaced by the immersed segment, and formation of mathematical models. Among the most commonly used data today are those of Dempster (1955). He weighed eight elderly male cadavers, dismembered them, weighed the segments, and determined the proportion of total weight for each segment. In addition, he located the center of gravity and specific gravity for each segment.

Using the same definitions of joint center used by Dempster, and using the segmental water volume values determined by Clauser (as cited in Plagenhoef et al., 1983), Plagenhoef and colleagues (1983) immersed the various segments of 135 subjects in water to determine segment weights as a percentage of total body weight. These data are presented in Figure 14.20 and Table 14.1. This research team then selected a smaller sample and again used the segmental immersion technique to locate the segmental centers of gravity as a percentage of the total segment length. These data are presented in Table 14.2.

With information on the proportionate mass of body segments and the location of the center of gravity of each segment, the center of gravity of the whole body in any plane may now be determined by making use of the principle of torques. The sum of the torques of the

TABLE 14.1 Location of the Segment Center of Gravity as a Percentage of the Segment Length

	Men (N = 7)		Women (N = 9)	
	Proximal	Distal	Proximal	Distal
Hand	46.8	—	46.8	—
Forearm	43.0	57.0	43.4	56.6
Upper arm	43.6	56.4	45.8	54.2
Foot	50.0	—	50.0	—
Shank	43.4	56.6	41.9	58.1
Thigh	43.3	56.7	42.8	57.2
Whole trunk[a]	63.0	37.0	56.9	43.1
Pelvis[b]	5.0	95.0	5.0	95.0
Abdomen	46.0	54.0	46.0	54.0
Thorax[c]	56.7	43.3	56.3	43.7
Head and neck[d]	55.0	45.0	55.0	45.0
Abdomen and pelvis[e]	44.5	55.5	39.0	61.0

[a]Hip joint to shoulder joint = 100%.

[b]Hip joint to plane of umbilicus = 100%.

[c]Pectoral line to shoulder joint (glenohumeral) = 100%.

[d]Top of the head to seventh cervical = 100%.

[e]Hip joint to T-11 = 100%.

Source: From "Anatomical Data for Analyzing Human Motion," by S. Plagenhoef, F. Evans, & T. Abdelnour, *Research Quarterly,* 54(2), 172, 1983.

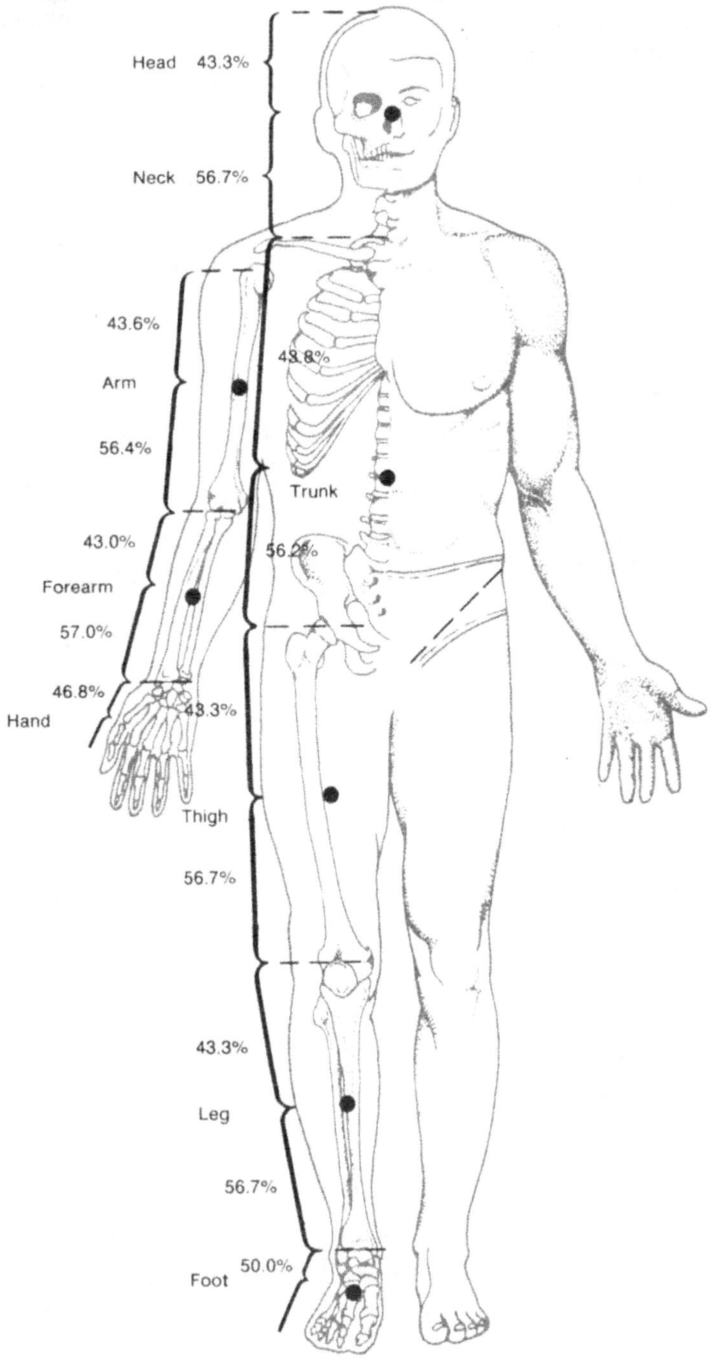

Figure 14.20 Joint centers and percentage distance of centers of gravity from joint centers in males. *Source:* Compiled from data in Plagenhoef et al., 1983; Hinrichs, 1990; and Dempster, 1955.

TABLE 14.2 Body Segment Percentages of Total Body Weight for Living Men and Woman

Segments	Men	Women
Hands	1.3	1.0
Forearms	3.8	3.1
Upper arms	6.6	6.0
Feet	2.9	2.4
Shanks	9.0	10.5
Thighs	21.0	23.0
Trunk (including head and neck)	55.4	54.0

individual segments about arbitrarily placed *x*- and *y*-axes will produce the location of the center of gravity of the whole body with respect to the *x*- and *y*-axes. This is because the total body weight acting at the center of mass is the resultant of the combined segment weights acting at their mass centers, and the resultant moment of the total body weight about the *x*-, *y*-axes is the sum of the individual segment torques about the same axes.

The segmental method for determining the center of gravity requires a considerable amount of measurement and calculation and therefore can be time consuming. The use of computer programs speeds up the process considerably, as does the use of motion analysis systems with built-in *x*-, *y*-coordinate systems.

Directions for locating the center of gravity using the segmental method follow.

Apparatus

1. Line drawing on graph paper taken from photographic image of subject (Figure 14.21).
2. Worksheet with Plagenhoef et al. proportions listed (Figure 14.22).

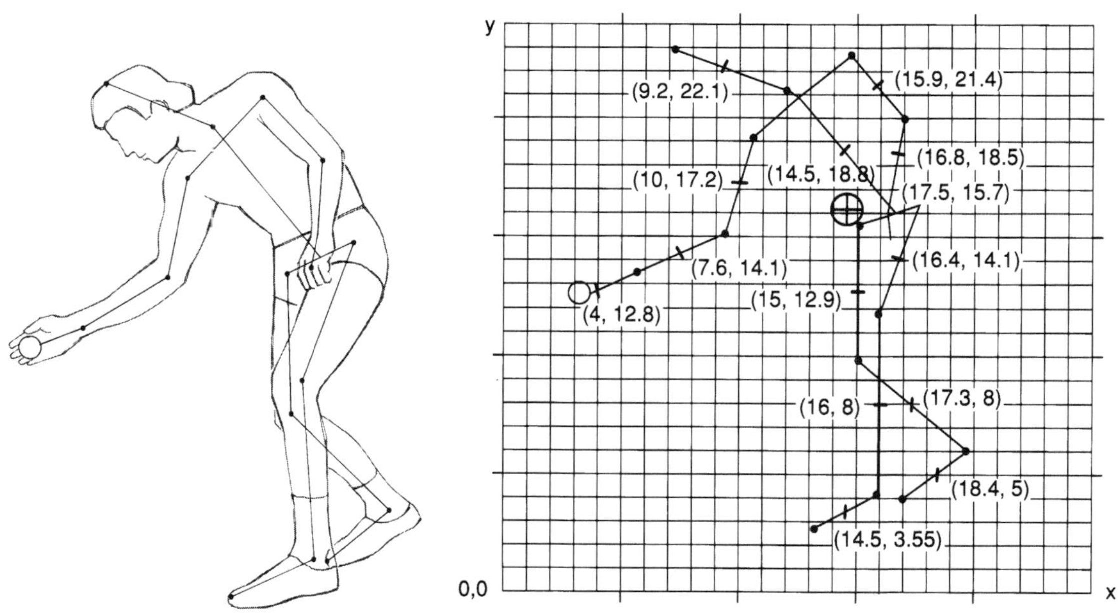

Figure 14.21 Segmental determination of the center of gravity. (a) Location of body segments. (b) The center of mass of each body segment is marked, and *x*-, *y*-coordinates are found using an arbitrarily placed *x*-, *y*-axis. With information on the proportionate mass of each body segment and the location of the center of mass of each segment, the center of gravity of the whole body may be determined using the principle of moments.

Body Segment	Proportion of Body Wt.	*x* Value	*x* Products	*y* Value	*y* Products
1. Trunk	.486	14.5	7.05	18.8	9.14
2. Head & Neck	.079	9.2	0.73	22.1	1.75
3. R. Thigh	.097	15.0	1.46	12.9	1.25
4. R. Lower Leg	.045	17.3	0.79	8.0	0.36
5. R. Foot	.014	18.4	0.26	5.0	0.70
6. L. Thigh	.097	16.4	1.59	14.1	1.37
7. L. Lower Leg	.045	16.0	0.72	8.0	0.36
8. L. Foot	.014	14.5	0.20	3.5	0.05
9. R. Upper Arm	.027	10.0	0.27	17.2	0.46
10. R. Lower Arm	.014	7.6	0.11	14.1	0.20
11. R. Hand	.006	4.0	0.02	12.8	0.08
12. L. Upper Arm	.027	15.9	0.43	21.4	0.58
13. L. Lower Arm	.014	16.8	0.24	18.5	0.26
14. L. Hand	.006	17.5	0.10	15.7	0.09
x - *y* Resultants (product total)			13.97		16.65

x Coordinate = 13.97

y Coordinate = 16.65

Figure 14.22 Worksheet for locating the center of gravity using the segmental method.

Directions

1. The locations of the extremities of the individual segments must be marked according to the link boundaries shown in Figure 14.20. This will result in marks at the end of the second toe, ankle, knee, hip, knuckle III of the hand, wrist, shoulders, seventh cervical vertebra, and top of the head. Where these points are obscured by other body parts, an estimate must be made. The upper trunk mark is the seventh cervical vertebra, located slightly above the midpoint of the transverse line joining the shoulders. The lower trunk mark is the midpoint of the transverse line joining the hips.
2. The extremity limits are joined to form a stick figure consisting of fourteen segments (see Figure 14.19a).
3. The mass center location for each segment length is found using the data provided in Table 14.1, where centers of gravity are located as a percentage of the distance between segment end points. The amount of

the percentage distance from one segment end point is multiplied by the picture length of the segment. The resulting product is the distance from the selected end point to the center of gravity of the segment. The distance is measured from the end point, and the center of gravity is marked by a short slash mark intersecting the segment line.

4. The *x*- and *y*-axes are drawn on the paper.
5. The *x*-, *y*-coordinates for each of the fourteen segment mass centers are determined and recorded on the diagram of the figure at the respective mass centers.
6. A worksheet such as that shown in Figure 14.20 is used to record the *x*-, *y*-coordinate values and the torques of those segments about the *x*- and *y*-axes. The individual torques are the products (col. 3) of the coordinate values (col. 2) and their related body segment proportions (col. 1).
7. The algebraic sum of the *x* products represents the *x*-coordinate of the total body's mass center, and the algebraic sum of the *y* products is the *y*-coordinate. These values are located and marked on the tracing (see Figure 14.19b).

This procedure has made it possible to locate the center of gravity of the handball player at the moment of contact with the ball. It must be remembered that this location is for one brief moment during the performance of the skill, and the position of the center of gravity will shift with body segment shifts.

While this may seem like a cumbersome process, the basic concept is still in use in many motion-capture systems. Through the use of the principles spelled out here, motion-capture systems can perform the calculations required to pinpoint the location of the center of gravity throughout the entire motion.

Students who desire to trace the path of the center of gravity during the execution of a dynamic skill, but who do not need the accuracy of the segmental method, may find the placement of a dot on the iliac crest to be a useful estimate for the location of the body's center of gravity (Figure 14.23). This technique should be used with caution, however. It is important to remember that the center of gravity will deviate appreciably from this location in some body positions (see Figures 14.1 through 14.4).

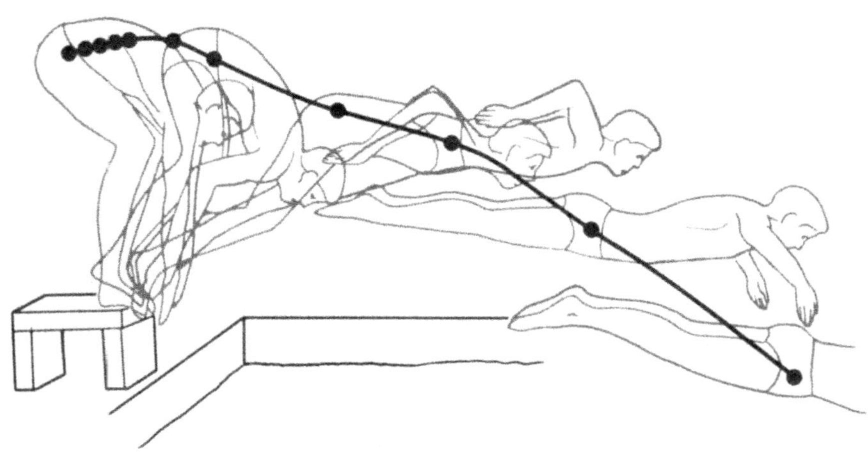

Figure 14.23 The iliac crest is used as an estimate of the location of the center of gravity of a swimmer during the execution of a racing dive. The tracking of the center of gravity of a dynamic skill is done through the use of tracings of individual video frames.

REFERENCES AND SELECTED READINGS

Bardy, B. G., Oullier, O., Bootsma, R., and Stoffregen, T.A. (2002). Dynamics of human postural transitions. *Journal of Experimental Psychology:Human Perception and Performance,* 28, 499–514.

Basmajian, J. V., & Deluca, C. J. (1985). *Muscles alive* (5th ed.). Baltimore: Williams & Wilkins.

Blackburn, J. T., Riemann, B. L., Myers, J. B., & Lehart, S. M. (2003). Kinematic analysis of the hip and trunk during bilateral stand of firm, foam, and multiaxial support surfaces. *Clinical Biomechanics,* 18, 655–661.

Bouisset, S., & Do, M. C. (2008). Posture, dynamic stability, and voluntary movement. *Clinical Neurophysiology,* 38, 345–362.

Dempster, W. T. (1955). *Space requirements of the seated operator.* Dayton, OH: Wright-Patterson Air Force Base (WADC TR 55–199).

Durkin, J. L., Dowling, J. J., & Andrews, D. M. (2002). The measurement of body segment inertial parameters using dual energy X-ray absorptiometry. *Journal of Biomechanics,* 35(12), 1575–1580.

Fiolkowski, P., Brunt, D., Bishop, M., & Woo, R. (2002). Does postural instability affect the initiation of human gait? *Neuroscience Letters,* 323(3), 167–170.

Forth, K. E., Metter, E.J., and Paloski, W.H. (2007). Age-associated differences in postural equilibrium contol: A comparison between Eqscore and minimum time to contact (TtC). *Gait and Posture* 25(1), 56–62.

Granata, K. P., & Lockhart, T. E. (2008). Dynamic stability differences in fall-prone and healthy adults. *Journal of Electromyography and Kinesiology,* 18, 172–178.

Haddad, J. M., Gagnon, J. L., Hasson, C. J., Van Emmerik, R. E. A., & Hammill, J. (2006). Evaluation of time-to-contact measures for assessing postural stability. *Journal of Applied Biomechanics,* 22, 155–161.

Henry, S. M., Fung, J., & Horak, F. B. (2001). Effect of stance width on multidirectional postural responses. *Journal of Neurophysiology,* 85(2), 559–570.

Hinrichs, R. N. (1990). Adjustments to the center of mass proportions of Clauser et al. (1969). *Journal of Biomechanics,* 23, 949–951.

Horak, F. B. (2006). Postural orientation and equilibrium: What do we need to know about neural control of balance to prevent falls? *Age and Ageing,* 35-S2, ii7–ii11.

Lovejoy, C. O. (2005a). The natural history of human gait and posture. Part 1. Spine and pelvis. *Gait and Posture,* 21(1), 95–112.

Lovejoy, C. O. (2005b). The natural history of human gait and posture. Part 2. Hip and thigh. *Gait and Posture,* 21(1), 113–124.

Plagenhoef, S., Evans, F., & Abdelnour, T. (1983). Anatomical data for analyzing human motion. *Research Quarterly,* 54, 169–178.

Pope, M. H., Goh, K. L., & Magnusson, M. L. (2002). Spine ergonomics. *Annual Review of Biomedical Engineering,* 4, 49–68.

Raymakers, J. A., Samson, M. M., & Verhaar, H. J. (2005). The assessment of body sway and the choice of the stability parameter(s). *Gait and Posture,* 21(1), 48–58.

Rougier, P.-R. (2008). What insights can be gained when analysing the resultant centre of pressure trajectory? *Clinical Neurophysiology,* 38, 363–373.

Visser, J. E., Carpenter, M. G., van der Kooij, H., & Bloem, B. R. (2008). The clinical utility of posturography. *Clinical Neurophysiology,* 119, 2424–2436.

Vuillerme, N., & Rougier, P. (2005). Effects of head extension on undisturbed upright stance control in humans. *Gait & Posture,* 21(3), 318–325.

Waterland, J. D., & Shambes, G. M. (1970). Biplane center of gravity procedure. *Perceptual Motor Skills,* 30, 511–514.

Winter, D. A., Patla, A. E., Riedtyk, S., & Ishac, M. (2001). Ankle muscle stiffness in the control of balance during quiet standing. *Journal of Neurophysiology,* 85, 2630–2633.

Wu, G., & MacLeod, M. (2001). The control of body orientation and center of mass location under asymmetrical loading. *Gait and Posture,* 13(2), 95–101.

LABORATORY EXPERIENCES

1. Define the following key terms and give an example of each that is not used in the text:
   Center of gravity
   Stability
   Base of support
2. a. Working with a partner, determine the position of your line of gravity using the reaction board method. Locate the point where this line intersects your base of support by marking it on a tracing of your feet.
   b. Determine the position of your line of gravity, leaning as far forward as possible with the body in a straight line from the top of the head to the ankles. Repeat, leaning as far backward as possible.
   c. Locate the line of gravity in the sagittal plane while leaning as far as possible to one side.
   d. Determine the height of your center of gravity with your arms at your side and then with them stretched over your head. What percentage of your total height is your center of gravity? How does this compare with averages for your sex?
   e. Choose an original position with a small or unstable base of support. Locate the point where the line of gravity intersects the base of support.
3. Make a tracing on graph paper of a picture of a person engaged in a motor skill. Locate the center of gravity using the segmental method.
4. Walk on a low balance beam and do the following:
   a. Look ahead at the wall.
   b. Look at a person who is in front of the balance beam doing a vigorous exercise such as a jumping jack.
   c. Walk with your eyes blindfolded.
   d. Walk along with a partner walking beside you. Without warning, the partner is to give you a slight but sudden sideward push. What measures do you take to maintain your balance? If you fail, explain why.
5. Build two columns of blocks, one with the blocks carefully centered one over the other, the second column with the blocks staggered but balanced. Grasping the lowest block of each column, slide the columns back and forth, changing the speed frequently and suddenly until the blocks tumble. Which column is the first to topple? Why?

PART III

Motor Skills: Principles and Applications

Introduction to Part III

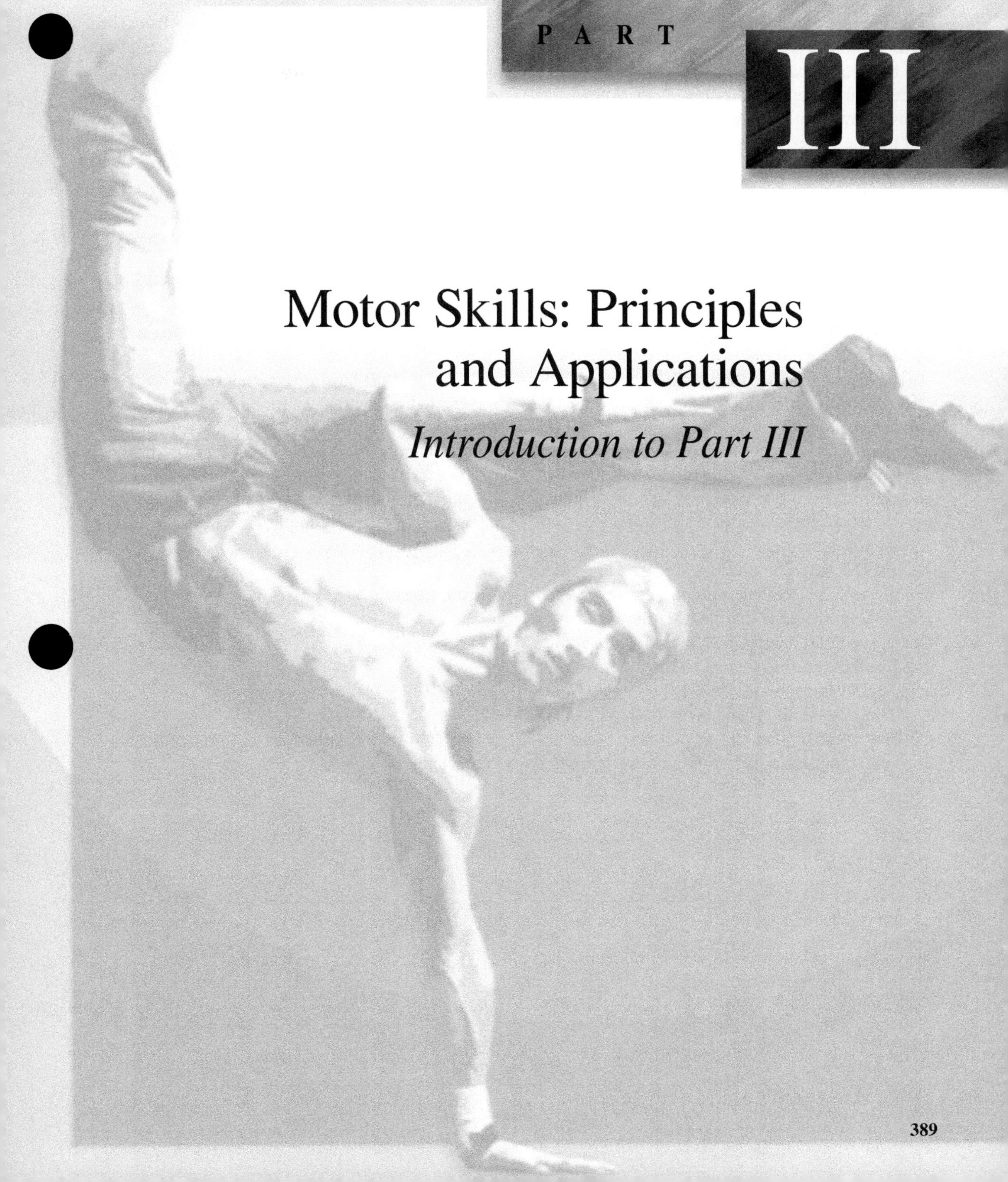

The most difficult aspect of the study of kinesiology is the application of anatomical and biomechanical concepts and principles so that students are able to generalize their knowledge across movement patterns and to apply it to new and unique patterns they may encounter. For students of human motion to be effective in applying their enhanced knowledge of kinesiological principles to improve performance, they must establish a logical framework for their analysis and engage in a systematic approach to critical observation and evaluation.

At the conclusion of Part III, students should be able to complete basic qualitative kinesiological analyses for all categories of skill classification. This means that they will have learned to observe and describe movements accurately, evaluate performance according to anatomical and mechanical principles, and prescribe corrective actions when needed. It also means that they will have developed the ability to select and evaluate the appropriateness of motor skills and exercises and related equipment.

Part III draws on the anatomical and mechanical information presented in Parts I and II. Analyses and applications that provide the framework for the successful performance of motor skills are presented based on the model for kinesiological analysis developed in Chapter 1.

The first seven chapters in Part III are organized according to the system for classification of motor skills (pp. 6–7) and are presented with the intent that the student progress from the study of relatively simple motions to more complex motions—that is, from static and dynamic postures through exercise and locomotion, to the giving of motion to external objects and the reception of impact. Included in each chapter is a brief description of the types of motion involved; outlines of anatomical and mechanical principles for effective, efficient, and safe performance; and an in-depth qualitative analysis of at least one motor activity.

Chapter 22 concludes Part III with a description of the instrumentation and methodology currently being used for motion analysis. It is becoming more and more likely that students at all levels will have direct experience with sophisticated equipment and methodology as early as their first kinesiology course. It is, therefore, important that they understand the significance of the contributions to our growing knowledge of human motion that have occurred through the expanding use of increasingly sophisticated analysis techniques and tools.

Assumption:

- Student understands the basic concepts in mechanics.

Review:

- Part II of this text provides an introduction to mechanics.

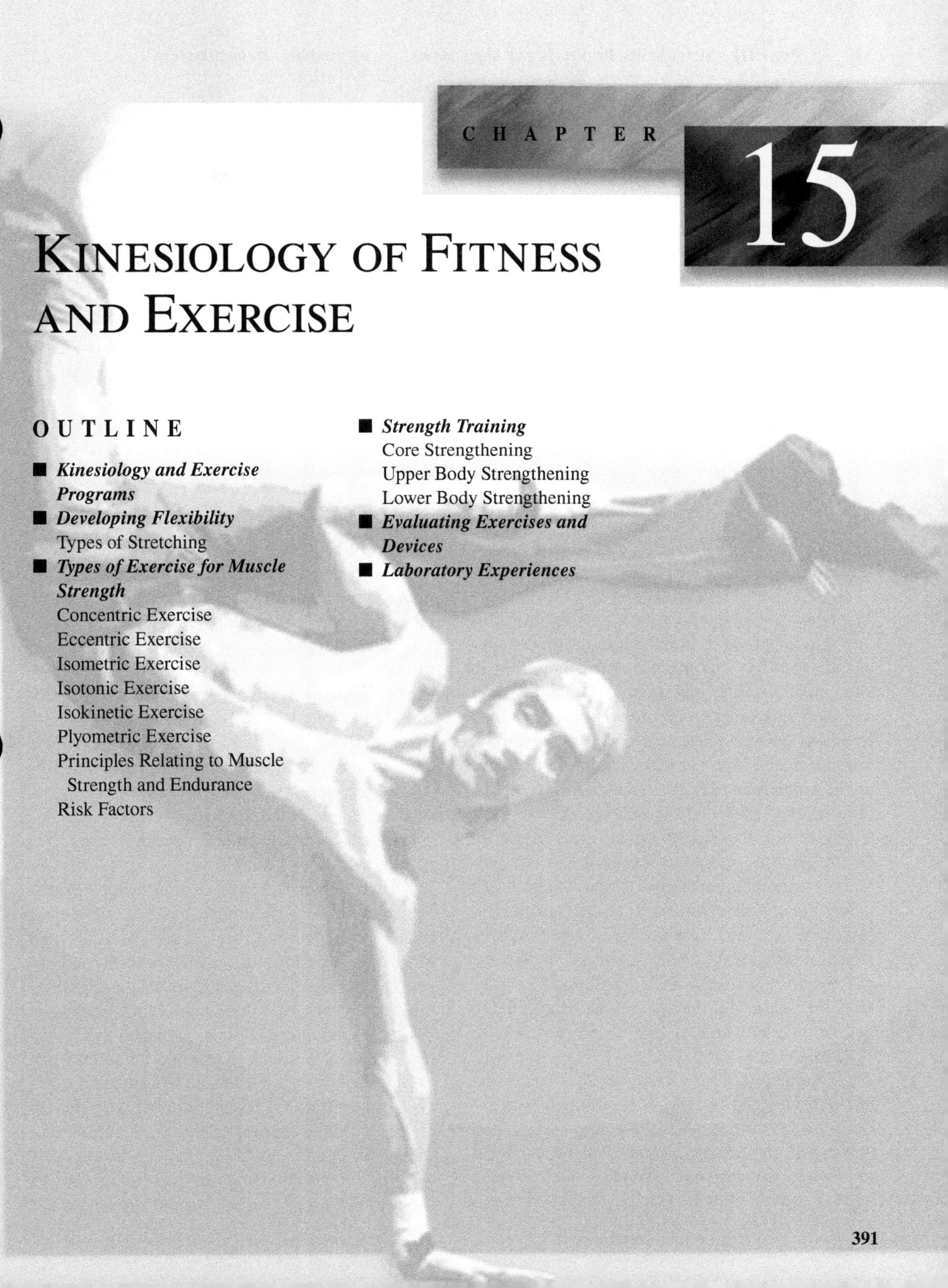

CHAPTER 15

KINESIOLOGY OF FITNESS AND EXERCISE

OUTLINE

OBJECTIVES

At the conclusion of this chapter, the student should be able to:

1. Define flexibility, muscular strength, and endurance, and state how each can be developed.
2. State the principles that should be followed when prescribing or engaging in exercises for flexibility.
3. Develop an appropriate exercise for improving range of motion in any joint.
4. Name and describe the four types of exercise programs used for muscle strength and development.
5. Identify the advantages and disadvantages of various types of muscle strength and endurance programs.
6. Develop a graded exercise series for strengthening each of three muscle groups. Justify the selection and order of the exercises using the outline for kinesiological analysis.

KINESIOLOGY AND EXERCISE PROGRAMS

The objectives of exercise programs are to facilitate musculoskeletal, circulatory, and respiratory adaptations that will make possible increases in strength, flexibility, and work capacity for safer and more enjoyable motion in work, play, and activities of daily living. In the twenty-first-century, exercise in any form has taken on new importance as the population changes. The sharp increase in the rate of obesity and the increase in active life span give new meaning to the idea of exercise for health. Exercise programs are used to ready athletes for competition, curb obesity, reduce falls in the elderly, decrease the incidence of musculoskeletal pain, and for a myriad of other reasons. Health professionals worldwide are sounding the call for an increase in levels of physical activity for all. It is the job of the movement specialist to help provide safe and effective means for exercise enhancement.

The interests of the exercise physiologist and the kinesiologist overlap in the realm of exercise. Both are concerned with the energy, work, and power aspects and the musculoskeletal and neuromuscular dimensions of exercise. They diverge in their concerns with the physiologist's focus on energy sources and demands and the kinesiologist's focus on forces causing the motion and analysis of technique. Knowing what to select for an appropriate conditioning or therapeutic exercise program requires knowledge of both exercise physiology and kinesiology. As might be expected, the discussion in this chapter is limited primarily to the kinesiology of selected exercises—namely, those designed primarily to increase flexibility, develop muscular strength and endurance, and improve core stability. Understanding the demands of a movement will help the individual select appropriate exercises to enhance performance or rehabilitate following an injury.

Exercise for the sake of improving flexibility, strength, and endurance has become a field in its own right. For this reason, a textbook in kinesiology cannot address all of the myriad aspects of exercise for fitness. This chapter provides the student with an overall sense of a kinesiological approach to the examination of exercise for fitness. There is not room in this text for an in-depth examination of exercise. Instead, the student is encouraged to read the research literature in the exercise areas of interest. Popular literature and exercise programs should be viewed with a critical eye. The selection and use of various exercises should follow a logical analysis to determine the safety, efficiency, and effectiveness of the movements involved.

DEVELOPING FLEXIBILITY

Flexibility is the ability of the tissues surrounding a joint to yield to stretching without interference or opposition and then to relax. The tissues to be stretched include not only the ligaments, fasciae, and other connective tissue related to the joints but, in many instances, the antagonistic muscles as well—that is, the muscles that oppose the movement in which the joint action is limited. For instance, the restriction in a person who is unable to bend over and touch the floor without bending the knees is more likely to be caused by tight tendons of the hamstring muscles than by tight knee ligaments. And the person who lacks the shoulder flexibility needed for raising the arms forward-upward and past the head is hampered at least as much, if not more, by tight pectoral muscles as by tight anterior shoulder ligaments.

Flexibility is joint—and activity—specific. The range of motion about a joint depends on the structure of the joint and the pattern of movement to which it has been subjected. The range of motion of the shoulder is far greater than that of most other joints. This being said, the demands on the shoulder joints of individual athletes may vary by sport. Swimmers and baseball players, for example, require greater shoulder flexibility than do basketball players or weight lifters. Moreover, a large degree of flexibility in one joint does not mean that there will be a large degree of flexibility in another joint. For example, weight lifters often have below-average flexibility in the shoulder and above-average flexibility in the trunk, whereas swimmers often have above-average shoulder flexibility and average trunk flexibility. Individuals participating in specific activities should know the joint range of motion demands necessary for optimum performance in the activity and select appropriate flexibility exercises for each involved joint.

An effective program of stretching has been shown to increase range of motion and muscle flexibility. There are some limitations, however, to the benefits of stretching. When the desired performance outcome is explosive power, acute stretching immediately prior to performance has been found to be detrimental. If the requirements of the activity demand a powerful contraction of muscle, greater muscle stiffness is required. This would be the case in explosive jumping or sprinting. On the other hand, good flexibility is important to performers who require a full range of motion or who are engaged in cyclic motion at low to moderate intensities. All can benefit from stretching during training, but consideration must be given to performance demands when using stretch as a warm-up activity (Cramer et al., 2005; Fletcher & Jones, 2004; Nelson et al., 2005; Shrier, 2004).

The relationship between stretching and injury is not yet clear. Although a number of investigators have found that static stretching reduces the occurrence of muscle strains, the same cannot be said for bone or joint injuries. Any link between stretching and delayed onset muscle soreness is also still open to debate. There is some evidence that stretching is ineffective in preventing the delayed onset muscle soreness that results from eccentric exercise (Amako et al., 2003; Gabbe et al., 2005; Small et al., 2008; Thacker et al., 2005).

Types of Stretching

Ballistic versus Static Stretching

The development of range of motion in a joint may best be accomplished using static stretching methods. In static stretching, the tissues are gradually stretched up to the point of discomfort, and the resulting position is held for a minimum of thirty seconds. Ballistic stretching methods, consisting of an active bobbing or bouncing action that makes use of the momentum of the moving body part to force the involved tissues to stretch, have been shown to be equally effective in developing flexibility, but the static stretch has become the preferred method because there is less danger of tissue damage through sudden overstretching, the energy requirement is less, and there is less postexercise muscle soreness. Another advantage is that a slow static stretch will reduce the stretch reflex contraction of the muscle being stretched. A hard ballistic stretch may trigger a phasic stretch reflex, which may then elicit a contraction of the muscle undergoing stretch. This adds to the potential for tissue damage. Despite the potential risks, ballistic stretching programs are more likely to develop dynamic flexibility, such as that demanded in most physical activity. Ballistic stretching programs should be structured with great care. Such a program should begin with static stretches to establish a base of flexibility. Next, slow, low-range motions should be incorporated. Gradually the program may be increased to fast, large-range motion stretches. Caution must be used to ensure that a solid base of flexibility is established before this level is reached (Alter, 1996).

Active and Passive Stretching

Stretching exercises may also be classified as active or passive according to the source of the stretching force.

Active stretching In active stretching, the antagonists of joint actions are stretched by the concentric contraction of the contralateral muscles. In the stretch shown in Figure 15.1, the muscles in the lower back and posterior leg are stretched due to the contraction of the extensors of the knee and ankle. In Exercise 3.1 of Appendix G, the pectoral muscles and anterior shoulder structures are stretched because of the contraction of the antagonists, posterior shoulder muscles, and scapular adductors.

Active stretch patterns may be used with almost any joint or segment of the body. Other examples might be side bending stretches (with motion occurring in the spine rather than hip joints) and stretch of the anterior muscles of the thigh produced through contraction of the hip extensors while in a prone position.

Active stretching may also be assisted. In active-assisted stretching, the force that produces the stretch is external. A common form of active-assisted stretching is partner stretch activity. Additionally, it is possible and popular to produce an active-assisted stretch using an external object as a point of fixation.

Passive stretching The passive exercise requires the help of another person or gravity unless the part of the body is one on which the subject can use another body part, such as the hands, to apply the stretch. *Except for conditions where the individual is unable to provide adequate force (as in paralysis), the assistance of another person is not a preferred method due to the danger of overstretching and injury.*

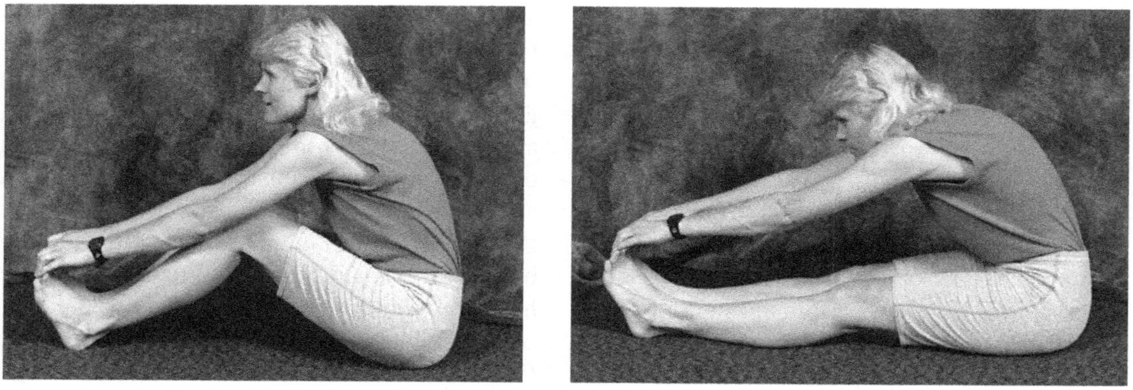

Figure 15.1 An example of active static stretching. The muscles of the lower back and posterior leg are stretched as a result of the contraction of the contralateral muscles of the legs.

Numerous exercises use the force of gravity as the stretching agent. A strong pectoral stretching exercise in which gravity does the stretching is passive hanging from a horizontal bar or pair of rings. For a somewhat greater stretch, swinging on a trapeze or pair of flying rings is usually enjoyable as well as effective. A still different kind of pectoral stretching exercise using gravity calls for the individual to stand in an open doorway with arms extended diagonally sideward and upward with the hands braced against the door frame. Keeping the hands and arms in that position, the subject leans forward from the ankles. The weight of the body in the slanting position puts the pectoral muscles and the anterior joint tissues on a stretch (see Exercise 3.1 in Appendix G).

Gravity also provides a stretch for the lower extremities in many exercises. In one example, the subject stands on a box or block while holding on to a bar or wall. With the feet kept parallel, the heels are lowered as far as possible in a position of dorsiflexion. This stretches the Achilles tendon as well as the posterior ligaments of the ankle. In the second exercise, as the subject leans toward the wall with the feet flat on the floor, the calf muscles crossing the posterior ankle are stretched by the downward torque of the body weight applied at its center of gravity. The weight of the body also forces the heel stretch in Exercise 3.2 (Appendix G).

The quadriceps stretching exercise shown in Figure 15.2 is a good example of a passive exercise in which the subject uses the hands to apply the force for the stretch. With the leg flexed at the knee, the ankle is grasped behind the body, and the anterior hip and thigh are stretched as the leg is pulled upward and posterior. Care must be taken not to apply any lateral or twisting forces, which may cause ligament, cartilage, or joint capsule damage to the knee.

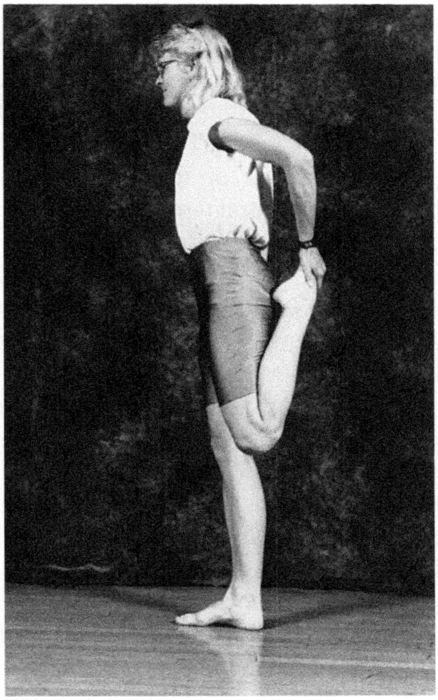

Figure 15.2 An example of passive static stretching. The anterior hip and thigh muscles are stretched by pulling up on the foot with the hand.

A second example is used to stretch the hamstrings. While lying on the back with one knee bent to the chest, the subject grasps the instep with the opposite hand. Maintaining this hold without twisting the foot, the subject pushes against the front of the knee with the other hand, attempting to straighten the leg in a vertical and upward direction. A third example applied to the hip is used for stretching in the direction of abduction and outward rotation. The subject assumes the position shown in Figure 3.8 in Appendix G and presses down on the knees.

Proprioceptive Neuromuscular Facilitation (PNF)

In proprioceptive neuromuscular facilitation (PNF) stretching, combinations of sustained static stretch and muscular contraction are used to increase range of motion. The basic concept in PNF stretching is to avoid triggering a stretch reflex contraction in the muscle to be stretched and to make positive use of the stretch reflex, the Golgi tendon organ (GTO) response, and reciprocal innervation to further relax the stretching muscle, although there is some controversy concerning the actual reflex involvement (Chalmers, 2004).

Several types of PNF stretches have been identified in the literature. Among these are the repeat contraction, slow reversal, slow reversal–hold, rhythmic stabilization, hold–relax, and contract–relax methods. There are, in addition, several combinations of these techniques. An example of the contract–relax style of a PNF stretch would be the hamstring stretch in a long sit position. While in the long sit position, the subject reaches forward slowly to grasp the ankles. In this stretch position, the subject then isometrically contracts the now-stretched hamstring muscle group to its voluntary maximum, holding the joints stationary. This static contraction should be held for approximately 5 seconds. Once this contraction is released, the quadriceps muscle group is contracted to produce further hip flexion while the subject uses the hands to attempt to pull the chest closer to the thighs. In this example, the sustained stretch of the hamstrings acts in the same manner discussed earlier. The contraction of the agonist hamstring muscles should produce sufficient tension in the muscle to stimulate the GTO, thereby initiating a reflex relaxation of the muscle. The following contraction of the quadriceps group further enhances this relaxation through reciprocal innervation. The PNF combination should allow for greater hip flexion than a simple static stretch.

The PNF stretch technique may be applied to any joint in the body. The key factor in PNF stretching is the active contraction of either the agonist muscle (GTO response) or the antagonist muscle (reciprocal innervation) or each in turn once the limit of range of motion has been reached. The short relaxation triggered by the two reflexes involved will allow additional stretch.

Whatever the method of stretching used, the instructor or therapist needs to be thoroughly familiar with the structure and function of the joint in question. Not only must the degree of limitation of motion be known, but the tissues responsible for the limitation must be known. The effect that the various reflexes may have and the conditions under which they are likely to be active must also be considered.

Types of Exercise for Muscle Strength

The one who selects exercises for muscular strength and muscular endurance must be aware of the meaning of each of these elements of physical conditioning and understand the relationship that exists between them. *Muscle strength* is the force a muscle or muscle group can exert against a resistance in one maximum effort. *Muscle endurance* is the ability to perform repeated contractions of the muscle(s) or to sustain a contraction against a submaximal resistance for an extended period of time. These elements are related so that training with an emphasis on strength will have an effect on endurance. However, different adaptations occur within the muscle, with different training emphases. For this reason, conditioning programs should be selected to be specific to the needs of a particular activity and should be patterned after the demands placed on the muscle in the activity. The most important factor in maximum strength development is the amount of resistance employed to overload the muscle. In endurance development, the emphasis is placed on the number of repetitions of the movement.

Concentric Exercise

As generally practiced, this form of exercise involves lifting weights—for example, dumbbells, kettlebells, disk weights, or stack weights, through a specified range of motion. The resistance to the contracting muscles is not only the actual magnitude of the weight lifted, but the product of the weight and length of the resistance arm of the anatomical lever involved. Hence the maximum resistance occurs only when the resistance force is acting at right angles to the lever.

Eccentric Exercise

The return movement of concentric-type exercises, when done in a slow, controlled manner, uses eccentric contraction of the antagonist muscles. Because a muscle can sustain more tension in eccentric contraction than it can develop in concentric contraction, exercise physiologists had thought that eccentric contraction exercises, or negative lifts, should be more effective in strength development than concentric exercises. The results of research to date do not support this theory. Eccentric exercises have been shown to be as effective as concentric exercises, and they do produce greater muscle hypertrophy. Eccentric exercise has been found to contribute significantly to delayed onset muscle soreness. With high repetitions or high loads, eccentric exercise may also lead to muscle damage. Strengthening the muscle concentrically has been found to reduce the negative effects of eccentric exercise. It is often the eccentric phase of lifting that produces the pain that leads to the saying, "No pain, no gain." In fact, microdamage to the muscle from lifting eccentrically does not contribute to muscle strength and may impair the ability of the muscle to develop adequate force in the short term. Intentionally damaging the muscle in the name of muscle strength or hypertrophy should be discouraged (Folland et al., 2002; Proske & Morgan, 2001).

Isometric Exercise

Because an isometric muscle contraction is defined as involving no change in muscle length, it follows that an isometric exercise is one that involves no motion either. Isometric exercise occurs when muscles contract in a static contraction in opposition to a fixed or immovable load. Isometric exercise, although providing some strength gain, does not increase strength throughout the range of motion. Further, not all of a muscle's fibers are activated during isometric contraction. This makes isometric exercise somewhat limited in application. A primary use for isometrics currently is in the rehabilitation of muscles surrounding injured joints.

There are many drawbacks and even potential hazards when using isometric exercises. Isometric exercises increase muscle strength only and are not effective for development of other fitness components such as flexibility and cardiovascular endurance. Moreover, the strength development achieved is greatest at the specific angle of the static contraction. If the objective is the development of strength throughout the range of motion, then the isometric exercise must be done at many joint angles spread over the entire range. Finally, a static contraction activates the slow-twitch muscle fibers predominantly and therefore does not act to enhance speed of movement in any way.

Isotonic Exercise

The term isotonic is a combination of the Greek words for "constant" and "tension." Hence, isotonic exercise is that in which muscular tension remains the same throughout the motion. In fact, this state is very difficult to produce and very difficult to measure. In most exercise forms, the tension produced in muscles will vary with muscle length, moment arm for the muscle, and with the variation in external torque. In other words, as the segment in motion moves through the range of motion, torque will vary with joint angle. A quick review of Chapter 13 will refresh the student's memory of why this is true. In the 1970s, fitness equipment companies started developing weight training machines to produce isotonic exercise. A number of systems employ an elliptical cam that provides a constantly changing resistance moment arm (Figure 15.3). The change in the resistance arm is calculated to coincide with both the changing muscle angle of pull and changing muscle length and is intended to provide for a constant resistance torque throughout the motion. This comes close to meeting the constant tension requirements of an isotonic exercise. Equipment of this type, designed to provide this very specific type of resistance, requires a separate machine for each muscle group and joint action.

Isokinetic Exercise

Isokinetic exercise is done with a constant rate of motion. An isokinetic exercise theoretically is one in which there is no acceleration and in which

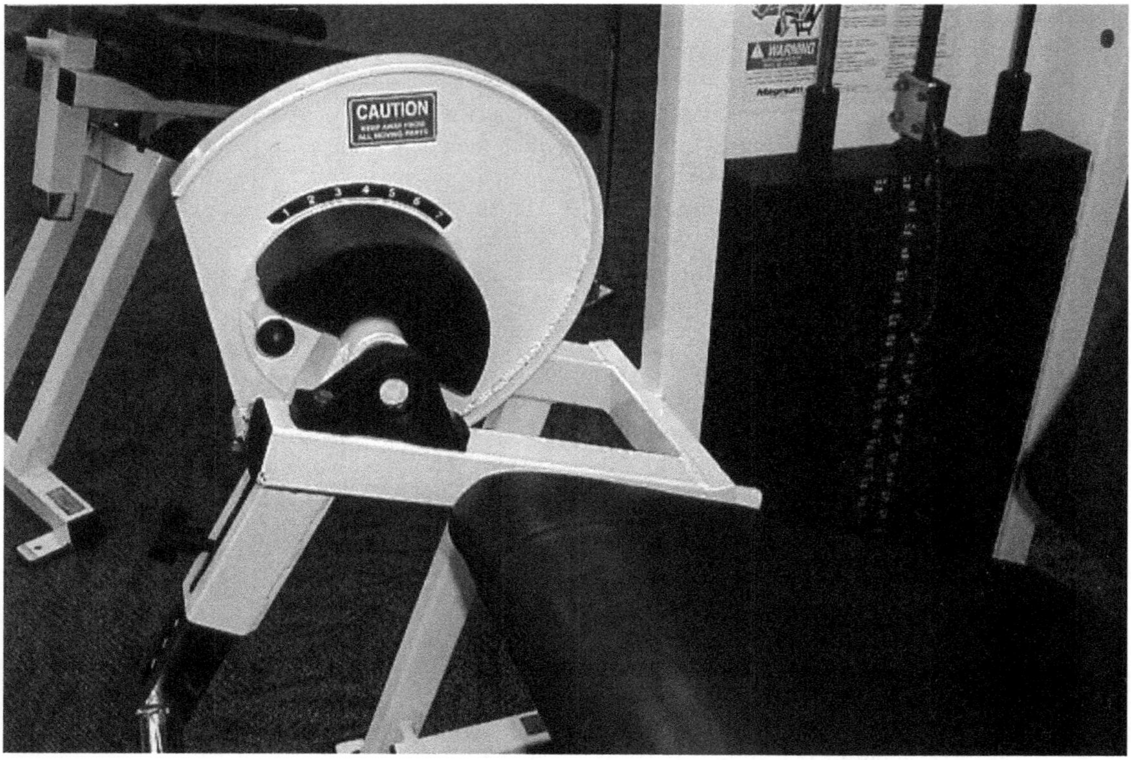

Figure 15.3 A resistance machine with an isotonic cam. The length of the resistance arm changes to vary the resistance as the muscle angle of pull changes.

the velocity remains constant. To accomplish this, machines such as the Cybex (Figure 15.4) have been developed. With such a machine, the angular velocity of segment motion may be preset to any selected rate within the limits of the machine. Because the machine accommodates to the force applied, it permits the individual to apply maximum force throughout the range of motion without increasing the velocity of the motion. Maximal resistance may be applied throughout the exercise without sudden acceleration or deceleration forces. Given that optimal training requires practice of a skill at the appropriate speed (often several thousand degrees per second), use of an isokinetic device permits maximum strengthening throughout the range of motion at required speeds without endangering joints. Isokinetic devices have proved valuable in the diagnosis and rehabilitation of athletic and other joint injuries. Such devices are also widely used in research.

Plyometric Exercise

Training programs for running, jumping, and throwing events have combined eccentric and concentric exercises into plyometric programs. These programs utilize eccentric contractions immediately followed by explosive concentric contraction. One example of a plyometric program is drop-jumping. In this exercise, the individual steps or drops off a bench, allowing flexion at the knees in a normal landing. Immediately following knee flexion, one or both legs extend in a maximum explosive jump. This training works on explosiveness by taking advantage of the stretch reflex, series and parallel elastic components of

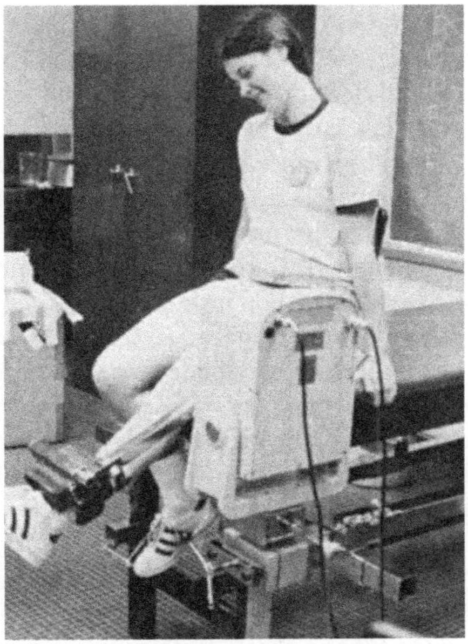

Figure 15.4 Isokinetic exercise for knee extensors using a Cybex machine.

muscle, and training for the synchronous firing of motor units. This combination results in a more forceful jump.

Any number of movements can be used as plyometric exercise. Besides the drop jump, countermovement jumps are a common technique. A countermovement jump is simply a vertical (or horizontal) jump using a rapid squat–extend motion. Almost any motion that involves joint motion in one direction followed immediately by joint motion in the other direction can become a plyometric exercise. The key is the rapid agonist stretch, followed immediately by the concentric agonist contraction. A higher-velocity eccentric contraction will lead to a greater plyometric response.

Plyometric training has been found to be a valuable tool for increasing both strength and power. In addition to increasing the ability of the muscle to generate force, plyometrics act on the neuromuscular system to ready the body for dynamic, changing situations or perturbations. This has been shown to help stabilize joints against injury (Myer et al., 2006; Toumi et al., 2004).

Principles Relating to Muscle Strength and Endurance

Overload

This principle has long been recognized as the essential physiological requirement for strength development: A muscle must be exercised at or near maximal strength and endurance capacity for a specified period of time if strength and endurance are to develop. The strength of a muscle exercised against normally encountered resistances will not increase.

Specificity

Strength or endurance training activities must be specific to the demands of the particular activity for which strength or endurance is being developed. The full range of joint action, the speed, and the resistance demands of the movement pattern should be duplicated in the training activity. It is preferable to do exercises that use multiple joints rather than to isolate a single joint.

Progressive Resistance

The resistance against which a muscle group is exercised must be increased in a planned manner, called periodization. A strength-training program may be periodized over a few weeks or a single day. The key is the variation in resistance. Because the overload program increases strength, the original overload eventually becomes inadequate and must be supplemented with progressive increases in resistance. The American College of Sports Medicine recommends that resistance be increased from 2 to 10% when the current load can be lifted one to two repetitions beyond the set number for that period. Strength-training programs should be designed based on individual abilities, needs, and goals (ACSM, 2009).

Training Dose

A regular program of exercises should be established and followed at least three to five times per week. For muscular endurance, the maximum number of repetitions used depends on the specific demands of the activity. The number of repetitions that an individual can do will depend on the actual work being performed. Because work performed will be based on repetitions, displacement, weight of the resistance, and weight of the segment, it will differ greatly from individual to individual.

The American College of Sports Medicine recommends that beginning and intermediate lifters train 2 to 3 times per week; advanced lifters may train as much as 4 to 5 times a week (ACSM, 2009). Other investigators have suggested that beginners lift 60% of their maximum capability, doing from 1 to 4 sets of each lift. Advanced lifters should work at 80% of their maximum (Bird et al., 2005; Peterson et al., 2005).

Mechanical Efficiency

Momentum Use of momentum to initiate motion in the resistance should be minimized. Where possible, the motion should be done in a slow, controlled manner using muscle force and not momentum. One must remember, however, that speed of motion is also related to specificity. Studies have shown that high-speed resistance training with light loads can lead to improvement in performance in ballistic movements such as throwing and running (McEvoy & Newton, 1998; Morrissey et al., 1995).

Resistance arm The longer the resistance arm, the more strenuous the motion. Segments should be kept close to the body until one is certain that individuals are capable of more strenuous effort. As an example, Figure 13.4 illustrates the manner in which moment arms can vary with varying bar positions in the squat.

Alignment and impact When the weight is supported by the feet, in an impact or nonimpact situation, the knees must always remain over the feet (the knee should never be twisted). If a resistance is used in a standing position, keep the knees slightly flexed to encourage posterior pelvic tilt. This will aid in proper alignment of the spine.

Open versus Closed Kinetic Chain

Most strengthening exercises are done in one of two conditions. If the distal end point of the limb, or kinetic chain, is fixed against something, the limb operates in a *closed kinetic chain*. As mentioned in Chapter 1, in this situation the segments moved by joint action will be the segments proximal from the joint, or closer to the body. For instance, if the feet are planted against the plate of a squat sled, when the knee and hip are extended, the whole body will move while the plate remains stationary. If, on the other hand, the participant is sitting on a bench with a weight strapped to the ankle, knee extension will produce motion only in the lower leg. This would be an *open kinetic chain*. In another example, a push-up would be a closed kinetic chain exercise, and a bench press would be an open kinetic chain. Both types of strength training exercises have been found to be effective. When selecting the appropriate kinetic chain exercise, it is important to consider joint stability or existing injury and investigate the different patterns of muscle activation for each kinetic chain type.

Exercise Order

The order in which strength training exercises are done should be carefully planned to achieve balanced conditioning while maximizing both workout effectiveness and safety. To effectively train muscle, both concentric and eccentric exercises should be included. When considering exercise order, multijoint exercises such as squats should be done before single-joint exercises, such as knee extensions. Large muscle groups, such as those in the lower extremity, should be exercised before the smaller muscle groups, such as those in the upper extremity. When exercise of varying intensities is to be performed, the higher-intensity exercise should be done first, followed by the lower-intensity work. Rest periods of from 1 to 3 minutes should be taken between sets, depending on the intensity and velocity of the exercise (Kraemer et al., 2002).

Warm-up

All muscle strengthening and endurance workouts should be preceded by warm-up and followed by cooldown exercises. The warm-up prepares the muscles and joint tissues by increasing their temperature and permits the neuromuscular system to adjust the threshold levels, thereby making the muscles and joints less susceptible to strains and tissue tears. The cooldown helps speed recovery, removing accumulated lactic acid.

Maintenance

Once muscular strength and endurance are developed, they may be maintained with less frequent workout sessions. The loss of strength and endurance progresses at a slower rate than its gain. Therefore, much will be retained for an extended time. Once the difficult development phase has been accomplished, retention of strength and endurance are possible with exercise sessions once every 1 or 2 weeks, provided maximum contractions are used.

Symmetry

An appropriate balance between joint flexibility and muscle strength must be maintained for each muscle and joint as well as a balance between agonist and antagonist muscle pairs. Imbalance can lead to injury or permanent deformity.

Anthropometry

Individual differences in anthropometry must be considered in exercise. Different limb lengths produce different angular kinematics. Consequently, all individuals should not be expected to perform to the same cadence. In the same manner, all equipment is not equally well fitted to all individuals. Care must be taken in working with weight machines to see that machine lever lengths are adjusted to match each individual. Many exercise machines are not designed to fit either very large or very small bodies.

Age

As resistance training becomes more popular for young people, care must be taken to prevent stress that may cause developmental problems or injury. As was discussed in Chapter 2, the skeletal structure is not fully formed until the late teen years. Those who work with children are cautioned that undue, high-resistance stress on soft epiphyseal growth plates can have long-term effects such as changes in normal growth patterns. Light weights and low repetitions are recommended.

On the other end of the age spectrum, resistance training has been shown to be beneficial in elderly populations. A variety of studies have shown that balance, strength, bone density, and mobility can all be improved through resistance training. When designing a resistance training program for the elderly, the movement specialist is encouraged to follow the guidelines set forth by the American College of Sports Medicine (Nelson et al., 2007). As discussed in the following text, risk factors that can cause problems in healthy adults may be magnified in the elderly, so caution should be used.

Risk Factors

Exercise, when properly used, is a powerful tool for positive health and well-being. It is the kinesiologist's role to understand and to properly evaluate exercise motions and to choose those that provide a safe, enjoyable, and appropriate exercise. Because exercise is most effective when the systems of the body are required to respond to stress, potential risk is involved in exercise programs for strength and endurance. To minimize risk, some motions should be avoided. In general, in choosing exercises for strength and endurance, the following guidelines should be followed:

1. *Avoid* motions that emphasize flexion and hyperextension in the cervical or lumbar regions to protect the vulnerable areas of the vertebral column. Therefore, when exercising, never hyperextend the trunk without stabilizing the pelvis and keeping the head in line with the neck.
2. *Avoid* combinations of motions in the vertebral column in more than one plane. Combination motions in more than one plane

executed simultaneously or in sequence increase the compression and shear forces applied to the discs.

3. *Avoid* forcing the knee joint into extreme flexion or hyperextension. Either action may weaken ligaments and other structures in the joint.
4. *Never* hold the breath while exercising. Breathe normally through the exercise to avoid increased undue stress on the cardiovascular system through increased intrathoracic pressure.

Strength Training

In many settings, expensive resistance training equipment is not readily available. Even without costly weight machines, it is possible to conduct a quality strength training program. A practical procedure is to modify familiar exercises in such a way that the resistance to be overcome can be progressively increased. Either or both of two ways can do this: (1) by increasing the length of the resistance arm of the involved lever and (2) by increasing the magnitude of the resistance. In many settings resistance machines, light hand weights, or free weights are becoming common. Strength training programs should be built around the principle of progressive resistance and should be varied enough to strengthen the entire musculoskeletal system. The exception to this would be in the rehabilitation of an injury. While many strengthening exercises indeed target the whole body, the following sections will be broken down into anatomical regions to simplify presentation and to highlight the particular concerns applicable to each group of joints and muscles.

Core Strengthening

The vertebral column and its supporting structures and musculature are commonly referred to as the core of the body. The primary concern in strengthening the muscles of the core region is to provide stability to the spine. Core strength provides stability not only for the maintenance of an upright posture, but for the manipulation of external loads. External loads can be extremely varied in nature, from an unexpected push to the very deliberate lift of a weight that challenges the individual's capability. The maintenance of sufficient core strength is considered by many to be invaluable in the ability to manage all potential loading situations in a safe, effective, and efficient manner.

Most core strengthening programs are focused primarily on the abdominal muscles and the muscles of the back. One must keep in mind, however, the importance of pelvic positioning on the stability of the spine (see Chapter 7). For this reason, some of the muscles of the lower extremity will also affect core stability.

Abdominal Exercises

It is important to remember that the primary function of the abdominal muscles is to flex and rotate the spine. They do not cross the hip joint and are, therefore, not active at the hip. With this in mind, exercises targeting the abdominals should focus on trunk flexion and rotation. Exercises that consist primarily of hip flexion do not use the abdominal muscles in a concentric-eccentric alternation. Rather, the abdominals are contracted statically to maintain the position of the pelvic girdle. While some abdominal strengthening may occur from this static contraction, it will not be as functional throughout the range of motion as strength gained through more dynamic contraction types.

A second important consideration in choosing an abdominal exercise that focuses on the abdominal muscles rather than the hip flexors is the protection of the low back. As discussed in Chapter 3, a muscle contracts toward its own center, pulling equally on both ends. In the case of the hip flexors, the pull would be equal on the thigh and on the pelvic girdle. The pull on the pelvic girdle will produce a torque toward anterior tilt. Anterior tilt, it will be remembered, is accompanied by spine hyperextension. As the hip flexor load increases, the torque producing anterior tilt increases (Figure 15.5). The resulting compression

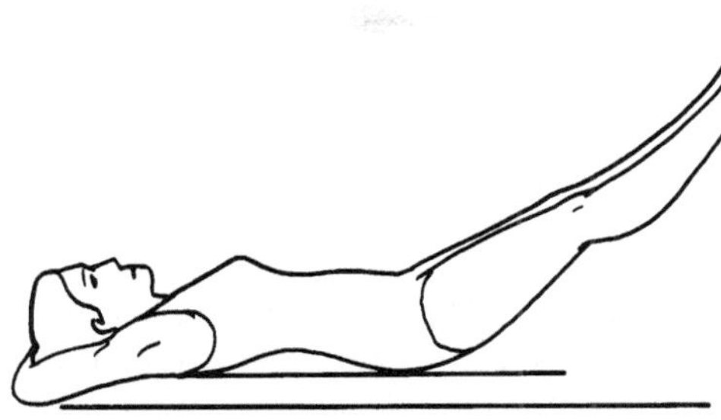

Figure 15.5 Straight-leg raising. Note the increased curve of the lumbar spine.

load is very difficult for the spine to support and may result in low back pain or injury. Hip flexion as an abdominal strengthening technique should be avoided. Research done over the years has indicated that the basic crunch remains one of the most effective abdominal strengthening exercises.

Principles for selecting abdominal exercises

1. The criterion for an abdominal exercise performed in the supine position is to prevent the tilting of the pelvis and the hyperextension of the lumbar spine. If the pelvic tilt and lumbar curve increase, it would seem to indicate the failure of the abdominal muscles to stabilize the pelvis and spine against the pull of the iliopsoas. Because the task is too great for these muscles, there is danger of straining them and stressing lumbar vertebrae and discs.
2. An objective in building a strong abdominal wall is to strengthen all four of the abdominal muscles: rectus abdominis, external oblique, internal oblique, and transversus abdominis. To do this successfully requires knowledge of the exercises in which these muscles participate and of the relative intensity of their action.
3. Individual differences and overall spine health must be taken into consideration when selecting an abdominal exercise. In those with disc problems, it may be important to maintain a neutral pelvis, whereas those with facet or impingement problems may benefit from an exercise with more pelvic and spinal mobility. All individual problems should be explored before prescribing a particular abdominal exercise (Escamilla et al., 2006).

The Basic Crunch

The crunch is a popular exercise for the development of core abdominal strength and endurance. Consequently much has been written about it, and considerable research has been done on muscle and joint participation during its execution. There are many forms of the crunch, some more rigorous than others and some more hazardous. Because of the many possible modifications, the exercise is easily adapted to form a series of safe, graded exercises once the related anatomical and mechanical factors are identified.

Starting position Supine lying position with hands resting lightly on thighs, feet flat on the floor, and knee joints flexed to approximately 90 degrees.

Movement The subject pulls in the chin and curls up to a half-sitting position. The action is then reversed, and the subject curls back down to the starting position.

Essential joint and muscle analysis The format used in Table 15.1 is presented as a model for the student who is just beginning to develop proficiency in movement analysis. The kinesiology student is encouraged to follow this procedure until comfortable with its use. Once the student becomes competent in this form of analysis, the level of detail may be decreased.

If the upward motion goes beyond about 30 degrees, the muscle action switches primarily to the hip flexors. The upward motion of the crunch should stop at this point to maintain a dynamic, concentric contraction of the abdominal muscles. The downward phase of the crunch is the reverse motion, extension in all named joints. In this phase, gravity is the force producing the

TABLE 15.1 Anatomical Analysis of the Crunch

Joint	Action	Segment moved	Force for Movement	Prime Movers	Contraction Type
Cervical spine	Flexion	Head and neck	Muscle	Sternocleido mastoid (SCM) Scalenes	Static
Thoracic and lumbar spine	Flexion	Trunk	Muscle	Rectus and oblique abdominals	Concentric
Hip	Flexion	Trunk	Muscle	Iliopsoas R. femoris Pectineus Sartorius	Static

motion. The same prime movers are active but are now contracting eccentrically.

In the initial stage of the crunch, the rectus abdominis and external oblique muscles are acting as movers to flex the spine; the iliopsoas and other hip flexors act as stabilizers to fix the pelvis against the pull of the abdominal muscles. The major abdominal muscle in a straight crunch is the rectus abdominis. If strengthening of the oblique abdominals is an objective, the crunch action should include rotation of the spine.

Progressive resistance series A set of abdominal exercises that are graded from easy to more difficult according to muscular effort necessary might be as follows. All exercises are performed with the feet unsupported and the legs flexed at the knees.

1. Eccentric crunch. Slowly curl down from sitting position with hands on thighs. Push back up to sitting position using hands. Repeat.
2. Crunch, hands under thigh to help pull up.
3. Crunch, hands resting lightly on thighs.
4. Crunch, fingertips on shoulders and elbows reaching forward.
5. Crunch holding weight; increase difficulty with increased weight, or move weight closer to the top of the head.
6. Crunch on inclined board. (Why does the incline increase the difficulty?)

Note: To support the neck, it may be more comfortable to place the hands to the side of the head, holding the head in position. The hands should never be used to pull the head up.

Discussion The crunch provides a clear-cut example of the effect that lengthening the resistance moment arm has on the effort needed (Figure 15.6). As the trunk is flexed, the action is resisted by the weight of the trunk applied at the center of gravity of the trunk. The downward torque to be overcome is greatest when the trunk is nearest the horizontal because the resistance moment arm is greatest at this point. Thus the muscular effort needed to move the trunk is also greatest at this part of the crunch.

Muscular effort may be increased throughout the range of the action if the resistance moment arm is increased in length by moving the center of gravity of the trunk closer to the head, either by moving the arms up or by adding weights (Figure 15.7).

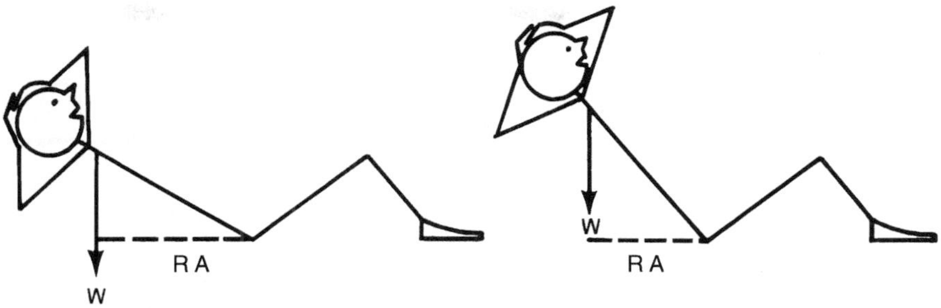

Figure 15.6 During the course of a crunch, the length of the resistance moment arm (RMA) changes, decreasing as the trunk moves toward the vertical and increasing as the trunk moves toward the horizontal.

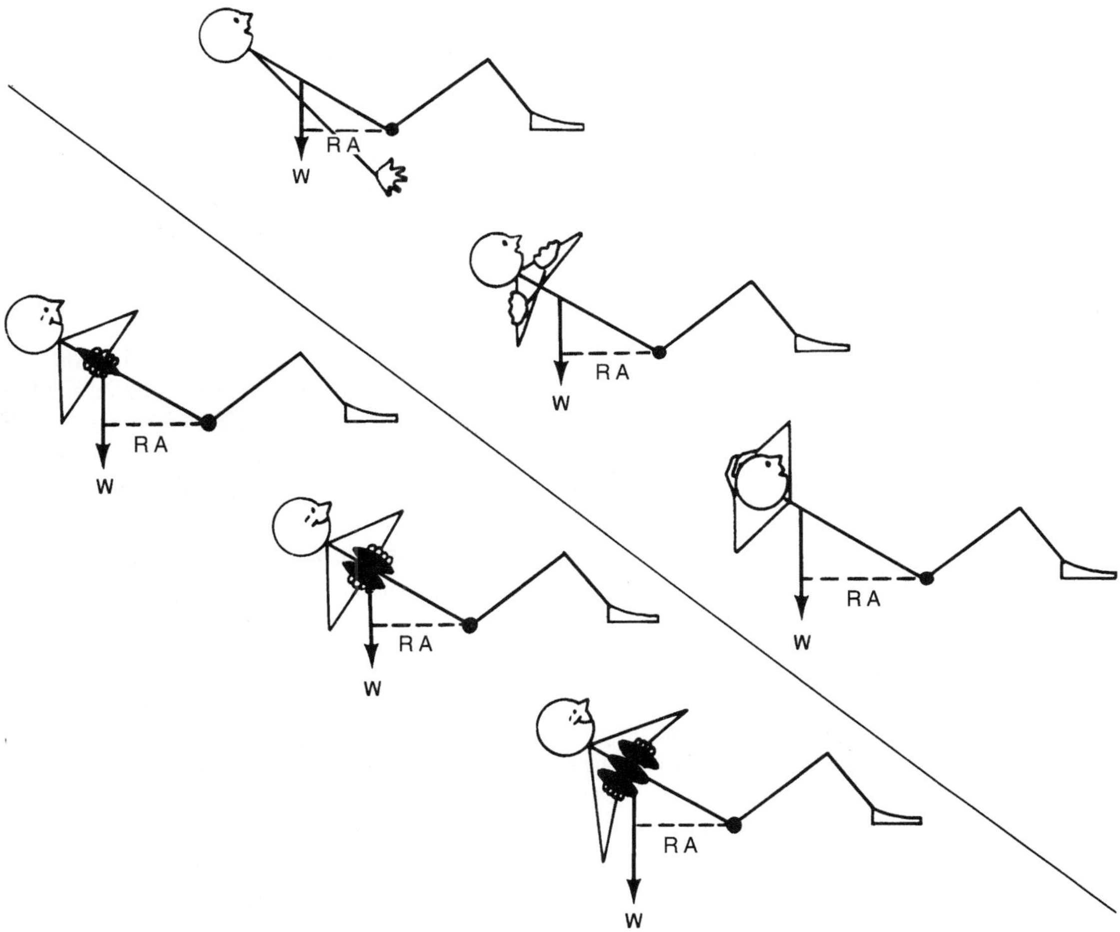

Figure 15.7 The crunch. (a) Increasing the effort requirement by lengthening the moment arm of the trunk (RA). By moving the arms higher, the weight line W is moved higher, thus making RA longer. (b) Increasing the effort requirement by increasing the magnitude of the weight W.

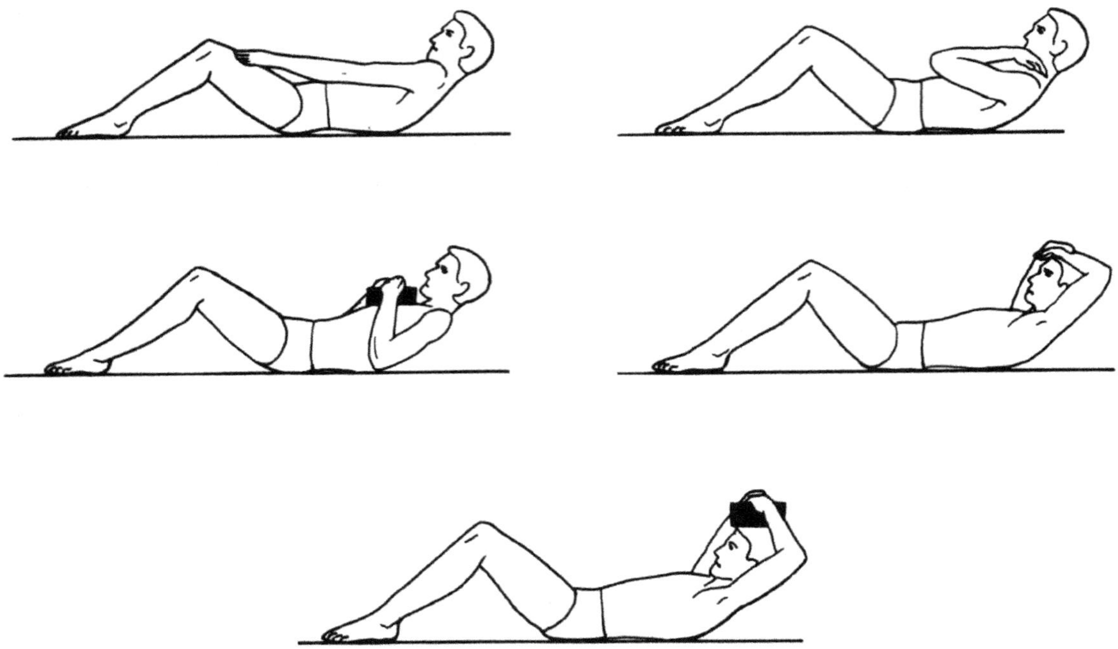

Figure 15.8 Partial crunch series for abdominal strength.

If the arms are moved and the magnitude of the weight increased, the demand made on the muscles will be increased markedly (Figure 15.8).

Nontraditional Abdominal Exercises

Strengthening of the abdominal muscles is easily accomplished using the resistance provided by body weight, with the muscles working against gravity. Less traditional forms of abdominal exercise are often performed with the aid of a device. These so-called ab exercisers are readily available, usually marketed as quick methods of conditioning the abdominal muscles. The movement professional should approach these devices with a critical eye. Careful evaluation of the exercise, the muscles involved, and any potential dangers must be undertaken before any device is recommended. Some abdominal exercisers may provide a greater activation of the abdominal musculature than crunches, whereas others may not. It is often difficult to make this determination with a cursory examination, and one should not hesitate to refer to the research to determine the efficacy of a given device. Special attention should be given to research findings on lumbar compressive forces. Exercise (stability) balls, for instance, have been found to increase abdominal muscle activity but may increase lumbar compression.

Strengthening the back

Since the muscles of the back have the primary purpose of extending the vertebral column, it would stand to reason that back extension exercises would be the most effective for strengthening these muscles. For the most part, this is an accurate assessment. Here again, however, one must be concerned with applying undue stress to the structure of the spine. In spine hyperextension, for instance, compressive loads on the posterior structures of the vertebrae will increase while the anterior portions of the vertebral structures will experience an increase in tension. This occurs due to the bending torque applied to the spine. For this reason, it is best to avoid exercises that emphasize spine hyperextension. This would include such exercises as prone leg or torso lifts (often known as "superman") A better choice would be to use some device such as a Roman chair or stability ball to first flex moderately, then return to neutral extension against gravity. That being said, exercises for back strength should also be designed to avoid extreme spine flexion, which produces high bending torques in the other direction. Extension done from moderate flexion provides adequate muscle activity while limiting excessive stress on the smaller structures of the spine.

In most multijoint exercises, good form will require cocontraction of the muscles of the core, including those of the back. Current thinking is that this activity can provide strengthening of the muscles of the back adequate for most things. The need for specificity of training should be kept in mind.

Upper Body Strengthening

Most upper body strengthening exercises are focused on the muscles of the shoulder and elbow. Because the upper extremity articulates with the torso through the shoulder girdle, stress in the upper extremity will be transmitted to the torso and thus the spine unless the torso is supported in some way. A key consideration in upper body strengthening is to maintain stability in the spine while providing resistance in the arms. As much as possible, the spine should be maintained in an extended (neutral) alignment with the head erect. This is most easily done when the spine is supported, as in the bench press, or in a closed kinetic chain exercise. In open kinetic chain exercises, such as the shoulder press with free weights, the muscles that provide stability to the spine should be contracted to hold the spine erect.

An example of a closed kinetic chain exercise for upper body strength is the push-up. In the push-up, the spine is not supported. In this situation, the muscles that provide stability to the spine must be used to control posture.

The Push-up

The push-up is an exercise for strengthening the elbow extensors and the anterior shoulder and chest muscles. The basic exercise is described and analyzed first, and then a graded series of variations of this activity is suggested.

Starting position The front-leaning rest position—that is, semi-prone with the body extended, the arms extended vertically toward the floor, and the weight supported by the hands and toes. The body is in a straight line from head to heels; there is no sag at the spine or hump at the hips. The hands are approximately shoulder width apart with the palms flat on the floor.

Movement With the body kept straight, the arms are allowed to flex at the elbow joints and the body is lowered until the chest almost touches the floor. By pushing the hands vigorously against the floor, the body is raised until it regains the starting position.

Because the hands are stabilized against the floor in a closed kinetic chain, the segments being moved are as follows: forearm acting about the wrist joint, the upper arm acting about the elbow joint, and the trunk acting about the shoulder joints. The force causing the motion is gravity when dipping and muscle when executing the push-up.

Essential joint and muscle analysis The dip phase of the push-up involves flexion at the elbow joint accompanied by a lowering of the body until it almost touches the floor (Figure 15.9b and Table 15.2).

The up phase of the push-up involves extension at the elbow joints until the body is again in the position shown in Figure 15.9a and Table 15.3.

Maintenance of straight alignment from head to heels is the same for both the dip and up phases of the push-up.

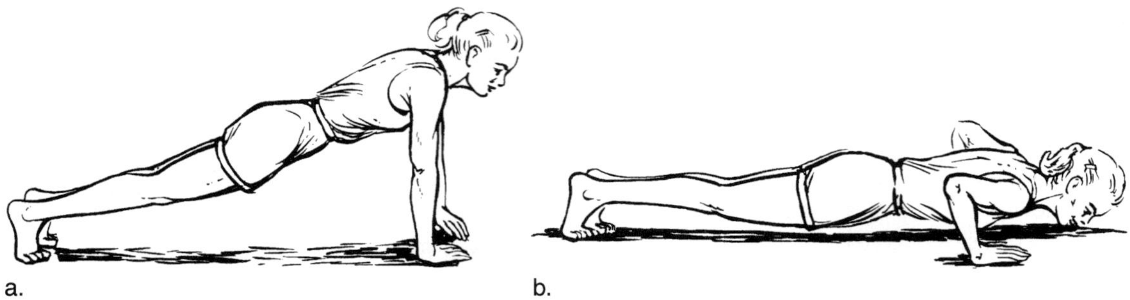

Figure 15.9 The push-up: (a) the starting and ending position; (b) the dip.

TABLE 15.2 Anatomical Analysis of the Push-up—Dip Phase

Joint	Joint Action	Segment Moved	Force for Movement	Prime Movers	Contraction Type
Shoulder joints	Horizontal abduction	Trunk	Gravity	Pectoralis major Anterior deltoid Coracobrachialis	Eccentric
Shoulder girdle	Adduction	Scapula	Gravity	Pectoralis minor Serratus anterior	Eccentric
Elbows	Flexion	Upper arm	Gravity	Triceps Anconeus	Eccentric
Wrists	Reduction of hyperextension	Forearm	Gravity	Extensor carpi radialis longus and brevis Extensor carpi ulnaris	Eccentric
MAINTENANCE OF STRAIGHT ALIGNMENT FROM HEAD TO HEELS AGAINST THE PULL OF GRAVITY:					
Head and neck	None	None		Cervical extensors	Static
Lumbar spine	None	None		Rectus abdominus Obliques	Static
Hips	None	None		Flexors	Static

TABLE 15.3 Anatomical Analysis of the Push-up—Up Phase

Joint	Joint Action	Segment Moved	Force for Movement	Prime Movers	Contraction Type
Shoulder joints	Horizontal adduction	Trunk	Muscle	Pectoralis major Anterior deltoid Coracobrachialis	Concentric
Shoulder girdle	Abduction	Scapula	Muscle	Pectoralis minor Serratus anterior	Concentric
Elbows	Extension	Upper arm	Muscle	Triceps Anconeus	Concentric
Wrists	Hyperextension	Forearm	Muscle	Extensor carpi radialis longus and brevis Extensor carpi ulnaris	Concentric

Progressive Resistance Series

In the push-up, the familiar form of the exercise represents the most difficult level in the series. Starting at what might be considered the lowest level and working up, the following push-up exercises are suggested.

1. Resting on hands and knees with legs flexed at right angles at hip and knee joints, dip and push up.
2. In semi-prone position with leg extended at the hip and weight supported by hands and knees, perform a half-dip and push-up (Figure 15.10a).
3. Same position as for 2, but complete the full dip and push-up.
4. Front-leaning rest position, facing stairs with feet on floor and hands on fourth or fifth step, body in a straight line from head to heels, dip and push up (Figure 15.10b).
5. Continue, placing hands on lower step until able to perform regulation push-up from floor (Figure 15.10d).

Discussion

A person may have to work up to a full push-up in any of the positions by first performing only the negative lift phase (letdown) or a half push-up; that is, a push-up from a half-dip position. Whatever type of push-up is practiced, the person should be able to repeat it several times in good form before being permitted to try a more advanced type.

Two common faults must be guarded against in the push-up. They are (1) a sagging back and (2) elevated hips. The latter fault is usually caused by an "overcorrection" of the first one—namely, maintaining a flexed position at the hips to prevent the back from sagging. The correction of both of these faults lies in strengthening the abdominal muscles and training them to prevent hyperextension of the lumbar spine when the body is in the extended position. Until the subject is kinesthetically aware of this position, the use of a mirror may be helpful.

The differences in difficulty among the forms of push-up shown in Figure 15.10 are primarily due to the length of the resistance moment arm in proportion to the effort moment arm. As the proportion of RMA to EMA increases in size, the effort in relation to the resistance also must increase ($E \times EMA = R \times RMA$). This can be demonstrated by placing a bathroom scale under each hand. An additional reason for the ease of the push-up from the knees (Figure 15.10a) is that less body weight (lower legs subtracted) is being pushed up.

The push-up from a half-dip is easier than the push-up from a full dip in any given position because the weight of the body is lifted through a shorter distance and because the joint positions permit the muscles of the elbows and shoulders to work to better advantage. The reverse dip is easier to execute than the push-up from any given level because the muscles are performing negative rather than positive work; that is, they are engaging in eccentric (lengthening) rather than concentric (shortening) contraction.

Lower Body Strengthening

In developing strengthening exercises for the lower body, one must keep in mind the vulnerability of the knee joint. The knee joint, it will be remembered, functions safely only in flexion and extension. Any varus or valgus loads applied to the knee will produce torque at the joint in the frontal plane. This is to be avoided, as the ligamentous structures that support the knee are not structured to resist such torques to any great extent. The knee is also vulnerable in flexion beyond 90 degrees. In flexion the knee is in an open state, and joint stability is dependent on soft tissue structures (see Chapter 8). Without the benefit of bony support, the structures of the knee are subjected to increasing levels of stress as flexion increases, putting these structures at risk for injury. It is suggested that knee flexion under load be restricted to less than 90 degrees.

As with the upper body, lower body strengthening exercises may involve the spine. The general guidelines offered in the upper body section hold true in this section as well.

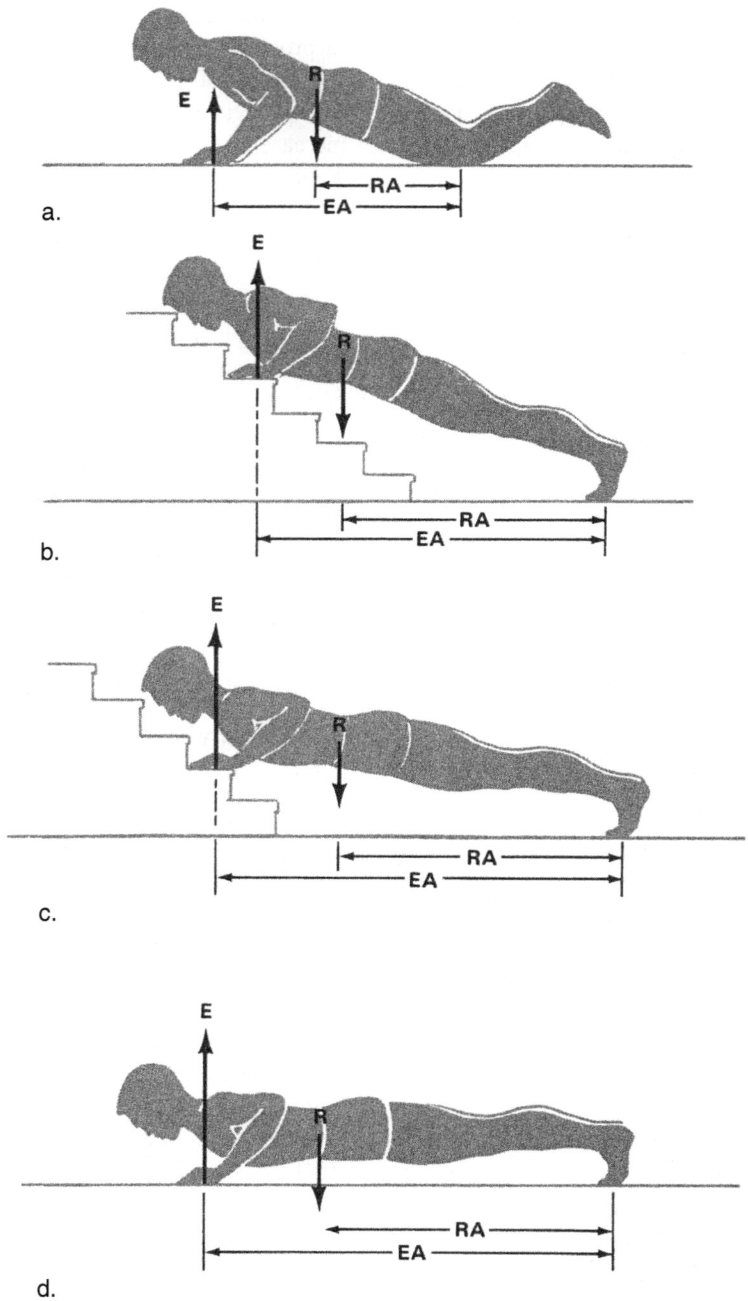

Figure 15.10 Push-up series for arm strength. As the ratio of the resistance moment arm (RMA) to the effort moment arm (EMA) increases in magnitude, the effort must also increase so that E × EMA is greater than R × RMA. Only then will the push-up occur. The order of increasing difficulty in this series is a, b, c, d.

Exercises to strengthen the lower body often involve simultaneous flexion or extension of the hip, knee, and ankle. It should be remembered that these sagittal plane motions are key for strengthening the muscles of the ankle and knee, but may not be adequate for the hip. While the ankle and knee move only in the sagittal plane, the hip is a triaxial ball-and-socket joint. To adequately strengthen all of the muscles of the hip, exercises must be designed in the frontal and transverse planes as well. Care must be taken in these two planes to protect the knee from undue lateral or rotational torques.

One common exercise for strengthening the leg extensors is the squat. Squats may be done with a load (weight) or by just using body weight. Common squat exercises are the free weight back squat, front squat, and single-leg squat. There are also closed chain squat machines or sleds. In addition, a common fitness exercise is the unloaded squat. The free weight back squat is presented here as a sample of a lower body strengthening exercise.

The Back Squat

Starting position The back squat starts with the weight bar across the shoulders, supported by the hands on either side. The body is erect and the feet approximately shoulder width apart. Stance width is often altered slightly to trigger greater or lesser activity in specific lower extremity muscles.

Movement Keeping the spine erect and the head up, the ankles, knees, and hips are allowed to flex simultaneously as the body is lowered into a squat position. The lower leg moves at the ankle, the thigh moves at the knee, and the torso, via the pelvis, is moved at the hip. The spine is maintained in an erect position by cocontraction of the trunk muscles. The force causing this motion is gravity.

When the lowest point of the squat has been reached, the ankle, knee, and hip are forcefully extended (triple extension), bringing the body back to the erect position (Figure 15.11). The essential joint and muscle analysis of the back squat is presented in Tables 15.4 and 15.5.

Progressive resistance series In the free weight squat, progressive resistance is produced through the addition of increased amounts of weight lifted. However, for the beginner there are squat exercises that can be used to increase leg strength before attempting a free weight squat.

1. Half squats holding onto the back of a chair are a good starting point.
2. Unweighted squats with no more than 70 degrees of knee flexion.

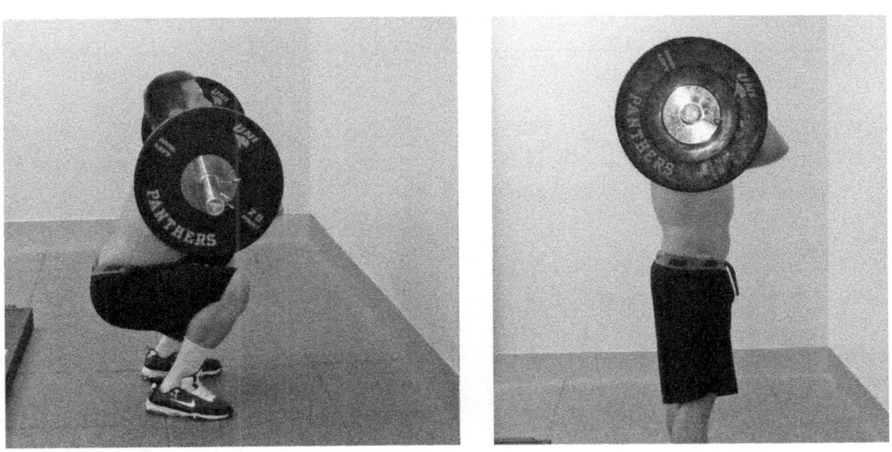

Figure 15.11 The back squat. (a) The squat. (b) The triple extension to stand.

TABLE 15.4 Anatomical Analysis of the Back Squat—Down Phase

Joint	Joint Action	Segment Moved	Force for Movement	Prime Movers	Contraction Type
Ankles	Dorsiflexion	Shank	Gravity	Gastrocnemius Soleus Peroneus longus	Eccentric
Knees	Flexion	Thigh	Gravity	Rectus femoris Vastus lateralis Vastus medialis Vastus intermedius	Eccentric
Hips	Flexion	Torso	Gravity	Biceps femoris Semimembranosus Semitendinosus Gluteus maximus	Eccentric

TABLE 15.5 Anatomical Analysis of the Back Squat—Up Phase

Joint	Joint Action	Segment Moved	Force for Movement	Prime Movers	Contraction Type
Ankles	Plantar flexion	Shank	Muscle	Gastrocnemius Soleus Peroneus longus	Concentric
Knees	Extension	Thigh	Muscle	Rectus femoris Vastus lateralis Vastus medialis Vastus intermedius	Concentric
Hips	Extension	Torso	Muscle	Biceps femoris Semimembranosus Semitendinosus Gluteus maximus	Concentric

3. Front squats with an unloaded weight bar held across the front of the shoulders. This form of the squat lift is easier on the knees than the back squat.
4. Back squat as described. Weight can be added to the bar as strength increases.

EVALUATING EXERCISES AND DEVICES

If the discussions and applications of exercises that have been presented in this chapter have helped give the student a sound basis for developing an effective exercise program, the chapter will have served its purpose. Exercise instructors who have a good kinesiological background should be able to analyze and evaluate exercises, not only those with which they are already familiar, but also those that are brought to their attention by their students or are seen on television or in popular magazines. They should be able to tell whether exercises are suitable for the inexperienced performer, a performer of moderate experience and ability, or an advanced performer. They should know whether the exercises have undesirable features such as the danger of straining ligaments, encouraging posture faults, or causing excessive tension. They should also recognize the mechanical problems that may be involved, such as problems of balance, leverage, or momentum. In brief, evaluation of exercises should be based on the answers to the following questions:

1. What is the purpose of the exercise?
2. Which joints and muscles are being targeted?
3. Which joints and muscles are actually being activated and to what degree?
4. Are any joints or muscles being placed at risk by the exercise or device? Why?
   a. Look for motion outside the anatomical range for the targeted joint(s).
   b. Look for excessive joint torques produced by inappropriate moment arms.
5. What are the intensity and difficulty? (Is it suitable for a beginner, a moderately experienced performer, or an advanced performer?)
6. Are there any elements of danger, injury, or strain against which precautions should be taken?
7. Is it likely to produce any undesirable or harmful physical responses against which the performer should be on guard?
8. If the exercise is difficult, what preliminary exercise would serve to prepare the performer for it?
9. What secondary or stabilizing actions must take place to support the exercise?

When the exercise instructor has acquired skill in answering such questions as these and in analyzing the individual needs of students, he or she will be well on the way to becoming a true kinesiologist. To assist in the achievement of this goal, the student should find it profitable to analyze as many exercises as possible. Table 1.1 and Appendix G should prove helpful in this connection.

References and Selected Readings

Alter, M. J. (1996). *Science of flexibility.* Champaign, IL: Human Kinetics.

Amako, M., Oda, T., Masuoka, K., Yokoi, H., & Campisi, P. (2003). Effect of static stretching on prevention of injuries for military recruits. *Military Medicine,* 168(6), 442–446.

American College of Sports Medicine. (2009). American College of Sports Medicine position stand. Progression models in resistance training for healthy adults. *Medicine and Science in Sports and Exercise,* 41(3), 687–708.

Bird, S. P., Tarpenning, K. M., & Marino, F. E. (2005). Designing resistance training programmes to enhance muscular fitness: A review of the acute programme variables. *Sports Medicine,* 35(10), 841–851.

Brindle, T. J., Nyland, J., Ford, K., Coppola, A., & Shapiro, R. (2002). Electromyographic comparison of standard and modified closed-chain isometric knee extension exercises. *Journal of Strength and Conditioning Research,* 16(1), 129–134.

Chalmers G. (2004). Re-examination of the possible role of Golgi tendon organ and muscle spindle reflexes in proprioceptive neuromuscular facilitation muscle stretching. *Sports Biomechanics,* 3(1), 159–183.

Cheung K., Hume, P., & Maxwell, L. (2003). Delayed onset muscle soreness: Treatment strategies and performance factors. *Sports Medicine,* 33(2), 145–164.

Chimera, N. J., Swanik, K. A., Swanik, C. B., & Straub, S. J. (2004). Effects of plyometric training on muscle-activation strategies and performance in female athletes. *Journal of Athletic Training,* 39(1), 24–31.

Cramer, J. T., Housh, T. J., Weir, J. P., Johnson, G. O., Coburn, J. W., & Beck, T. W. (2005). The acute effects of static stretching on peak torque, mean power output, electromyography, and mechanomyography. *European Journal of Applied Physiology,* 93(5–6), 530–539.

Escamilla, R. F., Babb, E., DeWitt, R., Jew, P., Kelleher, P., Burnham, T., et al. (2006). Electromyographic analysis of traditional and nontraditional abdominal exercises: Implications for rehabilitation and training. *Physical Therapy,* 86, 656–671.

Escamilla, R. F., Fleisig, G. S., Zheng, N., Lander, J. E., Barrentine, S.W., Andrews, J. R., et al. (2001). Effects of technique variations on knee biomechanics during the squat and leg press. *Medicine and Science in Sports and Exercise,* 33(9), 1552–1566.

Fletcher, I. M., & Jones, B. (2004). The effect of different warm-up stretch protocols on 20 meter sprint performance in trained rugby union players. *Journal of Strength and Conditioning Research,* 18(4), 885–888.

Folland, J. P., Irish, C. S., Roberts, J. C., Tarr, J. E., & Jones, D. A. (2002). Fatigue is not a necessary stimulus for strength gains during resistance training. *British Journal of Sports Medicine,* 36(5), 370–373.

Freeman, S., Karpowicz, A., Gray, J., & McGill, S. (2006). Quantifying muscle patterns and spine load during various forms of the push-up. *Medicine and Science in Sports and Exercise,* 38(3), 570–571.

Gabbe, B. J., Finch, C. F., Bennell, K. L., & Wajswelner, H. (2005). Risk factors for hamstring injuries in community level Australian football. *British Journal of Sports Medicine,* 39(2), 106–110.

Gillies, E. M., Putnam, C. T., & Bell, G. J. (2006). The effect of varying the time of concentric and eccentric muscle actions during resistance training on skeletal muscle adaptations in women. *European Journal of Applied Physiology,* 97, 443–453.

Gouvali, M. K., & Boudolos, K. (2005). Dynamic and electromyographical analysis in variants of push-up exercise. *Journal of Strength and Conditioning Research,* 19(1), 146–151.

Hunter, G. R., McCarthy, J. P., & Bamman, M. M. (2004). Effects of resistance training on older adults. *Sports Medicine,* 34(5), 329–348.

Marshall, P. W., & Murphy, B. A. (2005). Core stability exercises on and off a Swiss ball. *Archives of Physical Medicine and Rehabilitation,* 86(2), 242–249.

McEvoy, K. P., & Newton, R. U. (1998). Baseball throwing speed and base running: The effect of ballistic resistance training. *Journal of Strength and Conditioning Research,* 12, 216–221.

McGill, S. M., & Karpowicz, A. (2009). Exercises for spine stabilization: Motion/motor patterns, stability progressions, and clinical technique. *Archives of Physical Medicine and Rehabilitation,* 90, 118–126.

Monfort-Pañego, M., Vera-García, F. J., Sánchez-Zuriaga, D., & Sarti-Martínez, M. Á. (2009). Electromyographic studies in abdominal exercises: A literature synthesis. *Journal of Manipulative and Physiological Therapeutics,* 32, 232–244.

Mori, A. (2004). Electromyographic activity of selected trunk muscles during stabilization exercise using a gym ball. *Electromyography and Clinical Neurophysiology,* 44(1), 57–64.

Morrissey, M. C., Harman, E. A., & Johnson, M. J. (1995). Resistance training modes: Specificity and effectiveness. *Medicine and Science in Sports and Exercise,* 27, 648–660.

Myer, G. D., Ford, K. R., McLean, S. G., & Hewett, T. E. (2006). The effects of plyometric versus dynamic stabilization and balance training on lower extremity biomechanics. *American Journal of Sports Medicine,* 34(3), 445–455.

Nagano, A., Komura, T., Fukashiro, S., & Himeno, R. (2005). Force, work and power output of lower limb muscles during human maximal-effort countermovement jumping. *Journal of Electromyography and Kinesiology,* 15(4), 367–376.

Nelson, A. G., Kokkonen, J., & Arnall, D. A. (2005). Acute muscle stretching inhibits muscle strength endurance performance. *Journal of Strength and Conditioning Research,* 19(2), 338–343.

Nelson, M. E., Rejeski, W. J., Blair, S. N., Duncan, P. W., Judge, J. O., King, A.C., et al. (2007). Physical activity and public health in older adults: Recommendation from the American College of Sports Medicine and the American Heart Association. *Medicine and Science in and Sports and Exercise,* 39(8), 1435–1445.

Nobrega, A. C., Paula, K. C., & Carvalho, A. C. (2005). Interaction between resistance training and flexibility training in healthy young adults. *Journal of Strength and Conditioning Research,* 19(4), 842–846.

Peterson, M. D., Rhea, M. R., & Alvar, B. A. (2005). Applications of the dose-response for muscular strength development: A review of meta-analytic efficacy and reliability for designing training prescription. *Journal of Strength and Conditioning Research,* 19(4), 950–958.

Preuss R. A, Grenier, S. G., & McGill, S. M. (2005). Postural control of the lumbar spine in unstable sitting. *Archives of Physical Medicine and Rehabilitation,* 86, 2309–2315.

Proske, U., & Morgan, D. L. (2001). Muscle damage from eccentric exercise: Mechanism, mechanical signs, adaptation and clinical applications. *Journal of Physiology,* 537(Pt 2), 333–345.

Roig, M., O'Brien, K., Kirk, G., Murray, R., McKinnon, P., Shadgan, B., et al. (2009). The effects of eccentric versus concentric resistance training on muscle strength and mass in healthy adults: A systematic review with meta-analysis. *British Journal of Sports Medicine,* 43, 556–568.

Shrier, I. (2004). Does stretching improve performance? A systematic and critical review of the literature. *Clinical Journal of Sports Medicine,* 14(5), 267–273.

Siff, M. (2003). *Supertraining* (6th ed.). Denver, CO: Supertraining Institute.

Small, K., McNaughton, L., & Matthews, M. (2008). A systematic review into the efficacy of static stretching as part of a warm-up for the prevention of exercise-related injury. *Research in Sports Medicine,* 16, 3, 213–231.

Stensdotter, A. K., Hodges, P. W., Mellor, R., Sundelin, G., & Hager-Ross, C. (2003). Quadriceps activation in closed and in open kinetic chain exercise. *Medicine and Science in Sports and Exercise,* 35(12), 2043–2047.

Sternlicht, E., Rugg, S. G., Bernstein, M. D., & Armstrong, S. D. (2005). Electromyographical analysis and comparison of selected abdominal training devices with a traditional crunch. *Journal of Strength and Conditioning Research,* 19(1), 157–162.

Thacker, S. B., Gilchrist, J., Stroup, D. F., & Kimsey, C. D., Jr. (2005). The impact of stretching on sports injury risk: A systematic review of the literature. *Medicine and Science in Sports and Exercise,* 36(3), 371–378.

Toumi, H., Best, T. M., Martin, A., F'Guer, S., & Poumarat, G. (2004). Effects of eccentric phase velocity of plyometric training on the vertical jump. *International Journal of Sports Medicine,* 25(5), 391–398.

Trappe, S., Williamson, D., & Godard, M. (2002). Maintenance of whole muscle strength and size following resistance training in older men. *Journals of Gerontology. Series A, Biological Sciences and Medical Sciences,* 57(4), B138–B143.

Wolfe, B. L., LeMura, L. M., & Cole, P. J. (2004). Quantitative analysis of single- vs. multiple-set programs in resistance training. *Journal of Strength and Conditioning Research,* 18(1), 35–47.

Young, W., Clothier, P., Otago, L., Bruce, L., & Liddell, D. (2004). Acute effects of static stretching on hip flexor and quadriceps flexibility, range of motion and foot speed in kicking a football. *Journal of Science and Medicine in Sport,* 7(1), 23–31.

Zatsiorsky, V., & Kraemer, W. (2006). *Science and practice of strength training* (2nd ed.). Champaign, IL: Human Kinetics.

Laboratory Experiences

1. Turn to Appendix G. State the purpose and give the essential joint and muscle analysis for as many of the exercises as possible in Series 1 through 4.
2. Select from 3 to 10 exercises seen in popular magazines, newspapers, videos, or on television. Using the examples in this chapter as guides, analyze and evaluate these exercises and answer the nine questions in the last section of this chapter.
3. Observe someone doing a conditioning exercise. Analyze the exercise, using the examples in this chapter as guides.
4. Originate an exercise for stretching the hamstring muscles that will not tend to accentuate a round upper back.
5. In the straight-leg lowering exercise from supine lying, identify the resistance moment arm of the lever and also the rotary component of the resistance (see p. 333 and Figure 15.5). Under what circumstances, if any, would it be appropriate for an individual to do this exercise?
6. Devise an exercise for a swimmer who wants to increase ankle flexibility, especially plantar flexion. (*Note:* Merely plantar flexing the feet

volitionally is not forceful enough to increase the range of motion.)

7. Do an anatomical and mechanical analysis of a piece of "gimmick" exercise equipment. Determine to what extent the device fulfills its stated purpose. Apply each of the evaluation questions on page 413 to this device.
8. Devise an exercise for a person who is unable to get out of the deep end of a pool onto the deck without using the stairs. Validate its appropriateness by performing a complete kinesiological analysis following the outline presented in Chapter 1.
9. Perform a complete kinesiological analysis of an exercise selected from Appendix G, taking particular note of the purpose of the exercise, its classification, and the nature of the motion. Include also muscle participation, neuromuscular considerations, mechanical factors, and applicable principles and violations. Conclude the analysis with a prescription for improvement, including suggested methods for change and for the elimination of violations of principles.

CHAPTER 16

Moving Objects: Pushing and Pulling

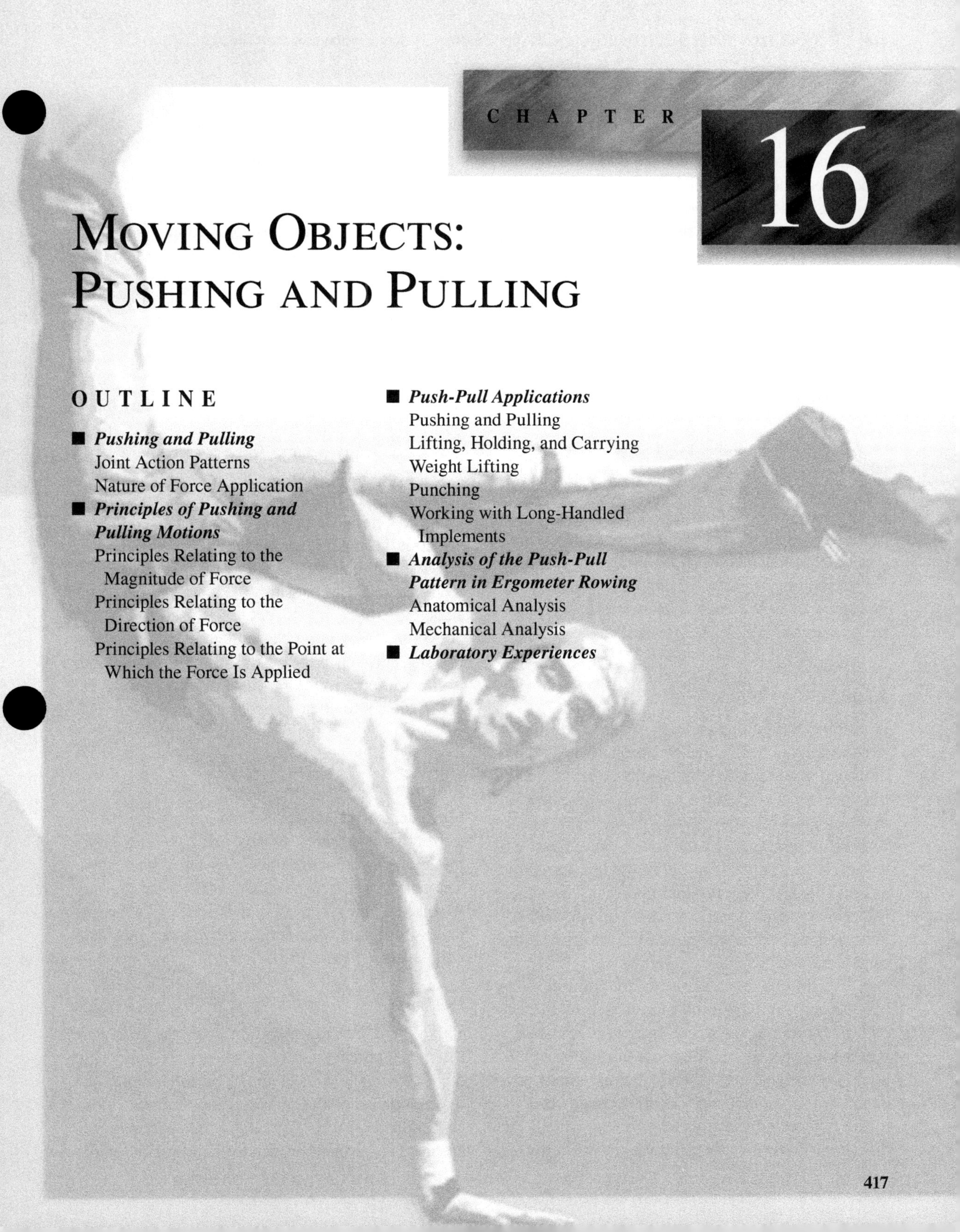

OUTLINE

- ***Pushing and Pulling***
  - Joint Action Patterns
  - Nature of Force Application
- ***Principles of Pushing and Pulling Motions***
  - Principles Relating to the Magnitude of Force
  - Principles Relating to the Direction of Force
  - Principles Relating to the Point at Which the Force Is Applied
- ***Push-Pull Applications***
  - Pushing and Pulling
  - Lifting, Holding, and Carrying
  - Weight Lifting
  - Punching
  - Working with Long-Handled Implements
- ***Analysis of the Push-Pull Pattern in Ergometer Rowing***
  - Anatomical Analysis
  - Mechanical Analysis
- ***Laboratory Experiences***

OBJECTIVES

At the conclusion of this chapter, the student should be able to:

1. Classify activities involving push or pull patterns according to the nature of the force application.
2. Name and discuss anatomical and mechanical factors and principles that apply to representative push or pull activities.
3. Analyze the performance of someone performing a push-pull skill under each of these force application conditions: momentary contact, projection, or continuous application. Follow the kinesiological analysis outline presented in Chapter 1.

PUSHING AND PULLING

A person pushes a table across the room, a boxer jabs at an opponent, a traveler lifts a suitcase onto an overhead rack, an archer shoots an arrow from a bow, and a schoolteacher lifts open a window. As widely diverse as these activities seem, they all have a common denominator: Each involves moving an external object, either directly by some part of the body or by means of an implement, in a pushing or pulling pattern.

Joint Action Patterns

In pushing and pulling patterns of motion, the basic joint actions are flexion and extension in one or more of the extremities. The joint actions in the upper extremities are characterized by flexion and extension in the elbow while the opposite movement is occurring in the shoulder. In the lower extremities, extension occurs simultaneously in the hip, knee, and ankle. This simultaneous and opposite joint action is a primary characteristic of push-pull patterns. All joint motions occur at the same time or very near the same time.

The simultaneous nature of the joint motions in push and pull patterns produces a rectilinear path of motion at the distal end point of the segments involved, as opposed to a curvilinear path. Such a rectilinear path means that all forces produced by segmental motion are applied directly to the object and that this force is applied in the direction of motion. Keeping this in mind makes it apparent that the primarily simultaneous push-pull patterns are of greatest value when it is important to apply a large force (overcome a large resistance) or to apply a force with maximum accuracy. All the forces involved are applied directly in line with the object being moved. There are no large-magnitude tangential forces.

A push, pull, or lift may be applied either directly or indirectly to an object. In the latter instance, the push or pull pattern is used to develop potential energy in an elastic device such as a bow or slingshot. When the elastic structure is released, it imparts force to the movable object, causing the arrow or shot to be projected into the air.

Nature of Force Application

Momentary Contact

Movements such as striking and hitting are characterized by momentary contact made with an object by a moving part of the body or by a held implement. The object itself may be either stationary or moving. A volleyball pass, a heading in soccer, and a fencing lunge are examples of momentary contact push and pull patterns (Figure 16.1).

Projection

This type of force application is characterized by the development of kinetic energy in a movable object that is held in the hand or hands, followed by the release of the object at the moment of desired speed or direction. Push and pull patterns are used for projection when the projected object

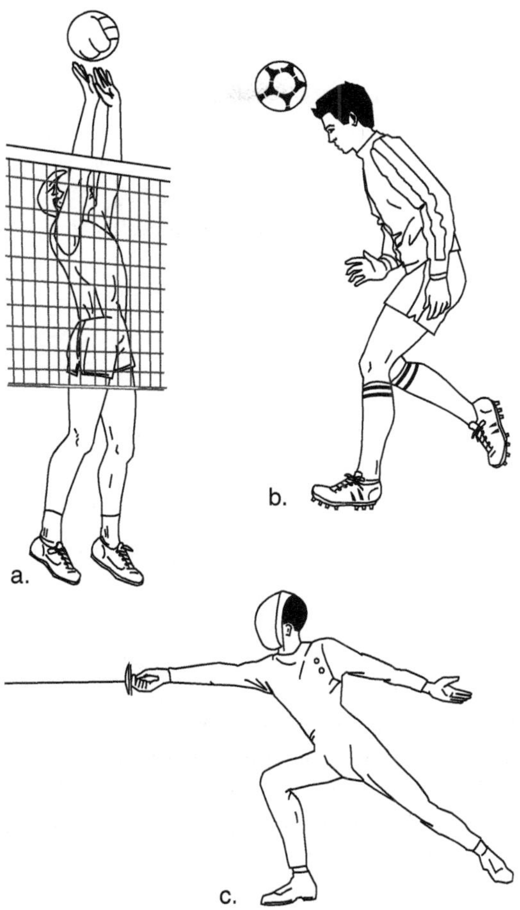

Figure 16.1 Push-pull patterns used in skills requiring momentary contact: (a) volleyball set; (b) heading in soccer; (c) fencing lunge.

has considerable mass (e.g., shot put) or when great accuracy is desired (e.g., free throw in basketball, chest pass, dart throwing, Figure 16.2).

Continuous Application

Movements in this category are characterized by the continuous application of force, usually by the hand or hands, but the legs may also be included. Most activities involving moving large resistance fall into this category (e.g., weight lifting, pushing heavy objects), although maintaining a push or pull position while waiting for release may also be classified as continuous (e.g., archery, Figure 16.3).

PRINCIPLES OF PUSHING AND PULLING MOTIONS

However motion is given, whether by hand, foot, head, or implement, it involves imparting force. And force, or effort, is described in terms of its magnitude, direction, and point of application. These three aspects of force provide the basis for the principles that apply to giving motion to external objects through pushing and pulling, the objects on occasion being other human bodies. Supplementing these aspects are the factors that relate to the stability of the body at the moment of giving motion; those that relate to the interaction between the body and the surface that supports it (for unless the body is stable when it is giving impetus, much of the force is wasted); and those that relate specifically to struck objects. The underlying mechanical principles have been presented in Part II. Stated briefly in descriptive terms, they are as follows.

Principles Relating to the Magnitude of Force

1. The object will move only if the force is of sufficient magnitude to overcome the object's inertia. The force must be great enough to overcome not only the mass of the object but also all restraining forces. These include (a) friction between the object and the supporting surface, (b) resistance of the surrounding medium (e.g., wind or water), and (c) internal resistance. Warming up helps prevent injury as well as decrease resistance. Increasing range of motion through training is also important and effective in reducing internal resistance.
2. Force exerted by the body will be transferred to an external object in proportion to the effectiveness of the counterforce of the feet (or other parts of the body) against the ground (or other supporting surface). This effectiveness depends on the counterpressure and friction presented by the supporting surface. The force applied to a ball thrown

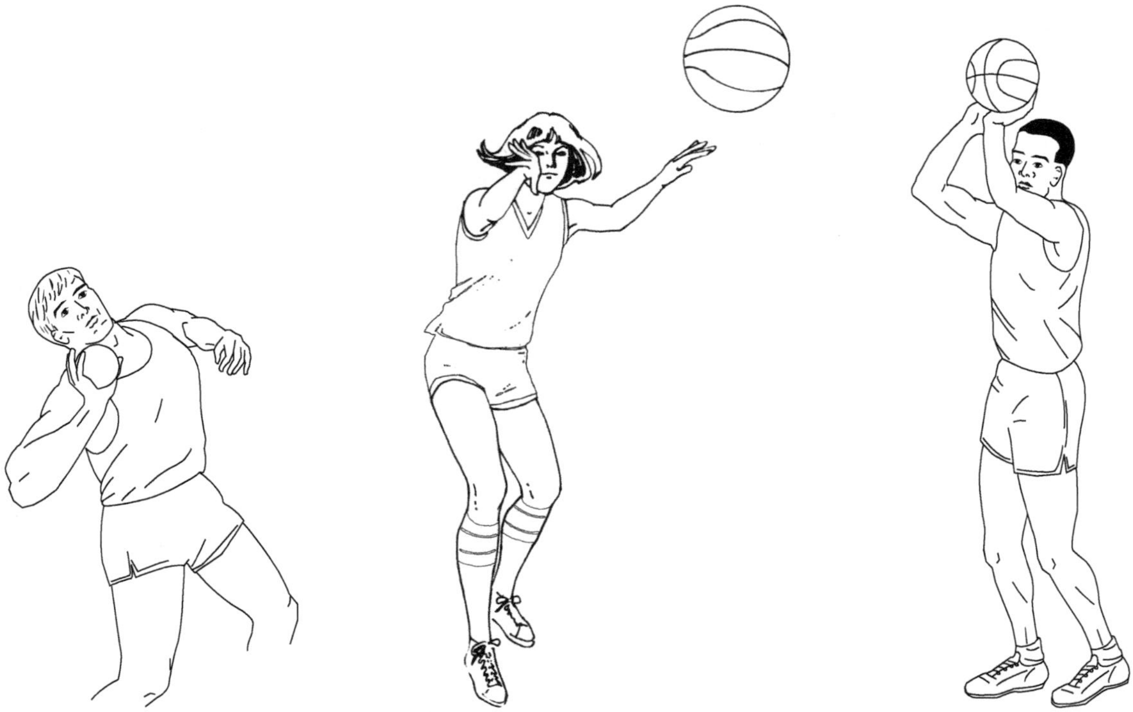

a. b. c.

Figure 16.2 Push-pull patterns used to project objects: (a) shot put; (b) chest pass; (c) free throw.

while in midair or while treading water is less than that applied to it while pushing against the ground.

3. Optimum summation of internal force is needed if maximum force is to be applied to move an object. The maximum number of segments that can safely be employed should be moved through the largest possible safe range of motion for maximum force production in a push or pull pattern.
4. For maximum accuracy, the smallest possible number of segments should be used through the smallest possible range of motion. The smaller motion limits the amount of error that is likely to be introduced into the rectilinear path.
5. For a change in momentum to occur, force must be applied over time (impulse). If maximum force is desired in projection-type activities, maximum muscle torques should be applied over as long a time as possible.

Principles Relating to the Direction of Force

1. The direction in which the object moves is determined by the direction of the force applied to it. If the force consists of two or more components, the object will move in the direction of the resultant of those components. After being projected or struck, the direction will be modified by gravity and air resistance.
2. If an object is free to move only along a predetermined pathway (as in the case of a window or sliding door), any component of force not in the direction of this pathway is wasted and may serve to increase friction.
3. When optimum force production is the purpose of the push or pull pattern, those segments involved should be aligned with the direction of intended force production. A misalignment of segments will produce high internal torque, thereby increasing the risk of injury.

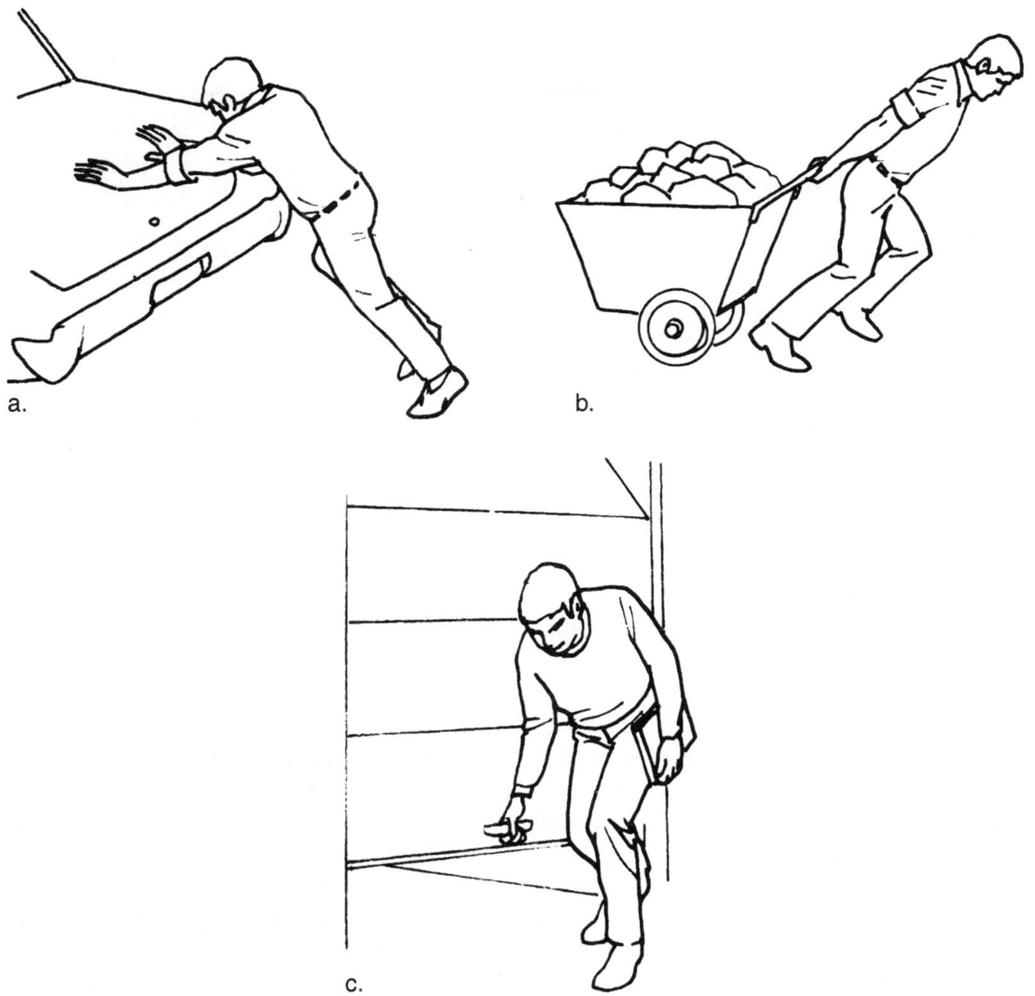

Figure 16.3 Push-pull patterns used in continuous application: (a) pushing a car; (b) pulling; (c) lifting.

Principles Relating to the Point at Which the Force Is Applied

1. Force applied in line with an object's center of gravity will result in linear motion of the object, provided the latter is freely movable.
2. If the force applied to a freely movable object is not in line with the latter's center of gravity, it will result in rotary motion of the object.
3. If the free motion of an object is interfered with by friction or by the presence of an obstacle, rotary motion may result, even though the force is applied in line with the object's center of gravity.

PUSH-PULL APPLICATIONS

Pushing and Pulling

The great majority of pushing, pulling, and lifting activities undoubtedly occur in everyday tasks. A number of sports, however, involve the continuous pushing or pulling of external objects. Archery is an interesting example because it consists of pulling with one hand while pushing with the other. The same is true of using a slingshot. Pushing is also used in football, and both pushing and pulling are used in wrestling. Weight lifting is the prime example of a sport activity involving lifting.

Rowing and paddling, although classified as forms of aquatic locomotion, may also be considered activities that involve external objects. Oars and paddles are both moved by continual pushing and pulling movements. Pole vaulting, rope climbing (previously classified as locomotor), and all suspension activities might also be included in the pushing and pulling category, provided one accepts activities that involve the moving of the body by means of pushing or pulling an external object, the object in such cases also serving as the means of body support.

The magnitude of the force used in pushing, pulling, and lifting can be increased in two ways. The immediate way is by using the lower extremities and, in some instances, the body weight to supplement the force provided by the upper extremities. In many, if not most, pushing and pulling activities the direction and point of application of force are interrelated. They both have an important bearing on the effectiveness of the force exerted and also on the economy of effort and avoidance of strain. Economy of effort is ensured when the force is applied in line with the object's center of gravity and in the desired direction of motion. When this application of force is not feasible, the undesirable component of force should be as small as possible. For instance, if one desires to push a heavy box across the floor, it would be difficult to stoop low enough to push with the arms or even the forearms in a horizontal position. One should stoop as low as conveniently possible, however, to reduce the downward component of force that would tend to increase friction. If it were necessary to move the box down a long corridor, it would be more efficient to tie a rope to the box and pull it. By using a long rope, the horizontal component of force would be relatively great and the vertical or lifting component relatively small. Some lifting component would be desirable, however, as it would serve to reduce friction.

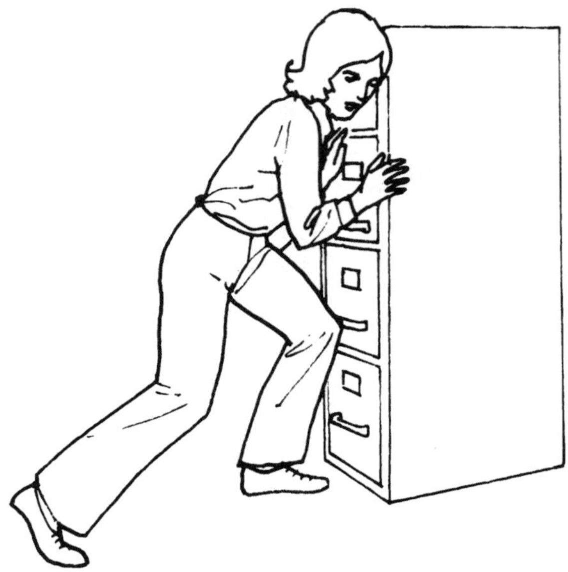

Figure 16.4 Using the lower extremities and body weight to supplement the upper extremities in a pushing task.

When friction is a major obstacle, as when pushing a tall object such as a filing cabinet across a carpeted floor, the horizontal push should be applied close to the cabinet's center of gravity at a point found by experimentation (Figure 16.4). When this point is found, it will be possible to push the cabinet without tipping it. When it does not seem practical to slide a heavy object along the floor, one may try "walking" it on opposite corners. This involves tipping the object until it is resting on one edge of its base and then, by a series of partial rotations, alternately pivoting it first on one corner and then on the other. The arms alternate in a lever action, one hand holding the upper corner that corresponds to the lower one that is serving as the pivot, and the other hand pushing the diagonally opposite upper corner forward.

When attempting to pull an object, the same general directions apply, but with this exception. As in the case of pulling the box with a rope, it may be advantageous to pull in a slightly upward direction because the lifting effect would help reduce friction. Nevertheless, unless one wishes to rotate the object, the pull should be applied in line with the object's line of gravity.

When applying a pull or a push to an object that must move on a track, such as a window or a sliding garage door or a weight on a weight machine, it is essential to apply the force in the direction that the track or runway permits. Force in any other direction is wasted and friction is increased. As an example, trying to open a heavy window or one that sticks can be done by standing with the right side next to it, the arm close to the body, elbow fully flexed, and the heel of the hand placed beneath a crosspiece of the frame, and then pushing vertically upward. If more force is needed, the knees and hips should be flexed and the hands placed against a lower crosspiece. The extension of the lower extremities then supplements the force exerted by the arm with little increase in the length of the resistance arm. If this action is inadequate, both hands can be used by twisting the trunk to face the window. In pulling the window down, one should face it, stand as close as possible, and use both hands, being careful to apply the force vertically downward.

Lifting, Holding, and Carrying

Lifting

Lifting is a form of pulling; it is pulling a movable object vertically or obliquely upward. The more nearly vertical the pull and the more in line with the object's center of gravity, the more efficient is the lift. The principle involved here is that of minimizing the resistance arm of a lever to reduce the amount of effort needed to lift a given weight. For instance, to give an extreme example, less effort is needed to lift and hold a heavy package close to the body than to lift and hold it at arm's length.

Of primary concern in lifting are the stresses applied to the lumbar region of the spine. Conventional wisdom has, for years, dictated that it is less damaging on the low back to lift from a squat position rather than from a stoop, or forward bending, position (Figure 16.5). Recently investigators have called this assumption into question. The change in resistance arm length between the two postures has been a major concern, but one must also take into consideration the nature of the stress produced during a lift. With this in mind, studies on shear stress (moving the vertebrae across each other), torque, and compression have found few differences between squat lifting and stoop lifting. Stoop lifting does produce greater shear

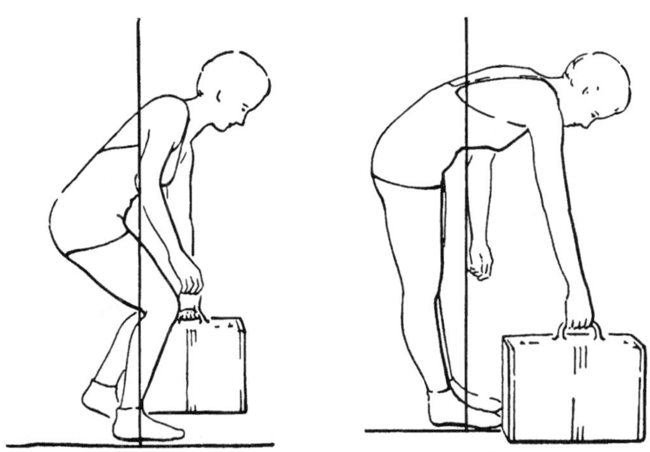

Figure 16.5 Picking up a suitcase: (a) semisquat; (b) stoop. Notice the position of the line of gravity.

forces, but squat lifting produces greater compressive loads. Torques produced in the two lift postures are within 5% of each other. Lift posture is often dictated by the requirements of the lift. A compromise lift technique using a semi-squat is proposed as the most efficient in terms of back stress. In many cases the semi-squat is the posture naturally adopted when no set posture is dictated (Burgess-Limerick, 2003; Kingma et al., 2004; Straker, 2003). Recent research continues to support the suggestions of Burgess-Limerick (2003), in which no significant difference was found between squatting and stooped lifting postures with regard to the lumbar moments (Hwang, Kim & Kim, 2009).

In addition to lift posture, a number of other factors must be considered when examining lifting motions for efficiency and safety. The velocity of the lift, foot position, load height, symmetry, and space constraints are among the factors that will affect the lift. A summary of the principles of lifting as adapted from Burgess-Limerick (2003) and Ferguson et al. (2002, 2005) follows:

- Greater mass requires greater force for motion, so reduce load mass as much as possible to reduce the stress on muscles and passive ligamentous structures.
- The lower the initial load to be lifted, the greater the flexion at spine, hip, knee, and ankle will be. Avoiding loads at floor level will reduce the initial extension loading on the joints involved.
- The farther the load is from the joints performing the lift, the greater the resistance arm. For this reason, loads should be kept as close to the body as possible. Reducing the resistance arm of the load will reduce the demands on the musculature and passive structures. To accomplish this, the feet must be kept as close to the load as possible. Ideally the feet can be placed on either side of the load.
- Maintaining the spine in a neutral posture will reduce both torque and shear stress on the spine. Compressive forces will still be present.
- Avoid trunk rotation while lifting. The lumbar spine is not structured to accept loading while in rotation. This motion will place undue stresses on the vertebral facets, discs, and ligaments. The muscles of the vertebral column are of insufficient size or strength to counteract these stresses.
- For the reasons stated previously, lateral flexion should also be avoided while lifting.
- While lifting, both feet should remain firmly on the supporting surface. The addition of an external load will change the location of the center of gravity with respect to the base of support; a solid base is necessary to maintain stability.
- Lift velocity should be held relatively constant. A constant velocity requires lower accelerations than sudden changes. Lower accelerations require less muscle contraction force and reduce the force on passive structures. The lifter should avoid "jerking" the load to start the motion. Velocity should be maintained throughout the lift motion if possible. Slowing and restarting the lift to change hand positions may introduce an unwanted acceleration.

Holding and Carrying

Although holding and carrying are not push-pull patterns, being static in nature, they are often related to the lifting motion just described. In holding, effort can be minimized by supporting the object from underneath, with only enough force applied to counteract the downward pull of gravity. Again, as in lifting, the closer the held object is to the line of gravity, the shorter the resistance arm, thus decreasing the torque produced by the object.

An object held in a pincerlike fashion between the fingers and thumb (Figure 6.30a) is an inefficient form for holding an object of any sizable mass, although it is excellent for fine control. The object held in this grip is supported by the relatively weak muscle of the thumb and hand, supplying sufficient pressure to maintain the level of friction required. As these muscles fatigue, the pressure between the object and the fingers is reduced, friction decreases, and the object falls because of the downward force of gravity. Holding positions that offer support against gravity or use of the larger muscle groups of the forearm are more effective and efficient (see Figure 6.30b, d, e).

The most efficient manner of carrying objects (the translation of a held object) is that which requires the least accommodation of the body's center of gravity. Objects may be carried in a variety of positions, such as on top of the head, in front of the body, to one side, or strapped on the back. In each case, the object becomes part of the moving body and therefore affects the location of the body's center of gravity. Therefore, the larger the mass of the object and the farther away from the body the object is located, the greater the change in the center of gravity of the total moving object–body system. The greater the change in the position of the center of gravity, the greater the necessity for segmental realignment of posture. As was discussed in Chapter 14, any postural deviation can increase stress on the body, often creating weakness or a predisposition to injury. Objects carried on top of the head raise the center of gravity of the moving system. The objects are also precariously perched on a relatively small, rounded base of support. This carrying position, however, places the object in line with the body's line of gravity, causing no relocation of the center of gravity in either the sagittal or frontal plane and producing little or no external torque on the vertebral column. In many cultures this is the preferred method of carrying. In some cultures, women have been found to carry as much as 60% of their body weight on their heads (Bastien et al., 2005).

Carrying loaded backpacks has become a concern for those working with schoolchildren. Children carry a variety of bag styles loaded with school books, school work, and personal belongings every day. It has been found that backpack carriage alters posture and can have an effect on the incidence of low back pain. To maintain stability and equilibrium, the combined center of gravity of the torso and backpack must be shifted forward over the feet. If this shift occurs in the spine or at the hips, as is most common, stress will be placed on the muscles and other structures of the region, usually due to increased torques. To minimize the effect of carrying a backpack, it is recommended that pack weight be no more than 10 to 20% of body weight, especially in children. Specifically, at loads of 20% of body, weight, changes have been noted in standing and walking conditions, and particular gait parameters are also affected. While wearing backpacks with 20% of body weight, children assumed a more forward lean when walking as compared to simply standing. In addition, during walking children demonstrated an increase in support time and a decrease in gait velocity. Caution should also be used when selecting a backpack. Shoulder carriage bags are popular, but carrying a load on one shoulder tends to produce an asymmetrical load on the spine, placing an unbalanced stress on one side and one set of muscles (Brackley & Stevenson, 2005; Cottalorda et al., 2003; Murray & Johnson, 2005).

A more commonly preferred method of carrying objects is to place equal loads on either side of the body. This creates a state of equilibrium within the system. Each separate load offsets the influence of the other without necessitating a change in posture or any realignment of the segments.

Whenever objects must be carried on one hip, in back, or in front, a postural adjustment must be made to maintain stability. To minimize stress on the joints, including the vertebral column, these adjustments should be made from the ankles. Thrusting the hips out or adjusting with the back may predispose one to injury unless compensation occurs by routinely altering the location of the load.

Weight Lifting

Lifting weights, whether done for strengthening and conditioning muscles or competitive lifting contests, involves the use of the levers of the body to overcome the inertia of relatively large masses. Depending on the lift being done, either a push or a pull pattern may be used. The key to safe and successful weight lifting is in arranging the various levers involved in such a way as to minimize the torque produced by the external resistance while maximizing the available muscle torques. To produce an efficient lift, one must first establish the location of the axis of rotation for the lift. The moving weight should be kept as close to this axis of rotation as possible, reducing the resistance moment arm. In the bench press, for example, it is much safer and more efficient to lift the bar directly over the shoulders than to allow the bar any horizontal motion. To further reduce the risk of injury, the axis of rotation should be well supported. In standing lifts, this means that the axis of rotation should be in line with the approximate center of the base of support. To allow the axis of rotation to move away from the base of support requires that postural torques be created for stability. These torques usually occur in the back and may lead to injury. The velocity of the lifting motion should be kept low. A high-velocity lift generates a great deal of momentum, requiring a large braking force. This braking force usually takes the form of an eccentric muscle contraction, which must act to decrease momentum.

Punching

Punches are simultaneous push-pattern motions. A punch is typically directed horizontally rather than vertically and usually terminates with contact to another body that provides the external resistance. Because the momentum of the punch is to be transferred to the opponent, it is desirable for punch velocity to be high. The purpose of the high-velocity punch can be to upset the balance of the opponent, as in boxing, or to cause injury to the opponent, as in karate and self-defense.

A boxing punch is typified by a long punch and a long follow-through. The force of the punch is transferred to the opponent over a broad area through the boxing glove. Punches to the head produce acceleration of the head and neck, which may lead to unconsciousness or may produce angular momentum, causing a loss of balance. A karate punch, on the other hand, is a shorter punch with little or no follow-through. The force of a karate blow is delivered to a very small area. Impact occurs at the peak velocity of the punch, and this impact can break bone and tear tissue. For this reason, karate is practiced as a noncontact sport and judged on correctness of form and accuracy. In addition, it is important that karate practitioners provide a stable platform from which this push-pull motion can be executed. Karate punches are a unique application of push-pull motion. When punching, a karate practitioner will push with the punching hand, but pull with the nonpunching hand. This helps to reduce the reaction force produced by the forward thrust of the punching hand. It has been shown that more experienced karate practitioners are able to stabilize their bodies better than novice practitioners when delivering a punch. Specifically, the center of gravity of experienced karate practitioners moved posteriorly less per unit of impulse than did that of the novice practitioners (Cesari & Bertucco, 2008).

The simultaneous nature of many karate punches and most boxing punches allows for maximum force production with a straight-line motion intended to give the opponent little or no time for defense. In both sports, quickness of the punch is vital, both for an effective offense and to allow for a rapid return to a ready position.

Working with Long-Handled Implements

Working with implements such as a hoe, rake, mop, or vacuum cleaner involves a combination of pushing, pulling, and, in some instances, lifting. The last is usually only for short distances, but it may occur with considerable frequency. One characteristic of working with implements such as these is that the body must maintain a more or less fixed posture for relatively long periods of time, causing tension and fatigue. Hence the chief problem is that of using the body in such a way that tension will be minimized and fatigue postponed for as long as possible. If the implement is used back and forth in front of the body, the tendency of the worker is to lean forward (Figure 16.6). This necessitates static contraction of the extensors of the spine to support the trunk against the downward pull of gravity. Because implements such as the rake and hoe are lifted at the end of each

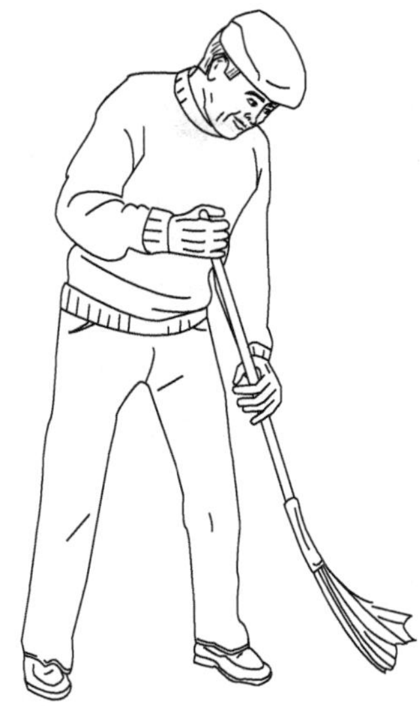

Figure 16.6 Long-handled implements may force a forward-leaning posture. The wider stride is beneficial.

stroke and carried to position for the next stroke, the force of gravity acts on the implement as well as on the worker's body. Although the implement may not weigh much in itself, its forward position means that the lever has a long resistance arm, the effect of which must be balanced by the muscles. This gives an added burden to the back muscles and not infrequently causes a backache. A better method is to stand with the side turned toward the worksite and the feet separated in a fairly wide stride, and work the implement from side to side. The reach can then be obtained by bending the knee of the leg on the same side as the implement and by inclining the body slightly to the same side. Those who are familiar with gymnastics will recognize this as a side lunge position. On the recovery, the knee and the trunk are both straightened. Thus there is an alternating contraction and relaxation of muscles and there is no necessity for any of the trunk muscles to remain in static contraction. Temporary relief can also be obtained by changing sides.

The use of a spade or snow shovel primarily involves the act of lifting. Because the load is taken on the end of a mechanical lever held in a more or less horizontal position, it is inevitable that the weight arm of the lever be relatively long. It can be shortened somewhat, however, by sliding one hand as far down the shaft as possible, using this hand as a fulcrum, and providing the force with the other hand by pushing down on the outer end of the handle. As a variation of this technique, when getting a particularly heavy load on a shovel, it is possible to bend one knee and brace the shaft against the thigh, thus using the thigh as a fulcrum. This is only for the initial lift, however; the hands must then be shifted to the position previously described to carry or throw the load.

Aside from taking and lifting the load on the spade, there is the factor of lowering the body to reach the load and of assuming the erect position for moving it. As in the case of stooping to lift a heavy object from the floor, the chief problems are economy of effort, maintenance of stability, and avoidance of strain. These problems are intensified by the additional factor of taking the load on a long-handled implement instead of directly in the hand. As before, separating the feet to widen the base of support, bending at the knees instead of bending from the waist to lower the body, and inclining the trunk forward only slightly will, respectively, increase stability, shorten the anatomical levers involved in the stooping, and divide the muscular work among the stronger knee, hip, and back extensors instead of making the weaker back muscles assume too large a share of the work. Because the lower back is easily strained by heavy shoveling, it is of great importance to protect it by observing the principles of good mechanics.

ANALYSIS OF THE PUSH-PULL PATTERN IN ERGOMETER ROWING

The motion used in the rowing ergometer mimics very closely the motion used to propel a rowboat or a sculling shell through the water. The rowing motion is a combination of leg pushing action and arm pull in a continuous cycle. The row can be broken down into two primary phases—the drive phase and the recovery phase. The rower starts with the ergometer slide in the forward position.

TABLE 16.1 Anatomical Analysis of the Drive Phase

Joint	Joint Action	Segment Moved	Force for Movement	Muscles Active	Kind of Contraction
Ankles	Plantar flexion	Shank	Muscle	Gastrocnemius Soleus	Concentric
Knees	Extension	Thigh	Muscle	Quadriceps femoris	Concentric
Hips	Extension	Trunk	Muscle	Hamstrings Gluteus maximus	Concentric
Shoulder joints	Extension	Upper arm	Muscle	Pectoralis major (sternal portion) Teres major Latissimus dorsi Teres minor	Concentric
Shoulder girdle	Adduction	Scapula	Muscle	Rhomboids Trapezius III	Concentric
Elbows	Flexion	Forearm	Muscle	Biceps brachii Brachioradialis	Concentric

The lower extremity is fully flexed while the arms are extended horizontally forward in front of the trunk.

Anatomical Analysis (Table 16.1)

Drive Phase

The rowing stroke begins with the initial catch. In the water, this is the point at which the oar is dropped into the water through a slight lifting of the hands. On the rowing ergometer, the catch marks the point at which the ergometer cable is fully retracted. At this instant the performer is in the starting position, with the knees and hips fully flexed, shoulders flexed, and elbows in extension. The spine should be erect.

The drive phase is initiated through extension of the lower extremity. The legs push strongly against the foot plate, pushing the body backward on the sliding seat. As the legs near full extension, the spine begins extension to maintain a smooth, continuous motion of the oar. The upper extremity now begins motion, with the upper arm pulling through shoulder horizontal abduction as the elbows flex. The stroke finishes with the knees in full extension, extension of the spine, full horizontal abduction of the shoulder, and complete flexion of the elbow. The joint motion of each extremity link system (upper and lower) is done simultaneously, although the lower body initiates the stroke and the upper body finishes it. Figure 16.7 presents the sequence of the rowing stroke from starting position through leg extension to the end of the drive phase.

Recovery Phase

The recovery phase of the stroke varies depending on the resistance setting. In the rowing ergometer the recovery motion of lower extremity flexion is produced by a fairly moderate concentric contraction of the flexor muscles (thus pulling the slide seat and body forward) while the forward motion of the upper extremity (shoulder horizontal adduction and elbow extension) is produced by similar contraction of the appropriate muscles, pushing the handle forward to the catch position. On the rowing ergometer, leg flexion is again produced by moderate contraction of the flexors, while arm motion may be produced primarily by the

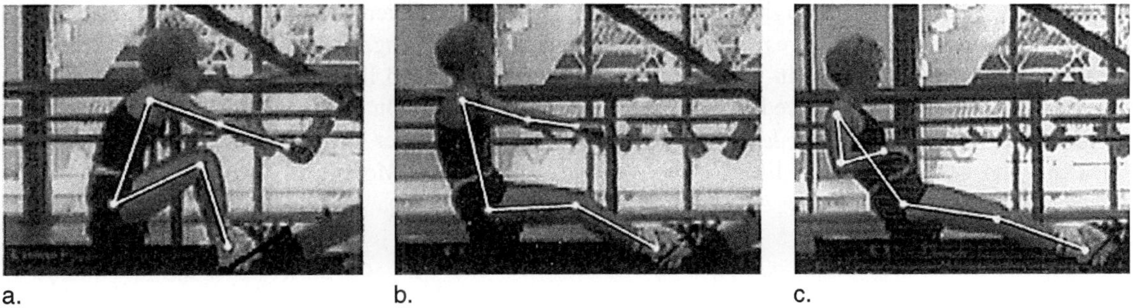

Figure 16.7 The rowing stroke from starting position through leg extension to the end of the drive phase.

retraction of the ergometer cable, although there is some activation of the tibialis anterior as the lower leg becomes vertical (Soper & Hume, 2004).

Mechanical Analysis

In rowing over water, the primary mechanical objective of the rowing action is to produce maximum power. The rower wants to generate the highest possible velocity in the boat. This is accomplished through the combination of stroke length and stroke rate. The most efficient and most effective performance is one in which the force can be applied to the water through the full range of motion allowed and the fastest possible stroke rate can be maintained. Stroke rates in rowing races in the Olympic Games, for instance, are often as high as 38 to 40 strokes per minute over a distance of 2.5 kilometers (Dawson et al., 1998).

Whereas the rower in a boat does work on the water to move the boat forward, the performer on the rowing ergometer is doing work against some form of machine resistance. However, the principal objective of producing maximum power through the optimum combination of stroke length and stroke rate still applies.

Force for motion in the rowing ergometer is provided through extension of the knees and hips. Lower extremity extension produces a ground reaction force in the foot plate, or stretcher. The force for extension is therefore reversed, producing motion in the seat. Approximately 65 to 75% of the oar velocity in the stroke is produced in this way. It is important that this force be applied in a smooth, consistent manner. Equally important is the transfer of these forces to the hands as the hips and knees reach extension. This usually occurs at about 70% of the drive phase. To effect this transfer efficiently, the trunk must be stabilized through hip and knee extension. The rower must be careful, therefore, not to begin the flexion of the lower extremities too soon. The force production in the drive phase should be maximized before the recovery phase begins. It has been found that the drive phase may be as much as twice the duration of the recovery phase. As stroke rate increases, this may change as drive time increases, but at no time should the recovery phase be rushed.

Forces applied to the handle in ergometer rowing are related to handle height as well as to muscle force in flexion. Studies have shown that pulling with the hands at the level of the navel produces greater force than when pulling with the hands at chest level. Peak force applied to the stretcher occurs before the peak force at the handle. The timing of this separation varies with skill level. The magnitude of the forces applied through the feet and the handle also vary with strength and skill (Soper & Hume, 2004).

Ergometer rowing differs somewhat from overwater rowing. In the recovery phase of overwater rowing, the oar blade must be lifted clear of the water by downward pressure on the grip, or inboard, end of the oar. The oar is then feathered, or rotated, as the hands are pushed forward so that the blade slices through the air parallel to the airflow. This requires hyperextension of the wrists, not necessary in ergometer rowing. The pull phase is then preceded by a "catch," as the hands are raised slightly, lowering the oars back into the water. There are likely to be other technique differences between overwater and ergometer rowing. As an example, ergometer rowers were found to lift the handle slightly at the end of the drive. On the water, this motion would drop the oars deeper into the water at an inappropriate time (Torres-Moreno et al., 2000).

REFERENCES AND SELECTED READINGS

Baker, D. G., & Newton, R. U. (2004). An analysis of the ratio and relationship between upper body pressing and pulling strength. *Journal of Strength and Conditioning Research,* 18(3), 594–598.

Bastien, G. J., Willems, P. A., Schepens, B., & Heglund, N. C. (2005). Energetics of load carrying in Nepalese porters. *Science,* 308, 1755.

Baudouin, A., & Hawkins, D. (2002). A biomechanical review of factors affecting rowing performance. *British Journal of Sports Medicine,* 36(6), 396–402.

Brackley, H. M., & Stevenson, J. M. (2005). Are children's backpack weight limits enough? A critical review of the relevant literature. *Spine,* 29(19), 2184–2190.

Burgess-Limerick, R. (2003). Squat, stoop, or something in between? *International Journal of Industrial Ergonomics,* 31, 143–148.

Cesari, P., & Bertucco, M. (2008). Coupling between punch efficacy and body stability for elite karate. *Journal of Science and Medicine in Sport,* 11(3), 353–356.

Chansirinukor. W., Wilson. D., Grimmer, K., & Dansie, B. (2001). Effects of backpacks on students: Measurement of cervical and shoulder posture. *Australian Journal of Physiotherapy,* 47(2), 110–116.

Chien-Feng, L., Wei-Hua, H., & Hui-Mei, L. (2007). Strength curve characteristics of rowing performance from the water and the land. *Journal of Biomechanics,* 40(52), S770.

Cottalorda, J., Rahmani, A., Diop, M., Gautheron, V., Ebermeyer, E., & Belli, A. (2003). Influence of school bag carrying on gait kinetics. *Journal of Pediatric Orthopaedics, Part B,* 12(6), 357–364.

Davis, K. G., & Marras, W. S. (2003). Partitioning the contributing role of biomechanical, psychosocial, and individual risk factors in the development of spine loads. *Spine Journal,* 3(5), 331–338.

Davis, K. G, & Marras, W. S. (2005). Load spatial pathway and spine loading: How does lift origin and destination influence low back response? *Ergonomics,* 48(8), 1031–1046.

Dawson, R. G., Lockwood, R. J., Wilson, J. D., & Freeman, G. (1998). The rowing cycle: Sources of variance and invariance in ergometer and on-the-water performance. *Journal of Motor Behavior,* 30, 33–43.

Dennis, G. J., & Barrett, R. S. (2002). Spinal loads during individual and team lifting. *Ergonomics,* 45(10), 671–681.

Elfeituri, F. E. (2001). A biomechanical analysis of manual lifting tasks performed in restricted workspaces. *International Journal of Occupational and Safety Ergonomics,* 7(3), 333–346.

Escamilla, R. F., Francisco, A. C., Kayes, A. V., Speer, K. P., & Moorman, C. T., III. (2002). An electromyographic analysis of sumo and conventional style deadlifts. *Medicine and Science in Sports and Exercise,* 34(4), 682–688.

Ferguson S. A., Gaudes-MacLaren, L. L., Marras, W. S., Waters, T. R., & Davis, K. G. (2002). Spinal loading when lifting from industrial storage bins. *Ergonomics,* 45(6), 399–414.

Ferguson, S. A., Marras, W. S., & Burr, D. (2005). Workplace design guidelines for asymptomatic vs. low-back-injured workers. *Applied Ergonomics,* 36(1), 85–95.

Forjuoh, S. N., Lane, B. L., & Schuchmann, J. A. (2003). Percentage of body weight carried by students in their school backpacks. *American*

Journal of Physical Medicine and Rehabilitation, 82(4), 261–266.

Hase, K., Kaya, M., Zavatsky, A. B., & Halliday, S. E. (2004). Musculoskeletal loads in ergometer rowing. *Journal of Applied Biomechanics,* 20, 317–323.

Holt, K. G., Wagenaar, R. C., Kubo, M., LaFiandra, M. E., & Obusek, J. P. (2005). Modulation of force transmission to the head while carrying a backpack load at different walking speeds. *Journal of Biomechanics,* 38(8), 1621–1628.

Hwang, S., Kim, Y., & Kim, Y. (2009). Lower extremity joint kinetics and lumbar curvature during squat and stoop lifting. *BMC Musculoskeletal Disorders,* 10, 15.

Jorgensen, M. J., Handa, A., Veluswamy, P., & Bhatt, M. (2005). The effect of pallet distance on torso kinematics and low back disorder risk. *Ergonomics,* 48(8), 949–963.

Jorgensen, M. J., Marras, W. S., Granata, K. P., & Wiand, J. W. (2001). MRI-derived moment-arms of the female and male spine loading muscles. *Clinical Biomechanics,* 16, 182–193.

Kingma, I., Bosch, T., Bruins, L., & Dieen, J. H. (2004). Foot positioning instruction, initial vertical load position and lifting technique: Effects on low back loading. *Ergonomics,* 47(13), 1365–1385.

Koukoubis, T. D., Cooper, L. W., Glisson, R. R., Seaber, A. V., & Feagin, A. J., Jr. (1995). An electromyographic study of arm muscles during climbing. *Knee Surgery, Sports Traumatology, Arthroscopy,* 3(2), 121–124.

Lafiandra, M., & Harman, E. (2004). The distribution of forces between the upper and lower back during load carriage. *Medicine and Science in Sports and Exercise,* 36(3), 460–467.

Lariviere, C., Gagnon, D., & Loisel, P. (2002). A biomechanical comparison of lifting techniques between subjects with and without chronic low back pain during freestyle lifting and lowering tasks. *Clinical Biomechanics* (Bristol, Avon), 17(2), 89–98.

McGorry, R. W., Dempsey, P. G., & Leamon, T. B. (2003). The effect of technique and shaft configuration in snow shoveling on physiologic, kinematic, kinetic and productivity variables. *Applied Ergonomics,* 34(3), 225–231.

Motmans, R. R., Tomlow, S., & Vissers, D. (2006). Trunk muscle activity in different modes of carrying schoolbags. *Ergonomics,* 49(2), 127–138.

Murray I. A., & Johnson, G. R. (2005). A study of the external forces and moments at the shoulder and elbow while performing everyday tasks. *Clinical Biomechanics* (Bristol, Avon), 19(6), 586–594.

Myer, G. D., & Wall, E. J. (2006). Resistance training in the young athlete. *Operative Techniques in Sports Medicine,* 14(3), 218–230.

National Institute for Occupational Safety and Health. (1997). *Musculoskeletal disorders and workplace factors: A critical review of epidemiological evidence for work-related musculoskeletal disorders of the neck, upper extremity, and low back.* Technical Report 97-141. Rockville, MD: Author.

Shibye, B., Søgaard, K., Martinson, D., & Klausen, K. (2000). Mechanical load on the low back and shoulders during pushing and pulling of two-wheeled waste containers compared with lifting and carrying of bags and bins. *Clinical Biomechanics,* 16, 549–559.

Smith, M. S., Dyson, R. J., Hale, T., & Janaway, L. (2000). Development of a boxing dynamometer and its punch force discrimination efficacy. *Journal of Sports Sciences,* 18(6), 445–450.

Soper, C., & Hume, P. A. (2004). Towards an ideal rowing technique for performance: The contributions of biomechanics. *Sports Medicine,* 34, 825–848.

Straker, L. (2003). Evidence to support using squat, semi-squat and stoop techniques to lift low-lying objects. *International Journal of Industrial Ergonomics,* 31, 149–160.

Tarkeshwar, S., & Koh, M. (2009a). Effects of backpack load position on spatiotemporal parameters and trunk forward lean. *Gait and Posture,* 29(1), 49–53.

Tarkeshwar, S., & Koh, M. (2009b). Lower limb dynamics change for children while walking with backpack loads to modulate shock transmission to the head. *Journal of Biomechanics,* 42(6), 736–742.

Torres-Moreno, R., Tanaka, C., & Penney, K. L. (2000). Joint excursion, handle velocity, and applied force: A biomechanical analysis of ergonometric rowing. *International Journal of Sports Medicine,* 21(1), 41–44.

OBJECTIVES

At the conclusion of this chapter, the student should be able to:

1. Classify activities involving sequential throwing, kicking, or striking patterns according to the nature of the force application.
2. Name and discuss anatomical and mechanical factors that apply to representative throwing, kicking, or striking activities.
3. Perform a kinesiological analysis of someone engaging in a sequential throwing, kicking, or striking skill under each of these force application conditions: momentary contact, projection, continuous application.

SEQUENTIAL MOVEMENTS

A baseball pitcher throws a baseball across the plate and the batter hits it to center field, an elderly man pitches horseshoes, a young person spikes a volleyball, a student practices driving a golf ball while a college athlete practices punting a football. Once more, as is the case with pushing and pulling, a widely diverse set of activities has a common denominator. Each of these activities involves sequential movement of the body segments resulting in the production of a summated velocity at the end of the chain of segments used. During the summation of velocity, it is important to note that changes are the result of an acceleration imparted through an unbalanced force. The magnitude of the unbalanced force as well as the time over which this force acts will determine the final velocity. This concept of the force and the time over which it acts effecting final velocity is called *impulse* (Chapter 12). Recall that the change in momentum is equivalent to the product of the force and time over which that force acts. The path produced by the end point of this chain of segments is curvilinear in nature.

Sequential segmental motions are most frequently used to produce high velocities in external objects. Depending on the objective of the skill, speed, distance, or some combination, modifications in the sequential pattern may be made. Greater or fewer numbers of segments may be involved, larger or smaller ranges of motion might be used, and longer or shorter lever lengths may be chosen. Regardless of the modifications, the basic nature of the sequential throwing, striking, or kicking pattern remains the same.

Joint Action Patterns

Broer was the first to call attention to the similarity of movement patterns used in seemingly dissimilar activities such as the baseball pitch, the badminton clear, and the tennis serve (Broer & Zernicke, 1979). Objective evidence of such similarities between throwing and striking activities within each of the three major upper extremity patterns (overarm, sidearm, and underarm) was originally revealed by the Broer and Houtz EMG investigations (1967) and confirmed by Moynes and colleagues (1986).

Atwater (1979) distinguished between the overarm and sidearm throwing patterns in terms of the direction in which the trunk laterally flexed. When lateral flexion occurred away from the throwing arm, an overarm pattern was used; lateral flexion toward the throwing arm indicated a sidearm pattern. The underarm pattern is distinguished by motion predominantly in a sagittal plane with the hand below the waist.

Each pattern involves a preparatory movement referred to as a backswing, or windup, followed by the establishment of a base of support prior to the initiation of the force phase and ending in a follow-through. The base of support in the direction of the force application (forward-backward) is a distinguishing feature of skill level. It has been well documented that more highly skilled individuals have longer strides. Once the base has been established, the more proximal segments begin the force application phase while the more distal segments complete the backswing. The purpose of the backswing is to place the segments in a favorable position for the force phase and exploit the stored elastic potential energy that is provided through the stretch-shortening cycle.

There are two primary benefits to including a backswing or windup phase in a sequential motion. The first of these is to take advantage of the impulse–momentum relationship. The backswing will increase the time over which the force can be applied, thereby increasing momentum. The second major benefit is to place the segments into a favorable position for a full range of motion force phase. The backswing lengthens the muscle groups that will be the agonists for the force phase, the stretch part of the stretch-shortening cycle (Grezios et al., 2006). Initiation of the concentric force phase utilizes the stored elastic energy to assist in the development of the contraction. This also evokes a phasic stretch reflex, further enhancing the force phase contraction.

Representative joint actions for each throwing pattern are as follows.

Overarm Pattern

This kind of throw or strike is characterized by rotation at the shoulder joint. In the backswing, or preparatory phase, the abducted arm rotates laterally, and in the forward, or force, phase the arm rotates medially. Some elbow extension, wrist flexion, and spinal rotation occur in the force phase. These movements are accompanied by rotation of the pelvis at the hip joint of the opposite limb, resulting in medial rotation of the thigh (Figures 17.1 and 17.2). An immature pattern (Figure 17.3) may be identified as using fewer segments, working more simultaneously rather than sequentially, and involving a more limited range of motion. This description is easily documented by referring to the developmental literature.

Underarm Pattern

This pattern consists of a forward movement of the extended arm in the sagittal plane, usually starting from a position of hyperextension and

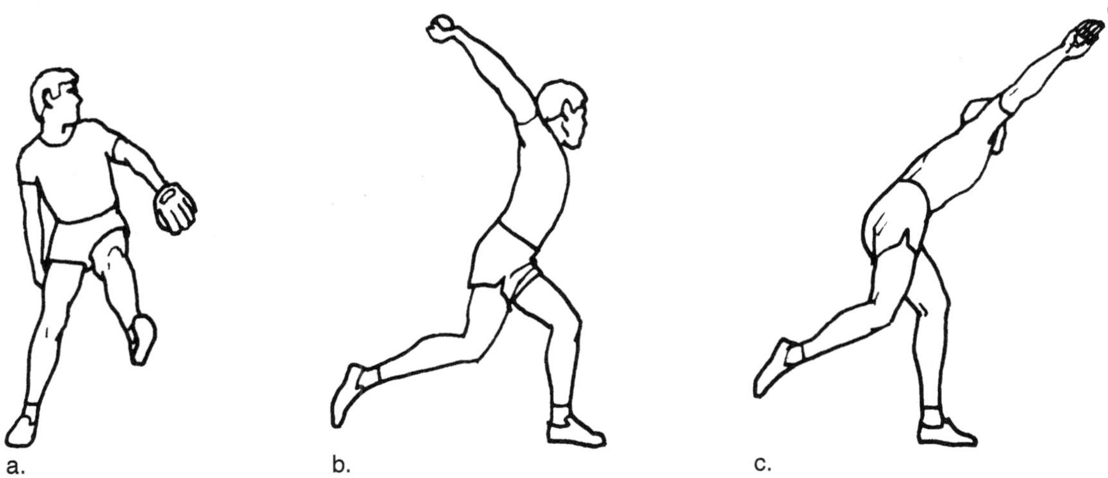

Figure 17.1 Overhand pattern applied in baseball pitch. The forward force phase is characterized by medial rotation of the arm, elbow extension, spinal rotation, and medial rotation of the pelvis at the contralateral hip joint.

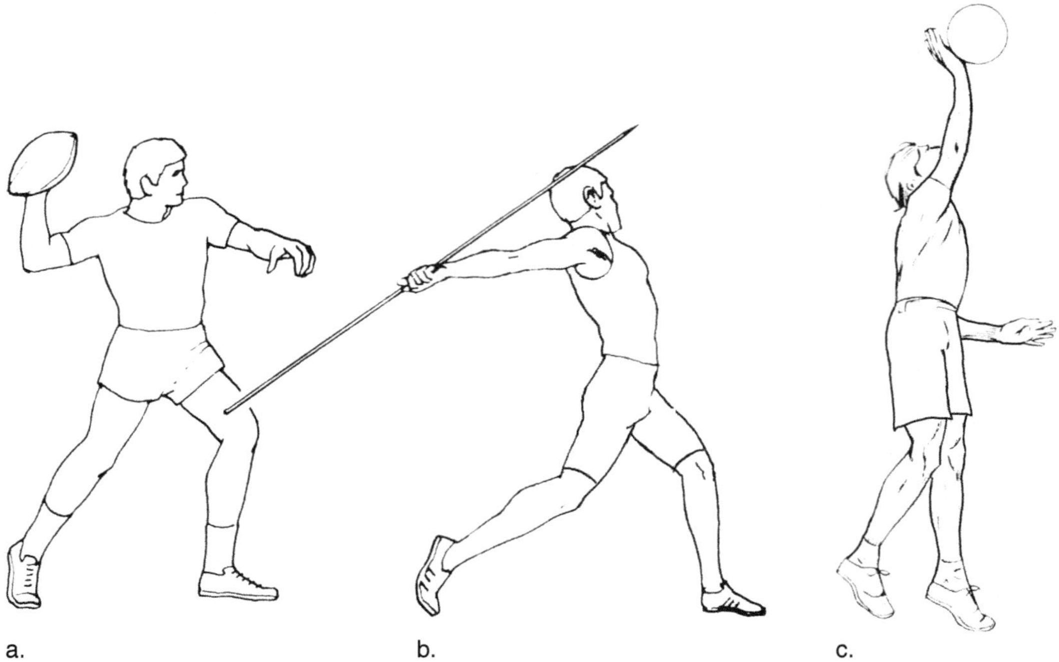

Figure 17.2 Examples of the overarm pattern: (a) football pass; (b) javelin throw; (c) volleyball serve.

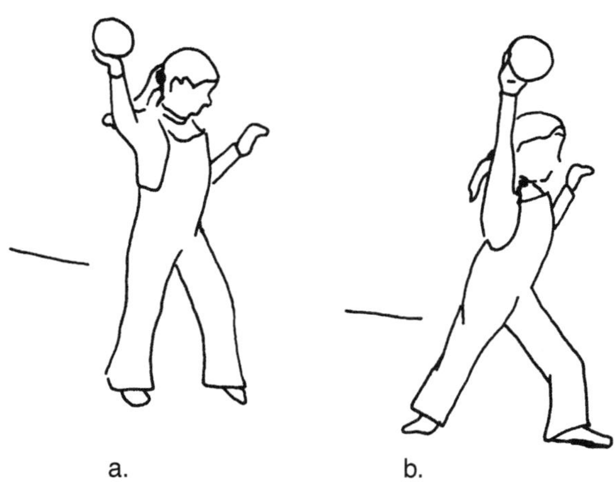

Figure 17.3 Overhand throw by a girl aged 3 years 10 months who had not been given any directions regarding how to throw. Note elbow extension, pelvic rotation, step, and weight shift.

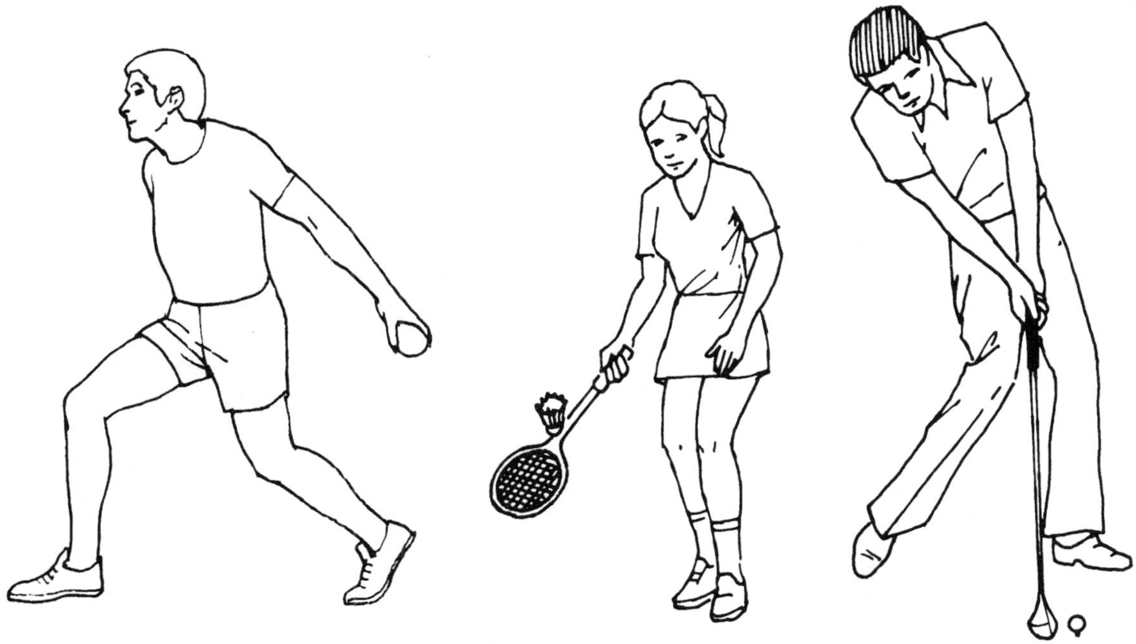

a. b. c.

Figure 17.4 Examples of the underarm pattern: (a) softball pitch; (b) badminton serve; (c) golf drive.

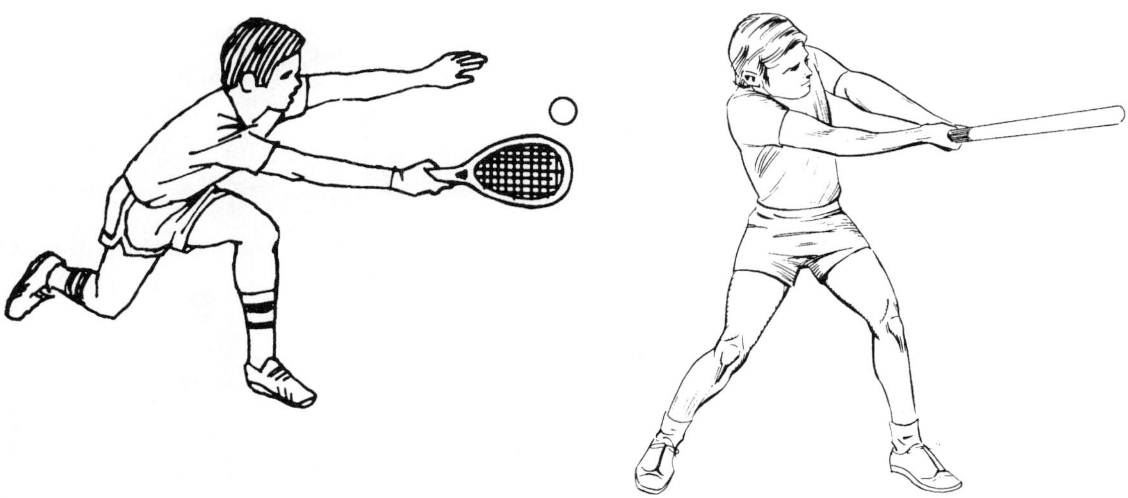

a. b.

Figure 17.5 Examples of the sidearm pattern: (a) racquetball drive; (b) softball swing.

ending in a forward reach. The basic joint action of the arm is flexion. The actions of the wrist, spine, and pelvis are the same as those observed in the overarm pattern (Figure 17.4).

Sidearm Pattern

In this pattern the basic movement is medial rotation of the pelvis on the opposite hip with the arm usually in an abducted position in the preparation phase. The arm is moved forward in a horizontal plane because of the pelvic action and spinal rotation. The spine also laterally flexes toward the throwing arm. The range of the upper extremity movement may also be enlarged by the addition of horizontal adduction at the shoulder during the force phase. The elbow is maintained in extension or is extended from a slightly flexed position, depending on the nature of the skill in question (e.g., basketball throw for distance, tennis forehand drive, or batting). Wrist flexion may also be part of the action in some techniques (Figure 17.5).

Kicking Pattern

Another form of sequential movement pattern involves use of the lower extremities and is referred to as kicking. This pattern is used, for example, when punting a football (Figure 17.6) or initiating a soccer kick. Kicking is a modification of a locomotor pattern in which force is imparted to an external object during the forward swing of the non-weight-bearing limb.

To initiate the kicking motion, the left foot (of a right-footed kicker) is stabilized. The pelvis is fixed over the thigh and rotated toward the left. The right non-weight-bearing limb lags behind, resulting in thigh abduction and hyperextension at the hip joint. The right thigh then begins to flex at the hip joint, followed by knee extension. This sequential segmental movement pattern results in the summation of forces and allows for maximum linear velocity of the foot at ball contact. The specific point of ball contact depends on the placement of the supporting foot and motion of the free-swinging limb during the backswing.

Nature of Force Application

Momentary Contact

Movements such as striking and kicking are characterized in sequential movement patterns by a momentary contact made with an object by a moving part of the body or by an implement held

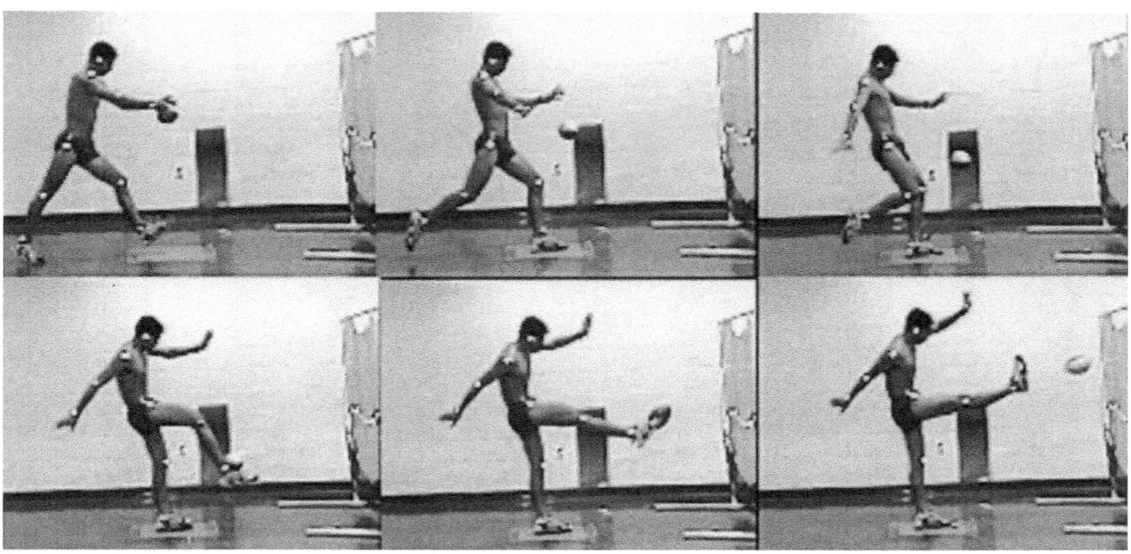

Figure 17.6 The kicking pattern as used in the football punt.

by or attached to a moving segment of the body. Baseball batting, golf, tennis, and soccer kicking are all examples of force imparted through momentary contact.

Projection

In sequential patterns, an object is given some velocity as the end point of a part of the body or as an implement attached to the body. At the desired point in the curvilinear path, the object is released to become a projectile. Throwing is an example of this type of projection, as are the projection of balls by implements as in lacrosse or jai alai.

PRINCIPLES RELATING TO THROWING, STRIKING, AND KICKING

Anatomical Principles

Regardless of which movement pattern is used, the following factors must be considered when imparting force to an object through the sequential use of body segments. To ignore the anatomical principles of sequential motion is to risk injury because sequential motion can generate extremely high velocities, as well as impart high braking forces.

1. Muscles contract more forcefully if they are first put on a stretch, provided they are not overstretched. This principle suggests the function of the windup in pitching and of the preliminary movements in other sport skills.
2. Unnecessary movements and tensions in the performance of a motor skill mean both awkwardness and unnecessary fatigue; hence, they should be eliminated.
3. Skillful and efficient performance in a particular technique can be developed only by practice of that technique. Only in this way can the necessary adjustments in the neuromuscular mechanism be made to ensure a well-coordinated movement.
4. The most efficient type of movement in throwing and striking skills is ballistic movement. Skills that are primarily ballistic should be practiced ballistically, even in the earliest learning stages. This means that from the beginning, the emphasis should be placed on speed and form rather than on aim. Accuracy of aim will develop with practice. If the emphasis is placed on accuracy in the learning stages, the beginner tends to perform the skill as a "moving fixation" or as a slow, tense movement. Once this pattern of movement is established, it is extremely difficult to change it later to a ballistic movement.
5. When there is a choice of anatomical leverage, the lever appropriate for the task should be used—that is, a lever with a long resistance arm for movements requiring range or speed, and a lever with a long effort arm for movements requiring strength. For example, kicking is an effective way to impart force to a football because the leg provides a lever with a long resistance arm, but, for the same reason, it is a poor way to move a heavy suitcase along the floor.

Mechanical Principles

Although many of the mechanical principles for throwing, striking, and kicking are similar to those cited for pushing and pulling, the applications of these principles are different. Whereas force application in push-pull patterns is maximized through using large numbers of segments simultaneously, force in throwing, kicking, and striking patterns is maximized through sequential transfer of momentum from large segments to less massive segments. To illustrate this, the mechanical principles involved in sequential movement patterns are given as they apply both to throwing and to striking.

Throwing

The efficiency of imparting force to a ball is judged in terms of the speed, distance, and direction of the ball after its release. The purpose of the throw determines which of these is given the greater emphasis. Both the speed and distance of the thrown ball are directly related to the magnitude of the force used in throwing it and to the speed of the hand at the moment of release. The speed the hand is able to achieve depends on the distance through which it moves in the preparatory part of the act and the summed angular velocities of the contributing body segments. Hence, the longer the preparatory backswing and the greater the distance that can be added by means of rotating the body, shifting the weight, and perhaps even taking a step, the greater the opportunity for accelerating. Approximately 50% of the ball speed is obtained from the forward step and body rotation. The remaining speed is contributed by the joint actions in the shoulder, elbow, wrist, and fingers. This is why the technique of a baseball pitcher is designed to allow maximum time and distance over which to accelerate the ball before its release. In addition, if the ground reaction force is to be maximal, the surface against which the thrower pushes must be firm and there must be no sliding between the ground surface and the foot. The more the direction of the body thrust is backward, the more important the friction becomes and the more the value of the cleated shoes is appreciated. If distance is a major objective of the throw, the angle of projection and the effects of gravitational force and air resistance must also be taken into consideration.

The accuracy with which a ball is thrown depends on accurate judgment of the distance and direction of the throw's target. The ball will leave the hand in the direction it is moving at the instant of release and continue in that direction except for modifications because of gravity and air resistance. Therefore, the effect of gravity, wind, and spin must be considered, as well as the release direction. If the hand is traveling in an arc at release, the ball will follow a path tangent to the arc, and the timing of the release is highly critical. Flattening the arc of the ball's path prior to release increases the margin of error by allowing more time over which the ball can be released in the desired direction. This may be done by taking a step and shifting the weight forward while flexing at the forward knee. The rotation of the pelvis and spine also helps.

The follow-through of any throwing motion is critical to the successful performance of a throw. In addition to the application of the impulse to the windup, impulse is employed during the follow-through as well. In the acceleration phase of a throw, the velocity of the ball is increased from zero to maximum velocity at ball release. Next, the arm must be decelerated to slow down the arm. The shorter the follow-through, the more force is required from the external rotators of the shoulder, particularly the rotator cuff muscles (especially the infraspinatus and teres minor).

When the object being thrown is other than a small ball, such as a javelin, discus, bowling ball, or horseshoe, the general principles are the same but must be modified according to the nature of the object and the regulations of the sport.

Principles

1. The object will move only if the force is of sufficient magnitude to overcome the object's inertia. The force must be great enough to overcome not only the mass of the object but also all restraining forces. These include (a) friction between the object and the supporting surface, (b) resistance of the surrounding medium (e.g., wind or water), and (c) internal resistance. Warming up helps prevent injury as well as decrease internal resistance. Increasing range of motion through training is also important and effective.
2. The pattern and range of joint movements depends on the purpose of the movement. If maximum force is not needed, the optimum movement pattern should be changed with respect to the range, speed, and number of joint actions until it is the most efficient for the task. Throwing a ball to a small child 10 feet away does not require the same pattern as does pitching a baseball.

3. Force exerted by the body will be transferred to an external object in proportion to the effectiveness of the counterforce of the feet (or other parts of the body) against the ground (or other supporting surface). This effectiveness depends on the counterpressure and friction presented by the supporting surface. The force applied to a ball thrown while in midair or while treading water is less than that applied to it while pushing against the ground.
4. Linear velocity is imparted to external objects as a result of the angular velocity of the body segments. The linear velocity at the end of any segment is the product of the angular velocity and the length of the segment. Thus, for a given angular speed, the linear speed imparted to a tennis ball with a tennis racket is much greater than that of a ball hit with the hand. On the other hand, more force is needed to move the longer of the two levers.
5. Optimum summation of internal force is needed if maximum force is to be applied to move an object. For the segment that will be releasing the projectile or making impact with an external object to reach maximum speed, the slower or heavier segments must start to move first and the lightest and quickest ones last. It is preferable for the slower segments to begin their forward movements while the faster segments are still completing the backswing. This timing pattern facilitates use of the stretch reflex and contributes to the humeral lag often associated with overhand throwing. (see Chapter 4).
6. For a change in momentum to occur, force must be applied over time (impulse). If maximum force is desired in projection-type activities, maximum muscle torques should be applied over as long a time as possible.
7. Force applied in line with an object's center of gravity will result in linear motion of the object, provided the latter is freely movable.
8. If the force applied to a freely movable object is not in line with the latter's center of gravity, it will result in rotary motion of the object.

Striking, Hitting, and Kicking

As in the case of throwing, the effectiveness of striking, hitting, and kicking is judged by the speed, distance, and direction of the struck ball. All the factors that apply to these aspects of a thrown ball apply similarly to a struck ball. There appear to be five major factors that apply to the speed of a struck ball. These are

1. The speed of the oncoming ball and the striking implement
2. The mass of the ball and the striking implement
3. The coefficient of restitution (elasticity) between the ball and the striking implement
4. The direction the ball and the implement are moving at the time of impact
5. The point of impact between the ball and the implement

The speed of the approaching ball and the speed of the striking implement may be further analyzed into secondary factors. For instance, the speed of the striking implement is determined by the magnitude of the force exerted and the time over which that force acts. The amount of time that the force can act depends on the distance of the preparatory backswing and the speed of the muscular contraction. The distance of the preparatory backswing further depends on the range of motion in the joints and the timing of the swing. Furthermore, the effectiveness of the force exerted by the body depends completely on a strong grip and a firm wrist for transmission of the force from the body to the striking implement, and a firm ground support for transmission of the normal reactive force to the body.

Objects that have been hit through their centers of gravity will have linear motion, whereas those that have been hit off center may curve because of a resultant spin. The more the striking

TABLE 17.1 Ball and Striker Velocities Before and After Impact and Time of Impact

	Ball Velocity (ft/sec)		Striker Velocity (ft/sec)		Time of Impact (sec)
	Before	After	Before	After	
Baseball	Hit from tee	128	103	90	1/800
Badminton	30 ft/sec	112	97.2	95	1/800
Football punt	0	92	60	39	1/125
Football kickoff	0	85	60	47	1/125
Golf, 7 iron	0	177	155	133	1/800
Golf drive	0	225	166	114	1/1,000
Handball serve	0	76	63	47	1/80
Paddleball	0	115	90	70	1/200
Soccer kick	0	85	58	42	1/125
Soccer, head	25	42	11	8.6	1/44
Squash, hard serve	0	160	145	111	1/333
Softball	Hit from tee	100	105	71	1/285
Tennis serve	0	167	123	107	1/250
Tennis forehand	0	93	71	41	1/200
Volleyball serve	0	72	65	45	1/100

Source: From *Patterns of Human Motion: A Cinematographic Analysis,* by Stanley Plagenhoef. Copyright © 1971, p. 59. Adapted by permission of Prentice Hall, Englewood Cliffs, New Jersey.

force is eccentric in its application, the less is the linear speed imparted to the ball. Furthermore, balls that hit a striking surface at an angle to the surface will rebound at an angle approximately equal and opposite to the striking angle. Some examples of ball and striker velocities before and after impact are presented in Table 17.1.

The force to bring about the changes in velocity noted in Table 17.1 can be rather large, as in this example using a baseball hit from a tee

$$\begin{aligned} \text{Mass of ball} &= 5 \text{ oz or } 1.42 \text{ kg} \\ v_i \text{ of ball} &= 0 \text{ m/s} \\ v_f \text{ of ball} &= 128 \text{ ft/sec or } 39.01 \text{ m/s} \\ \text{Time of contact} &= 1/800 \text{ sec or } 0.00125 \text{ sec} \end{aligned}$$

$$F \times t = (m)(v_f - v_i)$$

$$F \times (0.00125 \text{ sec}) = (0.142 \text{ kg})(39.01 \text{ m/s} - 0 \text{ m/s})$$

$$F = \frac{(0.142 \text{ kg})(39.01 \text{ m/s})}{0.00125 \text{ sec}}$$

$$F = 4{,}431.54 \text{ N} = 996.25 \text{ lb}$$

Therefore, if the time the bat contacts the ball is 0.00125 second, the bat impacts the ball with a force of 996.25 pounds (4,431 N).

Principles Those mechanical principles cited as pertaining to throwing patterns are also related to striking patterns. In addition, the following factors also must be applied when analyzing striking patterns.

1. The direction in which the object moves is determined by the direction of force applied to it. If the force consists of two or more components, the object will move in the direction of the resultant of those components. After being projected or struck, the direction will be modified by gravity and air resistance.
2. Momentum is conserved in all collisions. The momentum before impact must equal the momentum after impact, provided that none is lost through friction or other forces.
3. Any change in the momentum of colliding objects is related to the force and duration

of the collision. The greater the impulse (*Ft*), the greater will be the change in momentum. This is why the follow-through is important. The longer the missile can be carried along by the striking implement at its greatest velocity, the greater will be the change in velocity of the missile.

4. The greater the velocity of the approaching ball, the greater the velocity of the ball in the opposite direction after it is struck, other things being equal.
5. The greater the velocity of the striking implement at the moment of contact, the greater the velocity of the struck ball, other things being equal. Obviously, a full-powered swing will send the ball farther and faster than will a bunt. Both increasing the length of the lever and striking with a good follow-through help increase the velocity of the striking implement and therefore increase the force of impact.
6. The greater the mass of the ball, *up to a point,* the greater its momentum after being struck, other things being equal. A baseball will travel farther and faster than a softball. Nevertheless, an iron ball would offer too much resistance for the average batter using an average bat.
7. The greater the mass of the striking implement, *up to a point,* the greater the striking force, and hence the greater the speed of the struck ball, other things being equal. A good baseball player uses a heavier bat. Too heavy a bat, however, is inadvisable because of the difficulty in swinging it with sufficient speed and control.
8. The higher (closer to 1.00) the coefficient of restitution (elasticity) of the ball and of the striking implement, the greater the speed of the struck ball, other things being equal.
9. The direction taken by the struck ball is determined by four factors: (a) the direction of the striking implement at the moment of contact; (b) the relation of the striking force to the ball's center of gravity (an off-center application of force causes spin, and spin affects direction); (c) degree of firmness of grip and wrist at moment of impact; and (d) the laws governing rebound (see pp. 311–314).

Examples of Throwing and Striking

Analysis of the Overarm Throw

To give the reader a better understanding of the coordination pattern referred to as sequential segmental actions, the force phase of the overarm pattern is analyzed as applied in a forceful throw such as in pitching. This analysis includes joint actions, muscle activity, and mechanics for the upper extremity only.

The purpose of the backswing, or preparatory, motion is to place the segments in a favorable position for the force phase. There are many ways to execute the backswing while taking advantage of the stretch-shortening characteristics of muscle. Although some favor one method over another, any windup is appropriate that places the segments in the most advantageous position to maximize the number of segments and the time over which force can be applied. Such a windup, allowing the joints to be placed in an optimal position to involve the greatest number of segments, includes pelvic and trunk rotation in the opposite direction from the intended throw (right for a right-hander), horizontal abduction, and lateral rotation at the shoulder joint with elbow flexion and wrist hyperextension. This sequence of arm action continues as a forward step is taken with the opposite foot. This hand–foot opposition permits the greatest range of motion in the trunk and pelvis. It also allows for a large base of support over which the force phase can be applied while preserving balance.

No pause occurs between the windup and the force phases. The windup ends with a forward stride using the opposite leg. Establishment of a base of support is followed immediately by pelvic and then trunk rotation, accompanied by lateral flexion to the left (right-handed pitcher). The trunk motion causes increased horizontal abduction with continuing lateral rotation at the shoulder joint. Elbow joint extension is followed by the initiation of rapid medial rotation at the shoulder joint, forearm pronation at the radial–ulnar joint, and then flexion and often ulnar flexion at the wrist joint. The force phase ends with the release of the ball. The angle at the elbow joint at release is approximately 105 degrees. The follow-through includes the actions from ball release until the momentum developed in the arm can be safely dissipated as the arm continues across the body in a downward direction. In addition, a forward step is often used.

These actions proceed from the proximal (more massive) to the distal (lighter) segments. In characteristic sequential patterns, subsequent segments lag behind those preceding them. The subsequent segment is carried along, lagging behind until the more proximal segment attains its maximum angular velocity. The distal segment then accelerates because of a combination of the series elastic components, stretch reflex, and muscular contraction. This combination results in the reaction or slowing down of the preceding segment. Due to conservation of momentum, momentum (*mv*) is transferred from the more massive (proximal) to the less massive (distal) segments, significantly increasing their velocity. Therefore, the linear velocity at the end of the chain—that is, the ball at release—often can be over 90 miles per hour.

The legs play an important role in any successful throw. They provide the stable base over which the trunk and other segments act. In addition, the thrust they provide contributes significantly to the force of this movement. The transfer of momentum from proximal to distal, however, focuses the attention on the musculature of the upper extremity. Because this phase emphasizes the application of the force accelerating the limb, muscle contractions are mainly concentric preceded by a short eccentric phase because of the lagging of the distal behind the proximal segments.

Muscular Analysis of Upper Extremity (Table 17.2)

The lateral rotation preceding the medial rotation of the right shoulder joint is controlled by the eccentric contraction of the medial rotators of the

TABLE 17.2 Acceleration Phase (Initial Portion of Force Phase) of the Overarm Throw

Joint	Joint Action	Segment Moved	Force for Movement	Muscles Active	Kind of Contraction
Shoulder joints	Horizontal abduction	Upper arm	Muscle	Posterior deltoid Infraspinatus Teres minor	Concentric
	Medial rotation		Muscle	Subscapularis Latissimus dorsi Pectoralis major	Concentric
Shoulder girdle	Abduction	Scapula	Muscle	Serratus anterior Pectoralis minor	Concentric
Elbows	Extension	Forearm	Muscle	Triceps brachii	Concentric
Radioulnar	Pronation	Forearm	Muscle	Pronator teres Pronator quadratus	Concentric
Wrist	Flexion	Hand	Muscle	Flexor carpi radialis Flexor carpi ulnaris Flexor digitorum superficialis	Concentric

humerus followed by the concentric contraction of the same muscles, including the subscapularis, pectoralis major, and latissimus dorsi muscles. During the acceleration phase, the height of the humerus was controlled by a static contraction of the middle deltoid. The deltoid and supraspinatus muscles contract concentrically during the backswing to position the upper arm, and eccentrically during the follow-through to help decelerate the arm. The infraspinatus muscle was also very active (eccentric contraction) to assist in decelerating the arm during the follow-through.

The biceps brachii muscle activity reaches its peak as the elbow joint is flexed late into the backswing and at the beginning of the force phase. Marked activity again appears during the follow-through to protect the elbow joint in decelerating the forearm. The latissimus dorsi muscle, active during medial rotation, remains, active, eccentrically contracting during the follow-through to assist in controlling the arm motion across the body.

It is clear that the stretch reflex is an important facilitating mechanism in helping accelerate the lagging distal segment at the appropriate time. The more rapid the stretch (eccentric contraction), the greater will be the facilitating effect on the resulting concentric contraction of the same muscle. In this way, forces can be summated more appropriately. To gain the greatest facilitation from the stretch reflex, there should be no pause between the windup and force phases.

Because the trunk rotates under the stationary head (eyes focused on the target), the tonic neck reflex may facilitate the strong acceleration occurring during the force phase. The asymmetric tonic neck reflex facilitates the shoulder abductors and elbow extensors on the chin side. This is precisely the arm position at release.

The extensor thrust reflex may act on both the upper and lower extremities. Increasing pressure on the palmar side of the hand as the arm is being accelerated forward may facilitate the arm extensor muscles. Similarly, as the weight is transferred to the forward foot, the Pacinian corpuscles are stimulated by the increased pressure, resulting in a facilitation of the lower-limb extensor muscles. When accuracy is a factor, knee flexion must be maintained to flatten the arc through which the hand is carried. This flattening permits the tangential flight path of the ball to have a broader margin for error in the timing of the release while arriving at the same target point following release.

Analysis of the Forehand Drive in Tennis

Description

The forehand drive (Figure 17.7) is one of the fundamental strokes of tennis. Its objective is to send the ball over the net and deep into the opponent's court close to the baseline.

Starting position The player faces the net with the feet about shoulder width apart and the weight on the balls of the feet. The racket is held with an eastern or shake-hands grip.

Backswing The player pivots the entire body so that the shoulder and hips of the nonracket side are toward the net. At the same time, the racket is taken back at shoulder level in either a straight or a circular manner, with the head of the racket above the wrist and its face turned slightly down. The weight of the body is over the rear foot (racket side).

Forward swing and follow-through The player flexes at the knee joints to drop the racket and racket arm below the intended contact point (still keeping the racket head above the wrist with its face turned down) and steps toward the ball with the non-racket foot. The pelvis and spine rotate so the trunk faces forward, and the weight is shifted to the forward foot as the racket is swung forward and up. The racket face is perpendicular to the court at ball impact, thus imparting topspin to the ball as it swings through and up. The follow-through continues toward the intended target, with the racket arm swinging across the body and up toward the chin.

Anatomical Factors

The action in the forehand drive is ballistic in nature and, as such, is initiated by muscular force, continued by momentum, and finally terminated

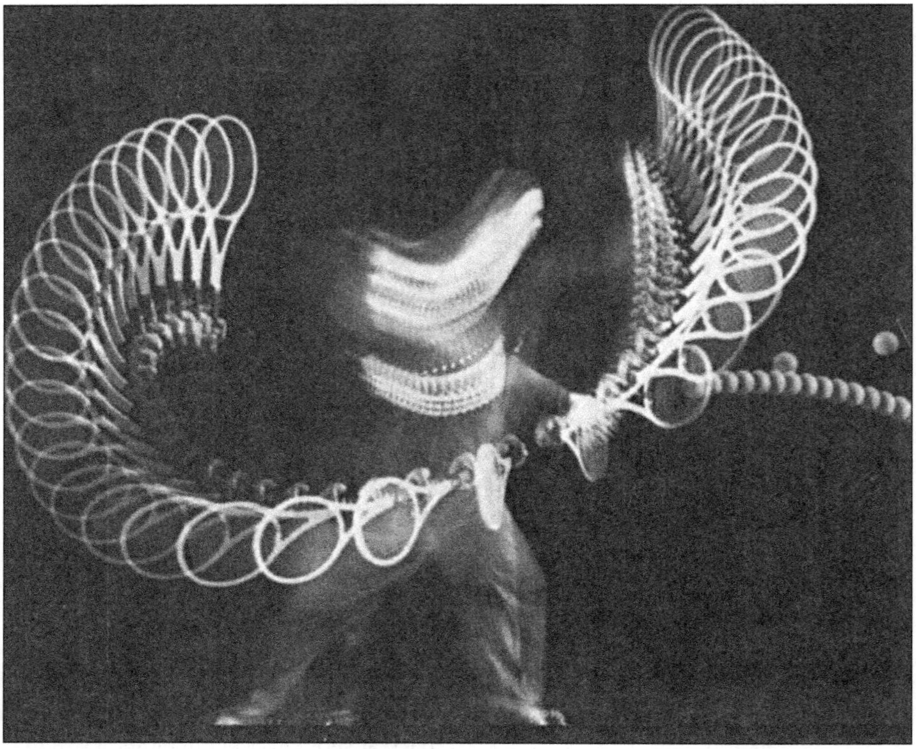

Figure 17.7 Tennis coach Vic Braden demonstrates loop forehand, 1977.

by the contraction of antagonistic muscles. The chief lever participating in the movement consists of the arm, trunk, and racket together with the fulcrum located in the opposite hip joint (see Figure 13.19), the point of force application at a point on the pelvis that represents the combined forces of the muscles producing the movement (mainly the gluteus medius and minimis and the adductor magnus), and the resistance point at the center of gravity of the trunk–arm–racket lever. At the moment of impact, however, the resistance point may be considered to be the point of contact of the ball with the racket face. The additional lever actions that are due to the rotation of the spine, the horizontal adduction at the shoulder, and flexion at the wrist, if present, should also be recognized.

Another important anatomical factor is the strength of the muscles responsible for keeping the arm abducted and for assisting in the forward swing as the arm is carried along by the rotating spine and pelvis. Those whose muscles lack the strength to swing the outstretched arm with speed are likely to flex the arm at the elbow or adduct the arm, bringing the racket closer to the trunk and thus shortening the resistance moment arm. Among the muscles that were tested by Van Gheluwe and Hebbelinck (1986) and found active in the forward swing of the forehand drive were the anterior deltoid, pectoralis major, latissimus dorsi, biceps, brachioradialis, and triceps, the latter in two short bursts, the first at the moment of impact, and the second during follow-through (Table 17.3). Lin et al. (2006) supported these findings, particularly with regard to the activity of the pectoralis major and anterior deltoid during adduction of the shoulder. The erector spinae, external oblique, and rectus

TABLE 17.3 Anatomical Analysis of the Forehand Drive in Tennis

Joint	Joint Action	Segment Moved	Force for Movement	Muscles Active	Kind of Contraction
Ankles	Plantar flexion	Shank	Muscle	Gastrocnemius Soleus	Concentric
Knees	Extension	Thigh	Muscle	Quadriceps femoris	Concentric
Hips	Extension	Trunk	Muscle	Hamstrings	Concentric
Trunk	Left rotation	Trunk	Muscle	Erector spinae Right external oblique Rectus abdominus	
Right shoulder joint	Horizontal adduction	Upper arm	Muscle	Anterior deltoid Pectoralis major Latissimus dorsi	Concentric
Right shoulder girdle	Abduction	Scapula	Muscle	Serratus anterior	Concentric
Elbow	Extension	Forearm	Muscle	Triceps	Concentric

abdominis are also active, with the erector spinae most active (Knudson & Blackwell, 2000).

Mechanical Analysis

The purpose of the forehand drive is to return the ball so that it will not only land within the opponent's court but also land in such a place and manner that it will be difficult to return. For the player to achieve this requires both high speed and expert placement of the ball. Hence, imparting maximum speed to the ball and, at the same time, placing it with accuracy are the two major skills that the player seeks to develop.

The force of impact is determined by the speed of the racket at the moment of contact with the ball, and maximum velocity can be obtained only when maximum distance is used for accelerating. The function of the backswing is to provide this distance. There are two types of backswing, the straight and the circular. The straight backswing has the advantage of greater ease in controlling the direction of the racket and in timing the movement, but the disadvantage of necessitating the overcoming of inertia to reverse the direction from the back to the forward swing. On the other hand, the circular backswing permits the arm to move in one continuous motion over a longer path, thereby providing more than twice the distance for building up momentum. For the more skillful player who is able to control both the direction of the racket and the timing of the entire movement, it is the more efficient method.

In considering the force involved in the forehand drive, it is important to distinguish between the force applied to the lever and the force applied by the lever to the ball. Whereas the force applied to the lever is muscular force, the force applied to the ball is the force of momentum. It is determined by both the mass and velocity of the implement that makes contact with the ball. These, in turn, are related to the distance of the point of contact from the fulcrum—in other words, the length of the temporary resistance arm of the lever ("temporary" because the distance from the fulcrum to the point of contact with the ball constitutes the resistance arm of the lever only for the brief moment of impact). In addition to the rotary movement of the trunk–arm–racket lever, the linear motion produced by the forward movement of the body (because of weight shift) adds to the force that meets the ball.

Starting with the pelvic rotation and weight shift and working out toward the racket, each movement in turn gets under way before the next one commences. If the timing is correct, the cumulative effect of these movements is to produce maximum velocity. If any of the movements is added to the preceding one either too early or too late, the potential velocity will not be realized.

Other important factors that contribute to the force applied to the ball, and therefore to the speed of the ball on its return flight, include the following:

1. The use of the arm in an almost fully extended position increases the length of the lever, thereby giving greater linear velocity to the racket head than would be the case if the upper arm were close to the body. This is only true, however, if the racket can be moved with the same angular velocity in both positions.
2. The effort needed to resist the force of the ball hitting the racket is less when the racket lever arm is shortened.
3. It takes less force to swing a shortened racket lever into the striking position than it does a fully extended one. (These first three related factors help explain why beginners and children bend the forehand elbow or choke up on the racket handle.)
4. The concentration of mass at the level of the shoulders moving forward at the moment of impact ensures maximum speed for striking.
5. A skillful player tends to use a relatively heavy racket because, other things being equal, the greater the mass of the striking implement, the greater the striking force (momentum) and, hence, the greater the speed of the struck ball.
6. A new ball and a well-strung racket ensure a good coefficient of restitution (elasticity), thereby increasing the speed of the struck ball.
7. The bending of the knees at the beginning of the forward swing followed by the extension of the legs and shift of weight as the racket is swung forward and up increases the ground reactive force imparted to the body and thus to the ball.
8. It has been generally accepted that a firm wrist and grip are essential for maximum impulse to be applied by the racket to the ball.
9. Placement of the ball is a matter of direction. It will be recalled that the direction taken by a struck ball is determined by four factors:
   a. The direction of the striking implement at the moment of impact.
   b. The relation of the striking force to the ball's center of gravity—in other words, the control of spin.
   c. Firmness of grip and wrist at the moment of impact.
   d. Angle of incidence.

The first of these factors is obvious. The beginner may be less aware of the importance of the other three. For successful placing of the ball, an understanding of the effect of spin and the skill of imparting the desired spin to the ball are essential. Firmness of grip depends on wrist and finger strength and is closely related to the angle at which the racket face makes contact with the ball. Because the angle of rebound equals the angle of incidence (actually slightly less than this in the case of tennis balls because of their compressibility), it will be seen that firmness of grip is therefore an important factor in the direction taken by the struck ball.

References and Selected Readings

Atwater, A. E. (1979). Biomechanics of overarm throwing movements and of throwing injuries. *Exercise and Sports Science Reviews,* 7, 43–85.

Bahamonde, R. E. (2000). Changes in angular momentum during the tennis serve. *Journal of Sports Sciences,* 18(8), 579–592.

Bahamonde, R. E., & Knudson, D. (2003). Kinetics of the upper extremity in the open and square stance tennis forehand. *Journal of Science and Medicine in Sport,* 6(1), 88–101.

Broer, M. R., & Houtz, S. J. (1967). *Patterns of muscular activity in selected sports skills.* Springfield, IL: Charles C Thomas.

Broer, M. R., & Zernicke, R. (1979). *Efficiency of human movement* (4th ed.). Philadelphia, PA: Saunders.

Chow, J. W., Shim, J. H., & Lim, Y. T. (2003). Lower trunk muscle activity during the tennis serve. *Journal of Science and Medicine in Sport,* 6(4), 512–518.

Escamilla, R. F., Fleisig, G. S., Zheng, N., Barrentine, S. W., & Andrews. J. R. (2001). Kinematic comparisons of 1996 Olympic baseball pitchers. *Journal of Sports Sciences,* 19(9), 665–676.

Gordon, B. J., & Dapena, J. (2006). Contributions of joint rotations to racquet speed in the tennis serve. *Journal of Sports Science,* 24(1), 31–49.

Grezios, A. K., Gissis, I. T., Sotiropoulo, A. A., Nikolaidis, D. V., & Souglis, A. G. (2006). Muscle-contraction properties in overarm throwing movements. *Journal of Strength and Conditioning Research,* 20(1), 117–123.

Hirashima, M., Kadota, H., Sakurai, S., Kudo, K., & Ohtsuki, T. (2002). Sequential muscle activity and its functional role in the upper extremity and trunk during overarm throwing. *Journal of Sports Sciences,* 20(4), 301–310.

Hong, D. A., Cheung, T. K., & Roberts, E. M. (2001). A three-dimensional, six-segment chain analysis of forceful overarm throwing. *Journal of Electromyography and Kinesiology,* 11(2), 95–112.

Knudson, D., & Blackwell, J. (2000). Trunk muscle activation in open stance and square stance tennis forehands. *International Journal of Sports Medicine,* 21(5), 321–324.

Lin, H. T., Guo, L. Y., Wu, W. L., & Wang, L. H. (2006). Using the change of angular momentum and muscle electromyography data to qualify the muscle function in tennis forehand volley. *Journal of Biomechanics,* 39(S1), S558.

Moynes, D. R., Perry, J., Antonelli, D. J., & Jobe, F. W. (1986). Gender differences in children's throwing performance: Biology and environment. *Research Quarterly,* 66, 1905–1911.

Nunome, H., Asai, T., Ikegami, Y., & Sakurai, S. (2002). Three-dimensional kinetic analysis of side-foot and instep soccer kicks. *Medicine and Science in Sports and Exercise,* 34(12), 2028–2036.

Nunome, H., Ikegami, Y., Kozakai, R., Apriantono, T., & Sano, S. (2006). Segmental dynamics of soccer instep kicking with the preferred and non-preferred leg. *Journal of Sports Sciences,* 24(5), 529–541.

Reid, M., & Elliott, B. (2002). The one- and two-handed backhands in tennis. *Sports Biomechanics,* 1(1), 47–68.

Van Gheluwe, B., & Hebbelinck, M. (1986). Muscle actions and ground reaction forces in tennis. *International Journal of Sport Biomechanics,* 2, 88–99.

Werner, S. L., Guido, J. A., McNeice, R. P., Richardson, J. L., Delude, N. A., & Stewart, G. W. (2005). Biomechanics of youth windmill softball pitching. *American Journal of Sports Medicine,* 33, 552–560.

Wight, J., Richards, J., & Halt, S. (2004). Influence of pelvis rotation styles on baseball pitching mechanics. *Sports Biomechanics,* 3(1), 67–83.

Yu, B., Broker, J., & Silvester, L. J. (2002). A kinetic analysis of discus-throwing techniques. *Sports Biomechanics,* 1(1), 25–46.

LABORATORY EXPERIENCES

1. Throw a tennis ball or baseball for distance:
   a. Standing still, facing in the direction of the throw.
   b. Standing with the left side toward the direction of the throw, with the feet apart and the weight evenly distributed, using a full arm swing and body twist with the throw.
   c. Same as in b, except with the weight on the right foot to begin with, shifting to the left as the ball is thrown.

   Compare the three methods for distance. Explain in terms of length of backswing, speed at moment of release, and total distance used in applying force to ball before releasing it.
2. If possible, observe a small child or an untrained youth and then a trained boy or girl throw a small ball as forcefully as possible at a target 20 or 30 feet away. Analyze the motions of each with reference to the pathway of the hand immediately preceding, at the moment of, and following the release. Explain the factors differentiating the good throws from the poor.
3. Observe slow-motion films of throwing, striking, and other forms of giving motion. Look for the application of the principles stated in this unit or for the lack of such application.
4. Perform a complete kinesiological analysis of a selected throwing, kicking, or striking skill, taking particular note of the purpose of the motion, its classification, the simultaneous-sequential nature of the motion, and its component parts. Include also muscle participation, neuromuscular considerations, mechanical factors, and applicable principles and violations. Conclude the analysis with a prescription for improvement, including suggested methods for change and the elimination of violations of principles.

CHAPTER 18

LOCOMOTION: SOLID SURFACE

OUTLINE

OBJECTIVES

At the conclusion of this chapter, the student should be able to:

1. Identify and classify motor skills belonging in the categories that fall under the heading of moving one's body on the ground or on another resistant surface.
2. Describe the anatomical and mechanical nature of motor skills representative of the major types of locomotor patterns.
3. Name and state anatomical and mechanical principles that apply to the locomotor patterns of walking, running, and jumping.
4. Evaluate performance of motor skills representative of the major locomotor patterns in terms of application of the related kinesiological principles.
5. Analyze the performance of someone performing a locomotor skill. Follow the kinesiological analysis outline presented in Chapter 1.

LOCOMOTION

Locomotion is the act of moving from place to place by means of one's own mechanisms or power. Locomotion in human beings is the result of the action of the body levers propelling the body. Ordinarily the propulsion is provided by the lower extremities, but it is occasionally provided by all four extremities, as in creeping, or by the upper extremities alone, as in walking on the hands or in suspension. It may involve the use of wheels, blades, skis, or other equipment attached to the feet, or it may involve a vehicle such as a bicycle or wheelchair, or a small craft such as a boat, canoe, or surfboard propelled by means of the arms or legs, with or without the use of a propelling implement such as oars, paddles, or poles. Locomotion may be on the ground or in the water but, at the present writing, not in the air without support. In all locomotion there must be a resistance against which the body part can push to generate a reaction force if motion is to occur.

All forms of locomotion performed on the ground constitute the category of motor skills of moving one's body on the ground or on other resistant surfaces.

On Foot
Walking
Running
Racewalking
Climbing (inclined plane, stairs, ladder)
Descending (inclined plane, stairs, ladder)
Jumping, leaping, hurdling
Skipping, hopping, sliding, sidestepping
Dance steps
Snowshoeing
Stilt walking

On Wheels, Blades, and Runners
Bicycling
Wheelchair propulsion
Skating and skateboarding
Alpine and cross-country skiing and snowboarding
Ice skating

On Hands and/or Knees or Hands and Feet
Walking on hands
Creeping and crawling
Crutch walking
Stunts

Rotary Locomotion
Cartwheels
Handsprings
Rolls

WALKING

To the casual observer, the movements involved in walking appear to be relatively simple, yet kinesiological analysis shows them to be exceedingly complex. The dovetailing of muscular action and the synchronization of joint movements beautifully illustrate the teamwork present in all bodily movements. Not even the most complex piece of machinery designed by the most skillful engineers exceeds the movements of the human machine in perfection of detail or in potential smoothness of function on a wide variety of terrain and in all conditions.

The work of Inman, Ralston, Steindler, Murray, and many others has served, over the course of the years, to emphasize the complexity of human walking (Rose & Gamble, 1994). In the past, researchers have been limited to studying gait and trying to compensate for those factors that often limited people in walking. Currently, a great deal of work is being done in the area of functional electrical stimulation (FES). Using computers and electrical currents, it is now possible to program the muscles of the disabled patient in such a way as to artificially stimulate the muscles of the lower extremity to reproduce the action of walking. Depending on the state of the neuromuscular system, those who once were forced to rely on wheelchairs, braces, and canes are now starting to walk with the aid of such computerized systems. Currently, whole-body vibration is showing real promise in the improvement of gait characteristics of individuals who have sustained a spinal cord injury (Ness & Field-Fote, 2009).

Description

Walking is accomplished by the alternating action of the two lower extremities (Figure 18.1). It is an example of translatory motion of the body as a whole brought about by rotary motion of some of its parts. It is also an example of a periodic, or pendulum-like, movement in which the moving segment (in this case the lower extremity) may be

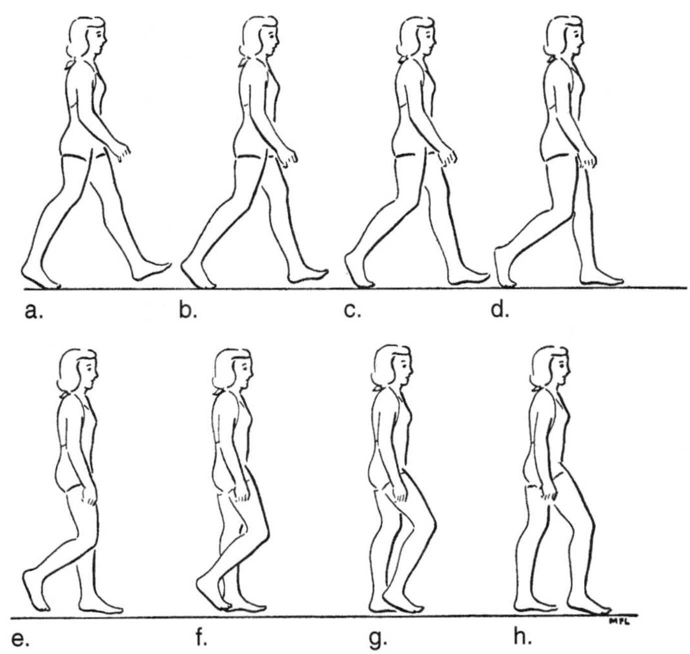

Figure 18.1 Walking is an example of linear motion of the body as a whole resulting from the angular motion of some of its parts.

said to start at zero, pass through its arc of motion, and fall to zero again at the end of each stroke. In walking, each lower extremity undergoes two phases: the swing or recovery phase and the support or stance phase. The support phase is further divided into foot strike, foot-flat, midstance, heel-off, and toe off phases. The toe-off phase of one leg overlaps the foot strike and foot-flat phases of the other leg, thus producing a period of double support when both feet are on the ground. This double support phase is characteristic of the walk and serves to differentiate it from the run.

The kinematics of the walking gait are often described in terms of strides and steps. A stride is one full lower extremity cycle. In walking and running, a stride is defined as being from foot strike on one leg to the next foot strike with the same leg. Stride length, then, is the distance covered during a single stride. A step starts with the foot strike on one leg and ends with the foot strike of the contralateral, or opposite, leg.

Gravity and momentum are the chief sources of motion for the swing phase; hence, this phase represents a ballistic type of movement, particularly when the individual is walking at a natural pace. The source of motion for the support phase is, for the first half, the momentum of the forward-moving trunk (provided by the propulsive action of the other leg) and, for the second half, the contraction of the extensor muscles of the supporting leg.

Anatomical Analysis

The six major components of walking have been defined as (1) pelvic rotation, (2) pelvic tilt, (3) knee flexion, (4) hip flexion, (5) knee and ankle interaction, and (6) lateral pelvic displacement. Each of these components is essential for efficient walking, and the loss of any one will cause an increase in the energy cost. Beyond the long-established six determinant theory, investigators have also developed the concept of dynamic optimization of gait. Dynamic optimization assumes that human walking is optimized to minimize energy consumption through the dynamic interaction of the complex kinetic link system (Vaughan, 2003).

The action taking place in the joints of the lower extremity consists essentially of flexion and extension. But, in much the same way that the shoulder girdle cooperates with the arm movements of the upper extremity, the pelvic girdle cooperates in movements of the lower extremities. The pelvis has the double task of transmitting the weight of the body alternately first over one limb, then over the other, and of putting each acetabulum in a favorable position for the action of the corresponding femur. The adaptations of the pelvic position are made in the joints of the thoracic and lumbar spine as well as in the hip joints. Thus, as first one foot and then the other is put forward, the flexion and extension movements of the thigh are accompanied by slight rotary movements and abduction and adduction at the hips, and by slight lateral flexion and rotation of the spine (Figures 18.2 and 18.3).

The muscular analysis presented here is a compilation of results from numerous studies on the walking gait. Walking, both normal and pathological, is one of the most widely studied of all human movement patterns. Movement specialists would be well advised to keep abreast of the on-going research in the area of gait analysis. Because of the relative importance and complexity of the walking gait, a complete discussion of the muscular involvement in walking is presented.

Swing Phase

The swing phase begins with toe-off and ends with foot strike.

Spine and Pelvis

1. *Movements:* Rotation of the pelvis toward the support leg and of the spine in the opposite direction; slight lateral tilt of the pelvis toward the unsupported leg. The simultaneous opposite actions help prevent excessive motion of the trunk. Pelvic rotation also lengthens the step and decreases the lateral deviation of the center of gravity of the body, whereas pelvic tilt decreases the elevation of the center of gravity.
2. *Muscles:* Semispinalis, rotatores, multifidus, and external oblique abdominal muscles on

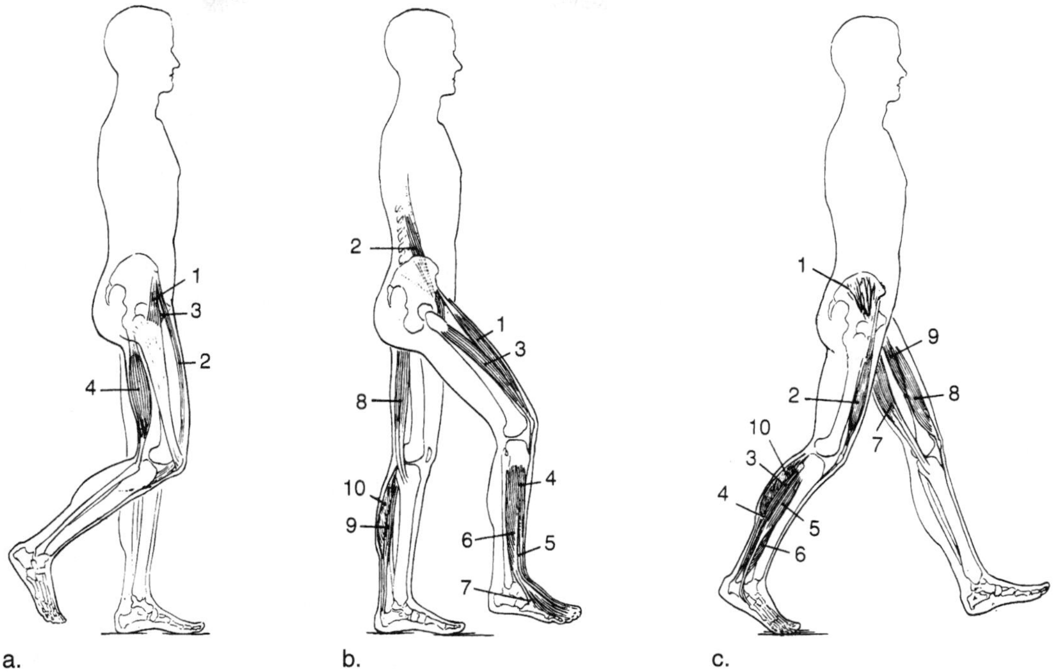

Figure 18.2 The muscles of the lower extremity used in walking. Key: a: 1. Tensor fasciae latae; 2. sartorius; 3. pectineus; 4. biceps femoris. b: 1. Rectus femoris; 2. iliopsoas; 3. vastus lateralis (medius and intermedius are not shown); 4. tibialis anterior; 5. extensor hallucis longus; 6. extensor digitorum longus; 7. peroneus tertius; 8. semitendinosus and semimembranosus; 9. soleus; 10. gastrocnemius. c: 1. Gluteus medius; 2. rectus femoris; 3. soleus; 4. tibialis posterior (underneath); 5. peroneus longus; 6. peroneus brevis; 7. semimembranosus and semitendinosus; 8. vastus medialis and intermedius (lateralis not shown); 9. adductor longus; 10. gastrocnemius.

side toward which the pelvis rotates. Erector spinae and internal oblique abdominal muscles on opposite side. (*Note:* Rotation of the pelvis to the right constitutes rotation of the spine to the left. See pp. 158–159.) The psoas and quadratus lumborum help support the pelvis on the side of the swinging limb, and the gluteus medius and minimus on the support-leg side support the pelvis against the pull of gravity.

Hip

1. *Movements:* Flexion; outward rotation (because of pelvic rotation); adduction at beginning and abduction at end of phase, especially if long stride is taken (also because of pelvic rotation, as well as stride length).
2. *Muscles:* The iliopsoas is the prime mover of the hip in the swing phase, with assistance from the rectus femoris, sartorius, gracilis, adductor longus, and pectineus, and the short head of the biceps femoris during the late part of the swing. The sartorius is active chiefly following toe-off.

In the latter part of the swing phase there is no appreciable action of the hip flexors in normal walking on level ground. This is consistent with the ballistic nature of the movement. The hamstrings contract with moderate intensity during the knee extension part of the swing, and the gluteus maximus and medius contract slightly at the very end of the swing. The adductors longus and magnus, and presumably brevis, contract slightly after the swinging limb has passed the halfway mark. The function of the adductor magnus is not clear. It may help

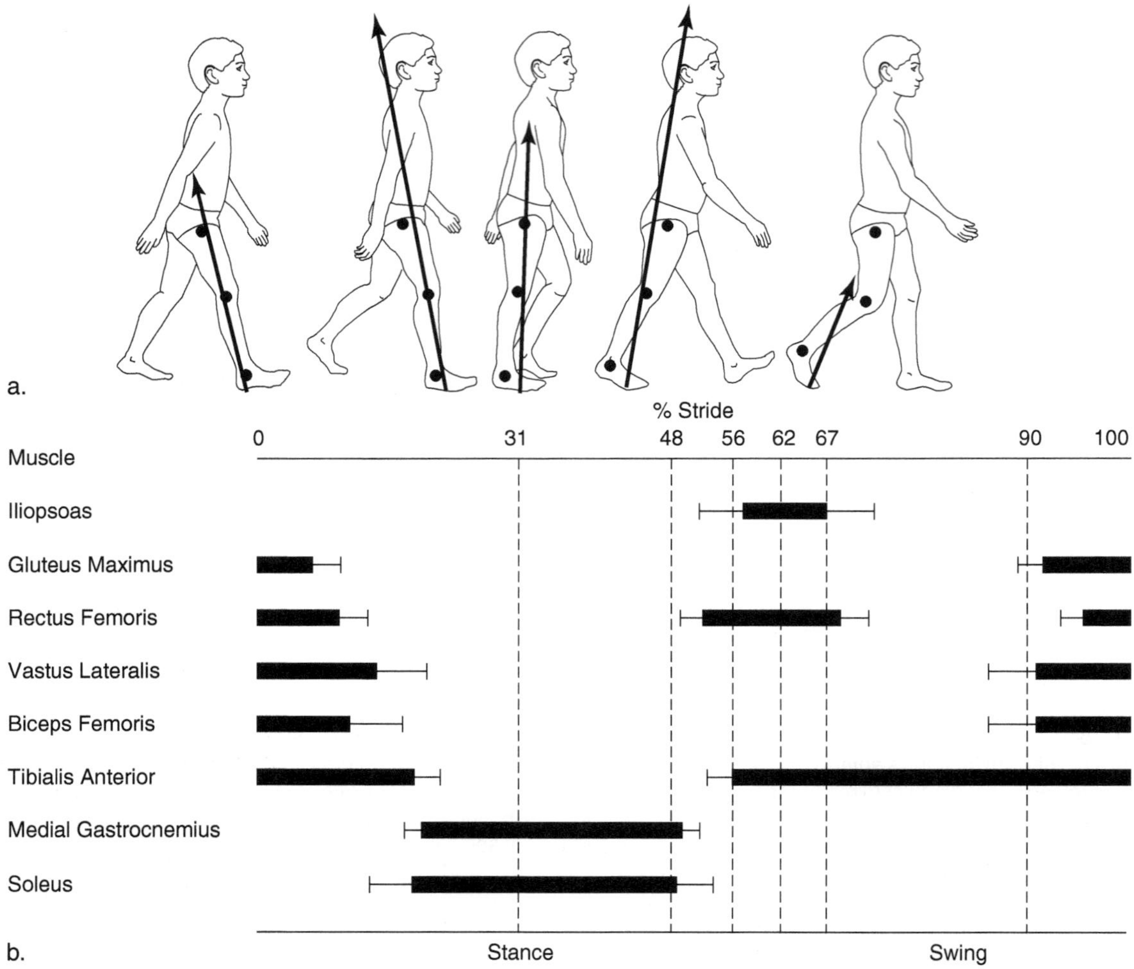

Figure 18.3 Right leg stance phase. The table indicates muscle activations during a particular percentage of the stride. The arrows indicate the magnitude and direction of the ground reaction force. *Sources:* (a) From "Theories of Bipedal Walking: An Odyssey," by C. L. Vaughn. *Journal of Biomechanics, 36,* 513–523 (2003); used with permission. (b) From "Energy Cost and Muscular Activity Required for Leg Swing during Walking," by J. S. Gottschall and R. Kram. *Journal of Applied Physiology, 99,* 23–30 (2005); used with permission.

steady and guide the forward-swinging limb. In any event, its action is extremely slight, even in rapid walking.

In rapid walking there is a noticeable increase in the activity of the sartorius and the rectus femoris and also a slight increase in that of the tensor fasciae latae.

Knee

1. *Movements:* Flexion during the first half; extension during the second half.
2. *Muscles:* As was true in hip flexion (and for the same reason), so also in knee flexion is there remarkably little muscular action in the swing phase of normal walking. The largest contributor to knee flexion during the swing phase is the flexion that is produced during toe-off as the knee extensors relax.

The quadriceps extensors contract slightly at the end of this phase. The action of the sartorius, a two-joint muscle, has already been mentioned in connection with the hip. The action of these muscles, as well as that of the medial hamstrings, increases in rapid walking. In an easy gait the movement appears to be initiated by gravitational force and continued by momentum. This force is sufficient to extend the leg at the knee, except perhaps at the very end of the movement. In more vigorous walking, the quadriceps femoris provides the force for leg extension.

Ankle and Foot

1. *Movements:* Dorsiflexion; prevention of plantar flexion.
2. *Muscles:* The tibialis anterior, extensor digitorum longus, extensor hallucis longus, and probably the peroneus tertius contract with slight to moderate intensity at the beginning of the swinging phase and taper off during the middle portion of this phase.

   Toward the end of the swing phase this group of muscles contracts again with considerable force in preparation for the foot strike. The plantar flexors are completely relaxed throughout the entire swing phase.

Support Phase

The support phase begins with foot strike and ends with toe-off. The portion between foot strike of the forward foot and toe-off of the other—that is, the rear foot—constitutes a period of double support that is characteristic of walking but does not occur in running.

Spine and pelvis Rotation of pelvis toward same side and spine to opposite side: lateral tilt away from support leg.

The lumbar portion of the erector spinae contracts at heel strike to stiffen the trunk for stability. There is also a low level of activity in the internal and external obliques, possibly to assist in trunk rotation in opposition to pelvic girdle rotation.

Hip

1. *Movements:* Extension through foot-flat to toe-off; reduction of outward rotation, followed by slight inward rotation; prevention of adduction of the thigh and dropping of pelvis to opposite side.
2. *Muscles:* During heel strike the gluteal muscles and the hamstrings contract statically with moderate intensity. These contractions then taper off during foot-flat and disappear at midstance. A number of EMG researchers have found evidence of gluteus maximus activity in the early part of the support phase (Anderson & Pandy, 2003; Kimmel & Schwartz, 2006). The gluteus minimus continues to contract moderately during the middle portion. The only muscles of the hip that contract appreciably during the last part of the support phase are the adductors magnus, longus, and possibly brevis.

   In rapid walking the gluteus maximus and minimus contract with appreciable intensity during the first part of the support phase, and the adductor longus during the last part. The hamstrings apparently have but a small part in the supporting phase of normal walking. Only the long head of the biceps contracts at all, and it contracts only slightly at the very beginning of this phase. In rapid walking both the long head of the biceps and the semitendinosus contract with greater intensity during the first half of the support phase.

Knee

1. *Movements:* Slight flexion from foot strike continuing into foot-flat, followed by extension from midstance until heel-lift when flexion for the swing phase begins. This flexion during the stance phase flattens the vertical path of the center of gravity of the body, thus increasing the efficiency of the gait.
2. *Muscles:* The quadriceps extensors contract moderately in the early part of the support phase, then gradually relax. They appear to control the slight flexion that occurs in the knee at the moment of foot strike. The vastii continue to contract throughout the first half of this phase. As the leg reaches

the vertical position, the knee apparently locks and makes contraction of the extensors unnecessary. The tension of the stretched hamstrings at the end of the swing phase, especially when a long stride has been taken, may well be the factor that initiates the slight flexion at foot strike. In rapid walking all of these muscles contract more strongly and for a longer duration. There is an abrupt increase in their action in the second half of the support phase, which would seem to indicate that the extension of the leg at the knee is much more forceful in rapid walking than in normal walking.

Ankle and Foot

1. *Movements:* Slight plantar flexion, followed by slight dorsiflexion; prevention of further dorsiflexion, which the body weight tends to cause. Plantar flexion of ankle and hyperextension of metatarsophalangeal joints at the end of the propulsive phase, especially in vigorous walking.
2. *Muscles:* There is considerable action of the tibialis anterior in the early part of the supporting phase, especially at foot strike. This action is likely related to the controlled lowering of the foot by eccentric contraction to prevent the foot from slapping down too hard. Contrary to earlier opinions, the tibialis anterior does not continue to show activity during the major weight-bearing period, but it becomes active again at toe-off. The extensor digitorum longus and hallucis longus follow a similar pattern. They reach their peak contraction almost at the moment of transition between the swing and support phases; they relax early in the support phase, commencing to contract slightly at the end of this phase.

   The gastrocnemius and soleus become active from midstance to heel-off, contracting eccentrically to control ankle dorsiflexion as the center of gravity continues moving forward. Peak activity in the plantar flexors is reached from heel-off to toe-off as the foot pushes against the ground to initiate the next step.

   The tibialis posterior is most active during the middle part of the support phase, one of its functions, according to Basmajian, being to prevent eversion (pronation) of the foot (Basmajian & DeLuca, 1985). He points out that the peroneus longus and tibialis posterior apparently cooperate in stabilizing the leg and foot in weight bearing. The gastrocnemius and soleus act to decelerate the lower leg and stabilize the knee at midstance. There is a sharp increase in gastrocnemius and soleus activity beginning after the heel lifts and continuing until the opposite foot contacts the ground, initiating the period of double support. Extension of the knee in the stance phase is always accompanied by calf muscle activity. In *rapid* walking, however, the calf muscle activity is much more pronounced. The peroneus longus follows a simple pattern but does not seem to contract quite so strongly as the others, except in rapid walking. The peroneus brevis does not start to contract until about the middle of the support phase, but it contracts more strongly than the longus. In rapid walking it starts earlier and contracts with intensity soon after the halfway point has been reached.

   The flexor digitorum longus contracts slightly during the middle portion of the support phase and increases abruptly to moderate contraction in the last portion. In rapid walking the contraction becomes strong. The flexor hallucis longus follows the same pattern, except that it does not start to contract until the middle of the phase.

   The toe muscles, flexor hallucis longus, flexor digitorum longus, and the short, intrinsic flexors of the toes contract in response to the pressure of the ground against the toes. In the propulsive phase, especially in vigorous walking, this contraction is intensified. In all parts of the support phase the contraction of the toe flexors is greater in barefoot walking than when shoes are worn. This is especially noticeable when walking on turf or sand.

Action of Upper Extremities in Walking

Unless restrained, the arms tend to swing in opposition to the legs, the left arm swinging forward as the right leg swings forward and vice versa. This reflex action is usually accomplished without obvious muscular action and serves to balance the rotation of the pelvis. When the arm swing is prevented, the upper trunk tends to rotate in the same direction as the pelvis, causing a tense, awkward gait.

In early research, Murray and colleagues (1967) used the technique of interrupted light photography to investigate the action of the upper extremities in walking. They noted "patterns of sagittal rotation of the shoulder and elbow," or flexion and extension of both joints. They found that, although the amplitudes of the arm-swing pattern varied considerably from one subject to another, each individual had a similar pattern in all trials, even at higher speeds. Furthermore, they noted that the increased amplitude accompanying the faster speeds was due mainly to increased shoulder (hyper-) extension in the backward swing and increased elbow flexion in the forward swing. Maximum flexion of both the shoulder and elbow joints occurred at the moment of foot strike of the opposite foot and maximum extension at the moment of foot strike of the foot on the same side. These findings have been corroborated by later investigators, who have found a consistent "coupling" between actions of the lower and upper extremities during walking (Dietz et al., 2001; Li et al., 2001). While the motions of the arms and legs have been said to be coupled (Dietz et al., 2001; Li et al., 2001), recent research has suggested that arm movements during gait are a compensatory action to the foot reaction moment (Park, 2008) and also decrease the metabolic cost of walking (Ortega et al., 2008).

Although the arms appear to swing without muscular effort in walking at a normal pace on level ground, actually their pendular action was caused by a combination of muscular activity and gravity. The middle and posterior deltoid and the teres major were the muscles found to be most concerned, the latter two being active mainly during the backward swing. The posterior deltoid also contracted toward the end of the forward swing, leading one to suspect that it was serving as a brake to check the movement. The middle deltoid was found to be active during both flexion and extension of the arm at the shoulder joint. As this muscle is primarily an abductor, it seems that its function might be to keep the arms from brushing the sides of the body as they swing past it.

Neuromuscular Considerations

Walking is an action that relies heavily on reflex; little conscious control is necessary. On the contrary, if too much attention is focused on any part of the gait, tension is likely to develop and the natural rhythm and coordination are disturbed. Reflexes control not only the movements of the limbs but also the extension of both the supporting limb and the trunk in resisting the downward pull of gravity. This extension serves to give stability to the body in the support phases of locomotion, a stability that provides for effective muscular action in producing the necessary movements. Thus, in walking, as in all the motions of the body, smooth, coordinated movement requires properly functioning reflexes, normal flexibility of the joints, and optimum stability of the body as a whole in the weight-bearing phases of the act.

Two reflexes that play prominent roles are the *stretch reflex* and the *extensor thrust reflex.* The stretch reflex may be involved at the extremes in motion, particularly at the shoulder and in the lower extremity, assisting with the change in the direction of joint motion. The extensor thrust reflex may facilitate the extensor muscles of the lower extremity as the weight rides over the foot on the support leg.

Anatomical Principles in Walking

Several key anatomical factors affect the efficiency of the walking gait. Key factors to consider in any analysis of a walking pattern are the following:

1. Alignment
   a. Good alignment of the lower extremities reduces friction in the joints and decreases the likelihood of strain and injury.
   b. The stability of the weight-bearing limb and the balance of the trunk over this limb are important factors in the smoothness of the gait. Both are improved with good alignment of the weight-bearing segments.
2. Unnecessary lateral movements decrease gait economy. Lateral movements are usually due to excessive motion in the shoulders or pelvis.
   a. Excessive trunk rotation may be caused by either exaggerated or restricted arm swing. Normally the arm swing exactly counterbalances the hip swing.
   b. The pelvis may drop on one side if the gluteus medius is not contracted for support. The result is an exaggerated hip sway.
   c. Pelvic rotation should be just enough to enable the leg to move straight forward. A straight sagittal plane action of the leg is ensured by keeping the knee and foot pointing straight forward in all phases of the gait. The feet should be placed in such a way that their inner borders fall approximately along a straight line. Deviation from this pattern of leg motion will produce a weaving, inefficient gait.
3. Normal flexibility of the joints (i.e., sufficiently long and flexible muscles, ligaments, and fasciae) reduces internal resistance and therefore reduces the amount of force required for walking.
   a. The tendons of the two-joint muscles of the lower extremity contribute to the economy of muscular action in walking.
4. Properly functioning reflexes contribute to a well-coordinated, efficient gait. Injury, disease, or substance abuse can interfere with the walking reflex.

Mechanical Analysis

Walking is characterized by the translation of the body's center of gravity forward as a result of the alternating pattern of the lower extremity joint movements during the stance and swing phases. The forces that control walking are the external forces of weight, normal reaction, friction, air resistance, and internal muscular forces. The direction and interaction of these forces determine the nature of the gait.

The inertia of the stationary body is overcome by the horizontal component of the propulsive force. Because periodic movement is characterized by an alternating increase and decrease of speed, the inertia must be overcome at every step, and the greater the weight of the body, the greater is the inertia to be overcome. As the center of gravity moves forward, it momentarily passes beyond the anterior margin of the base of support and a temporary loss of balance results. At this point the downward pull of gravity threatens a complete loss of equilibrium. A timely recovery of balance is effected, however, as the foot is placed on the ground. Thus a new base of support is established and a new support phase is begun. The downward force of the body's weight is counteracted by the vertical reactive force through the feet. If the vertical force exceeds that needed to balance the gravitational force at the time of push-off, an exaggerated lift to the body results, causing a gait characterized by a bounce or unusual spring.

When forward motion has been imparted to the trunk by means of the ground reaction to the backward thrust of the leg and foot, it tends to continue unless restrained by another force. Once the center of gravity passes beyond the base of support, it is essential to restrain the action of the trunk until a new base of support is established. Hence, as the foot is brought to the ground in front of the body at the close of the swing phase, a restraining, or loading, phase is constituted. This diminishes as the leg approaches midstance. During the period that the foot is in front of the center of gravity, there is a forward component of force in the thrust of the foot against the ground. This results in a *backward,* or braking, reactive force of the ground against the foot, which is transmitted to the leg and then to the trunk.

The degree to which the pressure of the foot actually imparts motion to the body in the propulsive phase and restrains it in the restraining phase is in direct proportion to the counterpressure of normal reactive force of the supporting surface. If the surface lacks solidity, as in the case of mud, soft snow, and sand, it offers too little resistance to give the needed counterpressure. The pressure of the foot results in slipping or sinking, and more pressure must be applied to achieve even a slow forward progress. Hence the efficiency of the gait depends on the right balance between the pressure of the foot and the counterpressure of the supporting surface (Figure 18.4).

Like counterpressure, friction is also an essential factor in the effective application of the forces needed in walking. Because of the diagonal thrust of the leg at the beginning and end of the support phase, friction between the foot and the ground is essential so that the counterpressure of the ground may be transmitted to the body. For efficient walking, friction must be sufficient to balance the horizontal component of force. If it is insufficient, the thrust of the foot results in a slipping of the foot itself rather than in the desired propulsion of the body. The greater the horizontal component of force (as when walking with a long stride), the greater the dependence on friction for efficient locomotion.

The forward-moving trunk meets with air resistance, which tends to push it backward. By inclining the body forward, the pull of gravity is utilized to balance the force of the air resistance. Under normal conditions this force is negligible and will not be noticed. When walking against a strong wind, it is necessary to incline the body farther forward to maintain balance. If the air resistance is not balanced by the force of gravity, it must be balanced by the contraction of the abdominal and other anterior muscles of the neck and trunk. If the body is inclined too far forward, however, the force of gravity acts too strongly on it and must be counteracted by tension of the posterior muscles. Thus the proper degree of forward inclination is a factor in muscular economy.

Mechanical Principles in Walking

A number of mechanical principles govern the walking gait. A mechanical analysis of walking should include all of these important principles.

1. A body at rest will remain at rest unless acted on by a force. The force for walking is ground reaction force produced by extension of the lower extremity against a resistive surface. Because walking is an alternating pendular motion of the lower extremities,

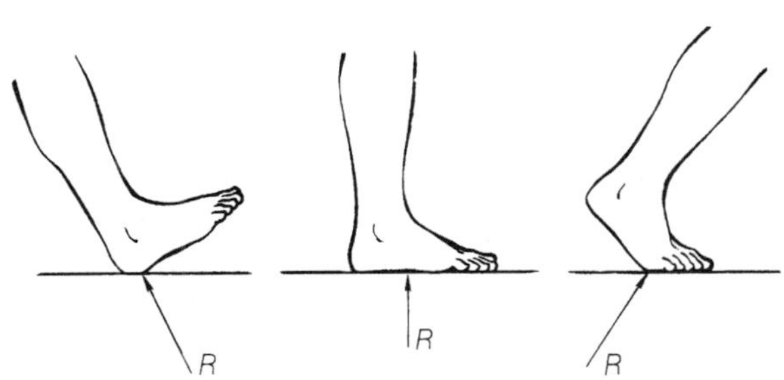

Figure 18.4 The ground reaction of force *R* is equal in action line and magnitude to the downward thrust of the foot during walking but is opposite in direction. The force is greater at heel strike than at midstance because of the body's momentum and is greater at push-off because of the plantar flexion thrust of the calf muscles driving the body forward. *Source:* From *Williams and Lissner: Biomechanics of Human Motion* (2nd ed.), by B. F. Leveau. Copyright © 1977, W. B. Saunders, Orlando, FL. Reprinted by permission.

the inertia of the body must be overcome at every step.

2. A body in motion will remain in motion until acted on by a force. Once motion is imparted to the trunk by the backward and downward thrust of the legs, the trunk has a tendency to continue in motion, even beyond the base of support. A brief restraining action of the forward limb serves as a brake on the momentum of the trunk.
3. Translatory movement of a lever is achieved by the repeated alternation of two rotary movements, the lever first turning about one end and then the other. In walking, the lower extremity alternates between rotating about the foot's point of contact (support phase) and the hip joint (swing phase). When muscles act to stop or start rotation at one end of the lever, power may be transferred to or absorbed from other segments. This power flow is cyclic in walking (Zajac et al., 2003).
4. Force applied diagonally has both horizontal and vertical components. The vertical component of the ground reaction force used in walking serves to counteract the pull of gravity. The horizontal component of this force serves to (a) check forward motion of the trunk during foot strike and (b) produce forward motion in the trunk during heel-off and toe-off.
5. The speed of walking is increased by increasing either the stride length or the stride rate, or both.
6. The speed of the gait is directly related to the magnitude of the pushing force and to the direction of its application. This force is provided by the extensor muscles of the lower extremity, and the direction of the force application is determined by the angle of the lower extremity when the force is being applied.
7. As propulsion of the body is brought about by the backward and downward push of the foot against the supporting surface, the efficiency of locomotion partially depends on the friction and ground reaction force provided by this surface.
8. The efficiency of gait is related to its timing with reference to the length of the limbs. The most efficient gait is one that is so timed as to permit pendular motion of the lower extremities.
9. Walking has been described as an alternating loss and recovery of balance (Steindler, 1973). This being so, a new base of support must be established at every step.
10. Stability of the body is directly related to the size of the base of support. In walking, the lateral distance between the feet is a factor in maintaining lateral stability. Average step width is about 10% of leg length.

Walking Variations

Individual Variations in the Gait

Although the basic analysis of the gait is valid for all physically normal people, individual characteristics are present to such a degree that people are often recognized by their gaits. These variations may be either structural or functional in origin. The structural differences include unusual body proportions as well as differences in the limbs themselves, such as knock-knees and bowlegs. Extreme variations in the angle between the neck and the shaft of the femur and in the obliquity of the femoral shaft are also responsible for atypical gaits.

Variations in the forward-backward distribution of weight and in the length of stride have already been mentioned. Other variations in movement patterns that are not structural in origin are often related to characteristics of the personality. This fact was brought home forcefully to Kay Wells (the original author of the text) when she attempted to help college students whose gaits were awkward. Almost invariably, the students who walked the most awkwardly were those who were extremely shy or lacking in self-confidence. A study investigating the possible relationship between the two might be rewarding.

Pathological gait Pain, disease, injury, or congenital deformity have all been shown to produce deviations from a normal gait pattern. The possible gait adaptations are far too numerous to categorize in this text. Joint injuries such as sprained ankles or cruciate ligament repairs in the knee will undoubtedly be followed by an asymmetrical, limping gait. A stroke may interfere with the ability of the neuromuscular system to produce a normal gait pattern. Cerebral palsy, multiple sclerosis, Parkinson's disease, and other neuromuscular conditions all produce gait variations that must be dealt with. It is important that the movement professional be well versed in the observation of gait patterns and offer any assistance required in the normalization of gait where possible. By recognizing deviations from a normal gait pattern, the student will be able to deduce the effects of gait variability and should be able to recommend appropriate remediation.

Age Age is also a factor in gait variations. As the human body ages, there is some decrease in both strength and flexibility as tissues change. Balance often becomes a significant concern. As a result of these changes, the gait of the elderly is often modified from that of a healthy young adult. Typically, the gait of a more elderly person will have the same cadence as that of a younger person, but the step length will be shorter. Along with the shorter step length, there tends to be a greater horizontal velocity component at foot strike with a longer time for weight acceptance and motion of the center of gravity over the support foot. Step width tends to be slightly greater and is more variable. In addition, more time is spent in the double support phase, and propulsive force is reduced. These changes in the gait pattern, although producing a slower gait, produce greater stability (Lockhart et al., 2003; Owings & Grabiner, 2004).

Obesity Obesity has also been found to have a negative effect on walking gait. While researchers have not found significant differences in sagittal or transverse plane movements, movements in the frontal plane between obese and nonobese individuals have been found to be significantly different. Hip and knee adduction angles are increased in the obese walking gait, as is ankle eversion angle. Obese individuals also tend to walk at a slower speed, with shorter strides, longer stance periods, and longer double support times. It is suggested that these changes in gait are an attempt to decrease the knee moments as well as energy expenditure. Interestingly, it has been found that obese individuals prcduce a smaller second ground reaction force peak, and smaller propulsive forces in comparison to nonobese walkers (Lai et al., 2008).

Walking Up and Down Stairs, Ramps, and Hills

In walking upstairs or up a ramp, the reactive force resulting from the push of the legs should be directed through the body's center of gravity and in line with the forward-upward slope. The most strain-free way of doing this is to incline the body forward in a straight line from the rear foot (Figure 18.5). The act of descending involves safely resisting the force of gravity on the body. The eccentric contraction of the muscles of the lower extremity enables the body

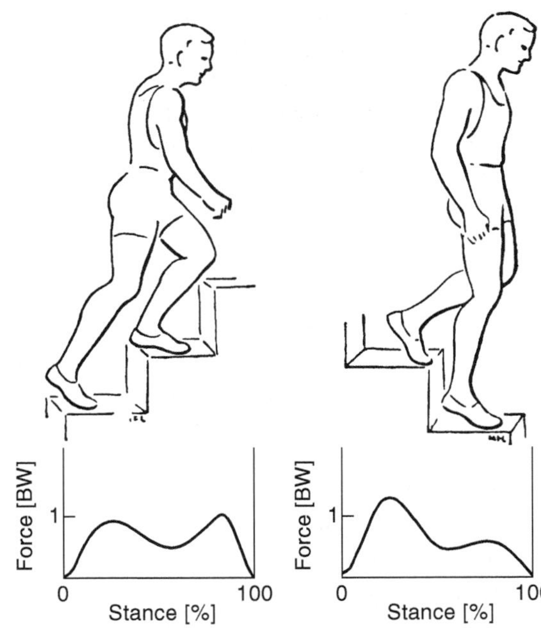

Figure 18.5 Going up and down stairs.

to be lowered at a controlled rate, and maintaining the line of gravity toward the back of the base of support prevents forward falls. In walking upstairs or up a ramp or hill, the swing phase is characterized by an increase in hip and knee flexion as well as ankle dorsiflexion. In addition, stride length is increased while going uphill (Leroux et al., 2002). According to Joseph and Watson, the hamstrings and tibialis anterior are the chief muscles involved (Basmajian & DeLuca, 1985). In the support phase, when the action is chiefly extension of the knee and hip, with the ankle being either slightly plantar flexed or else maintained in the midposition on the ball of the foot, they found the chief muscular action to come from the gluteus maximus, hamstrings, quadriceps femoris, and soleus, with the gluteus medius helping maintain stability at the hip joint.

The swing phase of walking downstairs starts with a slight lifting of the rear foot to clear the step. This movement involves slight knee flexion and dorsiflexion of the ankle. It is followed by slight hip flexion, then hip and knee extension and plantar flexion of the ankle as the foot reaches for the step below the one the supporting foot is on.

The support phase starts with the ankle in plantar flexion and the knee in extension. As the foot assumes the body weight, the ankle, knee, and hip are approximately in their neutral positions with the knee very slightly flexed. As the other foot swings forward, the supporting leg engages in slight hip flexion, increasing knee flexion and dorsiflexion of the ankle. In the brief period of double support, the knee and ankle flexion reach their maximum. The main muscular action of the supporting limb, according to Joseph and Watson, consists of eccentric contraction of the hamstrings, quadriceps femoris, and soleus, with the gluteus medius contributing to hip stability as it does in ascending (Basmajian & DeLuca, 1985).

Racewalking

The racewalking gait is an adaptation of walking intended to produce maximum walking speed without breaking into a run. Because the walk and the run are differentiated by the presence or absence of a double support phase, a racewalk must show a period of double support. A competitive racewalker attempts to minimize this double support period by increasing stride rate and decreasing stride length. In a normal walking gait, the stance phase accounts for 62% of the stride cycle and the swing phase makes up the other 38%. In the racewalk stance and swing phases, each accounts for 50% of the stride (Cairns et al., 1986). The peculiar straight-legged, hip-swing appearance of the racewalk gait is produced by a further stipulation in competitive racewalking that requires the knee of the support leg to extend fully during the stance phase (Figure 18.6).

The racewalk gait differs from the normal walking gait in several ways. In racewalking there is greater ankle dorsiflexion just prior to foot strike, and the leg is already fully extended at the knee when this contact occurs. The feet follow a line of progression closer to the midline of the body than in normal walking. There is a more exaggerated arm swing and therefore greater trunk rotation. Because of the straight support leg, there is greater lateral pelvic tilt as the pelvis rises above the support leg and drops on the swing side. The combined motion of the hip, trunk, pelvis, and arms acts to compensate for the lack of knee flexion in the support leg, producing little vertical motion.

RUNNING

Description

Easy running, like walking, is a pendulum type of movement. It is doubtful, however, whether running at top speed can be so classified. The most notable factors differentiating the run from the walk are the period of double support, characteristic of the walk but not present in the run, and the period of no support (a "sailing-through-the-air period"), characteristic of the run but not present in the walk. In the run the foot hits the ground in front of the body's center of gravity as in the walk, but not as far in front. As the speed of the run increases, the distance in front decreases until the foot contact is almost directly under the body's center of gravity. This position reduces the restraining part

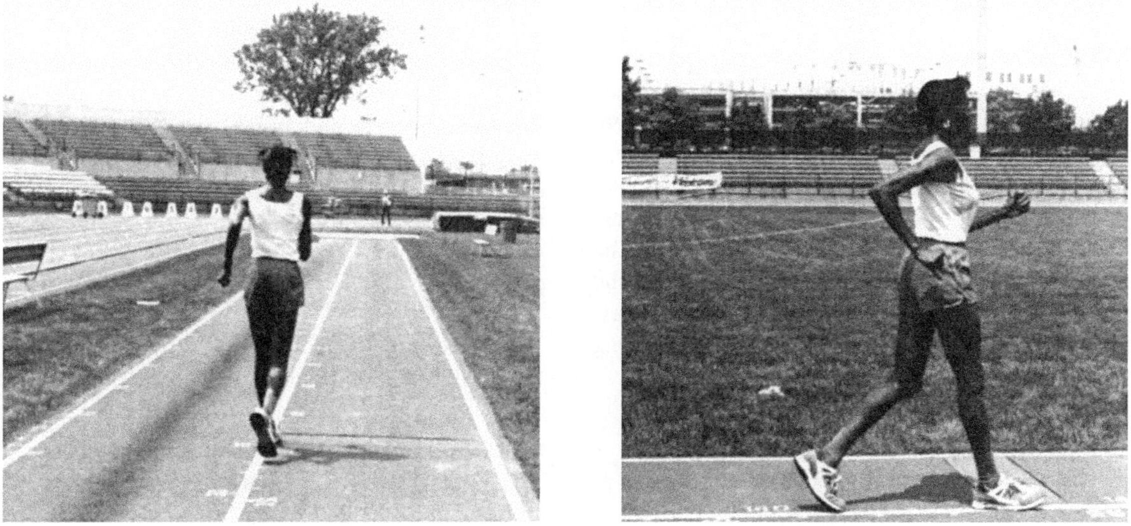

a. b.

Figure 18.6 Racewalk gait: (a) increased lateral pelvic tilt; (b) fully extended knee during support phase.

of the support phase and gives greater emphasis to the propulsive part. At maximum speed, the restraining part disappears completely. The use of the term *driving phase* for the support phase in running indicates its propulsive nature.

Speed in running is the product of stride duration and stride length ($v = d*t$). Variation in either stride duration or stride length will change the velocity of the run. Although it might seem that simply increasing stride length would be an effective way to increase running speed, it is important to keep in mind the preceding discussion of restraining, or braking, force. As stride length is increasing forward, the restraining force will increase, an inefficient trade-off. In modifying running speed it is critical to maintain running efficiency.

The transition from running usually occurs at about 2 m/s, with some variation. Investigators have found that just prior to this transition, the propulsive force seems to diminish. No single distinct trigger for the transition from walk to run (or from run to walk) has been found, but it is generally agreed that one will move to a new gait when the effort required to maintain gait speed becomes too great (Neptune & Sasaki, 2005; Prilutsky & Gregor, 2001).

There are two major types of running. The first is the kind of running done for its own sake, as in competitive races or jogging. The major concerns here are time and distance in one direction. The second is the type of running that is part of games and sports. Here it is necessary also to consider matters such as change of direction or pace and stability. The technique for a run varies with the purpose, but the basic anatomical and mechanical aspects are the same, regardless of the purpose.

Anatomical Analysis

The difference between the joint actions in walking and running is a matter of degree and coordination. The joint actions are essentially the same, but the range of motion in running is generally greater. This is especially apparent in the actions of the swinging leg. The difference in coordination is evident in the period of nonsupport and the absence of the period of double support.

Swing Phase

The swing phase begins with toe-off and ends with the foot landing (Figure 18.7). It is more muscular than pendular and is longer than the support phase. In fast running the initial foot contact may be the ball of the foot and, in slow running, the heel or the whole foot. The flexed leg in the swing phase brings the mass of the leg close to the hip, reducing the moment of inertia and increasing the angular velocity of the forward-swinging thigh, which in turn drives the center of gravity of the body forward (Table 18.1).

Support Phase

The support phase begins with the contact of the forward foot and ends at toe-off when the body is driven into the air (Figure 18.7b to d). During this time the knee and ankle "give" in flexion and then extend as the body passes over the foot and is driven into the air. The support time decreases as the speed of the run increases (Table 18.2).

Mechanical Analysis

The speed of running is governed by the length of the stride and the frequency of the stride. Better

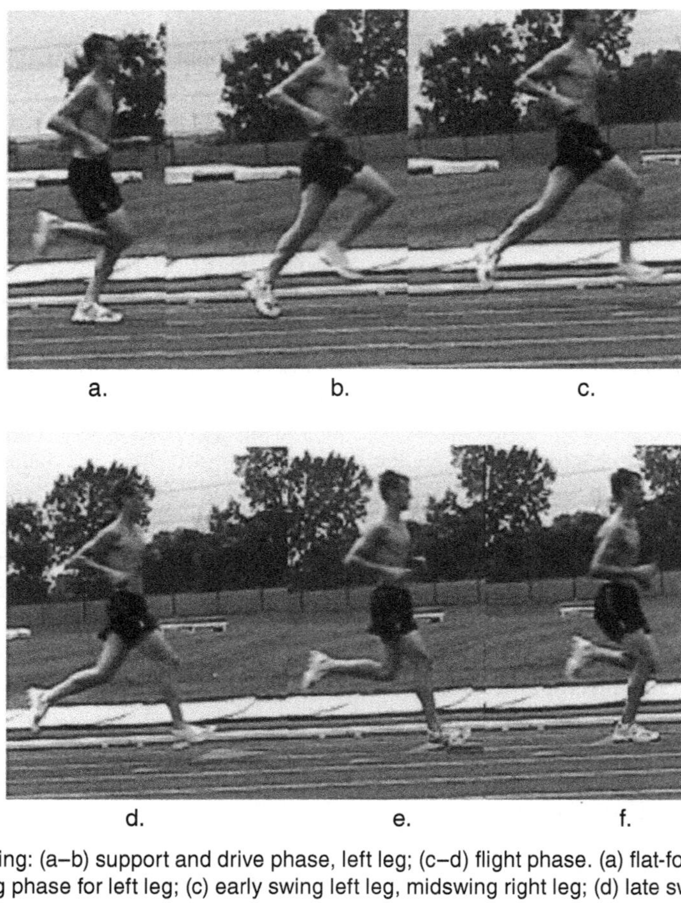

Figure 18.7 Running: (a–b) support and drive phase, left leg; (c–d) flight phase. (a) flat-foot; (b) toe-off and beginning of swing phase for left leg; (c) early swing left leg, midswing right leg; (d) late swing right leg; (e) heel strike, right leg; (f) flat-foot, right leg.

TABLE 18.1 Anatomical Analysis of Swing Phase in Running

Joint	Joint Action	Segment Moved	Force for Movement	Muscles Active	Kind of Contraction
Ankles	Dorsi flexion	Foot	Muscle	Tibialis anterior Extensor digitorum longus Extensor hallicus longus	Concentric
Knees	Flexion (fast, first ⅔ of swing)	Shank	Muscle	Reflex action and momentum	
Hips	Extension (last ⅓ of swing)	Thigh	Momentum	Hamstrings	Eccentric
	Flexion	Thigh	Muscle	Iliopsoas Rectus femoris	Concentric

Movements and muscular involvement in the spine and pelvis are the same as in walking but more vigorous in reaction to leg movements.

TABLE 18.2 Anatomical Analysis of Support Phase in Running

Joint	Joint Action	Segment Moved	Force for Movement	Muscles Active	Kind of Contraction
Ankles	Plantar flexion	Shank	Muscle	Gastrocnemius Soleus	Concentric
Knees	Flexion (initial support)	Thigh	Gravity	Quadriceps femoris	Eccentric
	Extension (at push-off)	Thigh	Muscle	Quadriceps femoris	Eccentric
Hips	Flexion	Trunk	Gravity	Gluteus maximus Hamstrings	Eccentric
	Extension	Trunk	Muscle	Quadriceps femoris	Concentric

Movements and muscular involvement in the spine and pelvis are the same as in walking but more vigorous in reaction to leg movements.

runners have a greater stride length per given pace than poorer runners. The length of the stride is determined by the length of the leg, the range of motion in the hip, and the power of the leg extensors, which drive the entire body forward. Like any projectile, the distance the body will move once it is driven into the air depends on the angle of takeoff (distance that center of gravity is ahead of takeoff foot), the speed of the body's projection, and the height of the center of gravity at takeoff and landing. The stride rate of the run is affected by the speed of muscle contraction and the skill of the performer.

In running, as in walking, the forces exerted to produce and control the movement are the internal muscular forces and the external forces of gravity, normal reaction, friction, and air resistance. There is no optimal speed in running because the energy needed to run is proportional to the square of the velocity. Therefore, whether the run is an easy jog or a full-speed sprint, economy of effort is a highly desirable objective. To achieve this it is essential that the runner observe the principles that apply to efficient running.

Mechanical Principles in Running

1. In accordance with the Law of Inertia, a body remains at rest unless acted on by a force. The force required to overcome inertia is greatest at takeoff and least after acceleration has ceased. The problem of overcoming inertia decreases as the speed increases.

2. In accordance with the Law of Acceleration, acceleration in the run is directly proportional to the force producing it. Hence, the greater the power of the leg drive, the greater the acceleration of the runner.

3. In accordance with the Law of Reaction, every action has an equal and opposite reaction. The force for the run is provided through the upward and forward ground reaction force in response to the downward, backward drive of the foot. The smaller the vertical component of this force, the greater the horizontal or driving component. In the most efficient run, vertical movements of the center of gravity are reduced to a minimum. There should be no bounce in running.

   In an efficient run, the foot should strike the ground as close as possible to the line of gravity. If the foot should strike ahead of the line of gravity, the reaction force to this forward and downward thrust will be a backward and upward force, acting to retard forward motion.

4. The more completely the horizontal force is directed straight backward, the greater its contribution to the forward motion of the body. Lateral motions are inefficient and detract from forward propulsion.

   The knees should be lifted directly upward and forward, with the motion of the entire lower extremity occurring within the sagittal plane. The arm swing should exactly counterbalance the twist of the pelvis and should not cause additional lateral motion.

5. Because a long lever develops greater speed at the distal end than does a short lever, the length of the leg in the driving phase should be as great as possible when speed is a consideration. Leg drive should be maximized as early as possible in the stance phase.

6. Resistance forces that are due to the moment of inertia of the free leg during the swing phase can be minimized. By flexing the free leg at the knee and carrying the heel high up under the hip, the leg is moved more rapidly as well as more economically. This high knee lift increases as speed increases.

7. The force of air resistance can be altered by shifting the center of gravity. A forward lean will work to counteract a head wind. A tailwind often enhances performance.

The Sprint Start

Because the object in sprint running is maximum horizontal velocity, sprint racers use the crouching start. This start enables the runner to exert maximum horizontal force at takeoff, providing maximum acceleration against inertia. In the sprint start, the runner pushes against starting blocks fixed to the track surface. The blocks provide a surface against which the foot can push horizontally while utilizing maximum hip, knee, and ankle extension. Moving the rear foot farther back in the blocks can increase the push-off force but decreases the time to apply the force, which may result in a smaller impulse (*Ft*). During the acceleration phase of the race immediately after the start, the horizontal component of the leg drive gradually diminishes until a constant level of speed is maintained, during which period horizontal velocity remains uniform. The period of acceleration is characterized by a gradual decrease in the inclination of the trunk, a lengthening of the stride (made possible by raising the center of gravity as the trunk becomes more erect), and a decrease of the knee thrust, resulting from the gradual straightening of the knee at the moment of foot contact with the ground (Figure 18.8).

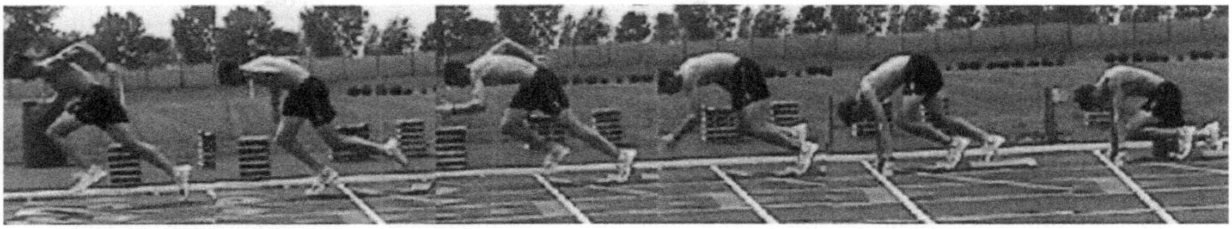

Figure 18.8 The sprint start. The period of acceleration is characterized by a gradual decrease in the forward inclination of the trunk and a lengthening of the stride.

JUMPING, HOPPING, AND LEAPING

Jumping, hopping, and leaping are forms of locomotion familiar from earliest childhood, whether engaged in as a simple expression of joy and exuberance, as a self-testing and competitive activity, or as an integral part of a sport. In each instance the goal is to propel the body into the air with sufficient force to overcome gravity and in the direction to accomplish the desired height or horizontal distance. Like any projectile, the path of the body in the air is determined by the conditions at the instant of projection. The differences between a hop, jump, and leap relate to the landing and takeoff. In the hop, the same foot is used for the takeoff and landing. In the leap, the takeoff is from one foot and the landing on the other. A jumper takes off from one or both feet and lands on both feet. Each of these types of projection may be initiated from a stationary position (vertical jump, standing long jump) or preceded by some locomotor pattern such as running (running long jump, triple jump, high jump, hurdle).

The total horizontal distance covered by the performer of these related patterns is the sum of three distances: (1) the horizontal distance between the takeoff foot and the line of gravity of the performer, (2) the horizontal distance the center of gravity travels in the air, and (3) the horizontal distance the center of gravity is behind the body part that lands closest to the takeoff point. The total height may be considered to be divided into the distance between the ground and the line of gravity at the moment of takeoff and the maximum distance the center of gravity is projected vertically. For some activities, such as the high jump and the pole vault, the vertical distance between the center of gravity and the crossbar may be an additional important unit of distance.

All forms of these activities share the problems of adequate muscle strength to project the body against the force of gravity and the coordination needed for utilizing what might be called secondary motions for achieving maximum height or distance. The force that projects the body is provided by the forceful contraction of the extensor muscles of the hips, knees, and ankles and, to a lesser extent, by the arm flexor muscles in swinging the arms forward and upward.

Mechanical Principles in Jumping, Hopping, and Leaping

1. For movement to occur, inertia must be overcome. One of the chief problems in jumping from a stand is overcoming inertia. A preliminary motion such as swinging the arms and upper body backward and forward, taking a hop or a step, or using a preparatory run helps overcome inertia in jumping.
2. Muscles can store elastic energy. When concentric contraction is preceded by a phase of active stretching, elastic energy stored in the stretch phase is available for use in the contractile phase. Work

done by the muscles that are shortening immediately after stretching is greater than that done by those shortening from a static state. For this reason the strong extension required for most jumping motions is usually preceded by a flexion phase. There should be no pause between this flexion and the thrust phase of the jump. This also makes full use of the phasic response of the stretch reflex.

3. Jumpers project themselves into the air by exerting force against the ground that is larger than the force supporting their weight. It is the reaction to the force that accelerates them upward. The faster and stronger the leg movements, the more force that is produced against the ground. Some of this downward force of the legs may itself be in reaction to upward motions of the upper extremities.
4. The upward thrust of the arms seen in the high jump accelerates the support leg downward, which in turn causes a reaction thrust from the ground. Trunk motion is also stabilized, allowing an increase in torque production at the knee. Additionally, the arm swing action in jumping has the effect of raising the center of gravity immediately prior to takeoff, which may result in increased jump height or distance (Ashby & Heegaard, 2002; Feltner et al., 2004)
5. The magnitude of the impulse that the jumper exerts against the ground is a product of the forces and the time over which they act. The vertical impulses in all jumps are those resulting from the swinging actions of the arms and the extension of the hip, knee, and ankle joints. The magnitude of the forces depends on the strength of the muscle, speed of joint actions, and coordination of the joint movements. The time for generating vertical impulse is greatest in jumps from a stationary start and in those jumps that have maximum height as their goal. The time required for the generation of impulse can also vary with the jumping style. In the high jump, for instance, the Fosbury flop style generally has shorter takeoff times than the straddle. Those jump styles with shorter takeoff times have generally produced higher jumps, apparently maximizing force production to produce a greater vertical impulse in less time.
6. The path of motion of a body's center of gravity in space is determined by the angle at which it is projected, speed of projection, height of the center of gravity at takeoff, and air resistance. The angle of projection varies depending on the purpose of the jump. In the long jump, where the goal is maximum horizontal distance, the optimum angle of projection is between 20 and 26 degrees. This angle is governed by the speed of the preparatory run and the vertical velocity generated at takeoff. The majority of the takeoff velocity is horizontal. Jumping at a 45-degree angle would require equal horizontal and vertical velocities. Because run velocities in the long jump are fairly fast, it would take a very large impulse to generate an equal vertical velocity. The long jump takeoff is too quick to allow for generation of this vertical impulse. Slowing the takeoff to the point where generation of equal velocities are possible would result in such low horizontal velocities that most of the jump distance would be lost. The most commonly quoted proportion between horizontal and vertical velocities is 2:1.

   In the high jump, the angle of projection is much greater. At the moment of takeoff the center of gravity should be as high as possible, and the vertical velocity should be maximum. In the running high jump, some horizontal velocity is necessary at takeoff to carry the performer forward over the bar.
7. Angular momentum may be developed by the sudden checking of linear motion or by an eccentric thrust (Figure 18.9).

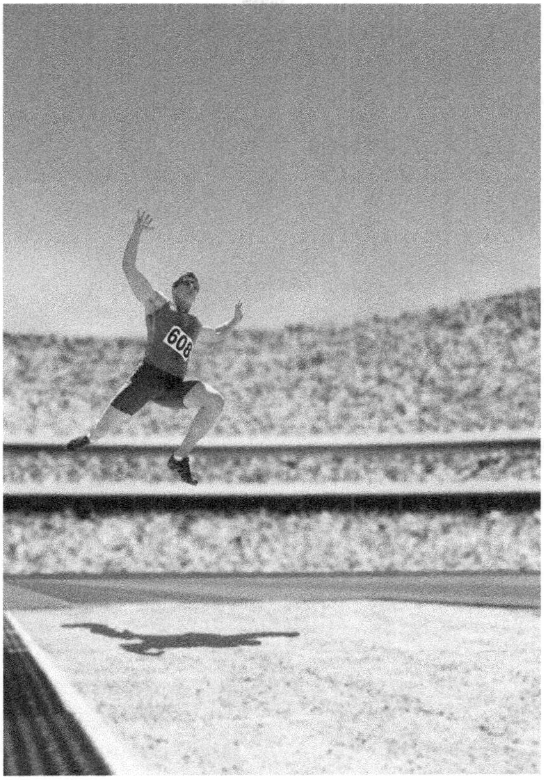

Figure 18.9 The long jump using the hang technique. The extended body position increases the moment of inertia about the horizontal axis, thus decreasing the undesired forward rotation developed at takeoff.

ADDITIONAL FORMS OF LOCOMOTION

Wheels, Blades, and Runners

Often, human locomotion over resistive surfaces is accomplished using the mechanical aids of wheels, blades, or runners. Devices such as bicycles, various types of roller skates, skis, and ice skates are designed to allow human beings to move farther faster for less effort, or to enable them to move quickly and easily over otherwise difficult surfaces. Unlike friction in locomotion involving a body segment in contact with dry, firm ground, friction using wheels, blades, and runners must usually be *minimized* in some respect rather than maximized. In using wheels for human-powered locomotion, friction in axles and rolling friction between wheels and ground must be kept to a minimum to avoid the heat and wear caused by excessive friction. With runners and blades, reducing friction between the mechanical device and the ice or snow surface is the primary concern.

Wheels

The most common form of human-powered locomotion, the bicycle, is also one of the most efficient in terms of transferring human muscle power to motion. Because the rider is constantly positioned over the center of gravity of the machine, the cycling motion has no braking or retarding phase. The continuous cyclic motion coupled with pedal and gear systems working on the principles of wheel and axles provide a mechanism in which little kinetic energy is wasted (Figure 18.10).

The speed at which the bicycle travels is determined by the gear ratio at which the bike is being operated, the pedal cadence of the rider, and the slope. The gear ratio of the bicycle determines the distance that can be traveled in each pedal revolution. A bicycle in first gear (smallest rear gear) need undergo only a single pedal revolution to cover the same distance as ten pedal revolutions in tenth gear, but it requires much greater force because of the shortened force arm in the wheel and axle configuration. On flat ground an efficient cyclist will use a small rear gear and forceful strokes to move the bike quickly. As the slope of the route increases, the cyclist will increase the size of the rear gear used, which will have the effect of maintaining the sense of effort at a relatively constant level but will decrease bicycle speed.

The force that produces pedal revolutions is provided by a cyclic extension–flexion motion of the lower extremities. The magnitude of the force that must be exerted depends on the gear ratio chosen. A lower gear, with a smaller force arm, requires greater pedal force but produces a greater distance traveled for each pedal revolution than do the higher gears with larger force arms. The pedal cycle itself has an extension, or power, phase and

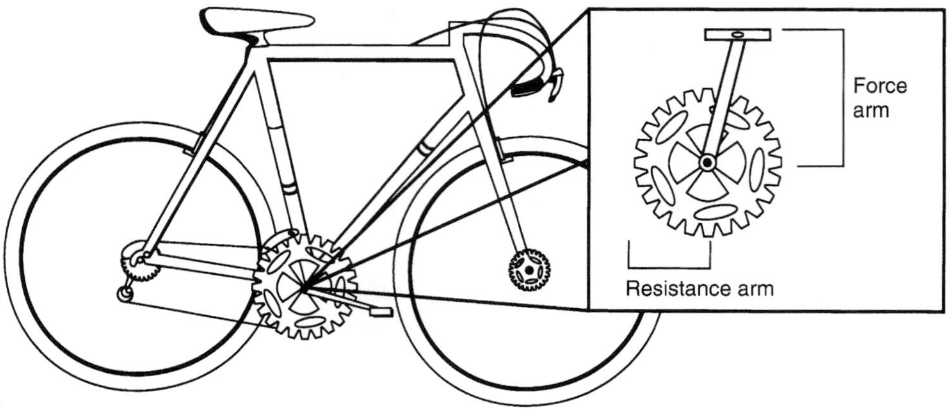

Figure 18.10 The longer force arm of the pedal crank makes the bicycle more efficient.

a flexion, or recovery, phase. Starting with the foot at the top of the pedal circle (top dead center, or TDC) and moving through the first 90 degrees of extension, the active muscles are the gluteus maximus, the rectus femoris, and the soleus, with the three vasti becoming active slightly before the rectus femoris. From 90 degrees to 180 degrees the hamstring group and the gastrocnemius become active. From 180 degrees back to TDC, muscle activity is primarily in the tibialis anterior with coactivation of the rectus femoris (Clarys & Cabri, 1993; Neptune & Herzog, 2000).

Although bicycling is an efficient form of locomotion when the system is in motion, kinetic energy is lost in stopping and starting. Each time the bicycle comes to a stop, kinetic energy is transferred to the braking system. To start the bicycle in motion, inertia must be overcome and kinetic energy reestablished. Along with inertia, rolling friction must constantly be overcome. This friction is inversely related to wheel diameter, which is why bicycles are more efficient than many other wheeled objects such as skateboards and roller skates. Rolling friction is greatest at the beginning of motion. As the wheel velocity increases, rolling friction decreases.

Increased velocity in bicycling produces increased air resistance acting against the cyclist. Drag increases as flow velocity increases. Often the cyclist will adjust the body position in an effort to reduce drag. The low handlebar position common in most racing and touring bicycles is an attempt to streamline the body, to reduce the surface area against which drag may act.

In most other forms of human-powered locomotion involving wheels, the movement involved is cyclic but not continuous as it may be in bicycling. In roller skating and in-line skating, for example, force is produced by each leg in turn, with a period of glide occurring between strokes. During this period of glide, there is a loss of velocity from friction. This means that some of the force expended on every stroke is used to regain lost velocity. Skateboards are similar but usually rely on only one leg for propulsion, the other leg maintaining constant contact with the moving board.

Wheelchair locomotion is similar to skating in that the motion involved is cyclic but not continuous. In most types of wheelchairs, the hand comes into contact with the push rim just before top dead center, then applies a propulsive force for an arc of 50 to 100 degrees. There is great variability in the propulsive stroke based on a variety of factors. These may include level of disability, type of chair, surface, slope, and velocity. In most cases, however, there is a brief period at the beginning of contact when the forces applied are braking forces rather than propulsive forces. This does decrease the efficiency of the wheelchair propulsive stroke (Kwarciak et al., 2009; van der Wooude et al., 2001).

Wheelchairs are now built for specific tasks. The day-to-day chair is very different from the racing chair pictured in Figure 18.11. Other chair styles have been created for sports like basketball, tennis, and rugby. A critical feature of most sport chairs is the cambered wheels. A cambered wheel is one in which the wheel is angled in toward the center of the chair rather than being oriented to the vertical. The effect of the camber is to bring the push rim closer to the shoulder, reducing the amount of shoulder abduction required. The reduction in shoulder abduction reduces the amount of push force directed laterally, making the propulsive stroke more efficient.

Both roller skates (or in-line skates) and skateboards are highly efficient during downhill motion. Velocity increases continuously because of gravity with no effort on the part of the human rider. Most will quickly remember, however, that in order to go down there must at some point have been an equivalent effort in the upward direction.

Blades

In ice skating, there is very little friction between the skate blades and the ice. This friction is reduced even further by a slight melting of the ice resulting from the pressure of the blade. Because of this extremely low coefficient of friction, it is not possible to push off in a backward direction as in running or walking. Instead, the skate blade is turned perpendicular to the direction of glide. The same pressure that produces the slight melting of the ice also causes the blade to sink slightly into the ice, allowing the blade to thrust against the ice as force is applied. Thus the slight depression in the ice provides the equal and opposite reaction necessary for forward motion (Figure 18.12). Besides the lateral push-off, ice skating differs from running in that little plantar flexion occurs in the push-off. Plantar flexion at this point of the skate stroke will probably scrape the skate toe along the ice, increasing friction.

As in other forms of human locomotion, speed in ice skating is based on stride length and stride rate. As velocity increases, the body also inclines forward to a greater degree and the feet separate. In speed skating the trunk may be inclined forward to a horizontal position to reduce drag. In figure skating, ice hockey, and recreational skating, this degree of lean is less common (Figure 18.13).

Runners

Similar to ice skating but using runners instead of blades is the sport of skiing. At present there are two basic forms of skiing: nordic, or cross-country, and alpine, or downhill. In addition, several other forms of sliding on snow are gaining in popularity and exposure. Ski jumping combines the speed of downhill skiing with aerodynamics and landing skills. Freestyle skiing uses the vertical velocity provided by small jumps or bumps to give the skier enough time in the air to perform a variety of gymnastic-style moves. Snowboarding, which replaces the familiar two skis with a single snowboard, is closely related to surfing and skateboarding.

Cross-country skiing is most closely related to walking, running, and ice skating in that an alternating stride pattern is frequently used for propulsion. The most common stride pattern in cross-country skiing is the diagonal stride, in which a backward thrust with one ski produces a forward glide on the forward or gliding ski. Ski poles are used to add additional thrust (Figure 18.14).

More recently, competitive skiers have been using a marathon skate stride or a V-skate stride. In both skating strides, the thrust is lateral, as in ice skating, rather than straight back. The marathon skate stride in cross-country skiing uses a single leg thrust, whereas the V-skate stride uses an alternating stride pattern. In both skate strides, the push from the rear ski is at a 30-degree angle to the glide direction.

Alpine or downhill skiing relies primarily on gravity for a propulsive force. The skier starts at the top of a slope (usually through mechanical transportation) and glides to the bottom. The movement problems encountered by the alpine skier revolve around changing directions and maintaining balance at high speeds while undergoing a variety of horizontal and vertical disturbances. In competitive alpine skiing, speeds are such that air resistance also plays a major role. The low crouch position assumed by most alpine

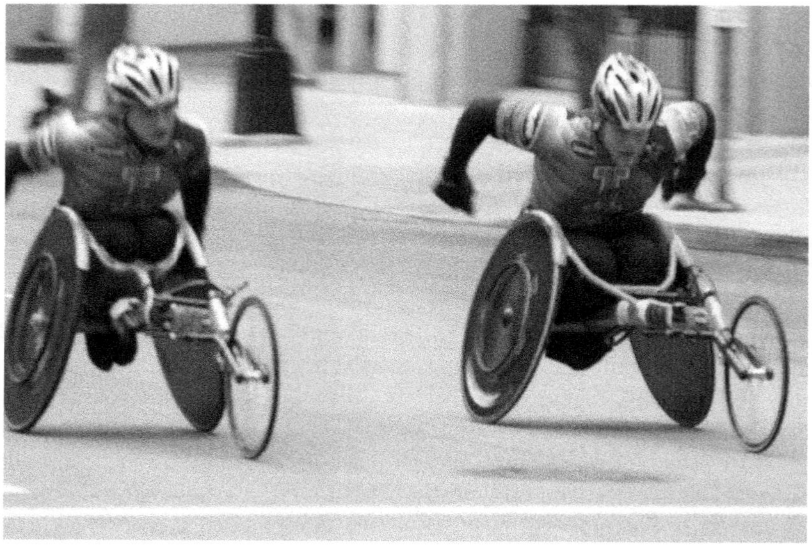

Figure 18.11

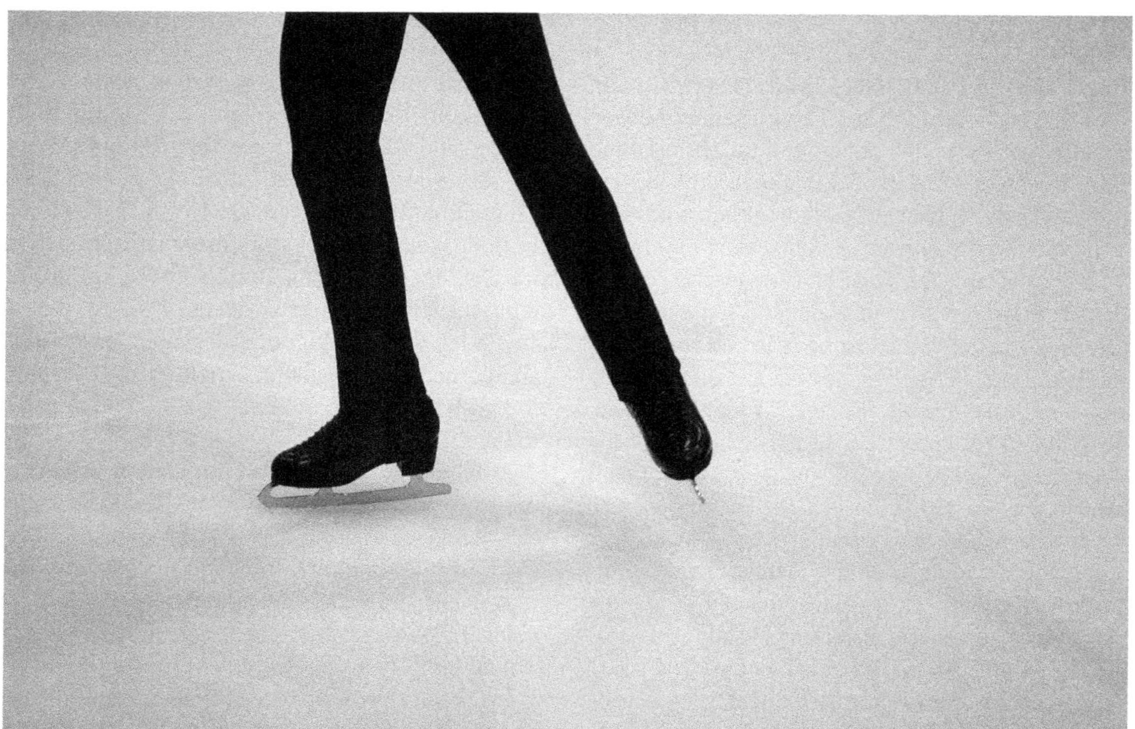

Figure 18.12 The straight back push-off in figure skating.

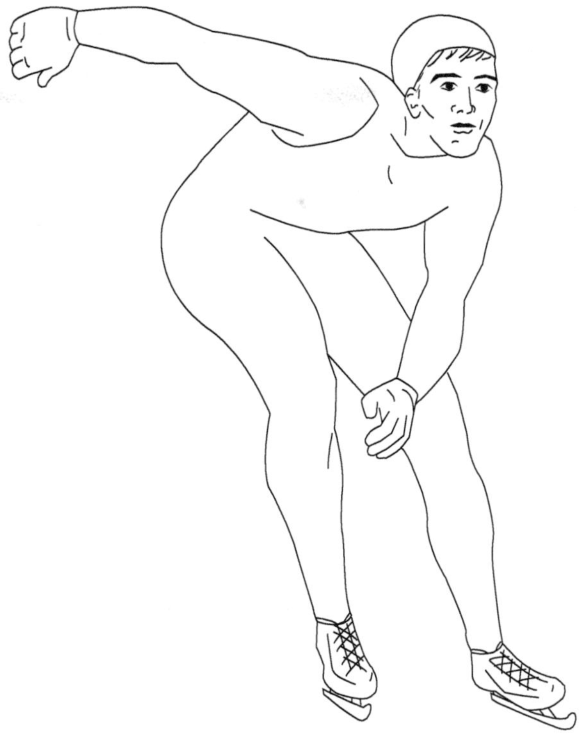

Figure 18.13 Body lean in the speed-skating stroke.

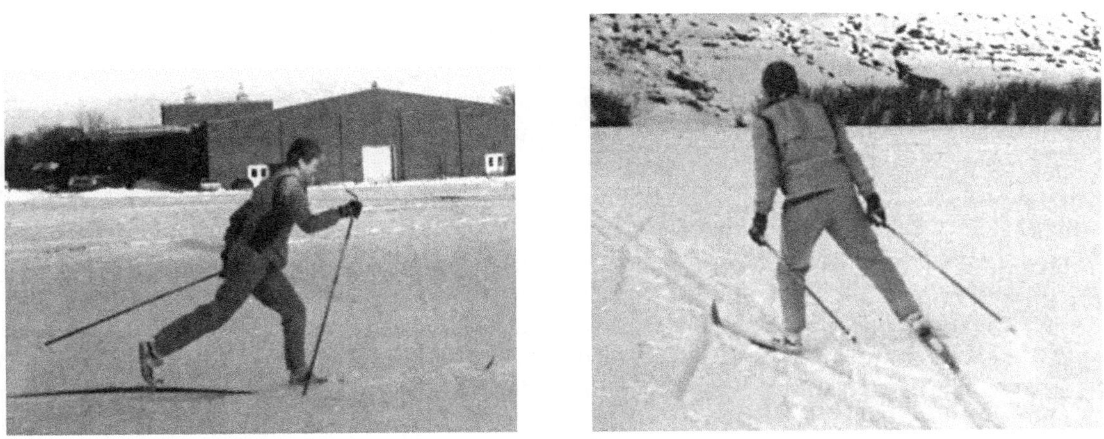

a. b.

Figure 18.14 The cross-country ski stride: (a) diagonal stride, (b) V-skate stride.

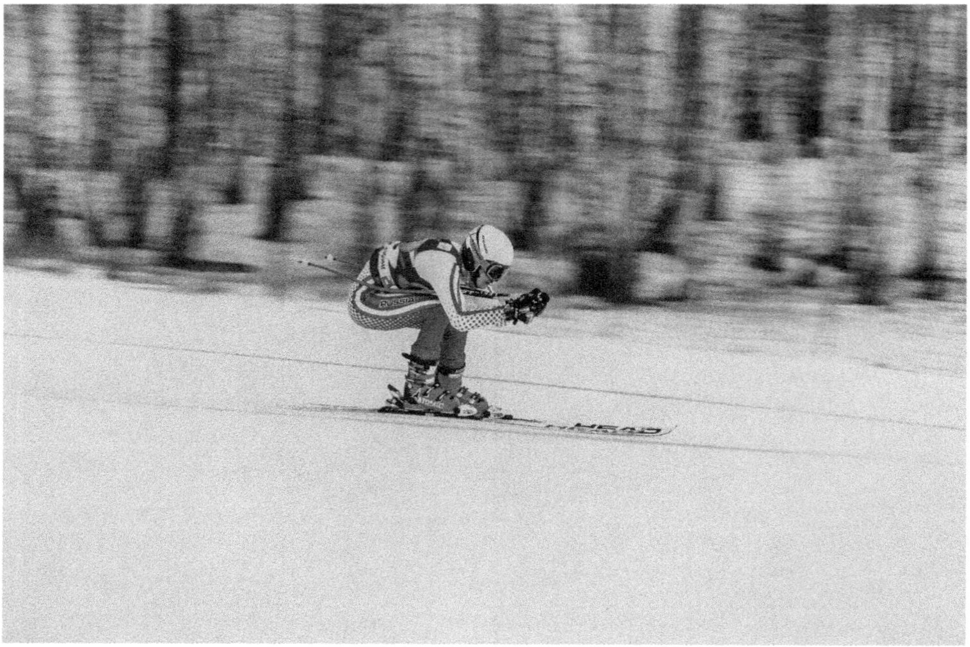

Figure 18.15 The aerodynamic low crouch position in alpine skiing.

racers reduces the surface area and thereby reduces form drag (Figure 18.15).

Rotary Locomotion

In general, the factors responsible for the successful performance of rotary locomotion are the magnitude, direction, and accurate timing of the forces contributing to the desired movement of the body, including the advantageous use of the force of gravity whenever possible.

The most common activities in this category are forward, backward, and sideward rolls, cartwheels, and handsprings. Each of these is achieved by rotating about the body's successive areas of contact with the supporting surface. In forward rolls, for instance, the body rotates about the hands, shoulders, rounded back, buttocks, and feet (Figure 18.16) and in cartwheels, about each hand followed by each foot with the body rotating laterally in a fully extended position. The impetus for the forward roll is given by the hands and feet, the direction of their thrust being a combination of backward and downward: backward to send the body forward, and downward to resist the downward pull of gravitational force on the head and trunk. When the hands and feet are no longer pushing, the head is tucked forward and the back is rounded with the knees bent close against the body to facilitate the roll. During the foot thrust, the hips are high, both for ensuring a stronger backward thrust with the legs and for making greater use of the force of gravity for the roll over the back.

Because a body at rest will remain at rest unless acted on by a force and a body in motion will continue in motion unless acted on by a force, it is important to keep the body moving in successive rolls and not let it come to a momentary halt following each roll. Even the briefest of interruptions necessitates overcoming inertia after each revolution. It takes velocity to acquire sufficient momentum to prevent these halts; therefore, each backward thrust of hands and feet against the ground should be as forceful as possible. Rotary movement is

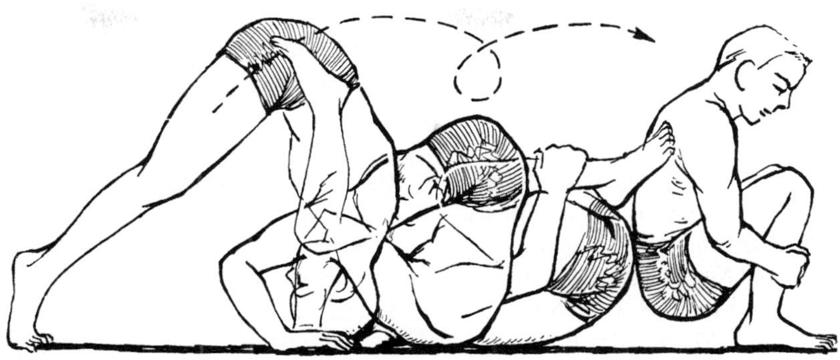

Figure 18.16 The body rotating around its points of contact with the supporting surface. *Source:* From *The Tumbler's Manual*, by William R. LaPorte & Al G. Renner. Copyright © 1938, p. 10. Adapted by permission of Prentice Hall, Englewood Cliffs, NJ.

accelerated by shortening the radius. In both forward and backward rolls, the radius is shortened by tucking the flexed lower extremities close to the body when the back is in contact with the floor.

Locomotion by Specialized Steps and Jumps

Other forms of ground-supported locomotion not involving the use of special equipment include two general categories. One of these consists of acrobatic stunts and athletic events, such as walking on the hands, successive jumping, and hurdling either with or without actual hurdles. The other category consists of activities used both in children's play and in forms of dance. It includes skipping, hopping, galloping, sliding, sidestepping, leaping, and standard dance steps, such as the polka and mazurka.

References and Selected Readings

Alexander, R. M. (2002). Energetics and optimization of human walking and running: The 2000 Raymond Pearl memorial lecture. *American Journal of Human Biology,* 14(5), 641–648.

Anderson, F. C., & Pandy, M. G. (2003). Individual muscle contributions to support in normal walking. *Gait and Posture,* 17, 159–169.

Anderson, F. C., Goldberg, S. R., Pandy, M. G., & Delp, S. L. (2004). Contributions of muscle force and toe-off kinematics to peak knee flexion during the swing phase of normal gait: An induced position analysis. *Journal of Biomechanics,* 37, 731–737.

Arnold, A. S., Anderson, F. C., Pandy, M. G., & Delp, S. L. (2005). Muscular contributions to hip and knee extension during the single limb stance phase of normal gait: A framework for investigating the causes of crouch gait. *Journal of Biomechanics,* 38(11), 2181–2189.

Ashby, B. M., & Heegaard, J. H. (2002). Role of arm motion in the standing long jump. *Journal of Biomechanics,* 35, 1631–1637.

Basmajian, J. V., & DeLuca, C. J. (1985). *Muscles alive* (5th ed.). Baltimore, MD: Williams & Wilkins.

Bus, S. A. (2003). Ground reaction forces and kinematics in distance running in older-aged men. *Medicine and Science in Sports and Exercise,* 35(7), 1167–1175.

Cairns, M. A., Burdett, R. G., Pisciotta, J. C., & Simon, S. R. (1986). A biomechanical analysis of racewalking gait. *Medicine and Science in Sport and Exercise,* 18, 446–453.

Chapman, A. R., Vicenzino, B., Blanch, P., Knox, J. J., & Hodges, P. W. (2006). Leg muscle recruitment in highly trained cyclists. *Journal of Sports Sciences,* 24(2), 115–124.

Clarys, J. P., & Cabri, J. (1993). Electromyography and the study of sports movements: A review. *Journal of Sports Sciences,* 11, 379–448.

Clarys, J. P., Alewaeters, K., & Zinzen, E. (2001). The influence of geographic variations on the muscular activity in selected sports movements. *Journal of Electromyography and Kinesiology,* 11(6), 451–457.

Cromwell, R. L., Aadland-Monahan, T. K., Nelson, A. T., Stern-Sylvestre, S. M., & Seder, B. (2001). Sagittal plane analysis of head, neck, and trunk kinematics and electromyographic activity during locomotion. *Journal of Orthopedic and Sports Physical Therapy,* 31(5), 255–262.

Den Otter, A. R., Geurts, A. C. H., Mulder, T., & Duysens, J. (2004). Speed-related changes in muscle activity from normal to very slow walking speed. *Gait and Posture,* 19, 270–278.

Dietz, V., Fouad, K., & Bastiaanse, C. M. (2001). Neuronal coordination of arm and leg movements during human locomotion. *European Journal of Neuroscience,* 14, 1906–1914.

Donelan, J. M., Shipman, D. W., Kram, R., & Kuo, A. D. (2004). Mechanical and metabolic requirements for active lateral stabilization in human walking. *Journal of Biomechanics,* 37, 827–835.

Duc, S., Villerius, V., Bertucci, W., Pernin, J. N., & Grappe, F. (2005). Muscular activity level during pedaling is not affected by crank inertial load. *European Journal of Applied Physiology,* 95(2–3), 260–264.

Dugan, S. A., & Bhat, K. P. (2005). Biomechanics and analysis of running gait. *Physical Medicine and Rehabilitation Clinics of North America,* 16(3), 603–621.

Feltner, M. E., Bishop, E. J., & Crisp, C. M. (2004). Segmental and kinetic contributions in vertical jumps performed with and without an arm swing. *Research Quarterly in Exercise and Sport,* 75(3), 216–230.

Ferber, R., Osternig, L. R., Woollacott, M. H., Wasielewski, N. J., & Lee, J. H. (2004). Bilateral accommodations to anterior cruciate ligament deficiency and surgery. *Clinical Biomechanics* (Bristol, Avon), 19(2), 136–144.

Frederick, E. C., Determan, J. J., Whittlesey, S. N., & Hamill, J. (2006). Biomechanics of skateboarding: Kinetics of the Ollie. *Journal of Applied Biomechanics,* 22(1), 33–40.

Gottschall, J. S., & Kram, R. (2005). Energy cost and muscular activity required for leg swing during walking. *Journal of Applied Physiology,* 99, 23–30.

Gushue, D. L., Houck, J., & Lerner, A. L. (2005). Effects of childhood obesity on three-dimensional knee joint biomechanics during walking. *Journal of Pediatric Orthopaedics,* 25(6), 763–768.

Hamel, K. A., Okita, N., Bus, S. A., & Cavanagh, P. R. (2005). A comparison of foot/ground interaction during stair negotiation and level walking in young and older women. *Ergonomics,* 48(8), 1047–1056.

Hardin, E. C., van den Bogert, A. J., & Hamill, J. (2004). Kinematic adaptations during running: Effects of footwear, surface, and duration. *Medicine and Science in Sports and Exercise,* 36(5), 838–844.

Hof, A. L., Elzinga, H., Grimmus, W., & Halbertsma, J. P. K. (2002). Speed dependence of averaged EMG profiles in walking. *Gait and Posture,* 16, 78–86.

Houdijk, H., de Koning, J. J., de Groot, G., Bobbert, M. F., & van Ingen Schenau, G. J. (2000). Push-off mechanics in speed skating with conventional skates and klapskates. *Medicine and Science in Sports and Exercise,* 32, 635–641.

Hunter, J. P., Marshall, R. N., & McNair, P. J. (2005). Relationships between ground reaction force impulse and kinematics of sprint-running acceleration. *Journal of Applied Biomechanics,* 21(1), 31–43.

Ivanenko, Y. P., Poppele, R. E., & Lacquaniti, F. (2004). Five basic muscle activation patterns account for muscle activity during human locomotion. *Journal of Physiology,* 556(Pt 1)1, 267–282.

Jonkers, I., Stewart, C., & Spaepen, A. (2003). The study of muscle action during single support and swing phase of gait: Clinical relevance of forward simulation techniques. *Gait and Posture,* 17, 97–105.

Kimmel, S. A., & Schwartz, M. H. (2006). A baseline of dynamic muscle function during gait. *Gait and Posture,* 23, 211–221.

Kivi, D. M., Maraj, B. K., & Gervais, P. (2002). A kinematic analysis of high-speed treadmill sprinting over a range of velocities, *Medicine and Science in Sports and Exercise,* 34(4), 662–666.

Korhonen, M. T., Mero, A., & Suominen, H. (2003). Age-related differences in 100-m sprint performance in male and female master runners. *Medicine and Science in Sports and Exercise,* 35(8), 1419–1428.

Kwarciak, A. M., Sisto, S. A., Yarossi, M., Price, R., Komaroff, E., & Boninger, M. L. (2009). Redefining the manual wheelchair stroke cycle: Identification and impact of nonpropulsive pushrim contact. *Archives of Physical Medicine and Rehabilitation,* 90, 20–26.

Kwon, O. Y., Minor, S. D., Maluf, K. S., & Muller, M. J. (2003). Comparison of muscle activity during walking in subjects with and without diabetic neuropathy. *Gait and Posture,* 18, 105–113.

Kyrolainen, H., Avela, J., & Komi, P. V. (2005). Changes in muscle activity with increasing running speed. *Journal of Sports Sciences,* 23(10), 1101–1109.

Lai, P. P. K., Leung, A. L. K., Li, A. N. M., & Zhang, M. (2008). Three-dimensional gait analysis of obese adults. *Clinical Biomechanics,* 23(51), 52–56.

Lay, A. N., Hass, C. J., & Gregor, R. J. (2006). The effects of sloped surfaces on locomotion: A kinematic and kinetic analysis. *Journal of Biomechanics,* 39, 1621–1628.

Leroux, A., Fung, J., & Barbeau, H. (2002). Postural adaptations to walking on inclined surfaces: I. Normal strategies. *Gait and Posture,* 15(1), 64–74.

Li, Y., Wang, W., Crompton, R. H., & Gunther, M. M. (2001). Free vertical moments and transverse forces in human walking and their role in relation to arm-swing. *Journal of Experimental Biology,* 204(Pt 1), 47–48.

Lockhart, T. E., Woldstad, J. C., & Smith, J. L. (2003). Effects of age-related gait changes on the biomechanics of slips and falls. *Ergonomics,* 46(12), 1136–1160.

Marks, R. (1997). The effect of restricting arm swing during normal locomotion. *Biomedical Sciences Instrumentation,* 33, 209–215.

McGraw, B., McClenaghan, B. A., Williams, H. G., Dickerson, J., & Ward, D. S. (2000). Gait and postural stability in obese and nonobese prepubertal boys. *Archives of Physical Medicine and Rehabilitation,* 81(4), 484–489.

Mero, A., Kuitunen, S., Harland, M., Kyrolainen, H., & Komi, P. V. (2006). Effects of muscle-tendon length on joint moment and power during sprint starts. *Journal of Sports Sciences,* 24(2), 165–173.

Modica, J. R., & Kram, R. (2005). Metabolic energy and muscular activity required for leg swing in running. *Journal of Applied Physiology,* 98, 2126–2131.

Mrachacz-Kersting, N., Lavoie, B. A., Andersen, J. B., & Sinkjaer, T. (2004). Characterisation of the quadriceps stretch reflex during the transition from swing to stance phase of human walking. *Experimental Brain Research,* 159(1), 108–122.

Muller, E., & Schwameder, H. (2003). Biomechanical aspects of new techniques in alpine skiing and ski-jumping. *Journal of Sports Sciences,* 21(9), 679–692.

Murray, M. P., Sepic, S. B., & Barnard, E. J. (1967). Patterns of sagittal rotation of the upper limbs in walking. *Physical Therapy,* 47, 272–284.

Nadeau, S., McFadyen, B. J., & Malouin, F. (2003). Frontal and sagittal plane analyses of the stair climbing task in healthy adults aged over 40 years: What are the challenges compared to level walking? *Clinical Biomechanics* (Bristol, Avon), 18(10), 950–959.

Neptune, R. R., & Herzog, W. (2000). Adaptation of muscle coordination to altered task mechanics during steady-state cycling. *Journal of Biomechanics,* 33(2) 165–172.

Neptune, R. R., & Sasaki, K. (2005). Ankle plantar flexor force production is an important determinant of the preferred walk-to-run transition speed. *Journal of Experimental Biology,* 208(Pt 5), 799–808.

Neptune, R. R., Zajac, F. E., & Kautz, S. S. (2004a). Muscle force redistributes segmental power for body progression during walking. *Gait and Posture,* 19, 194–205.

Neptune, R. R., Zajac, F. E., & Kautz, S. S. (2004b). Muscle mechanical work requirements during normal walking: The energetic cost of raising the body's center-of-mass is significant. *Journal of Biomechanics,* 37, 817–825.

Ness, L. L., & Field-Fote, E. C. (2009). Whole-body vibration improves walking function in individuals with spinal cord injury: A pilot study. *Gait and Posture,* 30(4) 436–440.

Nielsen, J. B., & Sinkjaer, T. (2002). Reflex excitation of muscles during human walking. *Advances in Experimental Medicine and Biology,* 508, 369–375.

Nilsson, J., Tveit, P., & Eikrehagen, O. (2004). Effects of speed on temporal patterns in classical style and freestyle cross-country skiing. *Sports Biomechanics,* 3(1), 85–107.

Ortega, J. D., Fehlman, L. A., & Farley, C. T. (2008). Effects of aging and arm swing on the metabolic cost of stability in human walking. *Journal of Biomechanics,* 41(16), 3303–3308.

Owings, T. M., & Grabiner, D. (2004). Variability of step kinematics in young and older adults. *Gait and Posture,* 20(1), 26–29.

Park, J. (2008). Synthesis of natural arm swing motion in human bipedal walking. *Journal of Biomechanics,* 41(7), 1417–1426.

Perry, J. (1992). *Gait analysis: Normal and pathological function.* Thorofare, NJ: Slack.

Pinnington, H. C., Lloyd, D. G., Besier, T. F., & Dawson, B. (2005). Kinematic and electromyography analysis of submaximal differences running on a firm surface compared with soft, dry sand. *European Journal of Applied Physiology,* 94, 242–253.

Prentice, S. D., Hasler, E. N., Groves, J. J., & Frank, J. S. (2004). Locomotor adaptations for changes in the slope of the walking surface. *Gait and Posture,* 20, 255–265.

Prilutsky, B. I., & Gregor, R. J. (2001). Swing-and support-related muscle actions differentially trigger human walk-run and run-walk transitions. *Journal of Experimental Biology,* 204, 2277–2287.

Riener, R., Rabuffetti, M., & Frigo, C. (2002). Stair ascent and descent at different inclinations. *Gait and Posture,* 15(1), 32–44.

Rose, J., & Gamble, J. G. (1994). *Human walking.* Baltimore, MD: Williams & Wilkins.

Salo, A., & Bezodis, I. (2004). Which starting style is faster in sprint running-standing or crouch start? *Sports Biomechanics,* 3(1), 43–53.

Stefanshyn, D. J., Nigg, B. M., Fisher, V., O'Flynn, B., & Liu, W. (2000). The influence of high heeled shoes on kinematics, kinetics, and muscle EMG of normal female gait. *Journal of Applied Biomechanics,* 16, 309–319.

Steindler, A. (1973). *Kinesiology of the human body.* Springfield, IL: Charles C Thomas, Lectures 37 and 38.

Van der Woude, L. H. V., Veeger, H. E. J., Dallmeijer, A. J., Janssen, T. W. J., & Rozendaal, L. A. (2001). Biomechanics and physiology in active manual wheelchair propulsion. *Medical Engineering and Physics,* 23, 713–733.

Vaughan, C. L. (2003). Theories of bipedal walking: An odyssey. *Journal of Biomechanics,* 36, 513–523.

Vaughan C. L., Davis, B. L., & O'Connor, J. C. (1999). *Dynamics of human gait.* Cape Town, South Africa: Kiboho.

Wakai, M., & Linthorne, N. P. (2005). Optimum take-off angle in the standing long jump. *Human Movement Sciences,* 24(1), 81–96.

Warren, G. L., Maher, R. M., & Higbie, E. J. (2004). Temporal patterns of plantar pressure and lower-leg muscle activity during walking: Effect of speed. *Gait and Posture,* 19, 91–100.

Zajac, F. E., Neptune, R. R., & Kautz, S. A. (2003). Biomechanics and muscle coordination of human walking. Part II: Lessons from dynamical simulations and clinical implications. *Gait and Posture,* 17, 1–17.

Zehr, E. P., & Stein, R. B. (1999). What functions do reflexes serve during human locomotion? *Progress in Neurobiology,* 58, 185–205.

Laboratory Experiences

1. Try this as a class exercise, working in pairs. A stands with heels against a wall with the feet otherwise in a comfortable, "natural" position in readiness to walk. B holds a ruler across the toes of A's feet and draws a line against the ruler. A then stands with feet parallel at right angles to the wall, and again B draws a line. Measure the distance between the two lines. This measurement is likely to vary from 0.5 cm to 2.5 cm in a sizable class. A and B now change places and repeat.

   Assume that you are to engage in a walking race of 1,000 meters; also assume that if you toed straight ahead, each step would be 1 meter long. It would therefore take you 1,000 steps to cover the distance. But suppose you toed out so that each step was (your measurement) __________ short. How many meters short of the finish line would you be when you had taken 1,000 steps? (Answer: If the distance between the two lines had been 0.4 cm, you would be 0.4 × 1,000 = 400 cm, or 4 meters, short.)

Implication: If you are walking against an opponent who walks at the same rate as you, but who toes straight ahead, you would be 4 meters behind when you cross the finish line. Yet, presumably you took the same number of steps.

2. Observe the gait of people on the street or campus, detect individual characteristics, and analyze them using anatomical and mechanical principles.
3. Get a subject to walk in each of the following ways. Observe and note differences in the movements of the head, shoulders, hips, and so forth.
   a. Place one foot directly in front of the other.
   b. Keep a lateral distance of 20 to 25 cm between the feet.
   c. Point the toes out.
   d. Point the toes in.
   e. Point the toes straight ahead.
   f. Take a short stride.
   g. Take a long stride.
4. Select four or five individuals who differ in leg length. Get them to practice walking until each one finds the stride and speed that feels most comfortable. Compare their strides and measure the distance between footprints for each individual.
5. Observe several individuals as they run. Look for the application of the principles listed. Which are "violated" and how?
6. Using the iliac crest as an estimate of the center of gravity, trace the path of the center of gravity on a sequence drawing of some form of jump (see Figure 14.23). Determine the percentage of the distance jumped that can be attributed to each of the following:
   a. Distance center of gravity is in front of takeoff point at the moment of takeoff.
   b. Distance center of gravity travels while body is unsupported.
   c. Distance center of gravity is behind landing point.
7. Compare the segment positions at several points during the execution of a standing long jump or vertical jump as done by several "poor" jumpers and several "good" jumpers. Identify the principles of concern in these jumps. Evaluate the performance by stating the related principles. On the basis of this information, try to improve the performance of the "poor" jumpers.
8. Choose a locomotor pattern not discussed in this chapter (hurdling, for example). Perform a complete kinesiological analysis, taking particular note of the purpose of the motion, its classification, and the nature of the motion. Include also muscle participation, neuromuscular considerations, and mechanical factors. Identify those principles that will help you determine whether someone performing this pattern is doing it correctly. Conclude the analysis with a prescription for improvement, including suggested methods for change and the elimination of violations of principles.

CHAPTER

19 LOCOMOTION: THE AQUATIC ENVIRONMENT

OUTLINE

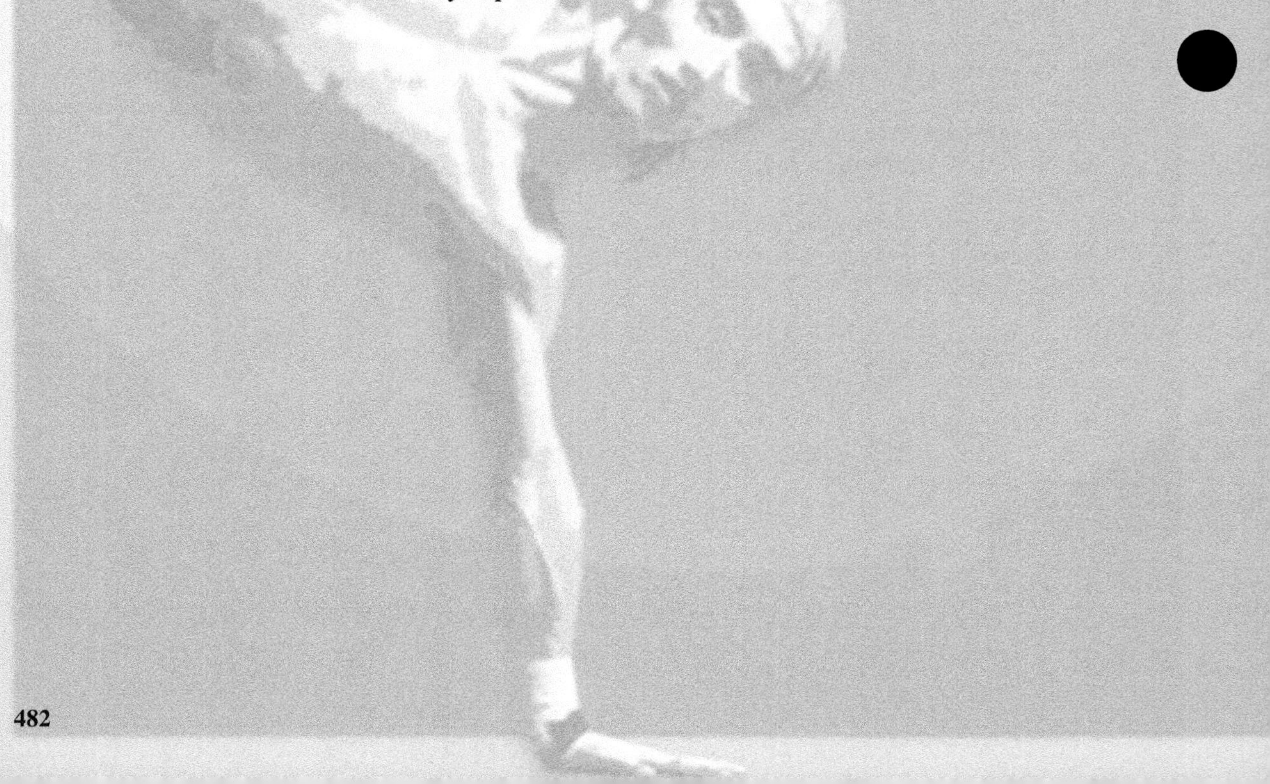

OBJECTIVES

At the conclusion of this chapter, the student should be able to:

1. Name those factors that contribute to the propulsion of a swimmer.
2. Name those factors that impede the progress of a swimmer.
3. Explain how the propulsive and resistive factors named affect the length or frequency of a swimming stroke.
4. Complete a kinesiological analysis of a swimming stroke by identifying the anatomical and mechanical factors important to success in the selected stroke, as well as those factors that appear to limit the particular performance.

AQUATIC LOCOMOTION: SWIMMING

The problem of moving the body through water is fundamentally not so different from that of moving it on land. As in walking, it is necessary to push against something to move the body from one place to another. The chief differences between locomotion in the water and locomotion on land are that (1) in the water the body is concerned with buoyancy rather than with the force of gravity, (2) the substance against which it pushes affords less resistance to the push, (3) the medium through which it moves affords more resistance to the body, and (4) as a means of getting the greatest benefit from the buoyancy and of reducing the resistance afforded by the water, it is customary to maintain a horizontal, rather than a vertical, position. (Review the discussion of buoyancy on pp. 314–316.) The practical problem in swimming is not to keep from sinking, as novices are inclined to believe, but to get the mouth out of the water at rhythmic intervals in order to permit regular breathing. This is a matter of coordination, not buoyancy.

In swimming, as in all motion, the initial mechanical problem is to overcome the inertia of the body. Once the body is in motion, the problem is to overcome the forces that tend to hinder it. In terrestrial locomotion the body exerts its force against the supporting surface, the ground, to overcome inertia. The forces resisting the progress of the body are the forces of gravity and air resistance. In aquatic locomotion the water is both the supporting medium and the source of resistance. In swimming the hands and feet depend on the reaction force of the water in order that the force may be transmitted to the body. At the same time, the body must overcome the resistance afforded by the water.

Swimming Speed

The speed obtained in swimming any stroke depends on the stroke length and stroke frequency. The length of the stroke is the result of the forces that move the swimmer forward in reaction to the movements of the arms and legs, and of the resistance of the water in the opposite direction. In the front crawl the arms are the primary source of power, whereas in the breaststroke the legs dominate. Regardless of the stroke, the actions of the arms and legs result in a combination of lift and drag forces that then propel the body forward.

Four different types of water resistance act to decrease the stroke length. *Form drag,* or pressure drag, is the resistance due to the surface area of the front of the body as it meets the oncoming water. This type of resistance has the greatest effect on the swimmer. Streamlining the body by changing its position in the water decreases form drag. *Surface drag* is caused by the resistance of the water next to the body. Although it has less effect on forward progress, swimmers have been known to shave the hair from their bodies as a means of decreasing skin friction. The introduction of new racing suits that mimic sharkskin or otherwise control surface drag have produced 3–5% increases in swimming speed. In a race decided by as little as 0.001 seconds, this can be significant (Mollendorf et al., 2004). A third form of drag is that which occurs at the surface as the body moves along, partially in water and partially in air. The resultant waves form an additional resistance to forward progress called *wave drag*. The amount of this resistance depends on both the speed and movements of the body as it progresses through the water. A fourth but minor resistance is turbulence that forms behind the body, causing it to pull some water along with it.

The *frequency* of the stroke depends on the amount of time spent per stroke cycle. This, in turn, is related to the nature of the stroke pattern and the muscle torques of the arms and legs. Thus the major problem in the mechanics of swimming is the minimization of the resistance that is due to the water, which is either pushed out of the way or dragged along, and the advantageous application of the force of the arms and legs. The swimmer reduces resistance by streamlining the body position through relaxing in the recovery phase of the stroke and by eliminating useless motion and tensions. The propulsive force is increased with improvements in technique and conditioning.

Mechanical Principles Applied to Swimming

1. *Less force is needed to keep an object moving than to overcome its inertia.* Force in swimming should be applied so that the progress through the water is even rather than consisting of cycles of speeding up and slowing down. In the front crawl, the beginning of one arm pull should start before the other arm finishes its pull. In strokes such as the breaststroke and sidestroke, too long a glide will result in a reduction in momentum and the need to expend extra energy to overcome inertia in starting up again.
2. *The body will move in the opposite direction from that in which the force is applied.* For instance, a backward thrust will send the body forward, downward pressure will lift it, and pressure to the right will send it to the left. In most strokes too much force at the beginning of the arc will have too great a downward component, thereby tending to lift the body. This increases resistance and is a needless expenditure of energy. In a similar manner, a wide recovery of the arm in the front crawl or back crawl will result in an opposite lateral reaction in the legs, and thus will cause additional resistance. In the breaststroke, the two arms balance each other; hence, too great an outward force at the beginning of the stroke or inward force at the end of the stroke does not produce lateral motion but results in a waste of energy.
3. *Forward motion in swimming is produced through a combination of drag force and lift force.* In all swimming strokes the hand follows an S-shaped path through the water, with an insweep and an outsweep. The function of this curved pattern is to produce water flow laterally over the hand, which creates lift perpendicular to the flow direction, usually forward, in the direction of motion. Drag force acts at the same time to resist motion against the direction of flow. This lift and drag combination acts to “anchor” the hand in the water, providing a somewhat stable “handle” over which the trunk is then pulled (Figure 19.1).
4. *Maximum force is attained by presenting as broad a surface as possible in the propulsive movements of the limbs and by exerting a backward pressure through as great a distance as possible, provided undesirable forces are not inadvertently introduced.* The full surface of the hand should be used in arm strokes. The hand, however, should not

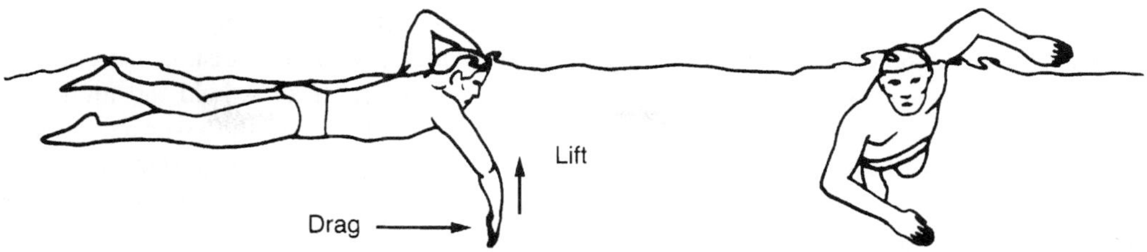

Figure 19.1 Drag and lift work together to "anchor" the hand during the pull phase of the front crawl.
Source: From *The Science of Swimming*, by James E. Counsilman. Copyright © 1968, pp. 61–65. Reprinted by permission of Prentice Hall, Englewood Cliffs, NJ.

enter the water so soon that it shortens the stroke unduly, nor pulled too far back.

5. *Momentum may be transferred from one body or part to another body or part as momentum is conserved.* If the breaststroker or backstroker checks the momentum of the arms at the end of the recovery, the momentum will be transferred to the body, forcing the head and body downward and thus setting up a bobbing stroke and additional resistance.
6. *The height of the body position in the water depends on the swimmer's buoyancy and speed of moving through the water.* The buoyancy of a swimmer is primarily determined by body composition and is not easily altered. Swimmers should not try to ride high in the water by raising the head or by pushing down, because each action will be followed by an opposite and equal reaction. However, it is possible to raise the legs somewhat by producing an efficient kick. The flutter kick contributes more to body position and stability than it does to forward propulsion.
7. *When a body is free in a fluid, movement of a part in one direction results in movement of the rest of the body in the opposite direction.* Swimming with the head out of the water, as in water polo, lifesaving, or synchronized swimming, causes the feet to drop. This position produces more frontal drag than the flat horizontal position and therefore requires more energy on the swimmer's part to overcome the additional resistance.
8. *A rapidly moving body in the water leaves a low-pressure area immediately behind it.* This creates a suction effect and tends to pull the body back. Although this backward pull (drag) cannot be entirely eliminated, it can be reduced by keeping the legs close together in the crawl strokes and during the glide phase of the resting strokes. Drag of this nature can also be reduced by maintaining a streamlined body position in the water.
9. *The more streamlined the body, the less the resistance to progress through the water.* Streamlining of the body can be accomplished by carrying the head so that the water level is near the hairline in prone strokes. The body should be parallel to the surface of the water with the buttocks just below the surface. In the flutter kick and the recovery portion of the resting strokes, the feet should be kept close together. In the same way, the hand should enter the water directly in front of or slightly inside the shoulder rather than to the outside.
10. *The drag on a body in any fluid increases approximately with the square of the velocity.* For this reason the recovery phase of the arm pull in breaststroke, sidestroke, or elementary backstroke and the entry of the recovery arm into the water in the crawl

stroke and the butterfly stroke should not be rushed. In these instances, the arm is moving in a direction opposite that which produces forward motion in the swimmer. A rapid recovery or entry will serve to increase the drag.

11. *The sudden or quick movement of a swimmer's body, or one of its parts, at the surface of the water tends to cause whirls and eddies. These create low-pressure areas that have a retarding effect on the swimmer.* The low-pressure areas can be reduced by slicing the hand into the water and by eliminating movements that do not contribute to forward progression. In the flutter kick, movements of the feet in the air do not contribute to the propulsion of the body; hence, the feet and legs should be kept just below the surface of the water.

Analysis of the Sprint Crawl

As an example of aquatic locomotion, the sprint crawl (Figure 19.2) has been chosen for analysis. The position of the head and trunk and the movement of the head in breathing are described briefly. The arm and leg strokes are described in somewhat greater detail, and their propulsive phases are analyzed anatomically.

The Head and Trunk

The head and trunk have three important functions in swimming, particularly in speed swimming. These are minimizing resistance, enabling the swimmer to breathe, and providing a stable anchorage for the arm and leg muscles to effect a maximum propulsive force. The position of the body is the key to reducing resistance. The body is as horizontal as possible, with the feet below the surface and the head breaking the water at hairline level. The flatter the body, the less drag there will be to decrease the swimmer's speed. The exact position of the body varies with the anatomical build and buoyancy of the individual, as well as with the speed of the stroke. The greater the buoyancy and speed, the higher the body will ride in the water. A common mistake is to lift the head too much. If the head is held too high or tipped back too far, it makes the swimmer's legs drop, causing a broader frontal surface and therefore more resistance. By static contraction of the rectus abdominis, the spine is held in a position of slight flexion—or at least of incomplete extension—and the pelvis in a position of slightly decreased inclination.

Lateral movements of the trunk will also increase the resistance to forward movements and should be minimized. Any circular movement of the arms or legs causes a countermovement in the rest of the body. A wide swing of the arms on recovery produces a lateral, opposite fishtail action of the legs. Lateral flexion of the head and neck also results in a counteraction. The turning of the head for inhaling must be accomplished with the least possible interference with the rhythm of the arm and leg action and with the progress of the body through the water. It is essential not to lift the head for breathing but rather to rotate it on its longitudinal axis while tucking the chin in close to the side of the neck. In this position the face appears to be resting on the bow wave, and the mouth is just above the surface of the water. After a quick inhalation, the face is again turned forward with the eyes in the horizontal plane and the nose and chin in the midsagittal plane of the body. Although breathing with every arm cycle is preferable in distance events, sprints are better swum with fewer breathing cycles because the turning of the head, even when done properly, causes additional resistance. This resistance is due primarily to the increased shoulder roll that occurs as the head is turned, making the stroke slightly asymmetrical.

To provide a firm base of attachment for the muscles of the arms and thighs, the trunk must be held steady. By the alternating action of the left and right oblique abdominals and spinal extensors, the spine and pelvis are stabilized against the pull of the shoulder and hip muscles. Thus they permit the latter to exert all their force on the limbs for the propulsive movements.

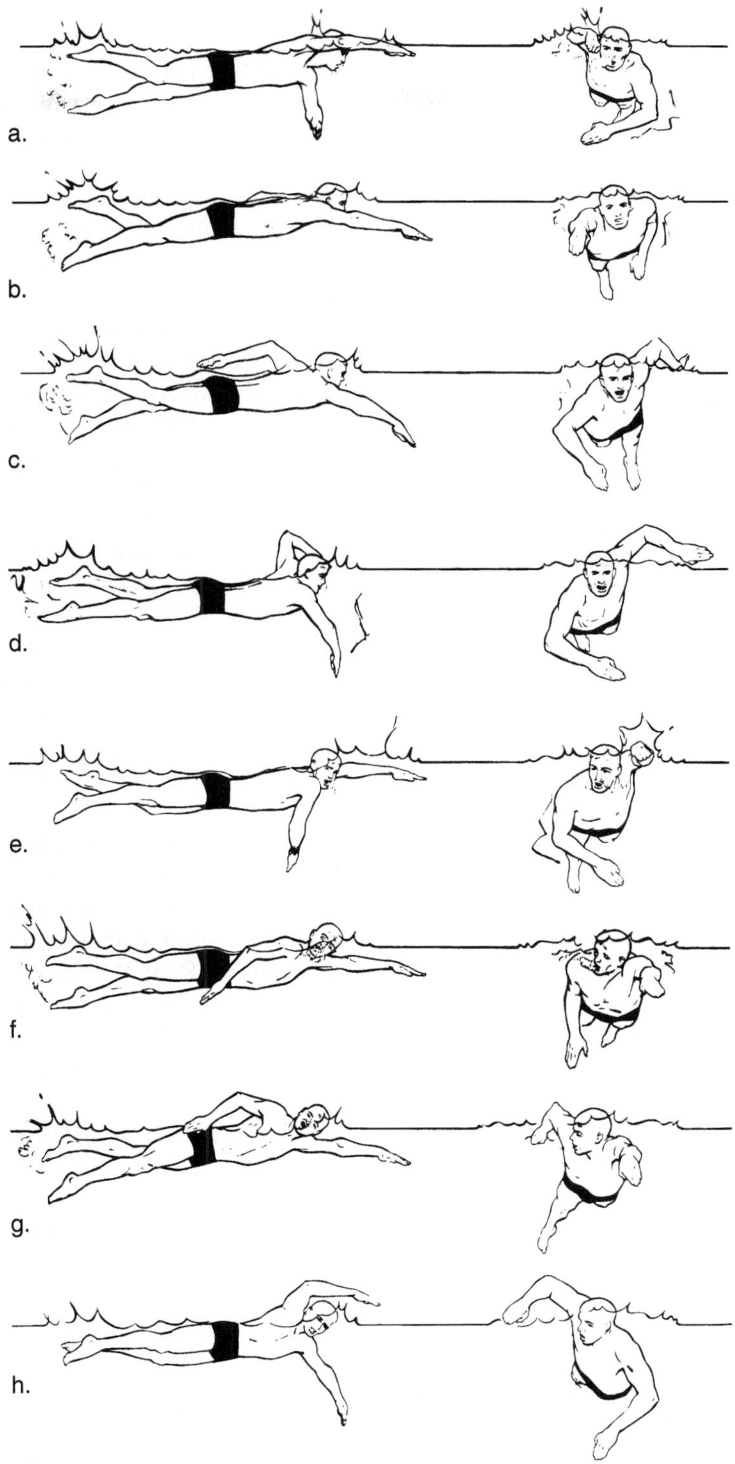

Figure 19.2 The crawl stroke. *Source:* From *The Science of Swimming,* by James E. Counsilman. Copyright © 1968, pp. 61–65. Reprinted by permission of Prentice Hall, Englewood Cliffs, NJ.

The Arm Stroke

Entry and support Because the arm stroke provides approximately 85% of the total power, the entry of the arm into the water should place it in the most advantageous position for exerting force that will be effective in driving the body forward. Its position on entry is with the forearm high and the elbow pointing to the side. The hand passes in front of the shoulder in preparation for the entry and then, reaching forward, it is driven forward and downward into the water directly in front of the shoulder. The elbow is slightly flexed at the beginning of the hand entry but extends during the entry. The brief moment between entry and the beginning of the chief propulsive action is known as the support phase, and its purpose is to keep the head and shoulders high in the water. The pressure of the forearm and hand is mostly downward and then backward, thus producing an upward and forward reactive force (Figure 19.2a, b).

Catch, pull, and push The moment at which the chief propulsive action changes from downward to backward constitutes the catch. The pull phase begins with the first backward movement of the hand. This occurs when the hand is 5 to 10 inches below the surface and involves a quick inward movement of the hand and arm that serves to bring the hand to a position in front of the axis of the body in such a way that the body weight is balanced above the arm. The upper arm is approximately vertical, a position that favors the large muscles (sternal portion of the pectoralis major and latissimus dorsi) for their task of pulling the arm downward and backward. Because the purpose of the stroke is to drive the body forward, it is essential to apply maximum force over the longest possible distance. This is best done by keeping the elbow high during the first part of the pull and by bending the elbow as the arm is pulled under the body (Figure 19.2c, d). The maximum bend occurs halfway through the pull, when the hand begins to push the water backward.

This elbow action assists in producing the S-curve, which allows for the creation of propulsive lift. Flexion at the elbow also reduces the moment arm of the upper extremity, reducing resistance to motion. In the pull phase the feel is as if the hand is being pushed backward through the water. In actuality, lift and drag act to stabilize the hand in the water. The body is then pulled forward over the relatively stationary hand.

The transition from pull to push occurs as the arm passes under the shoulder. The upper arm remains nearly vertical as the forearm gradually extends until it is in front of the hip, at which time the upper arm extends and the hand gives a quick push backward (Figure 19.2e, f). It would seem that the ideal direction of the swimmer's force should be directly backward for maximum forward horizontal movement. In actuality the path of the hand of most good swimmers is more like an inverted question mark. This apparent sculling motion constantly varies the angle between the surface of the hand and the direction of hand motion (angle of attack). The combination of drag forces and lift forces (see Bernouilli's principle, p. 318) that will be utilized for propulsion is extremely dependent on this angle of attack. By varying the angle of attack, the optimum lift and drag resultant for every position of the hand can be attained. This means that as the hand velocity direction shifts with the curvilinear path of the hand, the resultant of the drag and lift forces can still be maintained in line with the body's line of motion (Toussaint & Beck, 1992).

Brief anatomical analysis of propulsive phase of arm stroke Front crawl swimming is an excellent total body exercise. It has been estimated that at least 44 muscles act to produce the movements of the crawl. If all active muscles (antagonists, synergists, etc.) are considered, the estimate rises to 170 single muscles (Clarys & Cabri, 1993). For this reason, only the most active prime movers will be covered in this analysis (Table 19.1)

Release and recovery The elbow is now near the surface with the hand slightly lower and posterior to it and the palm facing mostly upward.

TABLE 19.1 Anatomical Analysis of the Propulsive Phase of the Arm Stroke

Joint	Joint Action	Segment Moved	Force for Movement	Muscles Active	Kind of Contraction
Shoulder joint	Extension Oblique adduction Medial rotation	Upper arm	Muscle	Posterior deltoid Latissimus dorsi Teres major Pectoralis major	Concentric
Shoulder girdle	Downward rotation Adduction	Scapula	Muscle	Rhomboids Pectoralis minor Trapezius	Concentric
Elbow	Flexion	Forearm	Muscle	Flexors	Concentric
Radioulnar	Pronation	Forearm	Muscle	Pronator teres Pronator quadratus	Concentric
Wrist	Held in midposition		Muscle	Flexor carpi radialis Flexor carpi ulnaris	Static
Fingers	Held in extension, adduction		Muscle	Flexors	Static

The pressure of the forearm and hand now being relaxed, the elbow and shoulder are raised until the hand is out of the water. The elbow leaves the water first and swings forward and upward with the hand trailing behind it, moving from a position near the hip to a position in front of the shoulder, preparatory to a new entry (Figure 19.2g, h). The movement of the arm from release to the completion of recovery is continuous. It is important that no break occur because this would mean a loss of momentum and would necessitate an additional force for overcoming inertia, or at least for regaining the lost velocity.

As the elbow is brought forward, it remains above the level of the hand throughout the recovery and entry, with the forearm virtually horizontal as the arm moves forward past the shoulder and the hand in line with the forearm. Finally, as the hand passes the head, the arm reaches forward in preparation for the entry, the shoulder girdle remains high, the tip of the elbow is above shoulder level pointing to the side, and the forearm then points downward from the elbow with the wrist slightly flexed, the palm facing the water, and the fingers aiming forward and downward into the water. Individual differences in style in the arm recovery are likely to occur. These variations are most likely due to differences in shoulder range of motion. Unless such variations interfere with other aspects of the stroke, they are most likely insignificant (Table 19.2).

The Kick

Nature of movement The leg stroke most often used in the sprint crawl is the flutter kick. Whether or not it contributes to the propulsive force has been questioned. It is generally acknowledged that the primary role for the kick is that of a stabilizer and neutralizer, and that therefore its timing with respect to the arm's action is critical. In this stroke the legs are relatively close together as they alternate in an up-and-down movement, with the feet attaining a maximum stride of about 1 to 2 feet. The width of the kick depends on such factors as the swimmer's build and strength and the speed of the stroke. In both the upstroke and downstroke, the movement, described as whip-like or lashing, starts at the hip joint and progresses through the knees to the ankle and feet. Unlike the arms, whose movements alternate between propulsion and recovery, both phases of the leg stroke are

TABLE 19.2 Anatomicazl Analysis of the Recovery Phase of the Arm Stroke

Joint	Joint Action	Segment Moved	Force for Movement	Muscles Active	Kind of Contraction
Shoulder joint	Hyperextension followed by horizontal adduction	Upper arm	Muscle	Posterior deltoid Latissimus dorsi Teres major Pectoralis major Anterior deltoid Coracobrachialis Biceps	Concentric
Shoulder girdle	Slight elevation	Scapula	Muscle	Trapezius	Concentric
	Upward rotation Abduction			Pectoralis minor Serratus anterior	
Elbow	Extension	Forearm	Muscle	Triceps Anconeus	Concentric
Radioulnar	Pronation	Forearm	Muscle	Pronator teres Pronator quadratus	Concentric
Wrist and Fingers	Relaxed until slight extension of hand at end of phase		Muscle	Extensor carpi ulnaris Extensor carpi radialis brevis Extensor digitorum indices Pollicis longus Intrinsic hand muscles	Concentric

propulsive, if anything. Flexibility in the ankles is important in the kick, and those with a greater range of plantar flexion have an advantage. In the downstroke the thrust is downward and backward and, in the upstroke, upward and backward.

Downstroke The downstroke begins with a downward drive of the thigh. The thigh flexes only slightly, and the knee, which was in a position of flexion at the completion of the upstroke, extends completely by the end of the downward movement. The ankle and foot remain in plantar flexion, probably being held in this position by the pressure of the water against the dorsal surface of the foot (Figure 19.2a, b). It seems likely that the dorsiflexors contract statically to stabilize the foot against this pressure. Throughout the downstroke the foot remains in a slight toeing-in position. The heels should not be allowed to drift apart in an attempt to facilitate the intoeing, because this would involve rotation of the thigh and would cut down on the driving power of the limb, as well as increase the form drag (Table 19.3).

Upstroke At the completion of the downstroke the thigh is in a position of slight flexion, the knee is completely extended, and the ankle is incompletely plantar flexed. The upstroke begins with thigh extension. Slight knee flexion develops near the end of the stroke at the same time the opposite leg is finishing the downstroke. The movements of the three major segments of the

TABLE 19.3 Anatomical Analysis of the Kick Downstroke

Joint	Joint Action	Segment Moved	Force for Movement	Muscles Active	Kind of Contraction
Hip joint	Partial flexion	Thigh	Muscle	Iliopsoas Tensor fasciae latae Pectineus Sartorius Gracilis	Concentric
Knee joint	Passive flexion due to water pressure until bottom of stroke, then forceful extension	Shank	Muscle	Quadriceps femoris	Concentric
Ankle joint	Incomplete plantar flexion probably caused by water pressure, stabilized by muscle contraction		Muscle	Tibialis anterior Peroneus tertius Extensor digitorum and hallucis longus	Static
Tarsal joints	Adduction Inversion	Foot	Muscle	Tibialis posterior Tibialis anterior Flexor digitorum and hallucis longus	Concentric

lower extremity are forceful in the upstroke but are under such good control that the foot stops just below the surface of the water. To break through the surface constitutes a major error, as it causes an immediate reduction in propulsive force (Figure 19.2d–f; Table 19.4).

Stroke Coordination

The front crawl consists of a six-beat leg kick for every complete arm cycle. This would imply that three leg beats occur for each arm. This uneven number of leg motions on each arm stroke acts to maintain the body in balance around the vertical axis while still allowing for the body roll necessary for breathing. Breathing occurs on one side of the body as the arm is lifted from the water. The head is turned with the chin tucked toward the axilla. The breath should be only an intake of air. Exhalation occurs underwater.

The arms would seem to be cycling in 180-degree opposition to each other. As one arm is in the entry and catch phase of the stroke, the opposite arm will be in release and recovery. In fact, this is true in a coordination currently referred to as opposition. As swim velocity increases, however, it is likely that the arm cycles will move closer together so that as one arm finishes the pull and moves to the push, the opposite arm is beginning the entry and catch phase. This coordination puts both hands in the water simultaneously for a brief instant. In the recreational swimmer, opposition coordination is the most common (Chollet et al., 2000; Seifert et al., 2005).

Additional Factors

Other factors of importance to the crawl stroke swimmer and to the coach are the rhythm of the stroke as a whole, the relaxation of the body, and the flexibility of the joints, particularly of

TABLE 19.4 Anatomical Analysis of the Kick Upstroke

Joint	Joint Action	Segment Moved	Force for Movement	Muscles Active	Kind of Contraction
Hip joint	Strong extension	Thigh	Muscle	Hamstrings Gluteus maximus	Concentric
Knee joint	Slight flexion against resistance	Shank	Muscle	Hamstrings Sartorius Gracilis Popliteus Gastrocnemius	Concentric
Ankle joint	Plantar flexion	Foot	Muscle	Gastrocnemius Soleus Peroneus longus and brevis Tibialis posterior Flexor digitorum and hallucis longus	Concentric
Tarsal joints	Plantar flexion	Foot	Muscle	Tibialis posterior Peroneus longus and brevis Flexor digitorum and hallucis longus	Concentric

the shoulders and ankles. Of these, possibly the last named is of greatest interest to the kinesiologist. The serious swimmer will want to know how to increase the range of motion in shoulder joints and ankles—that is, how to stretch the pectorals and anterior ligaments of the shoulders and how to gain greater plantar flexion of the feet. The kinesiology student should be able to originate several exercises that would accomplish this. One method that is frequently used is dry land exercise using various forms of elastic resistance.

Sample Analysis of a Common Fault in the Crawl Stroke

A **rigid flutter kick** is a common fault of beginners learning the standard crawl stroke. It is included in this text as an example of how the kinesiologist can analyze a common fault and use the analysis as a basis for making constructive suggestions in teaching.

Description In the rigid flutter kick the movement is one of alternate flexion and extension of the entire lower extremity, with the movement confined to the hip joint instead of being transmitted successively through the thigh to the knee joint and then through the leg to the ankle and foot. The knee joints are fully extended throughout the kick, and the feet and ankles are held in an unchanging position of plantar flexion, the exact degree of this flexion varying with individuals. This results in a narrower kick. A rigid flutter kick is obviously less efficient than the correct kick. In brief, the rigid flutter kick deviates from the correct form in that there is an absence of knee and ankle flexion, an absence of relaxation at the end of the downkick or beginning of the upkick, and an absence of fishtail action of the sole of the foot against the water.

Anatomical analysis In the correct downkick, the upward pressure of the water against the lower leg causes flexion at the knee. In the rigid kick, however, this is prevented by the tension of the quadriceps extensors. Normally, the slight flexion at the knee is followed by extension during the course of the downstroke but, when the knee is already rigidly extended, this extension cannot take place. Similarly, the reduction of the plantar flexion that should take place at the end of the downstroke fails to occur because of the continuous contraction of the plantar flexor muscles (soleus, peroneus longus and brevis, tibialis posterior, flexor digitorum longus, and flexor hallucis longus).

In the upstroke the tension of the quadriceps extensors again prevents the slight knee flexion that occurs when the kick is correctly performed (see Figure 19.2). Throughout the stroke the extensors of the lower back and the abdominal muscles contract to stabilize the pelvis against the pull of the hip flexors and extensors. Normally they relax momentarily just before the legs reverse their direction. The tension in the muscles of the lower extremities spreads to these, however, and the excess tension of these muscles causes interference with the action of the diaphragm. This, in turn, results in less efficient breathing and is an additional factor in causing fatigue.

Mechanical analysis The propulsive component of force that drives the body forward is that which pushes the water directly backward. In the downstroke this is provided most effectively by the instep of the foot, and in the upstroke, by the sole. The amount of propulsive force developed depends on the angle at which the instep and the sole of the foot are held with respect to the surface of the water. In the upstroke the best angle for the sole of the foot is possible only when the knee is flexed. In the rigid kick the knee is straight, and the sole of the foot is therefore not in the best position for providing propulsive force.

In the correct form each limb acts as a series of levers—thigh, lower leg, and foot—but in the rigid kick each limb acts as one long lever with the force arm extending from the distal attachments of the hip flexors and extensors to the axis of the hip joint. The resistance arm consists of the entire length of the lever from the instep or from the sole of the foot to the hip joint. The force acting on this lever comes solely from the muscles of the hip joints. The muscles of the knee and ankle do not contribute to the motion of this lever, but when the limb is used as a series of levers, they provide additional force. Inertia must be overcome with each reversal of direction in the kick. Because, in the rigid flutter kick, the stroke is shorter and faster than it should be, the muscles of the hip joint, which have the double task of overcoming both the inertia of the limb and the resistance of the water, are overburdened. They must work harder and faster to meet the demands made on them by the frequent changes of direction and the increased resistance of the water due to the speed of movement. Ordinarily the upstroke has an advantage over the downstroke because, when the stroke is performed correctly, the sole of the foot is in a better position to push back against the water than is the instep on the downstroke. In the rigid kick, this advantage is lost.

Teaching suggestions The rigid crawl flutter kick is associated with undue tension of the quadriceps extensors at the knee joint, and of the plantar flexors at the ankle joint during the changes of direction in both the downkick and the upkick. There may also be unnecessary tension of the abdominal muscles and the spinal extensors. Because the kick is inefficient, it is carried on at a faster rate and through a narrower arc than would be the correct kick for the individual swimmer. Conversely, a rapid, narrow kick tends to be a rigid kick. These factors aid in its recognition. In teaching the kick, it would seem the best procedure is to insist on a slow, deep kick in the student's first attempts, and to increase the rhythm gradually to the desired rate. Motivation should not be directed toward speed in the performance of the "kick glide" in the teaching progression. Also, one should not emphasize that the legs be held straight at the knees. The emphasis should be put on the increased action at the hips and at the ankles.

Aquatic Locomotion: Rowing, Canoeing, and Kayaking

Boating in its various forms has become a popular recreational activity for many people. In many parts of the world rowing, canoeing, and kayaking are among the most highly regarded of the Olympic sports. Activities that engage people in movement activities are always worthy of study, even when human power is used to produce locomotion of some other object, such as a boat. On the whole, the principles that apply to swimming apply also to rowing, canoeing, and kayaking. This is particularly obvious in canoeing and kayaking because the paddle is used in much the same way as are the arms in swimming. The use of the oars in rowing is more limited because they must be kept in the oarlocks at all times.

Rowing

In rowing, whether for pleasure or as part of a competitive crew, much of the propulsive force is generated by the legs. The analysis presented in Chapter 16 provides an overview of the rowing motion. The rowing stroke can be broken down into two distinct phases: the pull phase and the recovery phase. The force applied to the water by the oar blade during the pull phase is a primary determinant of the distance traveled by the boat during the stroke. The pull is initiated through extension of the flexed lower extremities in a pushlike motion, followed by trunk extension and then upper extremity pull.

In the recovery phase the oar blade is lifted clear of the water by downward pressure on the grip, or inboard, end of the oar. The oar is then feathered, or rotated, so that the blade slices through the air parallel to the airflow. During recovery the legs and trunk are flexed and the upper arms are horizontally adducted and elbows extended, pushing the oar into position for the next stroke (Figure 19.3). In competitive rowing, the motion in the lower extremities is enhanced through the use of a sliding seat.

In rowing, the oars are held to the gunwale (top edge) of the boat by an oarlock. This oarlock provides an axis of rotation for the oar such that forward motion of the inboard end of the oar results in backward motion of the oar blade and vice versa. For this reason, rowers row with their backs to the direction of forward motion.

Canoeing

The situation is somewhat different in canoeing. The paddle in canoeing is held in both hands, free of external support. The canoe paddle stroke is performed using primarily the arms, shoulders, and trunk with the lower body kept relatively quiet. The paddler in a canoe faces in the direction of canoe motion. The stroke with the paddle involves reaching out in either a forward or a sideward direction and pulling the paddle blade through the water.

In paddling, as in the arm movement of the crawl stroke, too much force at the beginning of the stroke has too great a downward component, and hence too great a lifting effect. Conversely, too much force at the end of the stroke has too great an upward component, and hence a depressing effect on the canoe. To make the canoe move smoothly in a horizontal direction without unnecessary bobbing up and down, it is essential to reduce these two components to a minimum and to emphasize the backward movement of the blade.

The techniques of steering the canoe are based on this same principle (Figure 19.4). One paddler paddling from the center of the canoe

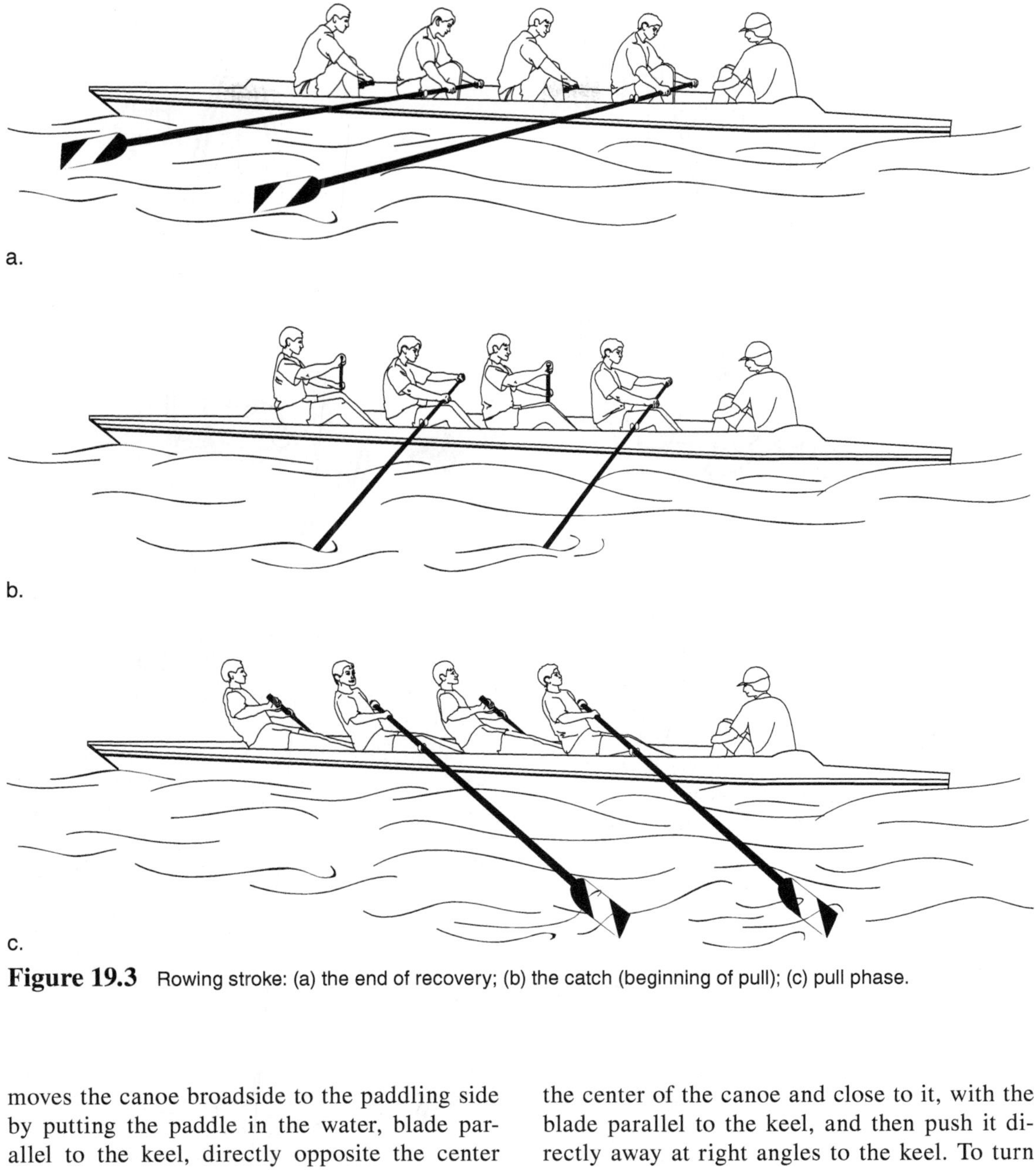

Figure 19.3 Rowing stroke: (a) the end of recovery; (b) the catch (beginning of pull); (c) pull phase.

moves the canoe broadside to the paddling side by putting the paddle in the water, blade parallel to the keel, directly opposite the center of the canoe, and as far out as can be reached conveniently and safely. The paddler then draws the blade squarely toward the canoe at right angles to the keel of the canoe. To move broadside away from the paddling side, the paddler would slice the blade into the water opposite the center of the canoe and close to it, with the blade parallel to the keel, and then push it directly away at right angles to the keel. To turn the canoe, the paddler would have to reach either forward or backward and press the blade toward or away from the canoe at a point as far from the canoe's center of buoyancy as can be reached conveniently. A drawing stroke nearer the bow would make the canoe turn toward the

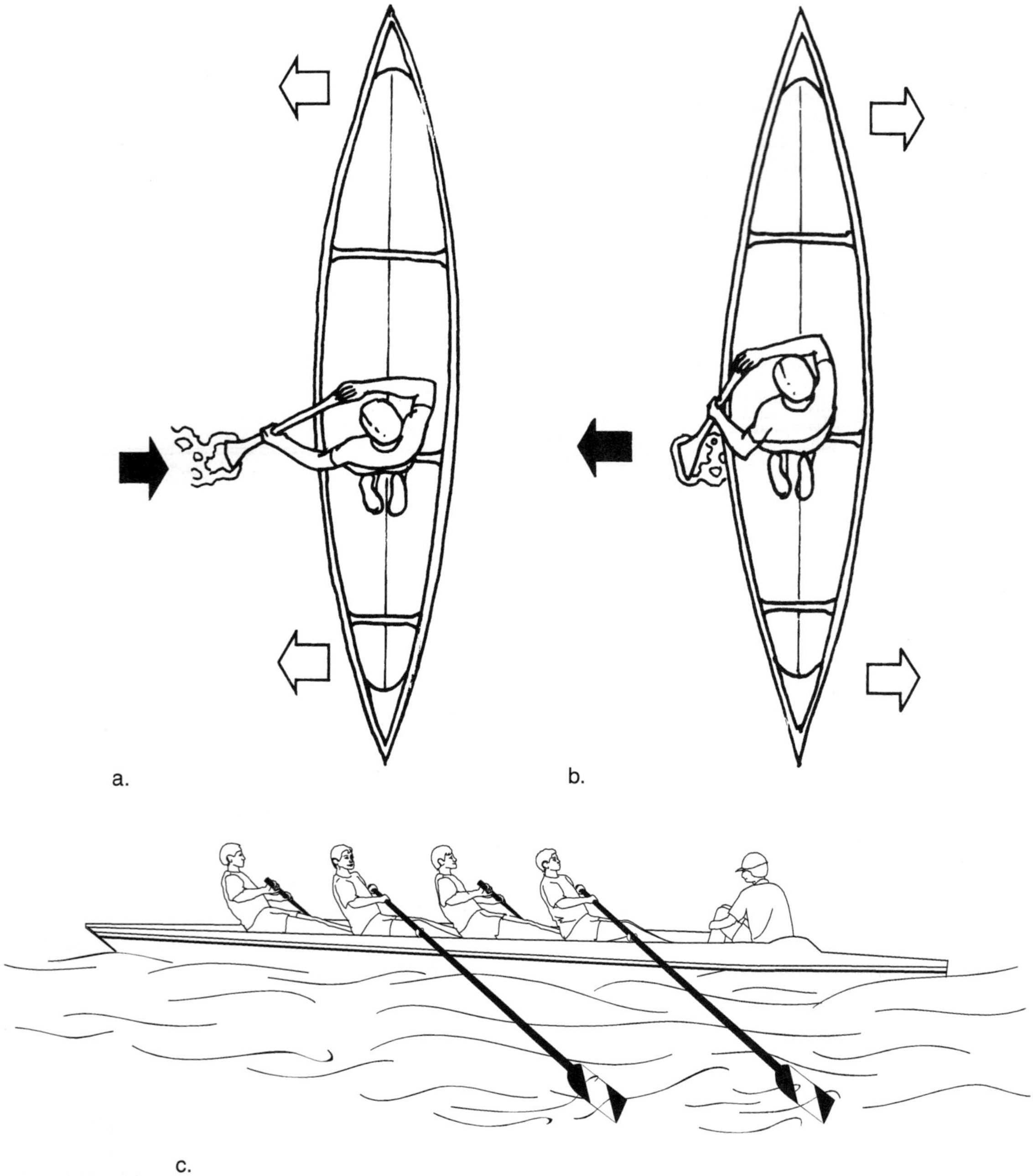

Figure 19.4 Movement in a canoe is in the direction opposite to that in which the force is applied. (a) Movement toward the paddling side occurs when the paddle is *drawn toward* the center of thw canoe. (b) The canoe moves away from lhe paddling side when the paddle is *pushed away* from the canoe. (c) The sweep stroke pushes the bow away from the paddling side and draws the stern toward it, causing the canoe to move forward in a sweeping turn away from the paddling side. (Black arrows indicate the path of the paddle, and white affows indicate the path of the canoe.)

paddling side; a drawing stroke nearer the stern would make the canoe turn away from the paddling side. (The direction taken by the canoe as a whole is stated in terms of the bow. As the stern of the canoe moves toward the paddling side, the bow moves away from it.) Steering a canoe is logical and simple when one remembers the principle that movement occurs in the direction opposite to that in which the force is applied and, at the same time, remembers that a canoe tends to rotate about its center of buoyancy when force is applied at any point other than one in line with this center.

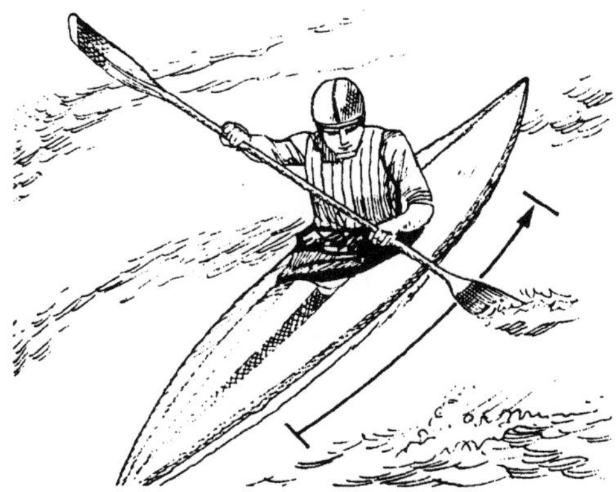

Figure 19.5 The kayak paddle stroke. Courtesy of the American Red Cross. All rights reserved in all countries.

Kayaking

The kayak is similar to the canoe. The kayak rides lower in the water than either the rowboat or the canoe and has covered decks rather than an open hull. Kayaks are often used in rough water such as oceans and whitewater rivers. A key difference between kayaks and other small craft is the use of a double-bladed paddle. The blades of this paddle are set perpendicular to one another so that the wrist and arm motion involved in the propulsion phase of the stroke on one side will cause the blade on the opposite side to feather during recovery. Using this paddle, the kayaker can effectively stroke on both sides of the boat in a cyclic fashion. While one blade of the paddle is in the recovery phase, the other blade is pulling. This continuous-stroke cycle eliminates the glide phase that occurs in other small craft during recovery so that little forward momentum is lost between strokes (Figure 19.5).

Because the kayak is long and slender, it is less stable in the water than the canoe, the rowing shell, or the rowboat. To increase stability, the kayaker sits low in the bottom of the boat with the legs extended forward, knees slightly flexed, and feet braced on a rib of the boat. The paddle stroke is produced primarily by the upper body in a continuous motion. It is important that the motion be continuous and that both sides of the body exert identical forces. Unequal forces between the two paddles cause the kayak to turn (unbalanced forces produce rotation). Varying the force applied by the two blades is how the direction of the kayak is controlled. The primary active muscles are those of the shoulder region, namely the upper trapezius, latissimus dorsi, rhomboid major, serratus anterior, and supraspinatus (Trevithick et al., 2007).

REFERENCES AND SELECTED READINGS

Berger, M. A. M., Hollander, A. P., & de Groot, G. (1999). Determining propulsive force in front crawl swimming: A comparison of two methods. *Journal of Sports Sciences,* 17, 97–105.

Chatard, J. C., & Wilson, B. (2008). Effect of cost of fastskin suits on performance, drag, and energy cost of swimming. *Medicine and Science Sports Exercise,* 40(6), 1149–1154.

Chollet, D., Chalies, S., & Chatard, J. C. (2000). A new index of coordination for the crawl: Description and usefulness. *International Journal of Sports Medicine,* 21(1), 54–59.

Chollet, D., Seifert, L., Leblanc, H., Boulesteix, L., & Carter, M. (2004). Evaluation of arm-leg coordination in flat breaststroke. *International Journal of Sports Medicine,* 25(7), 486–495.

Clarys, J. P., & Cabri, J. (1993). Electromyography and the study of sports movements: A review. *Journal of Sports Sciences,* 11, 379–448.

Laffite, L. P., Vilas-Boas, J. P., Demarle, A., Silva, J., Fernandes, R., & Billat, V. L. (2004). Changes in physiological and stroke parameters during a maximal 400-m free swimming test in elite swimmers. *Canadian Journal of Applied Physiology,* 29 *Suppl,* S17–S31.

Leblanc, H., Seifert, L., Baudry, L., & Chollet, D. (2005). Arm-leg coordination in flat breaststroke: A comparative study between elite and nonelite swimmers. *International Journal of Sports Medicine,* 26(9), 787–97.

Lerda, R., & Cardelli, C. (2003). Breathing and propelling in crawl as a function of skill and swim velocity. *International Journal of Sports Medicine,* 24(1), 75–80.

Meyer, J. (2003). Forget the "death grip": The proper push-pull technique, combined with torso rotation, will add efficiency to your stroke. *Canoe and Kayak* (Kirkland, WA), 31(3), 41.

Mollendorf, J. C., Termin, A. C., II, Oppenheim E., & Pendergast, D. R. (2004). Effect of swim suit design on passive drag. *Medicine and Science in Sports and Exercise,* 36(6), 1029–1035.

Potdevin, F., Bril, B., Sidney, M., & Pelayo, P. (2006). Stroke frequency and arm coordination in front crawl swimming. *International Journal of Sports Medicine,* 27(3), 193–198.

Psycharakis, S. G., & Sanders, R. H. (2010). Body roll in swimming: A review. *Journal of Sports Sciences,* 28(3), 229–236.

Salins, S. (2004). Sit up, reach up, choke up, finish up: Follow these pointers and get back to being a more powerful paddler this season. *Canoe and Kayak* (Kirkland, WA), 32(1), 35.

Seifert, L., Boulesteix, L., Carter, M., & Chollet, D. (2005). The spatial-temporal and coordinative structures in elite male 100-m front crawl swimmers. *International Journal of Sports Medicine,* 26(4), 286–293.

Seifert, L., Chollet, D., & Bardy, B. G. (2004). Effect of swimming velocity on arm coordination in the front crawl: A dynamic analysis. *Journal of Sports Sciences,* 22(7), 651–660.

Soper, C., & Hume, P. A. (2004). Towards an ideal rowing technique for performance: The contributions of biomechanics. *Sports Medicine,* 34, 825–848.

Toussaint, H. M., & Beck, P. J. (1992). Biomechanics of competitive front crawl swimming. *Sports Medicine,* 13, 8–24.

Trevithick, B. A., Ginn, K. A., Halaki, M., & Balnave, R. (2007). Shoulder muscle recruitment patterns during a kayak stroke performed on a paddling ergometer. *Journal of Electromyographic Kinesiology,* 17(1), 74–79.

Vennell, R., Pease, D., & Wilson, B. (2006). Wave drag on human swimmers. *Journal of Biomechanics,* 39(4), 664–671.

Yenai, T. (2003). Stroke frequency in front crawl: Its mechanical link to the fluid forces required in non-propulsive direction. *Journal of Biomechanics,* 36(1), 53–62.

Yenai, T. (2004). Buoyance is the primary source of generating bodyroll in front-crawl swimming. *Journal of Biomechanics,* 37(5), 605–612.

LABORATORY EXPERIENCES

1. Do the arm movement of the crawl stroke and deliberately press hard with the hand as soon as it enters the water. At the end of the stroke, instead of taking the hand out of the water at the proper time, continue the movement of the arm until the hand has pressed upward against the water. What is the effect of these two errors on the body?
2. Perform a kinesiological analysis of any of the standard strokes, such as the breast, side, elementary back, back crawl. Either observe or

practice the stroke before analyzing it. Use the outline for a kinesiological analysis described in Chapter 1.

3. Analyze other forms of aquatic locomotion, such as paddling and rowing. Either observe or practice each before analyzing it.
4. A qualified swimmer should perform this demonstration. Try to tip a floating canoe from each of the following positions:
   a. Lying supine on the bottom with arms at the side of the body and legs together.
   b. Sitting on the bottom with legs spread, arms at side of body.
   c. Kneeling in the center of the canoe, hands on gunwales.
   d. Sitting on center thwart, hands on gunwales.

   Explain your results for each of these attempts.
5. Analyze the following common faults kinesiologically and suggest coaching points for avoiding or correcting each fault: too wide a pull with the arms in the breaststroke; a short, choppy stroke in paddling; "catching a crab" in rowing (crew style).

CHAPTER

20

Locomotion: When Suspended and Free of Support

OUTLINE

- ***Suspension Activities***
  - Principles Related to Hanging and Hand-Traveling Activities
  - Principles Related to Swinging Movements
  - Suspension Analysis Example
- ***Nonsupport Activities***
  - Principles Related to Nonsupport Activities
  - Nonsupport Analysis Example
  - Free Fall
  - Weightlessness
- ***Laboratory Experiences***

OBJECTIVES

At the conclusion of this chapter, the student should be able to:

1. Explain how each of the following influences the action of swinging bodies: weight of the body, length of the pendulum, angular momentum, potential–kinetic energy, centripetal–centrifugal force, and friction.
2. Describe how to initiate pendular action, increase the height of a swing, alter the period, change grips, and dismount safely.
3. Explain how each of the following influences the flight path of unsupported bodies: angle of projection, vertical velocity, gravity, and angular momentum.
4. Describe how to initiate and control rotation of unsupported bodies.
5. Analyze the performance of a suspension and a nonsupport movement, following the outline for kinesiological analysis described in Chapter 1.

SUSPENSION ACTIVITIES

Climbing, hanging, swinging, and other suspension activities were more commonly engaged in by our early ancestors than by members of more recent generations. The modern version of these brachial activities is seen in the trapeze activities of the aerial artist at the circus, in gymnastics events on the high bar, parallel bars, uneven bars, and rings, and in various forms of hanging on ladders and ropes in the gymnasium and on the playground. Success in suspension activities depends on considerable strength and endurance, particularly of the hand, arm, and shoulder musculature, and the ability to adjust body positions to counteract or take advantage of the forces acting on the body (Figure 20.1). Ladder, rope or rock climbing, and brachial locomotion are modifications of locomotion. Where swinging movements of a suspended body are involved, the principles of a pendulum, angular momentum, and centripetal–centrifugal forces are major considerations.

Principles Related to Hanging and Hand-Traveling Activities

1. *In hanging activities the muscles of the arm and shoulder girdle must contract to protect the joints.* The pull of the body's weight puts stress on the joints by tending to separate them.
2. *Hand traveling is a locomotor pattern governed by the principle of action and reaction.* As in walking, force applied against a supporting surface in one direction causes the body to move in the opposite direction. Hand traveling sideward on a bar or rail without swinging is achieved by alternately moving one hand away from the other hand and then moving the second hand toward the first. As the first hand moves, the second hand pushes laterally against the apparatus. Both hands share the weight equally for a moment, then the second hand is released and brought toward the first hand while the first hand is pulling laterally on the apparatus.
3. *The action used in hand-climbing activities is essentially a pull-up action.* In rope climbing, for instance, either with or without the use of the legs, the body is raised through a forceful pull-up action of the arms. The rock climber uses a similar motion to advance up the rock face. The gymnast using a kip motion to mount a bar or the rings uses this same pull-up action to raise the body toward the hands. This action is then often converted to a push-up type of motion, ending in a straight-arm support position.

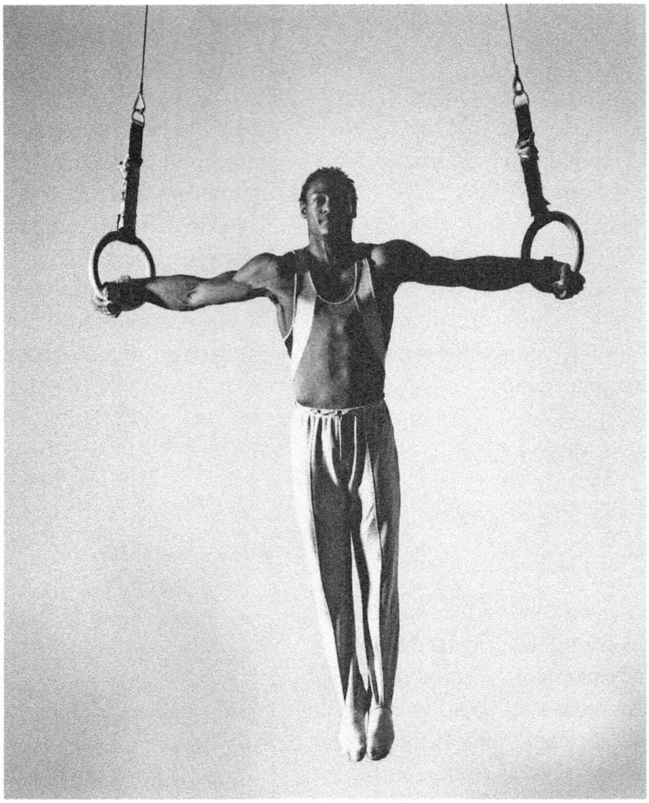

Figure 20.1 Movement of the body in suspension. This maneuver on the still rings illustrates the need for good muscular development in the shoulders.

4. *In accord with Newton's Law of Inertia, sequential hand-support movements should be continuous. The momentum of one action contributes to the next action.* In the kip movement of the gymnast, there should be no pause between the pulling phase and the pushing phase of the hands and arms. Similarly, the rock climber tries to use the motion produced by the upward pull of one arm to contribute momentum to the next upward pull.

Principles Related to Swinging Movements

1. *The movement of a pendulum is produced by the force of gravity.* This statement presupposes a starting position in which potential energy is present. In other words, the pendulum must be moved from its resting position before the force of gravity can make it swing downward.

The initial problem of the child on the swing and of the gymnast on the rings is that of being given potential energy. Without the help of an assistant, the swinger must find a way to be put into a position with potential energy. This is usually done in one of three ways. The performer may move the apparatus to some position other than its normal position of rest before being suspended (i.e., the swing is pulled back and up); the performer may initiate the swing with a push of the feet against the floor or with small running steps; or a pumping action may be used to get started. For the gymnast swinging on the rings, the last alternative involves bending the legs up in front of the body and then extending them as high as possible. The range of the arc of motion may be increased by the repetition of this procedure on the forward-upward phase of the swing. The child in the swing accomplishes the same result by inclining the trunk backward and raising the feet forward while pulling the ropes toward the body and pressing forward against the seat.

2. *As the pendulum swings downward, gravity causes its speed to increase; as it swings upward, gravity counteracts its speed, diminishing it until the zero point is reached.* Hence the pendulum's speed is greatest at the bottom of the arc and least (zero) at each end of the arc.

   Caution must be exercised to maintain a firm grip on the supporting surface (rings, bar, or ropes), particularly at the bottom of the swing where the tendency to fly off is the greatest.

3. *The upward movement of a pendulum is brought about by the momentum developed in the downward movement.* The swinging body moves through an arc, first in one direction and then in the reverse direction (one-half the arc's distance is called the *amplitude*). Thus it undergoes partial rotation about a center of motion. Because this rotation takes place in a vertical plane, the influence of gravitational pull must be taken into consideration. Whereas the force of gravity *produces* the downward swing, it *opposes* the upward swing. Nevertheless, it is indirectly responsible for the latter, inasmuch as the upward swing is caused by the momentum that was built up in the preceding downward swing.

   This relationship is especially important in skills performed in gymnastics when long, swinging actions are involved. The higher the position from which the downswing is initiated, the higher will be the upswing. The range of a swing depends on the height from which the movement is initiated.

4. *The potential energy of the pendulum is greatest at the height of the swing and least at the bottom.* Conversely, kinetic energy is greatest at the bottom and zero at the top. In a perfect mechanical system, a pendulum would continue to swing with a constant amplitude with the required energy supplied by the perpetual conversion from potential to kinetic energy. Most of the potential energy is converted to kinetic energy in the downswing and reconverted on the upswing. Some is lost, however, to friction and air resistance, and a pendulum left to its own devices will gradually decrease in amplitude and stop.

   To make up for the lost mechanical energy, supplemental energy in the form of properly timed muscular action of the swinger must be used. Maximum repetitions of a pendulum left to its own devices will occur if the initial height is maximum and friction is minimized.

5. *The centripetal–centrifugal force in pendular movements increases as the mass or velocity increases and decreases as the radius increases* $\left(C_F = \frac{mv^2}{r}\right)$. The centripetal force is greatest at the bottom of the swing, where the velocity is the greatest, and decreases to zero at the height of the swing. However, bodies develop proportionately more centripetal force and need more strength to maintain a grasp and counteract the opposing centrifugal force than do those of less weight. When centripetal force ceases to act on a swinging performer, the body will obey Newton's first law and will fly off tangent to the arc of the swing at that instant.

   The grip must be the most secure at the bottom of the swing, where the tendency to fly off is the greatest. Centripetal force has been calculated to be four to five times body weight as the body swings under the bar in a giant swing. To resist the equal and opposite outward-pulling centrifugal force, strong hands and arms are essential. The bottom of the swing is the point where the beginner or the novice is most likely to lose contact with the bar.

Although actions requiring release and regrasp of a bar or ring should be done at the peak of the swing, the same is not always true of dismounts. Dismounts and cutaways should be timed to occur at a point where the tangent of the arc at the instant of release coincides with the desired line of flight.

6. *When a pendulum reaches the end of its arc, just before it reverses its direction, it reaches a zero point in velocity.* At this precise moment, the force of gravity is momentarily neutralized by the upward momentum.

   The performer can take advantage of this situation by using this moment to perform position changes such as changing grips, reversing direction, and performing dismounts and cutaways. A release move on the high bar is best executed if the grip is released and the regrasp occurs at the top of the swing, during the instantaneous period of weightlessness.

7. *The height of a swing may be increased by lengthening the radius of rotation on the downswing and decreasing it on the upswing* (Figure 20.2). Shortening the radius on the upswing decreases the moment of inertia and therefore increases the angular velocity. This occurs because the angular momentum is conserved and, because angular momentum equals $I\omega$, a decrease in I requires an increase in ω. The increased angular velocity is accompanied by an increase in kinetic energy, and consequently more height results. The increased height for the start of the downswing and the lengthened radius of rotation produce a gain in angular momentum on the downswing because gravity has a longer time to act on the body before it reaches the bottom of the swing. When the shortening of the radius occurs for the next upswing, the increased momentum is

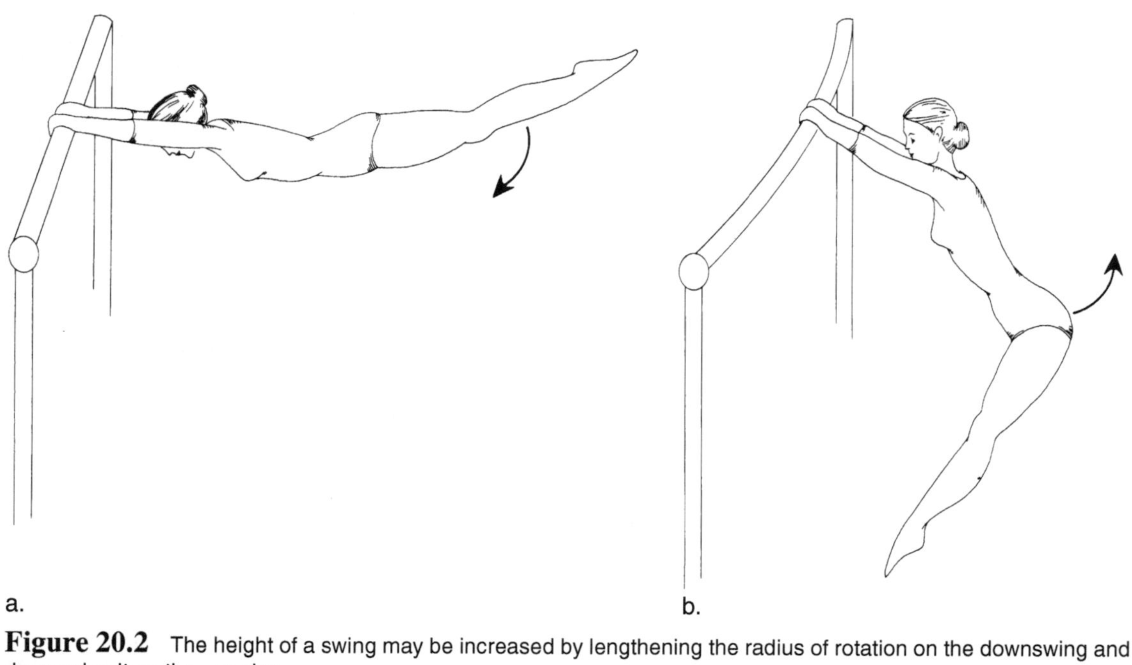

a. b.

Figure 20.2 The height of a swing may be increased by lengthening the radius of rotation on the downswing and decreasing it on the upswing.

conserved and, once again, there is an increase in angular velocity. The equation for angular momentum, $I\omega$, also shows that the greater the angular velocity on the downswing, the less the body has to be shortened to decrease I to reach its desired height on the upswing.

A swinging performer may shorten the radius of rotation by moving body parts toward the axis of rotation. This may be done by flexing at the hips, hunching the shoulders by depressing the shoulder girdle, or arching the back. A performer in the giant swing depresses the shoulder girdle and flexes at the hips on the upswing and may also arch the back slightly. In a circle from a front uprise, the head is thrown back to shorten the radius on the upswing.

8. *To increase height, the decrease in radius should be initiated at the moment the center of gravity of the body is directly under the axis of rotation.* In the movement of a pendulum, speed is greatest at the bottom of the arc. Shortening the radius at this point accelerates its angular velocity more than at any other position.

   In the backward hip circle on the uneven parallel bars, for example, the movement is started with the body extended and the hips on the bar. This gives the longest possible radius of rotation on the downswing. At the moment the legs pass under the hands (the axis of rotation), the hips are flexed to shorten the radius on the upswing, thereby decreasing the moment of inertia and increasing the angular velocity.

9. *The time taken by the pendulum to make a single round-trip excursion (known as its period) is related to the length of the pendulum.* The longer the pendulum, the more slowly it swings. Specifically, the period of the pendulum is proportional to the square root of its length.

   When the hands are the axis of rotation, such as in the preparatory moves for a giant swing, the period is longer than in swings about a hip axis or a knee axis.

10. *The period of the pendulum is not influenced by its weight.* A heavy body will swing no faster than a lighter one, and vice versa. This is consistent with the behavior of freely falling bodies.

    Trapeze artists take advantage of this principle. A performer swinging from one trapeze knows that an empty trapeze of the same length, swung from an opposite platform of the same height and at the same time as the trapeze artist's, will have the same period. Consequently the performer also knows that it is safe to let go of the original bar at the height of its swing and turn around in midair, because the empty bar will be right there to be grasped, also at the height of its swing.

11. *When a body consisting of two segments reaches the vertical with the proximal segment leading on the downswing, the distal segment will accelerate relative to the other segment and precede it into the upswing.* If, on the other hand, the distal segment reaches the vertical first, the reverse will occur. The distal segment will decelerate, and the proximal segment will lead into the upswing (Figure 20.3).

    Action at the bottom of a swing that forces the hips through in front of the feet increases the acceleration on the upswing owing to hip flexion in shortening the radius. Such swings are called "beat" swings. Beat swings are used to set up release–regrasp skills on apparatus such as the uneven and even parallel bars, the high bar, and the still rings.

12. *The rotation of the hands about a bar is opposed by frictional forces.* This accounts for some loss in swinging energy as it is converted into heat energy. Evidence of this is the appearance of friction blisters and skin irritations on a gymnast's hands. These friction forces tend to strengthen the gymnast's grip when the swing is in the direction the palms are facing and weaken it when the swing is in the reverse direction.

    Gymnasts reverse their grasps when the swing is reversed. This is usually done

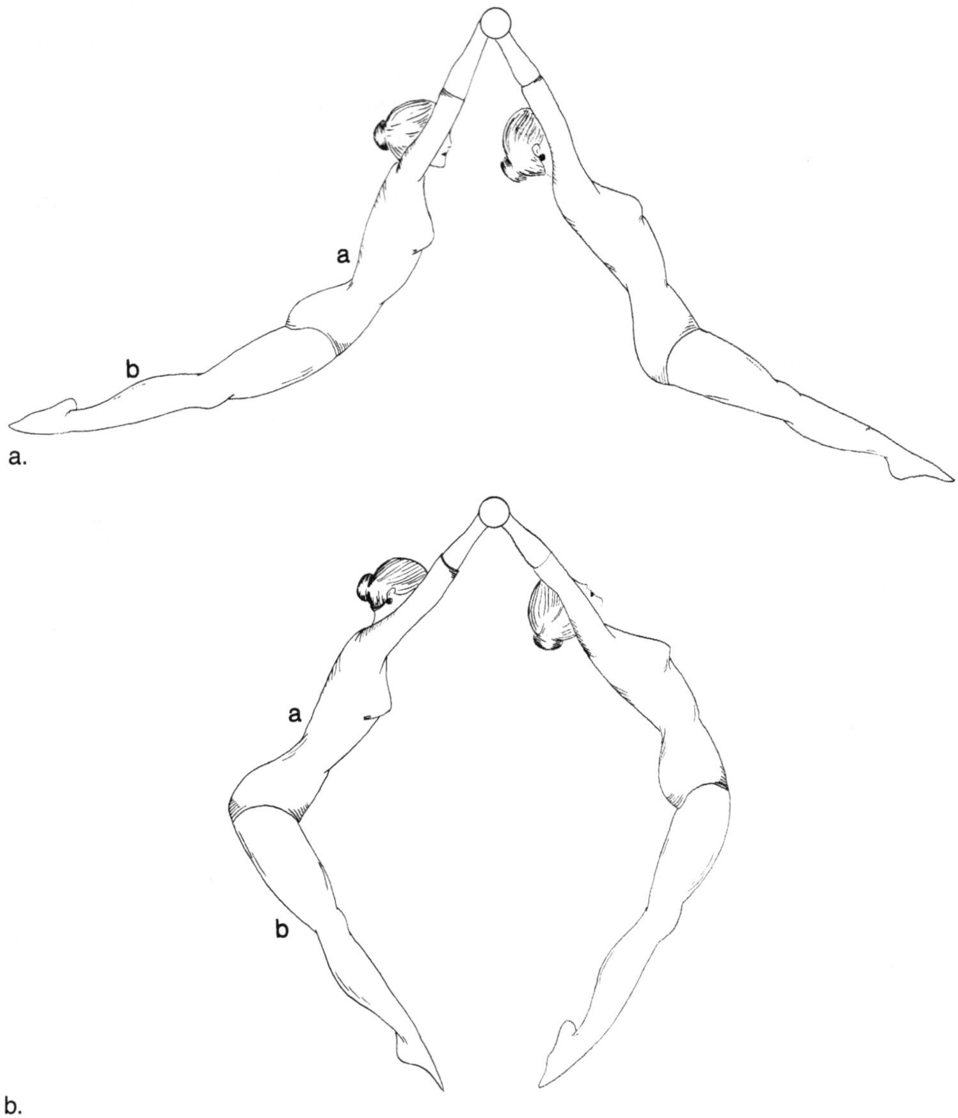

Figure 20.3 (a) Double pendulum swing. If segment *a* precedes segment *b* to the vertical, segment *b* accelerates and precedes *a* in the upswing. (b) When segment *b* precedes *a* to the vertical, *a* will lead into the upswing, but the whole pendulum decelerates.

at the peak of the swing at the point of "weightlessness," when the pressure on the hands is at a minimum. Gymnasts also sand the bar before each performance to ensure its smoothness and to minimize the friction on the hands.

13. *In all mounting exercises involving swinging, the center of gravity must be brought as near as possible to the center of rotation.* This is usually done when the center of gravity is directly under the bar on the downswing.

In the glide kip on the unevens, for instance, the performer swings the body forward and back, alternately flexing and extending to gain momentum. At the end of the glide the gymnast flexes fully at the hips so that the feet are near the bar. This sharp flexion increases the angular velocity by decreasing the moment of inertia. As the center of gravity passes under the bar on the downswing, the hips are extended vigorously. This movement raises the body and places the center of gravity close to the bar, thus further decreasing the moment of inertia and enabling the body to rotate until it is in a front support position with the center of gravity located at the fixed point of the grip.

14. *In support swings the center of gravity should be at the point of support.* Hip circles forward or backward require the center of gravity of the body to be close to the hand supports. In this position it takes less effort to keep the body against the bar while turning because the torque between the center of gravity of the body and the axis of rotation is kept at a minimum.

Suspension Analysis Example

Half-Turn Flying Hip Circle with Hecht Dismount—Uneven Parallel Bars

Gymnasts who perform on the uneven parallel bars have numerous combinations of movements from which to choose. Each routine starts with a mount and concludes with a dismount. In between the gymnast selects from a series of movements, including those characterized as circling, swinging, and flight elements. Within these broad categories turns around the long axis, grip changes, releases, and saltos should be included. Difficulty is rated from A to G. In the nine difficulty elements, each of the five element categories should be included. The moves shown in Figure 20.4 and described here are B-level moves (Fédération Internationale de Gymnastique, 2006). The gymnast starts in a handstand position on the high bar (a). As she begins to swing downward, she performs a half-twist so that she faces in the direction of the swing (b, c). At the bottom of the swing, she begins to flex at the hips in preparation for continuing in a back hip circle around the low bar (d, e). Toward the end of the hip circle, she extends at the hip joint and dismounts forward over the low bar in a move called a *Hecht* (f, g). She lands with her back to the bars (h).

Mechanical essentials In starting the downward swing from the handstand position, the gymnast pushes against the bar. Because of action–reaction, the bar pushes back in the opposite direction. The give of the bar adds to the reactive force and thus increases the total energy of the system. The push of the gymnast backward and the accompanying stretch increase the distance between the center of gravity and the axis of rotation and thus increase the torque on the downward swing. The time for gravity to act on the downward-swinging body is also increased. The half-twist is performed at the beginning of the downswing when the forces acting on the hands are minimal and the grip change can be accomplished with ease (Figure 20.4b). At the bottom of the swing the gymnast flexes at the hips, thus shortening the radius of rotation and increasing her angular velocity on the upswing. This piked position also enables her to "wrap" around the low bar as she moves into the backward hip circle (Figure 20.4d). There should be no pause between one movement and the next. Any slowing down would require more energy to pick up again (Law of Inertia) and fluidity would be lost. As the gymnast's hands leave the high bar, she pushes up and forward, causing the reactive force to add to the downward trunk rotation (Figure 20.4e).

The hip circle should be accomplished with the hips close to the bar so that the center of gravity is near the axis of rotation. Otherwise, centrifugal force would tend to pull the body away from the bar. Toward the completion of the hip circle, the gymnast forcefully extends by lifting the upper trunk and arms forward and upward (Figure 20.4f). This action causes several things

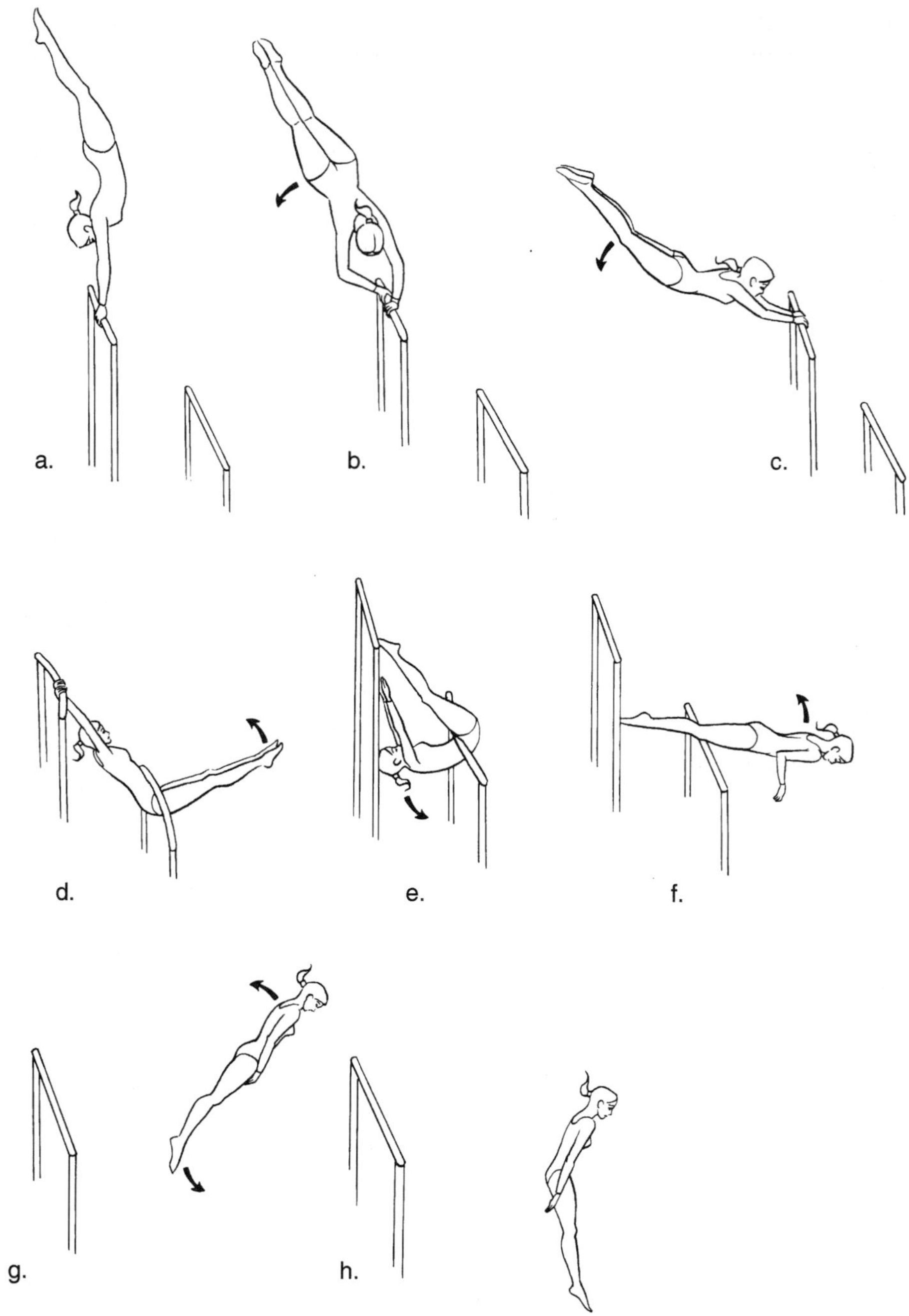

Figure 20.4 Half-turn flying hip circle with Hecht dismount.

to happen. In reaction, the legs also extend so that the whole body is straight. The moment of inertia about the transverse axis is increased, and the rate of rotation decreases. The body pushes down and back against the bar, causing the bar to push the body forward and up. All of this results in the body rotating up and away from the bar for the dismount. Once the body has left the bar, the back should be arched to again decrease the radius slightly and aid in the rotation of the body, allowing the feet to move slightly ahead of the center of gravity at the moment of landing (Figure 20.4h). The success of the hecht dismount depends on sufficient angular momentum being developed in the downswing and hip circle and a forceful, properly timed extension of the body at the end of the hip circle.

Anatomical essentials The anatomical essentials for successful performance in this movement series are strength and flexibility. Strength of shoulders, arms, and hands is especially important for swinging movements. Grip strength is essential, and until one is sure of such strength, certain swinging movements should not be attempted without the assistance of a spotter. Arm and shoulder strength can be checked by testing oneself with push-ups and pull-ups. Strong abdominal and back extensor muscles are also important. These muscle groups play a significant role in maintaining and changing the trunk position in the downward swing, the hip circle, and the Hecht dismount as shown here. Range of motion is also needed for these movements, particularly in the shoulder during the swing, and in the hip and lower back during the pike of the hip circle. In the absence of EMG data, these general statements must be sufficient. Any joint-by-joint anatomical analysis would be based on implied muscle actions deduced from joint motions and forces.

NONSUPPORT ACTIVITIES

The unsupported body moves through the air along a pathway determined prior to the beginning of flight. The flight path of the body may be primarily horizontal, as in a long jump, mostly vertical, as in springboard diving or high jumping, or somewhere in between, as in vaulting and tumbling events. Principles governing the flight path of the body relate to those of the projectile. Additional principles explaining the effect of the body's lean at the moment of takeoff and the twisting movements in the air are derived from Newton's third law, the Law of Action–Reaction and the Conservation of Angular Momentum.

Principles Related to Nonsupport Activities

1. *The path of motion of the body's center of gravity in space is determined by the angle at which it is projected into space, the force of the projection, and the force of gravity.* Nothing a diver or a gymnast can do will alter the pathway of the center of gravity once the feet have left the push-off surface. The horizontal velocity of the body remains constant and the path of the center of gravity is a parabola determined by the initial force and gravity. Without the application of an external force, this path cannot be altered. For this reason, the initial path must be suited to the desired result. The diver must allow for clearance of the board and sufficient air time for stunts, the gymnast must either produce a vertical path to land on a trampoline, balance beam, or vaulting horse or must produce sufficient air time for stunts on the floor.

2. *The time a body remains unsupported depends on the height of its projection, which is governed by the vertical velocity of the projection* (Figure 20.5). The more complicated or lengthy the stunt a diver or gymnast wishes to perform, the higher the peak of projection must be. A diver must emphasize vertical rather than horizontal distance.

3. *Most rotary movements are initiated before the performer leaves the supporting surface.* To possess angular momentum

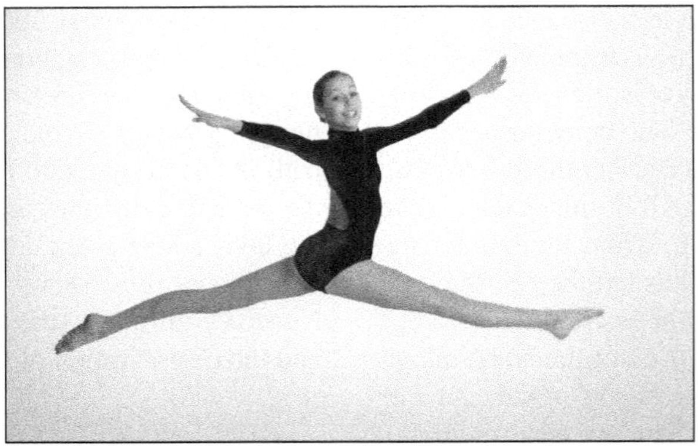

Figure 20.5 Movement of the body in the air. The height of projection depends on the vertical velocity of the takeoff.

during a nonsupport activity, an eccentric force must be used for takeoff. In a front somersault, for example, the center of gravity must be in front of the feet at the moment of takeoff for torque to exist. In a somersault with a twist (Figure 20.6), the push must be sideways as well as diagonally backward as the upper body leads the twist in the opposite direction. In keeping with Newton's third law, the direction of the twist is opposite to the direction in which the feet push against the supporting surface.

4. *The angular momentum* (Iω) *of an unsupported body is conserved. It cannot be increased or decreased.* A performer executing a somersault may increase the angular velocity by decreasing the moment of inertia. This is done by decreasing the radius of rotation, that is, by increasing the amount of tuck. A tuck somersault has a smaller moment of inertia than a pike somersault, and a pike

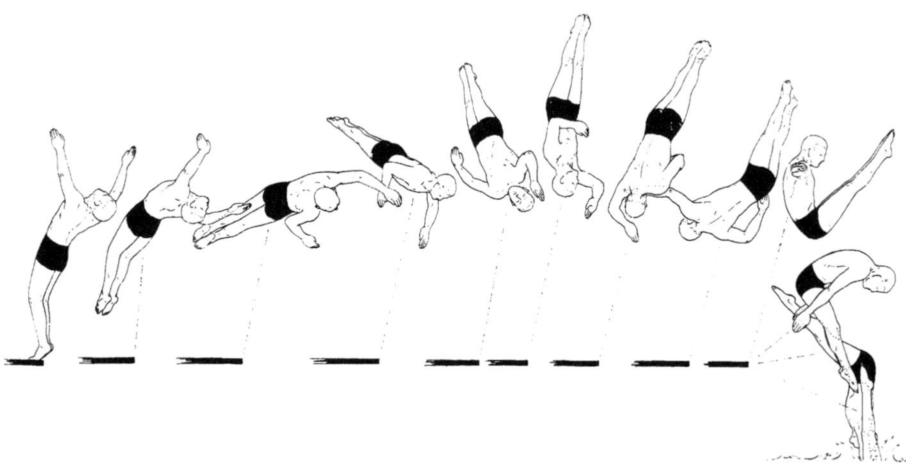

Figure 20.6 Back one-and-one-half somersault, one-and-one-half twist, free. *Source*: From *Swimming and Diving* (5th ed.), by D. A. Armbruster et al. Copyright © 1968, C. V. Mosby, St. Louis. Reprinted by permission.

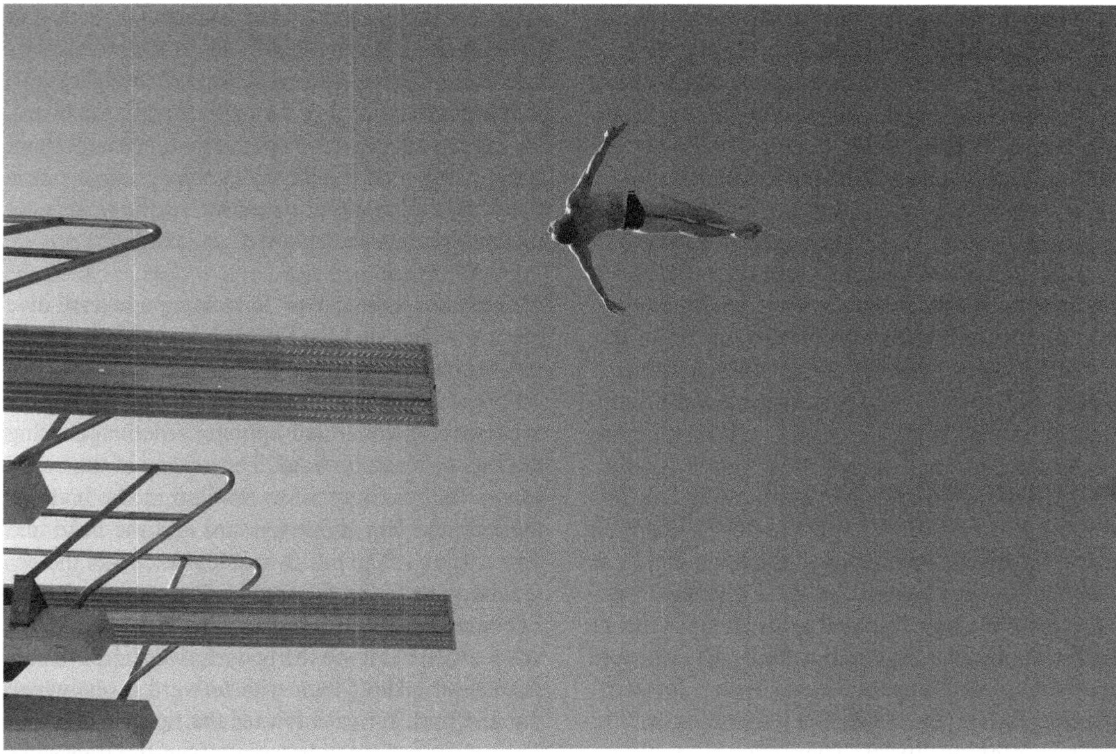

Figure 20.7 Diving.

somersault has less than a layout. To stop rotation in anticipation of landing or entry into the water, the moment of inertia is increased, thereby decreasing the angular velocity.

If a somersault starts with a twist from the push-off surface, the twist can be increased by decreasing the arch or the pike of the spin and by moving the arms closer to the body. Each of these moves decreases the moment of inertia and increases the angular velocity of the twist.

5. *When a body is free in space, movement of a part in one direction results in movement of the rest of the body in the opposite direction.* In a back dive in the pike position, the diver should wait until the legs have rotated past the vertical before the pike is opened. As the trunk and arms move back, the legs will react in the opposite direction and therefore move back to the vertical position.

   A reverse layout dive with a one-half twist may be performed by initiating the twist in the air rather than from the board. The diver will cause the body to twist to the opposite direction by moving one arm across the chest after the body is in a layout position in the air. The arm must then be moved overhead, keeping it close to the body so that another equal and opposite reaction does not occur. This method for initiating a twist is slow and is not usually used for more than a half-twist.
6. *A performer who is rotating about a horizontal axis in the air may initiate a twist*

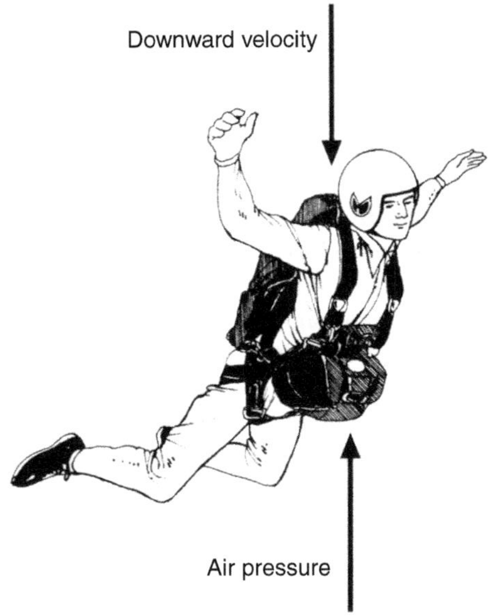

Figure 20.9 The spread-eagle position used to increase air pressure in skydiving.

"spread-eagle" position reduces the terminal velocity to 100 mph, reached in about 15 seconds. By manipulating the shape of the body in this way, the rate of descent can be partially controlled. Direction can also be modified by flexing and extending the extremities on one side of the body. Arm and leg flexion will decrease drag on that side of the body, producing a sideslipping or sideways motion. Reducing drag at one point of the body will produce rotation (Figure 20.9).

Weightlessness

Once human beings ventured into space, dealing with a gravity-free environment became a matter for serious study. With the planning and construction of orbiting space stations, more and more people will be confronted with the necessity of living and working in weightless conditions. Students of movement in the first few decades of the twenty-first century will most likely be the generation that devises exercise programs and sports for a three-dimensional, gravity-free environment. With this in mind, the concepts of mechanics take on a whole new meaning.

One critical fact must always be remembered in dealing with human motion in weightless conditions: *The laws of motion still apply.* Objects still possess inertia based on mass or momentum, acceleration is still directly related to force and mass, and every action has an equal and opposite reaction. The only difference is that the force of gravity no longer provides a constant downward acceleration. In a weightless environment the terms *down* and *up* are relatively meaningless.

The implications of a gravity-free environment deserve some attention in any study of human motion. In such an environment a force equal to or greater than the mass of an object or body is still required to start that object in motion. A force equal to the product of mass and acceleration is also required to stop a body in motion. A ball thrown in space requires the same throwing force and will strike the catcher's hand with the same force as on earth. However, because of a lack of gravity pulling downward, it will travel in a straight line, not a parabolic path.

Of great concern in manned spaceflight is the loss of bone mineral that occurs with prolonged weightlessness. In an environment with gravity such as that experienced on earth, humans must constantly resist the effects of gravity. In a weightless environment, this stress is removed. Because bone reacts to the stresses placed on it, a reduction of stress produces a reabsorption of bone material. For this reason, researchers and other space scientists are working to devise exercise programs that will continue to stress the musculoskeletal system in a weightless environment. A major obstacle to providing adequate exercise programs is the lack of adequate resistance. In space, if the astronaut pushes against something, such as a treadmill in running, there is still an equal and opposite reaction. Because the astronaut is not subject to the pull of gravity, rather than push off into a running step, the astronaut will push completely off the treadmill. Likewise, lifting weights is as likely to move the astronaut down as to move the weight up. A number of devices have been tested or are being considered to enable astronauts to do quasi-weight-bearing exercise in space. Treadmills with elastic tethering systems provide some resistance and hold the astronaut against the treadmill. Centrifugal acceleration systems that use centrifugal force to produce a simulated "gravitational" environment are also a potential mechanism for combating the disuse atrophy that is a result of space travel (Clement & Pavy-Le Traon, 2004; di Prampero & Narici, 2003).

Because of the lack of gravity, the concept of up and down has little meaning in space. Once a position is assumed through concentric muscle contraction, the segment or body remains in the new position unless moved by another force, such as further muscle contraction, or through contact with an external force. Reflexes are greatly affected by weightlessness. The extensor thrust reflex is less important because no deep pressure is experienced by the Pacinian corpuscles. Also, in the absence of gravity, information from the proprioceptors is confusing, resulting in disorganization within the system. Until the individual adjusts, this disorganization often results in nausea, a serious problem in space travel.

Microgravity

Not all space travel involves weightless conditions. At this writing, humans are in the process of considering travel to Mars and well as the moon. Working and living on these bodies will subject astronauts to microgravity conditions. Most space travel as we know it takes place in microgravity. There will be some gravity, but it will be only a fraction of the gravity on earth, based on the size of the planet or moon. In microgravity normal human motion will be modified. As an example, it has been predicted that it will be more economical to run than to walk on Mars, with walking speed being 30% slower and the walk-to-run transition occurring sooner (Hawkey, 2005).

REFERENCES AND SELECTED READINGS

Blajer, W., & Czaplicki, A. (2001). Modeling and inverse simulation of somersaults on the trampoline. *Journal of Biomechanics,* 34(12), 1619–1629.

Brancazio, P. J. (1984). *Sport science.* New York: Simon & Schuster.

Clement, G., & Pavy-Le Traon, A. (2004). Centrifugation as a countermeasure during actual and simulated microgravity: A review. *European Journal of Applied Physiology,* 92(3), 235–248.

Courtine, G., Papaxanthis, C., & Pozzo, T. (2002). Prolonged exposure to microgravity modifies limb-endpoint kinematics during the swing phase of human walking. *Neuroscience Letters,* 332(1), 70–74.

di Prampero, P. F., & Narici, M. V. (2003). Muscle in microgravity: From fibres to human motion. *Journal of Biomechanics,* 36(3), 403–412.

Fédération Internationale de Gymnastique. (2006). *Code of points—women's artistic gymnastics.* Retrieved from http://www.fedintgym.com/rules/

Fédération Internationale de Natation. (2005). *Rules and regulations: FINA diving rules 2005–2009.* Retrieved from http://www.fina.org/rules/english/diving.php

Hawkey, A. (2005). Physiological and biomechanical considerations for a human Mars mission. *Journal of the British Interplanetary Society,* 58(3–4), 117–130.

Hiley, M. J., & Yeadon, M. R. (2003). Optimum technique for generating angular momentum in accelerated backward giant circles prior to a dismount. *Journal of Applied Biomechanics,* 19, 119–130.

Hiley, M. J., & Yeadon, M. R. (2005). The margin for error when releasing the asymmetric bars for dismounts. *Journal of Applied Biomechanics,* 21(3), 223–235.

King, M. A., & Yeadon, M. R. (2004). Maximising somersault rotation in tumbling. *Journal of Biomechanics,* 37(4), 471–477.

Miller, D. I., & Sprigings, J. (2001). Factors influencing the performance of springboard dives of increasing difficulty. *Journal of Applied Biomechanics,* 17, 217–231.

Pendrill, A. M., & Williams, G. (2005). Swings and slides. *Physics Education,* 40(6), 521–533.

Sprigings, J., Lanovaz, J. L., & Russell, K. W. (2000). The role of shoulder and hip torques generated during backward giant swings on rings. *Journal of Applied Biomechanics,* 16, 289–300.

Trappe, S., Costill, D., Gallagher, P., Creer, A., Peters, J. R., Evans, H., et al. (2009). Exercise in space: Human skeletal muscle after 6 months aboard the International Space Station. *Journal of Applied Physiology,* 106, 1159–1168.

Yeadon, M. R., & Brewin, M. A. (2003). Optimised performance of the backward longswing on rings. *Journal of Biomechanics,* 36(4), 545–552.

Yeadon, M. R., & Kerwin, D. G. (1999). Contributions of twisting techniques used in backward somersaults with one twist. *Journal of Applied Biomechanics,* 15, 152–165.

LABORATORY EXPERIENCES

1. Hang motionless from a rope or a pair of rings. Now start swinging without the help of anyone else. How was the swing accomplished? Explain.
2. Swing on a pair of rings without attempting to get much height. Perform the following movements. Explain the results by stating the underlying principles. Be sure to have mats placed under the swinging area.
   a. Reverse the grasp of one hand. At which point in the swing is this accomplished most easily?
   b. Dismount at various positions along the arc of the swing. Note the effect on the body.
3. Perform the following movements in the water and explain the actions by stating underlying principles. (Except for the factor of increased resistance, the actions simulate those of an unsupported body.)
   a. Lie on the side and swing both legs forward vigorously, keeping the knees straight. Note the effect on the trunk.
   b. Lie on the back with the arms in a side horizontal position. Keeping the elbows straight, swing both arms in a clockwise direction across the surface of the water in a 90-degree arc as you roll to the right into a prone float. Note the direction in which the feet now point compared with the starting position.
4. Perform a complete kinesiological analysis of a selected swinging or airborne activity, taking particular note of the purpose of the motion, its classification, and the nature of the motion. Include also muscle participation, neuromuscular considerations, mechanical factors, and applicable principles and violations. Conclude the analysis with a prescription for improvement, including suggested methods for change and the elimination of violations of principles.

CHAPTER 21

IMPACT

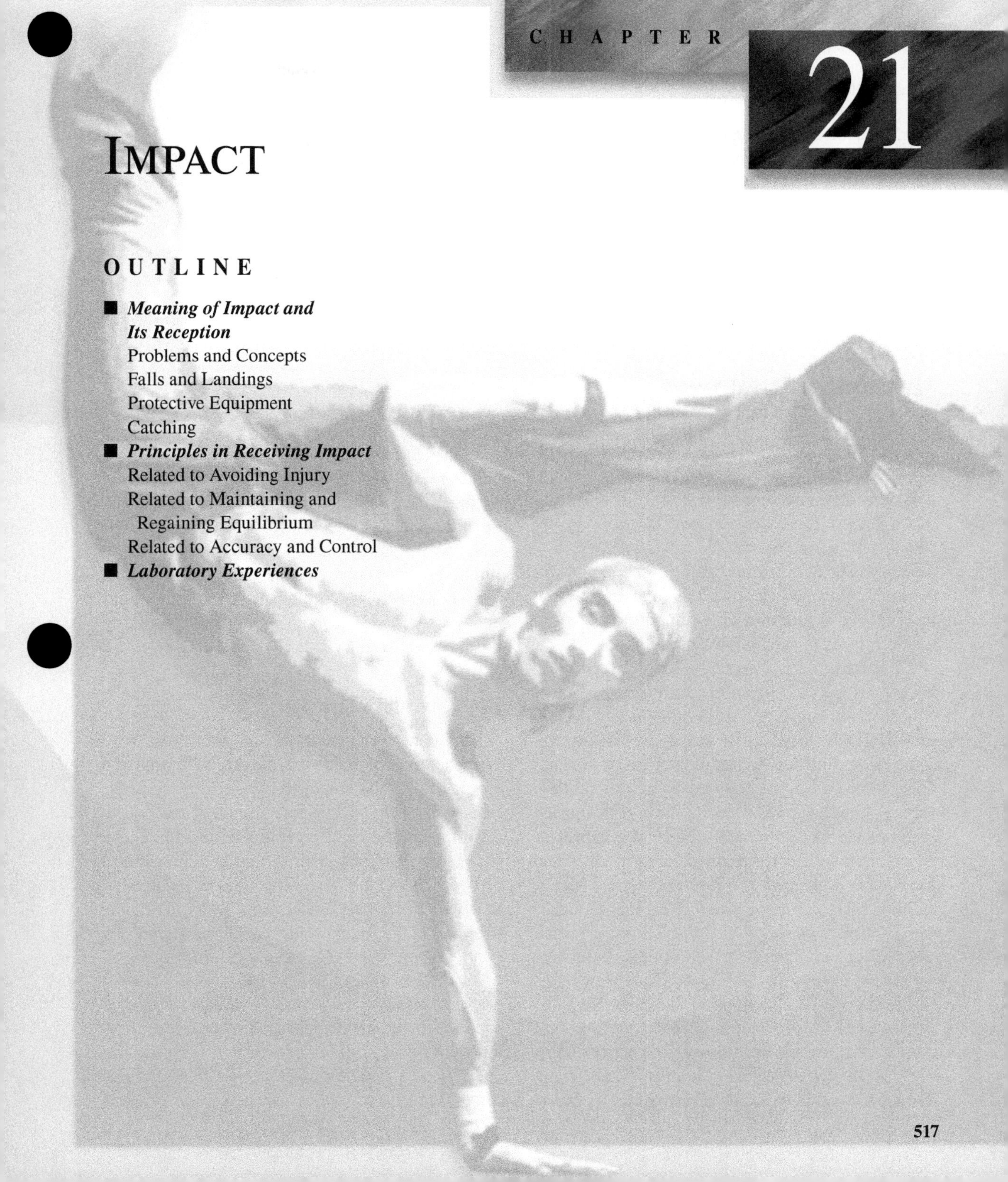

OUTLINE

OBJECTIVES

At the conclusion of this chapter, the student should be able to:

1. Name the common problems associated with the diverse forms of receiving impact.
2. Explain how the work–energy, impulse–momentum, and pressure–area relationships apply to receiving the impact either of one's own body or of external objects.
3. State the principles related to avoiding injury while receiving impact, and furnish an application for each.
4. State the principles related to maintaining and regaining equilibrium while receiving impact, and furnish an application for each.
5. State the principles related to accuracy and control while receiving impact, and furnish an application for each.

MEANING OF IMPACT AND ITS RECEPTION

The word *impact* is derived from the Latin word *impingere,* "to press together." Impact is further defined as force of contact, violent collision, striking together. Receiving impact is opposing or resisting in some manner the force with which a moving body tends to maintain its speed and direction. Impact may be from one's own body, as in landing from a jump or fall, or imparted by external objects, as in catching or spotting.

Impact of one's own body is experienced following any fall through space. Such falling motion, which occurs subsequent to a jump, a dive, or an accidental fall, has a rapidly increasing velocity because of the uniform acceleration effect of gravitational force. When the body lands on a supporting surface, impact has been said to occur. The impact is felt as the force of contact. Likewise, impact is experienced in a horizontally moving body when the motion is stopped as a result of contact with a resisting surface, such as a wall or another obstacle.

Examples of receiving impact from external objects are commonly seen in sports. Baseballs are caught or fielded with the hands, hockey balls and pucks are received with a stick, soccer balls are trapped with the feet, and blows from an opponent's fist are received by various parts of the body. Examples of receiving impact are also seen in industry and in daily life. Cartons and tools are tossed from one person to another, red-hot rivets are caught in tongs, and victims from a fire are caught in nets or air bags.

Impact generally has a negative connotation, but there are benefits to controlled impacts, such as mechanical loading of bone during walking. Specifically, it is widely accepted that bone will adapt to the mechanical stresses placed upon it. Intuitively, it is apparent that the bones of adults and adolescents will not adapt in the same manner, yet the bones of both groups are altered by mechanical loading (Ruff et al., 2006).

Problems and Concepts

What are the particular problems involved in these diverse forms of receiving impact, and what are the principles that enable us to solve these problems satisfactorily? In the reception of the body's own impact, the chief problems seem to be those of *avoiding injury* and *regaining equilibrium promptly.* Three problems appear to be involved in receiving the impact of external objects: (1) *avoiding injury,* (2) *maintaining equilibrium,* and (3) *receiving the object with accuracy and control.*

Whether the moving object is one's own body or an external object, the basic concepts enabling us to understand and solve these problems are the same. The first concept is the *kinetic energy–work relationship: When a body or object is "received," it has work done on it equal in amount to the change in kinetic energy of the moving body* (see Chapter 12). If, for example, velocity of an object is reduced to zero, all of its kinetic energy would be used to do work on the receiver. Because work equals the product of force and distance, the work done in receiving may consist of any combination of force and distance as long as the product of the two is equivalent to the kinetic energy lost by the moving object.

The second applicable concept is the *momentum–impulse relationship* (see pp. 303–305): *Any change in momentum requires a force applied over a period of time (impulse) and is equal to the product of that force and the time.* Again, the reduction in momentum of any object can be accomplished by any equivalent product combination of force and time. Both impulse and kinetic energy are proportional to the mass and velocity (momentum) of any object and will change if the momentum does.

The third concept involves *pressure* and is especially important with respect to avoiding injury: *The pressure that any part of the body must absorb is inversely proportional to the area over which the force is applied.*

Falls and Landings

The abrupt loss of motion resulting from collision with an unyielding surface is likely to cause an injury in landing after falls and landings. To avoid injury, it is necessary to find some means of losing the body's kinetic energy more gradually. This is achieved by increasing the distance and time over which the kinetic energy and momentum are lost. Landing on "giving" surfaces, such as mats or sand, controlled flexion at the joints of the landing extremities through eccentric contraction of the antagonist muscles, and rolling are important contributors to the gradual decrease in momentum without injury. Landings are often categorized as "soft" or "stiff" based on joint involvement. The knee is a major contributor to force dissipation in most landings. Limiting or stiffening the knee can lead to undue forces in the frontal plane, a direction in which the knee is not intended to move. In soft landings, the involvement of both the ankle and the hip increase. In stiff landings, the contribution of the ankle is greater while the contribution of the hip decreases. A similar pattern occurs with landings from different heights. As the height of landing increases, the involvement of both the hip and the ankle increase (McNitt-Gray, 1993; Zhang et al., 2000). In all cases, the muscles that will control the landing are activated before landing. The pre-activation serves to prepare the muscle for the upcoming stretch that will occur as the feet contact the ground. Drop height will affect the levels of pre-activation as well as muscle activation at contact.

Another factor in injury that should not be overlooked is the relationship of the force of impact to the size of the area that bears the brunt of the impact. A force of 450 N concentrated on 1 square centimeter of body surface, for instance, is likely to cause more serious injury than the same amount of force spread over an area of 50 square centimeters. Hence the solution is to increase the size of the area that receives the force of the impact. This is especially important when there is limited opportunity for increasing the distance over which the kinetic energy is lost.

Athletes in activities involving landing from substantial heights adopt a variety of landing strategies based on the requirements of the sport. Jumpers such as high jumpers and pole-vaulters decrease the trauma to the body by landing on very deep crash pads. Gymnasts, on the other hand, land on mats of varying thickness, based on the event. As mat thickness decreases, the gymnast uses an increased angle of hip and knee flexion on landing to increase the time over which kinetic energy is lost (McNitt-Gray et al., 1993).

The problem of regaining equilibrium in falling and landing is largely a problem in controlling the placement of the limbs in preparation for landing, because equilibrium is regained when an adequate base of support is established. This requires sufficient control to place the feet, or perhaps both the hands and the feet, in a position that will provide a favorable base of support. The problem of regaining equilibrium is closely related to that of avoiding injury because establishing an adequate base depends on the integrity of the bones and joints that receive the force of impact.

Various methods of falling are taught in classes in tumbling, martial arts, and modern dance. Perhaps one of the most effective measures for the prevention of injury in accidental falls is this kind of instruction, followed by the practice of a variety of falls until the techniques have been mastered. Practice helps establish the right patterns, patterns that will be followed automatically when accidental falls occur.

Protective Equipment

The goal of most protective equipment is to take a blow from a relatively small point of contact and dissipate or distribute that force over a greater surface area or to use a compressible material to dissipate or absorb the shock of the impact. The giving material will increase the time over which the striking object will be in contact with the protective equipment and thus will decrease the peak force that is imparted to the protective equipment. This is another example of impulse. By increasing the time over which the force is applied, a smaller force is required to bring about the same change in momentum.

Helmets

Helmets are designed to protect the head and, in particular, the brain. Helmets are broadly classified as single-impact helmets (motorcycle or bicycle helmets) and multi-impact helmets (football, hockey, and lacrosse helmets). Single-impact helmets must be replaced after every significant impact, whereas multi-impact helmets are designed to sustain repeated impacts before needing replacement.

Bicycle helmets are a single-impact helmet. Once a bicycle helmet has sustained damage, it cannot be used safely again. Bicycle helmets use interior foam to dissipate the energy of an impact. By crushing the interior foam, the speed of the skull can be brought to rest over a slightly longer period of time than if no helmet was worn. This application of impulse is highlighted by the fact that the change in momentum of the head will be nearly the same with and without the helmet (except for the mass of the helmet); however, by increasing the time over which the head is brought to rest, the force required to bring about such a change can be diminished.

Recently, much attention has been paid to the rate of concussion in American football. All football helmets worn in high school, college, and professional American football must adhere to the demands of the National Operating Committee on Standards for Athletic Equipment (NOCSAE). Fortunately, rule changes and better helmet designs have decreased the occurrence of concussion. However, due to the devastating long-term effects of concussion, research continues. The most notable, recent advance in football helmet design addresses the findings that concussions are often the result of side head impacts. Manufacturers have addressed this newly identified injury mechanism by increasing the hard shell coverage of the helmet and redesigning the interior padding arrangement to attenuate side shocks with greater effectiveness (Collins et al., 2006).

Forces imparted to a head wearing a helmet can be particularly devastating. Helmets help to attenuate these forces through compression of the interior foam. The purpose of the interior foam is to increase the time over which the head is brought to rest. This helps to dissipate the energy transmitted during the collision. This energy is converted to heat and is used in the compression of the interior foam.

A natural assumption would be to suggest that more foam is better. However, more foam moves the hard shell further away from the skull and leaves the head and neck susceptible to greater rotational forces. The foam needs to be soft enough to be comfortable but dense enough so as not to completely flatten out during an impact.

Body Protection

Shoulder pads dissipate force over a greater surface area, thus decreasing the stress on the body beneath. If the surface area over which that force is transmitted can be increased, the force per unit area will decrease, thus diminishing the peak force at any one given contact point. It is important for padding to fit properly with no significantly higher contact points so that no point will be forced to withstand a larger portion of the impact force.

Elbow and knee pads use foam surrounding the joint, thus increasing the surface area over which the force is dissipated. Energy is absorbed in deforming the foam. The stiffer the foam, the more energy required to deform it. The foam should not be so thick and dense as to restrict movement, yet be thick enough to withstand a direct blow. It should be pointed out that however hard one hits the ground while diving for a volleyball or a line drive, the ground is going to hit back just as hard. The protective padding is being asked to respond to the loading that comes from inside the material and from the external impact. Therefore, the outside layer of the protective padding must be rugged enough to withstand the frictional forces associated with sliding across the floor or the ground, yet the inside material must be soft enough to prevent significant damage to the underlying joint or anatomical structure.

Catching

As in the case of receiving the impact of one's own body, avoidance of injury in catching or receiving external forces is achieved by increasing the distance over which the object's kinetic energy is lost. When catching a fast-moving baseball, the experienced player will not hold the hands rigidly in front of the body but will give with the ball. By moving the hands toward the body through a distance of 10 to 20 inches as the ball is received, the catcher is making it possible for the ball's kinetic energy to be lost gradually. This same principle is likewise true for the player who is reaching for a high ball with one hand. The extended arm acts as a lever, the force being applied by the impact of the ball on the palm. The torque is therefore the product of the force of impact and the perpendicular distance from the shoulder joint to the ball's line of flight at the instant it is caught. If the line of flight is perpendicular to the outstretched arm, the torque is the product of the force of impact and the length of the arm. Catching a fast ball with the arm extended can put a tremendous strain on the shoulder joint, as well as endanger the bones of the hands. To avoid injury, the player should give by reaching somewhat forward for the ball and drawing the arm back at the moment of impact and by rotating the body and stepping back if the force is sufficiently great. If the elbow flexes slightly, the lever of the arm will be shortened and the torque reduced.

Another factor in avoiding injury when catching fast balls is the position of the hands. Beginners often reach with outstretched arms and point their fingers toward the approaching ball. This leads to many a "baseball finger." The fingers should be pointed either down or up, according to whether the ball is below or above waist level. Balls approaching at approximately waist level can be caught above the waist if the player bends the knees.

The second problem in receiving the impact of external objects—that of maintaining equilibrium—is often neglected. The receiver should prepare for it in advance because a fast ball or a sudden blow can easily cause anyone caught off balance to lose equilibrium. The stance is of great importance here. The base of support needs to be widened in the direction of the ball's flight, thus making it possible for the catcher to shift the weight of the body from the forward to the rear foot at the moment of impact. This action not only increases the chances of maintaining equilibrium but also contributes to the gradual reduction of the ball's motion. Widening the stance in a direction at right angles to the flight of the approaching ball does little to increase the catcher's stability.

The third problem—that of receiving the ball or another object with accuracy and control—is perhaps the one given the most emphasis in game situations. As in the attempt to avoid injury, one of the key factors is the gradual loss of the object's kinetic energy. This reduces the danger of the ball's bouncing off the hands. Accurate vision, judgment, and positioning of the body are of vital importance. "Keeping the eye on the ball" is essential to judging its speed and direction, and hence to adjusting the position of the body. Thus accurate judgment depends on accurate vision, and accurate adjustment of the body depends on both of these, as well as on agility and smoothness of neuromuscular response. Together, these factors make up what is known as "hand–eye" and "foot–eye coordination." To a certain extent this is innate, but it is also developed and improved by practice.

Intercepting a ball or a puck is another illustration of receiving impact. Ice hockey, field hockey, soccer, basketball, and football are all games in which a player tries to intercept a pass. The same principles that apply to catching apply to intercepting, but with this difference: Whereas in catching there is usually time to place oneself in a favorable position and to use one's arms, hands, or feet advantageously, in intercepting, one must take advantage of the opportunity when it comes. There is no time for preparation. The important principle to observe is to give with the hands, feet, or stick the moment that contact is made with the ball or puck in order to keep control of it; otherwise, it is likely to bounce off.

In receiving both the impact of one's body and that of external objects, an important factor to be considered is the subsequent movement one expects to make. It may be the determining factor in deciding what stance to assume. For instance, if a run is anticipated, a forward–backward stance will be more favorable than a lateral one. Furthermore, it will be desirable to have the weight over the forward foot. If a catch is to be followed immediately by a throw, the movements used for giving may be blended into the preparatory movements of the throw. These are fine points that have much to do with the degree of one's skill in an activity.

A summary of the principles to observe in receiving impact, both that of one's own body and that of external objects, is presented in the next section, together with some representative applications of these principles.

Principles in Receiving Impact

Related to Avoiding Injury

1. *The more gradual the loss of momentum (or kinetic energy) of the moving body or object, the less the force exerted on the body.* In other words, increasing either the time or the distance used in stopping the motion will decrease the forces imparted in the deceleration. When landing from a jump, for instance, the performer should use eccentrically controlled flexion in the ankles, knees, and hips to increase both the time and the distance for losing momentum (Figure 21.1). High jumpers and pole-vaulters often increase the time and distance even more through the use of thickly padded landing pits. Any amount of padding, whether by fatty or muscle tissue such as in the buttocks, or artificial padding such as in shoe insoles, uniform padding, or on playing surfaces, helps reduce the forces of impact. If the hands and arms must be used in the landing, care must be taken to allow the joints to give into flexion to avoid injury.

Often in falling, there is horizontal as well as vertical momentum to be absorbed. Using a roll or a series of rolls is an effective

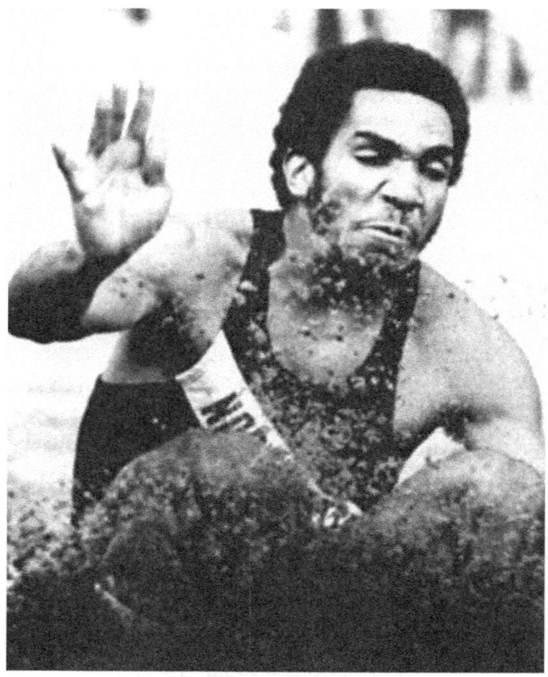

Figure 21.1 Landing from the running long jump. The momentum of the moving body is decreased through the controlled flexion at the ankles, knees, and hips and the "give" of the landing surface. Courtesy of Northeastern University.

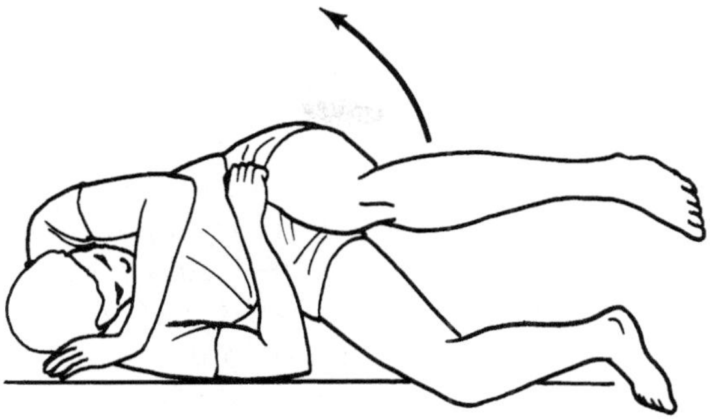

Figure 21.2 To avoid injury when landing from a jump or fall, the horizontal motion should be decreased gradually. An effective technique is the shoulder roll. The action is controlled by landing and rolling on the more heavily padded parts of the body.

way to increase the time and distance over which this momentum is lost (Figure 21.2). Rolls are commonly taught in the martial arts as falling techniques. If a roll is not possible, a few running or hopping steps may serve the same purpose.

When catching a ball or receiving a blow, giving with the impact will increase the time and distance over which momentum is transferred to the body. In catching a ball, the performer gives by pulling the arms back toward the body at the moment of impact and, if necessary, shifting the weight backward or taking a backward step or two. The speed of the joint motion due to the momentum of the incoming object will be controlled by eccentric contraction of the antagonist muscles. If the ball is caught with only one hand, the arm should be allowed to move horizontally backward and the body should rotate. This catching motion may be adapted to serve as the preparatory phase in a subsequent throw. A similar giving action is used when absorbing blows to the head or body. Moving the body or body part in the same direction as the motion of the blow will decrease the force of the blow.

As in landing and falling, any padding that can be added to the catching or striking surface will aid in the gradual decrease in momentum, as well as increasing the area over which stress is absorbed. The gloves and pads worn by softball and baseball players, boxers, and some karetekas (martial arts performers) all help reduce impact forces (Figure 21.3).

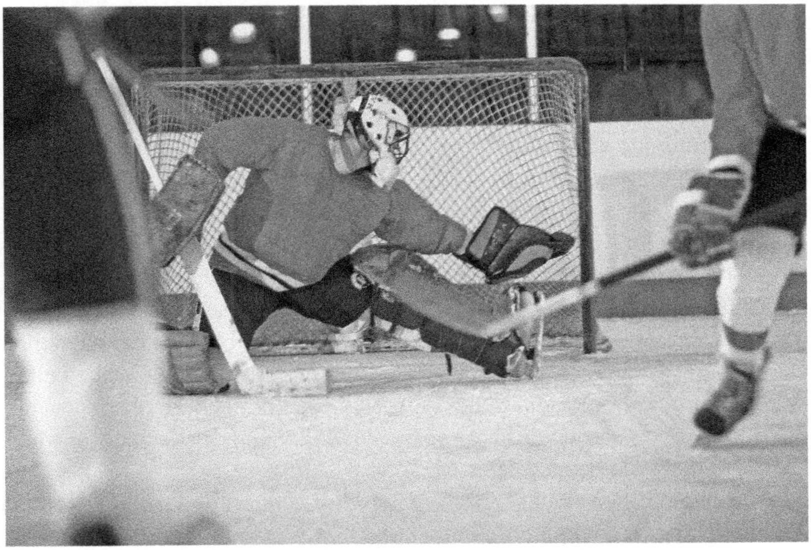

Figure 21.3 The padding on the hockey goalie increases the area of impact, thereby reducing the shock against the part of the body receiving the impact.

2. *The larger the area receiving the impact, the less will be the force per unit of surface area.* Falls in the martial arts often include slapping motions with the arms. The arm slap increases the surface area over which the fall is broken, thus reducing the force on any given area. Turning during a fall in order to land on a broad area such as the back (with the head tucked), the thighs, and buttocks, or rocking onto the chest are all methods of increasing the surface area for impact.
3. Repeated impacts, such as in running, gymnastics, aerobic exercise classes, and other activities may lead to overuse injuries. Repeated impact landings should be "soft" whenever possible. Attention should also be given to the nature of the landing surface. Energy-absorbing surfaces are preferable for repeated impacts.

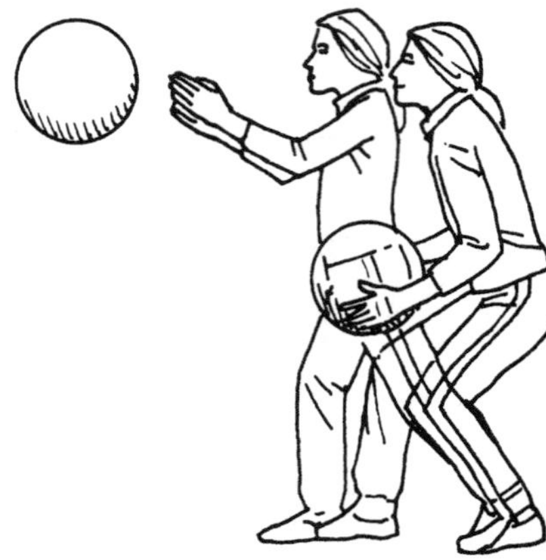

Figure 21.4 Catching a medicine ball. The principles of stopping a heavy object are demonstrated. The feet are separated in the direction of the oncoming ball; the line of gravity is forward in preparation for catching the heavy ball; there is a gradual "give" in the joints of the arms and legs and a backward weight shift so that the momentum of the ball may be reduced gradually; the stability of the receiver is improved by lowering the center of gravity.

Related to Maintaining and Regaining Equilibrium

4. *Other things being equal, the larger the base of support in the direction of the impetus, the greater will be the body's equilibrium.* In any jump or fall, the body's equilibrium is temporarily lost. To gain prompt control of the body upon landing, a favorable base of support can be established by adjusting the position of the feet prior to landing in such a way that they will provide an adequate base when the landing is made. This foot position should be such that it will facilitate equal distribution of the body weight over the two feet. If the force of the landing makes it difficult to establish an adequate base of support with the feet alone, one or both hands may be used to temporarily broaden this base long enough for equilibrium to be established. In any case, the larger dimension of the base of support should be parallel with the horizontal direction of movement. This is exemplified by the forward lengthening of the stride, which occurs almost automatically when one trips while running or walking.

   When preparing to receive an external impetus, the base of support should be widened in the direction of the expected force. This can be applied to catching a heavy object, maintaining standing balance on a moving vehicle such as a train or bus, or receiving a push, pull, or blow (Figure 21.4).
5. *At the moment of impact, the line of gravity should be centered above the base.* This position will provide maximum distance in any direction should it be necessary to adjust for any horizontal forces upon contact. To provide maximum distance for the establishment of balance after landing from a forceful horizontal movement, the line of gravity should be located close to the near edge of the base of support at the moment of landing. In the same way, the line of gravity should be near the front edge of the base of support and the knees should be bent in preparation for receiving an object with large horizontal momentum. In this way, the horizontal distance over which the center of

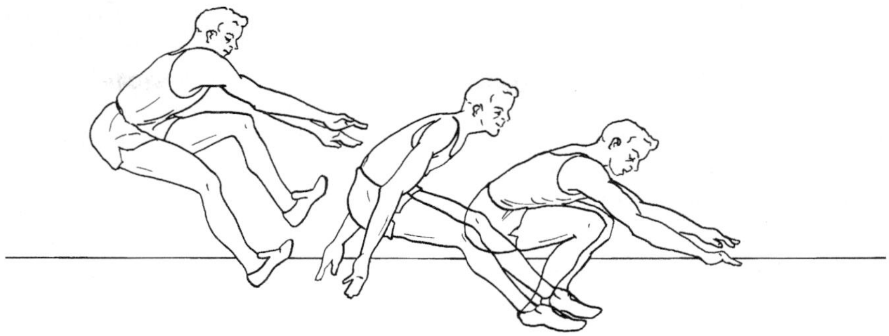

Figure 21.5 Stability in landing is increased by lowering the center of gravity and moving the line of gravity toward the front edge of the base of support.

gravity can move and still stay over the base of support is maximal (Figure 21.5).

Related to Accuracy and Control

6. *The more gradually the velocity of an external object is reduced, the less likely is the object to rebound when its impact is received.* All the methods suggested for avoiding injury and maintaining equilibrium when receiving the impact of external objects also apply to preventing rebound.
7. "*Keep the eye on the ball.*" Whether the object whose impact is about to be received is a ball, carton, or fist, keeping the eyes on it will enable one to judge its speed and direction and to respond accordingly. The tendency of some novices to shut the eyes should be corrected at the outset.
8. *Catching an external object with accuracy and control depends largely on the position of the catcher relative to the direction of the approaching object.* Putting oneself in the most favorable position possible is an essential objective for accurate catching. This precaution applies also to such everyday tasks as lifting a heavy suitcase or carton down from a high shelf, as well as to catching objects that are approaching more or less horizontally (Figure 21.6). This is basic to the prevention of injury and the maintenance of equilibrium.

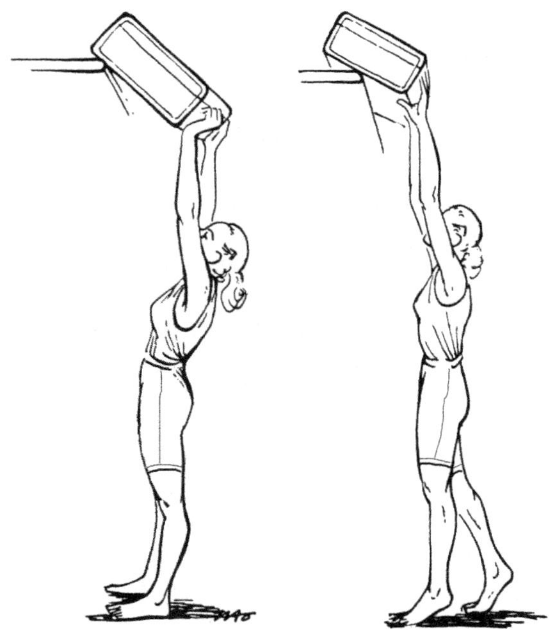

Figure 21.6 Lifting a suitcase down from a high shelf: (a) inefficiently; (b) efficiently. In (b) the woman is prepared to take a step backward if necessary and to bring the suitcase down close in the front of her body. The base of support is widened in the direction of the force being received, and the center of gravity is located over the front edge of the base of support.

References and Selected Readings

Collins, M., Lovell, M. R., Iverson, G. L., Ide, T., & Maroon, J. (2006). Examining concussion rates and return to play in high school football players wearing newer helmet technology: A three-year prospective cohort study. *Neurosurgery,* 58(2), 275–286.

DeGoede, K. M., & Ashton-Miller J. A. (2002). Fall arrest strategy affects peak hand impact force in a forward fall. *Journal of Biomechanics,* 35(6), 843–848.

Gruneberg, C., Nieuwenhuijzen, P. H., & Duysens, J. (2003). Reflex responses in the lower leg following landing impact on an inverting and non-inverting platform. *Journal of Physiology,* 550(Pt 3), 985–993.

Hui, S. K., & Yu, T. X. (2002). Modeling the effectiveness of bicycle helmets under impact. *International Journal of Mechanical Sciences,* 44, 1081–1100.

Hwang, L K., Kim, K. J., Kaufman, K. R., Cooney, W. P., & An, K. N. (2006). Biomechanical efficiency of wrist guards as a shock isolator. *Journal of Biomechanical Engineering,* 128(2), 229–234.

James, C. R., Bates, B. T., & Dufek, J. S. (2003). Classification and comparison of biomechanical response strategies for accommodating landing impact. *Journal of Applied Biomechanics,* 19(2), 106–118.

McIntosh, A., & Janda, D. (2003). Evaluation of cricket helmet performance and comparison with baseball and ice hockey helmets. *British Journal of Sports Medicine,* 37(6), 325–330.

McIntosh, A., McCrory, P., & Finch, C. F. (2004). Performance enhanced headgear: A scientific approach to the development of protective headgear. *British Journal of Sports Medicine,* 38(1), 46–49.

McNitt-Gray, J. L. (1993). Kinetics of the lower extremities during drop landings from three heights. *Journal of Biomechanics,* 26, 1037–1046.

McNitt-Gray, J. L., Yokoi, T., & Millward, C. (1993). Landing strategy adjustments made by female gymnasts in response to drop height and mat composition. *Journal of Applied Biomechanics,* 9, 173–190.

Naunheim, R. S., Standeven, J., Richter, C., & Lewis, L. M. (2000). Comparison of impact data in hockey, football, and soccer. *Journal of Trauma,* 48(5), 938–941.

Parkin, P. C., & Howard, A. W. (2008). Advances in an examination of four common outdoor activities. *Current Opinions in Pediatrics,* 20(6), 719–23.

Pollard, C. D., Sigward, S. M., & Powers, C. M. (2010). Limited hip and knee flexion during landing is associated with increased frontal plane knee motion and moments. *Clinical Biomechanics,* 25, 142–146.

Robinovitch, S. N., Inkster, L., Maurer, J., & Warnick, B. (2003). Strategies for avoiding hip impact during sideways falls. *Journal of Bone Mineral Research,* 18(7), 1267–1273.

Ruff, C., Holt, B., & Trinkaus, E. (2006). Who's afraid of the big bad Wolff: "Wolff's law" and bone functional adaptation. *American Journal of Physical Anthropology,* 129, 484–498.

Santello, M. (2005). Review of motor control mechanisms underlying impact absorption from falls. *Gait and Posture,* 21, 85–94.

Shiratori, T., & Latash, M. L. (2001). Anticipatory postural adjustments during load catching by standing subjects. *Clinical Neurophysiology,* 112(7), 1250–1265.

Viano, D. C., & Pellman, E. J. (2005). Concussion in professional football: Biomechanics of the striking player—part 8. *Neurosurgery,* 56(2), 266–280.

Yokota, H., & Tanaka, S. M. (2005). Osteogenic potentials with joint-loading modality. *Journal of Bone Mineral Metabolism,* 23, 302–308.

Yu, B., Lin, C. F., & Garrett, W. E. (2006). Lower extremity biomechanics during the landing of a stop-jump task. *Clinical Biomechanics* (Bristol, Avon), 21(3), 297–305.

Zhang, S., Clowers, K., Kohstall, C., & Yu, Y. J. (2005). Effects of various midsole densities of basketball shoes on impact attenuation during landing activities. *Journal of Applied Biomechanics,* 21(1), 3–17.

Zhang, S. N., Bates, B. T., & Dufek, J. S. (2000). Contributions of lower extremity joints to energy dissipation during landings. *Medicine and Science in Sports and Exercise,* 32, 812–819.

LABORATORY EXPERIENCES

In each of the following Experiences, select the preferable method of executing the movement. Justify your selection by citing the anatomical and mechanical principles demonstrated, as well as those that are violated.

1. Jump from a low bench to the floor, landing on both feet.
   a. Landing with minimum give (stiff landing)—that is, with as little flexion at the ankles, knees, and hips as possible.
   b. Landing with maximum give (soft landing)—that is, allowing the ankles, knees, and hips to flex to a full squat position. The head should be kept erect.
   c. Landing as in b but looking down at the feet.
   Which method is preferable? Why?
2. Trip on the edge of a mat and fall forward, landing first on the knees, then on the hands.
   a. Keeping the arms rigid, elbows straight.
   b. Letting the elbows flex, arching the back, rocking down onto the abdomen and chest, with the head turned sideways.
3. Jump down from a table or gymnasium box, using the parachute landing technique—that is, landing on the toes with the feet together, bending the knees slightly and turning sideward, rolling onto the side of the leg, thigh, and hip, then onto the back of the shoulder, keeping the arms close in front of the chest and the head flexed forward.
4. Catch a medicine ball thrown straight toward your chest.
   a. With your arms rigidly outstretched.
   b. With your hands held close in front of your chest.
   c. With your arms outstretched at first but brought in toward your chest at the moment of impact.
   Which method is preferable? Why?
5. Receive a hard drive in field hockey (a) with and (b) without giving with the stick. Compare the results of both as to control of the ball and sensation in the hands.

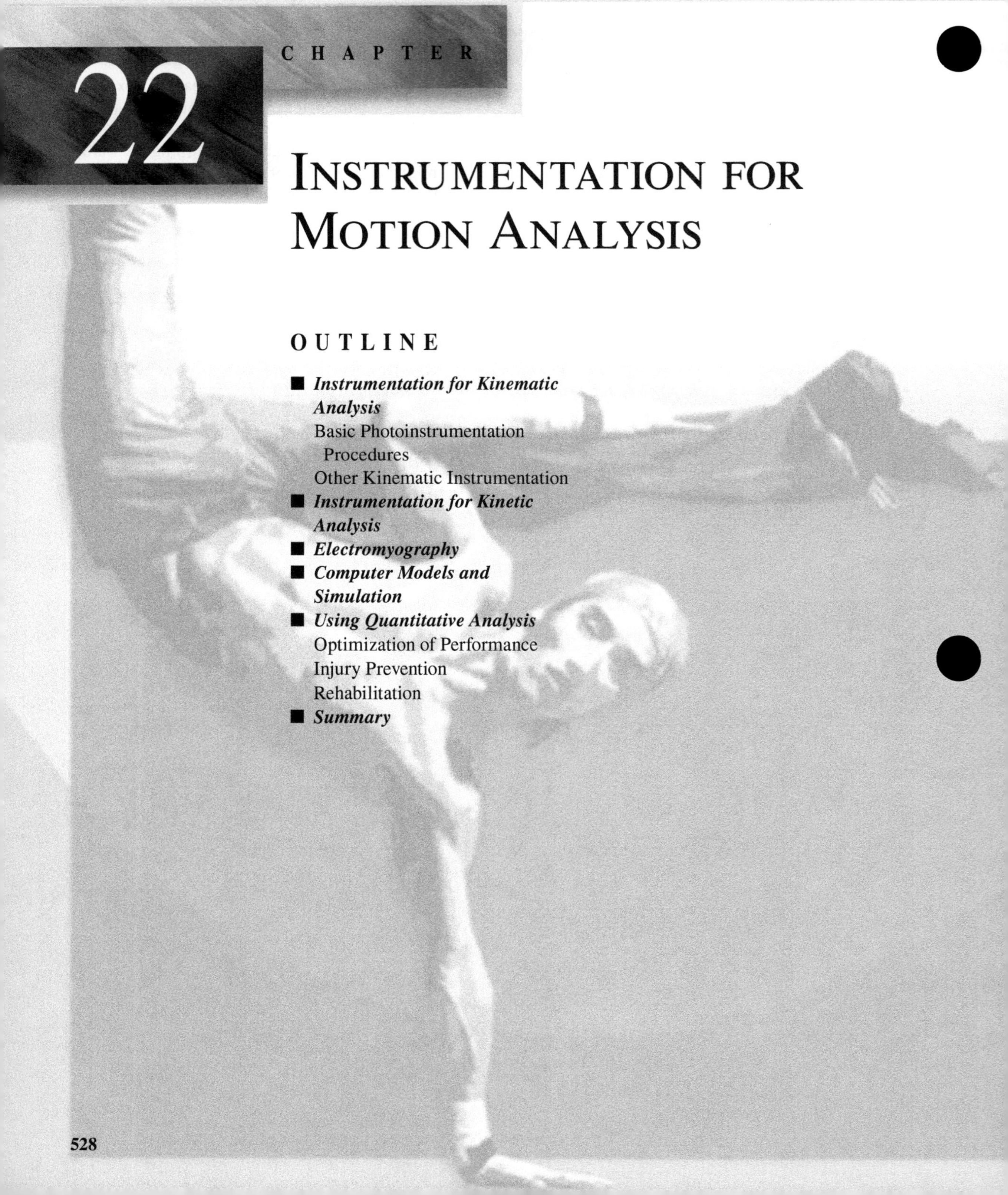

CHAPTER 22

Instrumentation for Motion Analysis

OUTLINE

- ***Instrumentation for Kinematic Analysis***
  - Basic Photoinstrumentation Procedures
  - Other Kinematic Instrumentation
- ***Instrumentation for Kinetic Analysis***
- ***Electromyography***
- ***Computer Models and Simulation***
- ***Using Quantitative Analysis***
  - Optimization of Performance
  - Injury Prevention
  - Rehabilitation
- ***Summary***

OBJECTIVES

At the conclusion of this chapter, the student should be able to:

1. Identify and discuss instrumentation for the collection and analysis of kinematic data in human movement.
2. Identify and discuss instrumentation for the collection and analysis of kinetic data in human movement.
3. Discuss the limitations of biomechanical instrumentation.
4. Critically examine the research literature in the field of human movement with an understanding of the methodologies used.

The scholarly study of people in motion has interested scientists for centuries, and their contributions have established the foundation for the advances that continue to be made in kinesiology and biomechanics research in the twenty-first century. Methodology has progressed from exclusive dependence on observations by the naked eye to the use of sophisticated photographic and electronic equipment for analyzing and quantifying the anatomical and mechanical nature of human performance. Although the student in the undergraduate course in kinesiology is not expected to have much experience using some of the more sophisticated equipment and methodology, much of the technology used in movement analysis is readily available. Because of this increased availability of analysis technology and the increased interest in undergraduate research, the student should be aware of the available instrumentation and more advanced approaches to movement analysis. In addition, the principles and methods utilized in the more sophisticated systems are based on some basic principles that can be implemented with much less sophisticated devices.

There are two broad areas of study in the field of biomechanics: kinematics and kinetics. As noted in Chapter 10, kinematics is the description of motion without consideration of the forces involved. Kinematic variables include position, displacement, time, velocity, and acceleration—all of which are discussed in Chapter 11. Kinetics is the study of the forces that produce motion. Kinetic variables include force and torque, among others. Kinetic variables are the focus of Chapters 12 and 13. Information about each of these variables is gathered through the collection of data. There are three primary categories of biomechanical data collection. The first of these is motion capture data, which are valuable for the study of kinematics. Commercially available motion capture systems vary widely in complexity and cost. Motion capture may be based on video, electromagnetic systems, or electrogoniometry. In kinematic studies, measures of position and time are used to calculate the derivatives velocity and acceleration (Chapter 11). Kinematic data from motion capture systems may be linear or angular or both. The second primary category of data collection includes force measuring systems. Force measures are collected through the use of force transducers that convert pressure, stress, or energy to a digital signal. Finally, muscle activity is measured through the use of electromyography (EMG), as mentioned in Chapter 3. Electromyography measures the minute electrical signals generated by active muscle and can provide information on the contraction state of muscle.

INSTRUMENTATION FOR KINEMATIC ANALYSIS

Kinematic data, or data that describe a motion, are collected with a variety of instruments ranging from still cameras through high-speed film and video to sophisticated motion-tracking systems.

The primary purpose of all such instrumentation is to enable people to analyze motion beyond the capabilities of their own physical senses. The human eye, for instance, can take in information at a rate of only ten to twelve items per second. When you are looking at motions that take less than 1 second to complete, a great deal of the visual information is lost (Morrison et al., 2005). By "freezing" sequential pieces of the movement artificially, it becomes possible to analyze any given movement pattern in detail, including those bits of information that may be lost to the human eye or quickly forgotten by the brain.

One of the simplest and least expensive forms of kinematic instrumentation is the still camera. Still cameras are useful in motion analysis when used with special adaptations. For example, if the camera shutter is left open during the filming, and the exposure is controlled by a flashing strobe light, multiple images on a single picture are the result (see Figure 17.7). Another technique is to attach tiny lightbulbs to the joints and extremities. When photographed in a dark room with an open shutter, the motion appears as a light streak and the nature of the movement pattern is revealed.

Similar results may also be obtained by attaching a motor drive to a camera, allowing for rapid film advancement and exposure. Simple forms of motor-driven cameras are available, whereas other cameras may require the addition of an external motor drive unit. Although simple still camera techniques are not commonly used in research today, they are still an inexpensive and effective tool for undergraduate study Figure 22.1).

For many years the most frequently used kinematic research instrument was the high-speed motion picture camera coupled with a stop-motion film analyzer. Cameras with speeds up to 500 frames per second and variable shutters provide an ample number of clear data points for analyzing the fastest of human motions. Cameras with speeds up to 20,000 frames per second are often used to study projectiles and impacts. Such a camera can freeze a bullet in flight or at impact and can photograph the lighting of a match as several dozen individual pictures.

Historically, quantitative analysis of movement captured on high-speed film required a projector that presented one frame at a time, so that measurements could be made of that image in that frame. These measurements were completed with a process known as digitizing, which is the identification and assignment of *x*-, *y*- (and often *z*-) coordinates to specific points within the image. Over time, paper-and-pencil digitizing was replaced with digitizing tablets and eventually computers. Now, quantitative analysis of movement is conducted almost entirely by computers.

In some cases, video files are uploaded and computer processing is conducted. In some of the more advanced systems, the processing is done within each camera and the *x*-, *y*-, and *z*-coordinates of specific points are sent to the computer, rather than the image. The computer then uses these coordinates to calculate linear and angular kinematic variables, through the same processes noted in Chapters 10 and 11. Three-dimensional analysis techniques require that each marker or location of interest be recorded by at least two synchronized cameras. The more cameras that capture a marker, the more accurate the calculations for that marker will be. A number of free or low-cost computer programs are available that allow the observer to manually digitize the locations of anatomical landmarks for quantitative analysis. Furthermore, simply being able to observe movement frame by frame has a tremendous advantage over watching a movement in real time (Figure 22.1).

In addition to the optically based systems, electromagnetic systems (often referred to as "flock of birds") also capture motion in three dimensions. These systems produce real-time, three-dimensional models but are often constrained to the laboratory. The reader may be familiar with the "virtual reality" images that are sometimes produced using such systems.

The use of digital video opens up a number of possibilities for motion analysis. Most computer systems have some basic level of digital video processing. This allows the movement professional to create short clips of motion for practice or to export single frames as photos and draw lines and

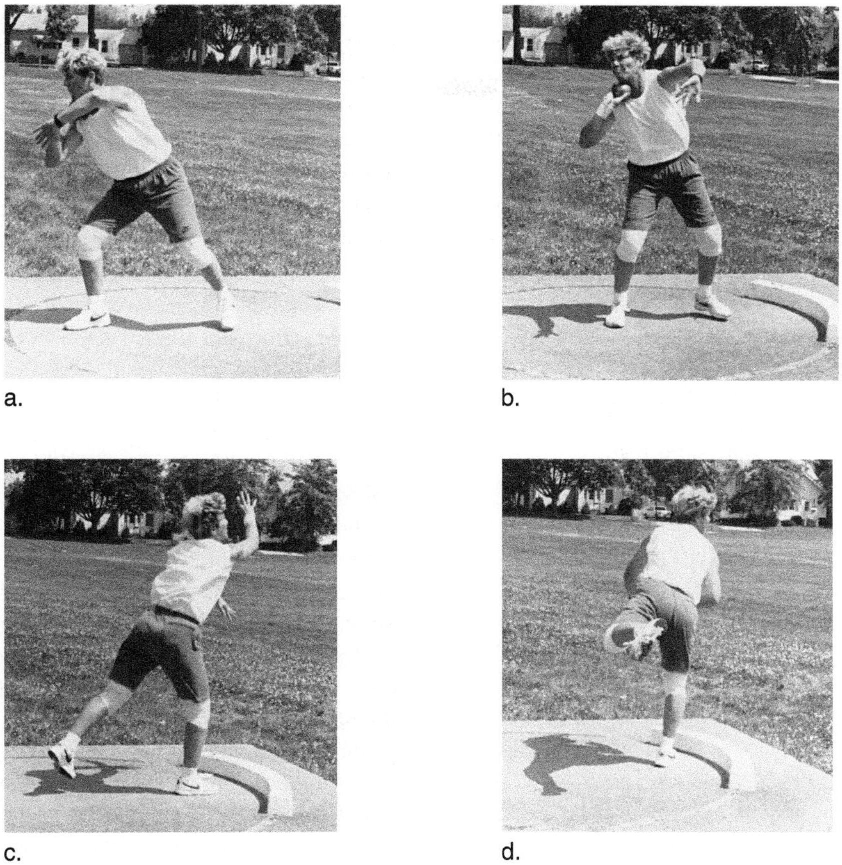

Figure 22.1 Movement pictures using a motor-driven still camera.

angles, do measurements, and highlight phases of the motion. More extensive software may allow basic kinematic analysis, side-by-side analysis, or comparison with expert models (Figures 22.3 and 22.4). The student is encouraged to become familiar with as many digital tools as may be available. When using visual images, adhere to the procedures of good photoinstrumentation.

Basic Photoinstrumentation Procedures

In any consideration of kinematic motion analysis, some fundamental procedures must be followed regardless of the instrumentation that is to be used. Because the basic measurements in kinematics are time and displacement (both angular and linear), care must be taken to ensure maximum accuracy in these two measurements.

The measurement of time in most photographic instrumentation is based on the frame rate, or the rate at which images are photographed or captured. In still photography this rate is controlled by the rate at which the light source is emitted (stroboscopic) or at which the motor drive operates. In cinematography and videography, frame rate is the rate at which the film moves through the camera or the data are captured. The typical home video camera has a frame rate of 30 frames per second. High-speed movie cameras and video cameras can have frame rates as high as 20,000 frames per second. The rule of thumb for determining the rate at which the motion should be captured is based upon the

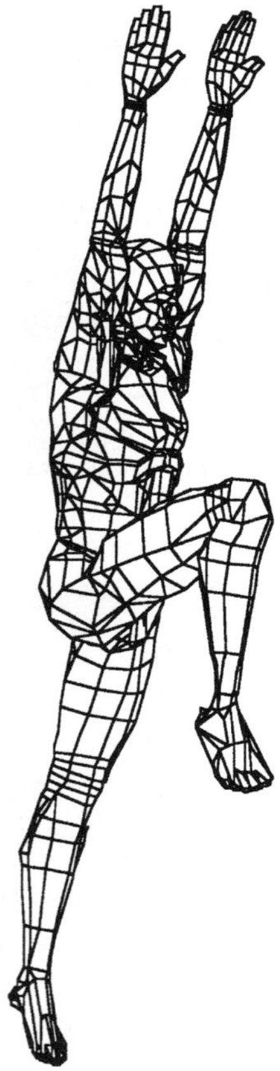

Figure 22.2 Representation of a three-dimensional human form in motion as seen by a computer.

Nyquist sampling theorem that says the data collection rate should be at least two times greater than the greatest frequency of the movement. Adhering to this theorem will help prevent aliasing or the missing of pertinent data. For example, in Chapter 16 it was noted that Olympic rowers can achieve stroke rates greater than 40 strokes per minute. To record this motion, the stroke rate in cycles per second (in hertz, abbreviated Hz) is calculated. In this case, 40 strokes per minute is equal to a stroke rate of 0.667 Hz. To ensure that all of the motion is captured, the acquisition rate should be two times greater than 0.667, or about 1.5 data points per second. Since standard video captures frames at 30 Hz, it is clear that standard video would be fast enough to adhere to this requirement. In any movement to be analyzed, it is important to determine which aspect of the motion will be the focus of the analysis. The data capture rate is then set for the frequency of this aspect of the motion. In the golf swing, for instance, the motion in the legs is a very slow-frequency motion of low amplitude. The motion of the club, on the other hand, may reach much higher frequencies. In the swing pictured in Figure 11.16, the elapsed time for the two frames before contact with the ball is only 0.013 seconds. The frequency of this part of the swing, therefore, is 74 Hz. A video camera with a frame rate of 30 Hz would capture a blur at this point in the motion. Most human motion can be filmed at 60 to 100 Hz. If the analysis is to

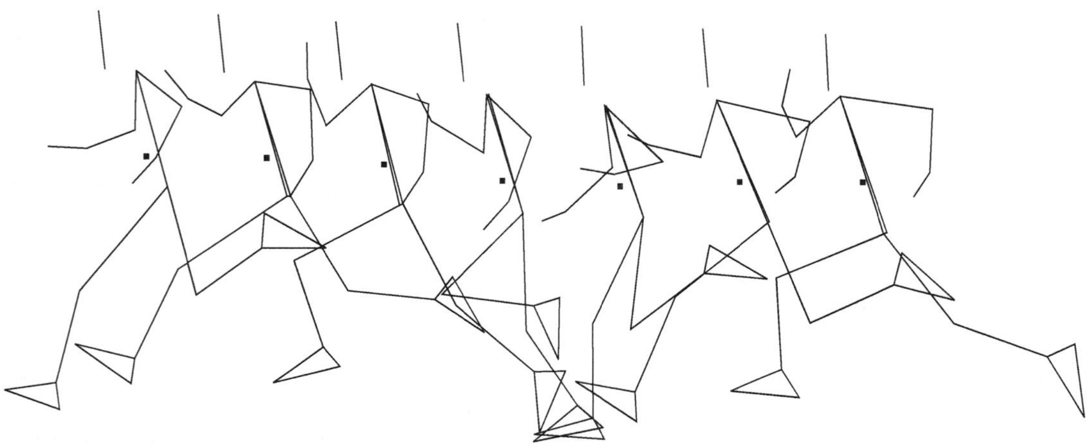

Figure 22.3 Computer-generated stick figure of running.

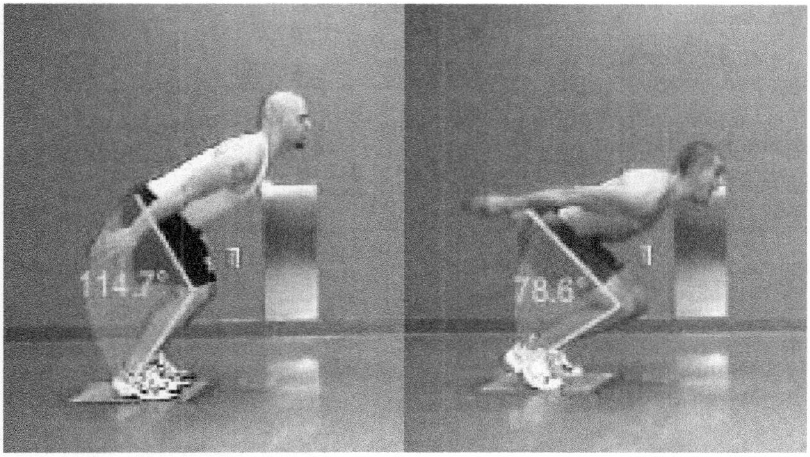

Figure 22.4 Side-by-side comparison of digital video images.

include an impact of some sort or the release of an object, frame rates need to be higher—from 300 to 500 Hz. Once frame rate has been established, the time elapsed between frames or the time over which displacement occurs is equal to the frame rate divided into 1 second. At a frame rate of 60 Hz, therefore, the frame time would be 1/60 of a second, or 0.017 seconds.

The second basic kinematic measure is displacement. To accurately measure displacement, there are two primary concerns. First, when working in two dimensions, care must be taken to place the camera in a position exactly perpendicular to the plane of the motion. If the camera is placed at an angle to the motion, parallax errors will occur. To see what a parallax error looks like, hold a pencil in front of you so that you are able to see its full length. Now rotate the point of the pencil slowly away from you. Note how the pencil seems to grow shorter. This foreshortening is due to parallax. Filming anywhere other than perpendicular to the plane of motion can produce similar effects that cause large errors in measures of displacement.

The second consideration in measuring displacement is to have some scale reference in the picture. It is necessary to have some way of relating the image size on film to real-life distances. A simple way to do this is to place a meter stick in the field of view of the camera in such a way that it is in the same plane as the motion and the same distance from the camera. This may be done by photographing the meter stick first, before the performance or at the end of the film. This scale reference could also be taped on a floor, a wall, a goalpost, or some other surface. Any known length can be used. Reference measures should be done in all planes in which the motion will occur. For instance, in a two-dimensional analysis, reference measures should be done both horizontally and vertically (Figure 22.5).

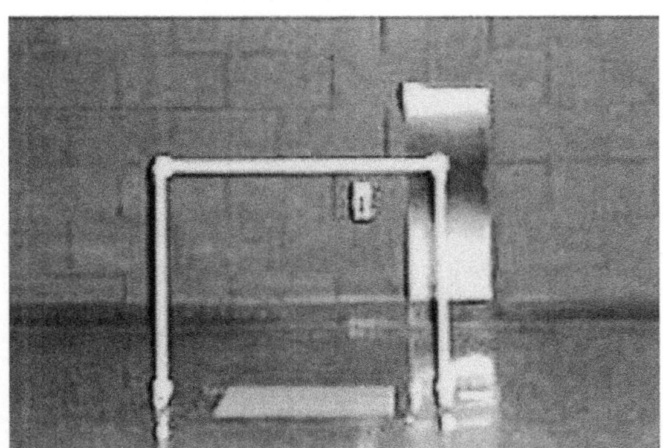

Figure 22.5 A reference frame consists of known distances in the *x* (horizontal) and *y* (vertical) directions.

Once the scale reference has been photographed, it should be measured again on the image. This measurement is then divided into the real length of the scale reference to produce a conversion factor. For example, if the scale reference is actually 1 meter long but measures only 11 cm on the video or film image, the conversion factor would be 1/11 or 0.091. The conversion factor is a constant and has no units. This means that all linear measures (done in centimeters) taken from the film in this example need to be multiplied by 0.091 to give real-life displacements in meters. Scale references and conversion factors are not necessary for angular measurements. The angles viewed in any given frame remain constant regardless of image size.

When using cameras for motion analysis, it is important that the camera be kept still and level. Furthermore, it is imperative that the camera not be moved or bumped once it has been calibrated. Any movement of the camera will require recalibration. For this reason, a tripod and a level are necessities.

The accurate calculation of displacement from frame to frame requires the ability to consistently identify a location of interest, for example, the elbow. Choosing a slightly different location from one frame to another will introduce an error into the displacement measures. This error will be magnified by the frame rate when calculating velocity, and again when calculating acceleration. To reduce error as much as possible, it is advisable to mark the locations of interest in some way that is easily visible on the recorded video. Reflective markers are most often used for this. The small marker spheres are coated with reflective tape or paint. A light source is then aimed at the subject, and the reflected light seems to make the markers glow. Since light will reflect off these markers at the same angle at which it initially strikes the surface, the light that is used should be as close to the camera lens as possible. Figure 22.6 is an example of reflective markers in place on a subject. Marker locations will depend on the nature of the analysis to be done. For a simple analysis in two dimensions, it is common to mark joint centers, establishing these locations through palpation. For more complex three-dimensional and computer or real-time systems, marker locations are determined by the program to be used. Systems can require forty or more markers for accuracy. It should also be mentioned that simple motion analysis may be done by marking the key joints and landmarks with athletic tape or markers.

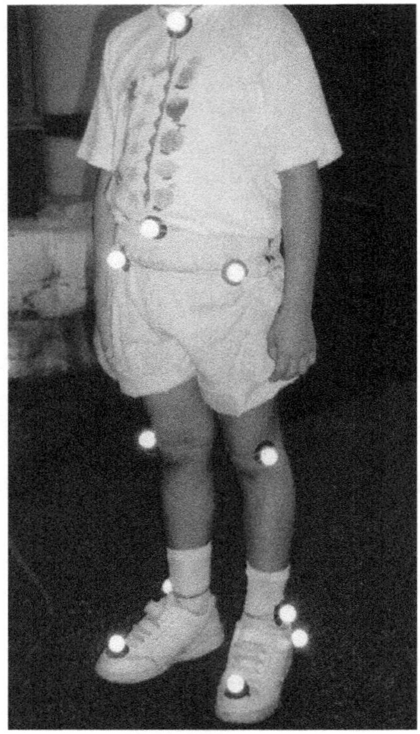

Figure 22.6 Reflective markers are used with a number of optoelectronic data collection systems.

Optoelectronic systems

Motion capture systems that use passive markers such as ink, tape, or reflective markers are susceptible to having the markers blocked (or occluded) as limb segments or clothing may block the markers from the camera view. In addition, when automatic digitizing programs are used, the software could confuse marker identification. For example, if the hand were to pass by the hip during a gait analysis, the software might frequently switch the wrist and hip markers. To overcome this limitation, optoelectronic systems were developed with active markers consisting of LEDs (light-emitting diodes). These systems do not record images, but rather the location of the LEDs in space. The advantage of these active markers is that they are illuminated in a predetermined order, so marker confusion can be eliminated. The cameras are sensitive to these light sources and transmit their locations in space to a computer as a series of *x*-, *y*-coordinates. Kinematic calculations are done on the basis of changes in these coordinate locations. In this type of system the pictorial output usually takes the form of a stick figure or computer-generated model rather than an actual video picture. Most optoelectronic systems are used in laboratory settings rather than in field-based studies because lighting must be very carefully controlled.

Three-Dimensional (3-D) Systems

Both photoinstrumentation systems and optoelectronic systems are commonly configured to collect data in three planes, or three-dimensional data. To conduct a three-dimensional analysis of motion, it is necessary to have more than one camera. The simplest configuration for this analysis method is to position two cameras such that the two camera axes are close to perpendicular. Because kinematic calculations are based on both position and time, it is important that the two cameras' frame rates be carefully synchronized. This is usually done through a generator lock (genlock) mechanism connecting the two cameras. This "black box" locks the two cameras' operating systems together. In addition, the system must be calibrated in three dimensions. The simple meter stick calibration that was described previously is not sufficient in this case. In most three-dimensional systems, calibration is done using a cube or a multiarmed device. Reflective markers are placed on the calibration device at carefully measured points. These makers are then recorded by the system and their locations are input to the computer. The computer can then use these known locations to perform kinematic calculations. The area in which this calibration is correct is called the capture volume. Only movements that happen within this capture volume can be reliably analyzed.

Each camera used in a three-dimensional analysis records marker positions in two dimensions only. Conversion of these data from two-dimensional data into three-dimensional data is done by combining data from all cameras mathematically. The process used for this conversion is referred to as direct linear transformation (DLT). It is an advanced process that involves construction of a series of matrix equations that are then programmed into the computer of the motion analysis system.

Real-Time Systems

As previously mentioned, three-dimensional analysis requires at least two captured images to construct a point in space. Older camera-based systems would use larger computer servers to collect the images and allow software to scan the images for the bright spots on the images made by the reflective makers (Figure 22.6). Due to advances in processing power, specialized cameras now do the searching for the reflective markers and then send only the *x*, *y*, and *z* marker locations to the central computer that is controlling and synchronizing the cameras. Because this process has eliminated the image step, the construction of the marker location in space can happen in what is considered real time. These systems use calibration tools constructed of reflective markers to define the capture volume, as noted above.

Electromagnetic Systems

Electromagnetic systems, also known as "flock of birds" systems, have become more popular due to real-time data collection ability. These systems work by using a transmitter to "construct" a capature volume comprised of electromagnetic field lines. Sensors that are tethered to the computer are attached to the limb segments of interest on the participant. As the sensors move through the field lines, the computer is able to map the location and movement of the sensors. The advantage of such systems is that the signal to the computer is not blocked by the motion of the extremities, as often happens in film or videotape. These virtual reality systems show a great deal of promise for rapid and accurate collection of three-dimensional data.

Regardless of the nature of the transmitter/sensor devices in real-time motion tracking, these systems are all capable of analyzing motion with six degrees of freedom. The term *degrees of freedom* refers to the number of unique directions in which a system can move. In human motion, six degrees of freedom account for motion in each of the three planes and around each of the three axes.

Many real-time, six-degree-of-freedom systems are primarily used in laboratory settings, with subjects connected to the computer and sensor system by cables. Some newer systems are using small, individual transmitters attached to the body, freeing subjects from cable systems. As technology in this area progresses, this system will become more accessible and more adaptable. The student of kinesiology in the next several years is quite likely to encounter one of these real-time motion tracking systems.

Excellent examples of kinematic data collection systems are easily found on the Internet. The student who wishes to view these systems, see examples of the analysis that can be done, or, in some instances, interact with sample data from such systems is advised to spend some time online perusing the large number of sites available.

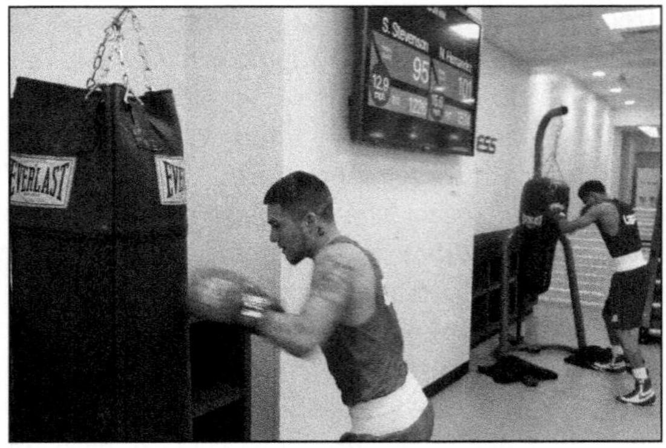

Figure 22.7 3-D accelerometers attached to the wrists, measuring frequency, force and effort exerted. Measurements displayed on screen.

Other Kinematic Instrumentation

Two other instruments sometimes used in kinematic measurement are the electrogoniometer, or elgon, and the accelerometer. The elgon is a double-arm goniometer (see Figure 2.7) with a potentiometer for an axis. A potentiometer, acting like a light dimmer switch, converts changes in angular displacement to changes in electrical current. These changes in electrical current are then recorded by the computer, and through calibration, are converted to an angular measure through which the segment has swept. An elgon recording provides no information concerning movement other than joint angle changes over time. Elgons can be constructed to measure movement in one or all three planes.

The accelerometer is an instrument that, when used singly, measures linear acceleration (Figure 22.7). These measurements are based on variations in electrical current in response to pressure changes caused by the inertia of the accelerometer. Accelerometers are most frequently used to study impact, where objects or limbs undergo rapid, high levels of acceleration. Accelerometers are often used to study levels of physical activity by simply recording the number of accelerations produced by the motion of stepping. Such measures are very rough and provide little information about the mechanics or magnitude of the activity. More precise accelerometry data are often used to study the effects of impact when impact accelerations tend to be very high. The crash test dummies used in automobile testing are equipped with this type of accelerometer, as are the head forms used for helmet testing.

With the availability of signals from global positioning satellites (GPS), released for public use in 2001, the use of GPS receivers to measure displacement and altitude change over time has increased. This technology has been found to be easily portable and fairly accurate (Witte & Wilson, 2005). Although GPS receivers do not provide detailed analysis of movement, they are of value in the examination of displacement and velocity data over a longer period of time or over a great distance.

Both accelerometers and elgons are rigid items that must be attached to the body. Elgons also may have wires leading to the output device or to a radio transmitter also worn on the body. Because of these necessary attachments, both forms of instrumentation may interfere with the performance of the movement skill. For this reason elgons are most often used in laboratory situations for experimental research.

INSTRUMENTATION FOR KINETIC ANALYSIS

Kinetic data are usually collected through the use of dynamometers or force transducers. Dynamometers are primarily spring-and-cable tension instruments that measure static muscle strength, or strength in a single position. Examples of dynamometers are the grip-strength dynamometer and the leg-strength dynamometer.

Force transducers are a common tool in kinetic analyses. One example of a force transducer frequently used in kinetic studies is the strain gauge. In the strain gauge, altered resistance due to strain on the mechanism, which may be made of wire or a semiconductor substance, produces a change in output voltage, which may then be recorded by an output device. Strain gauges can be manufactured to fit almost any analysis situation. Strain gauge systems have been fabricated to measure forces on uneven parallel bars, impact on a tennis racket, the strain in a hammer throw chain, and many other applications. Strain gauges or piezoelectric force transducers (which respond to pressure) have been used extensively in gait analysis. The small transducers are placed at strategic points on the sole of the foot, and the force present during gait is measured.

Two types of adaptable pressure-sensing materials that are used in kinetic analysis are piezoelectric film and force-sensing resistors (FSRs). Both sensors come in a variety of sizes and configurations and can easily be adapted to a variety of movement problems (Figure 22.8). Each is also easily connected to a computer containing an

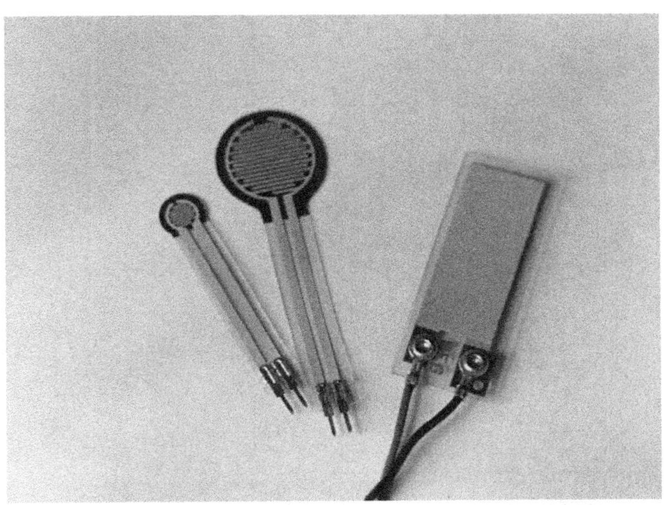

Figure 22.8 Force-sensing resistors (FSRs) and piezoelectric film used to collect force and pressure data.

analog-to-digital converter. This type of technology is highly affordable and easy to work with. For this reason the student is cautioned to carefully examine data produced by these devices. Both piezoelectric film and FSRs are difficult to calibrate. It is best to look at these data as being relative to some known measure, such as body weight.

Perhaps the most common use of force transducer technology in kinetic motion analysis is the force plate. This force, or pressure-sensing, instrument is placed in the floor, ground, or wall so that ground reaction forces may be recorded in all six possible modes (vertical, two horizontal, and about each of the three axes) while walking, running, jumping, landing, or making any of a vast number of movements. As the foot or any other body part lands on the platform, linear forces and torques acting at the point of impact are identified through output to a computer system (Figure 22.9). From data generated in this

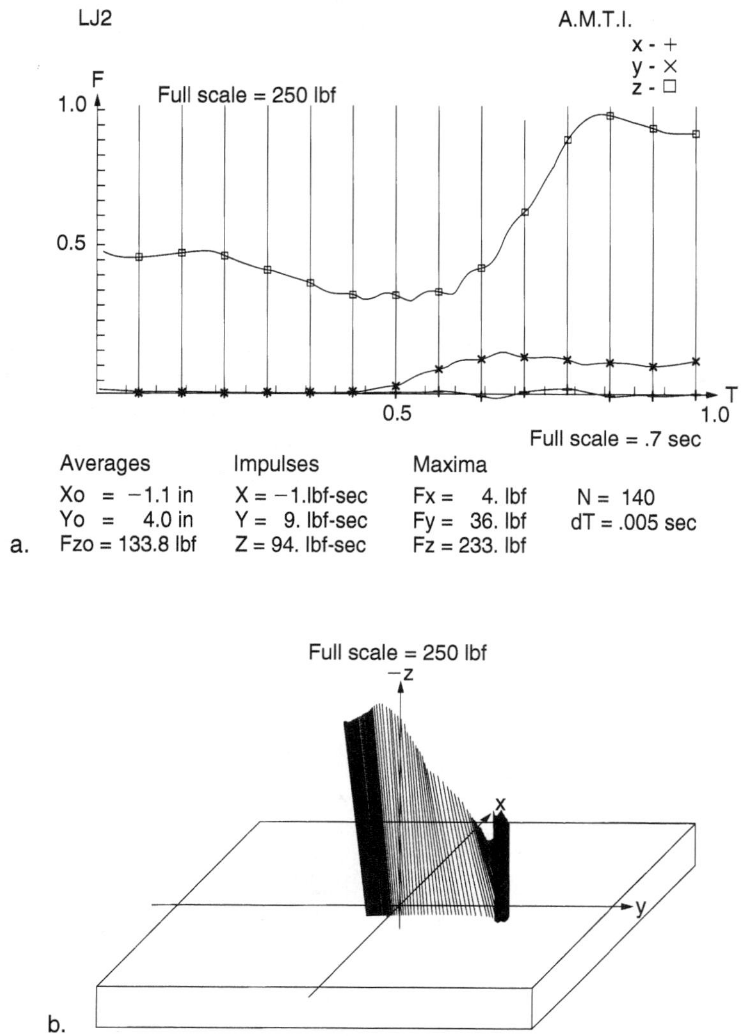

Figure 22.9 Force-time data collected by a force plate and computer: (a) force-time history of the takeoff in a standing long jump; (b) force vector diagram of the same jump.

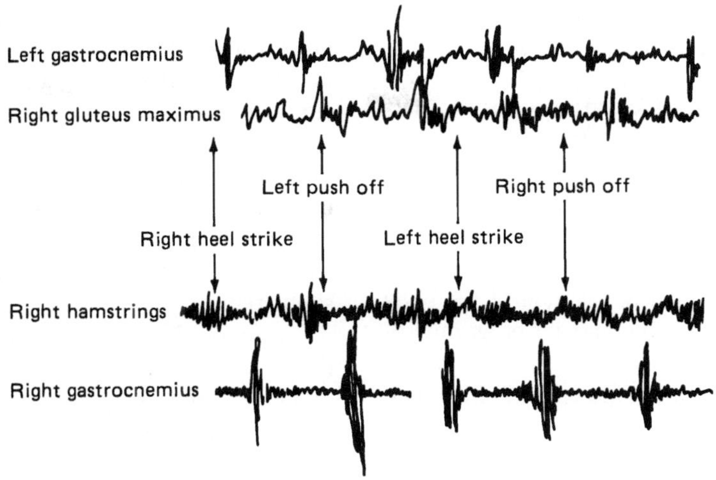

Figure 22.10 EMG trace of muscles of the legs during walking.

manner, especially when combined with kinematic data, a mathematical process referred to as inverse dynamics may be used to calculate joint forces and torques that are acting throughout the motion.

ELECTROMYOGRAPHY

Most studies to determine muscle activity during any given movement have been done using electromyography. In electromyography (EMG), the electrical activity generated by the differences in action potential between two sites on the same muscle is measured through the use of electrodes, which are sensitive to changes in electrical current. These electrodes may be small metallic plates attached to the skin, or they may be indwelling needle or fine wire electrodes (see Figure 3.13). The action potentials from the muscles are sensed by these electrodes, and the signal that is generated is amplified and transmitted to a computer. An analysis of the recorded EMG signal can then provide information on the intensity of muscle contraction and the temporal and sequential order of muscle activation. Such information can provide great insight into the muscular demands of specific activities. Figure 22.10 is a sample of the EMG data.

Although EMG is an excellent tool for determining the existence of muscle activity at any given point in time, the recorded data are simply indicative of action potential. EMG data provide no information concerning the type of muscular contraction (static, concentric, or eccentric) or the force produced by the muscle contraction. The primary purpose of EMG for the movement specialist is to identify and verify the presence or absence of muscle activity in a given muscle at a given point in time.

Some quantitative analysis of EMG signals is done by "normalizing" the EMG output. This technique involves the transformation of the EMG signal during activity to a percentage of the signal recorded for a maximum voluntary contraction of the muscle being investigated. This normalizing technique is often used to compare the changes that occur in muscle activity with changes in activity conditions such as load, muscle angle of pull, joint angle, movement speed, and fatigue. The student is cautioned, however, to remember that many factors can affect EMG output, and conclusions based on EMG results should be carefully examined.

COMPUTER MODELS AND SIMULATION

Kinematic, kinetic, and electromyographic data about human motion are often compiled and synthesized into sets of equations that describe the motion mathematically. These sets of equations are referred to as mathematical models or, more frequently, as computer models. A computer model is a mathematical description of the body in motion compiled into a computer program. Often these equations are used to produce a graphic representation of motion. Figures 22.2, 22.3, and 22.11 are examples of the graphic representations of computer models.

When a computer model is manipulated experimentally by changing the value of the variables, the result is a computer simulation. Computer simulations allow for the exploration of the limitations and capacities of human movement systems without endangering human subjects. The values for the variables one wishes to test are entered into the computer program, and the computer simulates the desired motion using the given values. As an example, several angles of takeoff may be simulated for the long jump without the necessity of using an actual jumper. These simulations may be done quickly and optimal performance predicted once an accurate computer model has been designed. Computer simulations have been used to predict limits to human performance that are even now being challenged by athletes. Figure 22.12 illustrates a simple computer simulation.

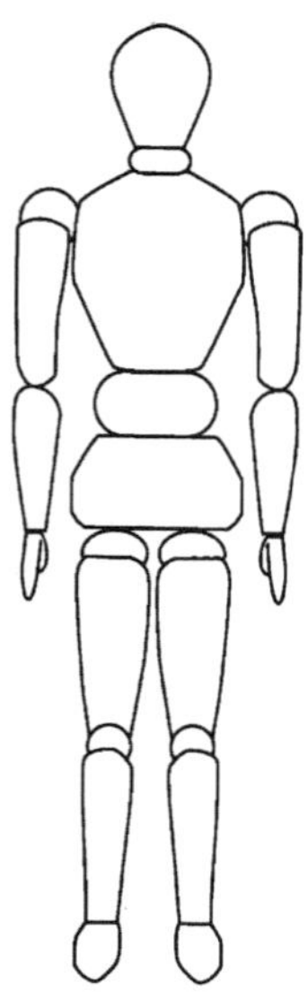

Figure 22.11 Computer model of the human body represented as a series of segmental levers.

One of the more forbidding challenges in the work of computer modeling and simulation of human movement is to represent accurately the complexity of the human body in the model. When one considers the makeup of the human system, with all the possible combinations of joint and muscle, the task seems overwhelming. Most computer models, therefore, use greatly simplified representations of the various biological components of any given motion. An example of this is the way in which muscle action is frequently simulated. When analyzing closely the action of a given muscle, one must consider not only the contractile element of the muscle but also the elastic components. A simplified model of muscle might be somewhat like that depicted in Figure 22.13, consisting of a contractile element, a series elastic component, and a parallel elastic component. Each of these components must then be assigned a value based on the researcher's knowledge of the body. This simple muscle model then gains rapidly in complexity if it is applied to each of the muscles that might be active in a given motion. For this reason, computer simulations often vary greatly from what one might expect from actual human performance. Still, they provide the movement specialist with increased knowledge about the movement potential of the human body. Computer modeling continues to advance in aid of the complex problem of modeling human movement. A technique that is becoming more widely used is the construction of finite element mesh (FEM) models. In FEM models a complex system is deconstructed into a set of finite elements, each having structural properties to match the material

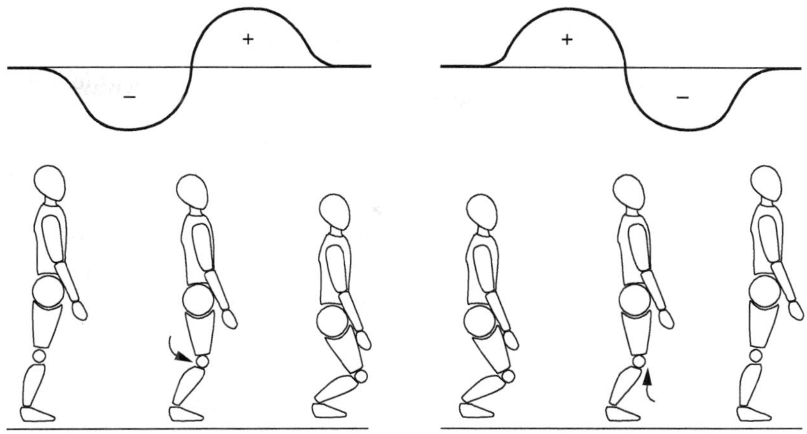

Figure 22.12 Computer simulation of unweighting skis through fast flexion and extension. *Source*: From *Biomechanics of Human Movement,* by Marlene A. Adrian & John M. Cooper. Copyright © 1989, Benchmark Press. Reprinted by permission of Times Mirror Higher Education Group, Inc., Dubuque, IA. All rights reserved.

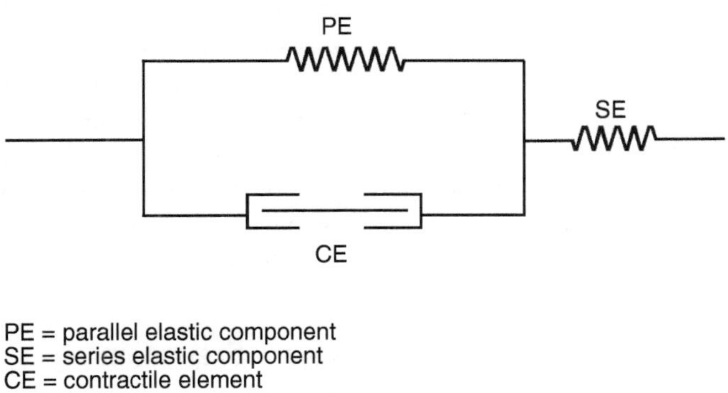

Figure 22.13 A simplified model of the contractile properties of muscles, as represented in a computer-generated model of human movement.

being modeled. Each element contains several "nodes," often where elements join. As stresses are applied to the nodes in the model system, the response of the collective elements helps to predict the effects of the stress in real life. A common use for FEM models is in shaping and manufacturing artificial joints.

In the very near future, it is likely that software for simulating various human movements will become readily available. However, one must remember that the computer simulation, although useful, cannot yet completely model human neurology, physiology, or psychology. Regardless of the complexity of the model used to produce a computer simulation, such simulations are still simplifications of actual motion.

USING QUANTITATIVE ANALYSIS

As the task of collecting data on human movement becomes easier and more automated, there is a risk of producing such data for their own sake, with no thought toward application. When one sets out to collect movement data, there should be some clear purpose in mind. It is the purpose of the analysis that will determine the type of data that need to be collected and the methodology and instrumentation to be used. A sound plan is to base the collection of biomechanical data on a carefully designed analysis plan, using a model such as that introduced and used throughout this text. The analysis that one undertakes should be aimed toward some end result.

In the various fields that deal with human movement, there are several purposes to which the collection of movement analysis data might be directed. Examples of the purposes for performing a movement analysis include such things as the optimization of performance, the prevention of injuries, and rehabilitation.

Optimization of Performance

Often, when considering the efficiency and effectiveness of performance, the maximum is not the most desirable. For instance, in shooting free throws, the basketball player who applies maximum force is more than likely to overshoot the target, resulting in a missed shot. The long jumper who generates maximum horizontal velocity may have trouble converting to a vertical velocity. The computer operator who types at the fastest possible speed may find many errors. In instances such as these and countless others, what is needed is an *optimum* performance. Optimal performance implies that all the factors that make up the motion are combined in such a way as to produce the most effective result. The optimization of human performance has been the goal of much of the quantitative biomechanical analysis that has been done.

Quantitative biomechanical data are useful in the process of optimizing performance in that they provide a mathematical description of the relationships between various factors that comprise the performance. As an example, it is well known that running speed depends on the combination of stride length and stride frequency. At first glance it would seem that producing the longest stride length of which an individual is capable and taking these strides as fast as possible would generate the fastest running speed. In actuality, there is a point where increased stride length simply adds to the braking force of the stride by producing too much horizontal force in the wrong direction. It is possible, through kinematic motion analysis and force plate studies, to determine the stride length at which the individual produces the greatest possible impulse in the desired direction. This, then, becomes the optimum stride length. Once this stride length is mastered, further increments in running speed will be due to increases in stride frequency. Stride frequency might be enhanced by examining the quantitative data on the angular velocities that are generated as the swing leg is brought forward on each step. As will be remembered from earlier chapters, the velocity of the swing leg can often be improved by decreasing the moment of inertia of the lower extremity through greater hip and knee flexion. Thus the running stride has been optimized to produce the best possible performance for that individual runner.

Injury Prevention

Injuries are often the result of forces applied to the body in excessive or inappropriate ways. Torques that are too great in magnitude or that are applied in the wrong direction, high acceleration forces, impact, and sudden forceful stretch can all produce injuries. Quantitative data collection can provide valuable information about the risk of injury in any movement. Most people are now familiar with the impact studies that have been done by the automobile industry. By using heavily instrumented crash test dummies to quantify the force acting on the human body during an automobile accident, newer and more effective safety devices have been developed. The same sort of studies have been done on football and bicycle helmets, playing surfaces, mats and landing pads, and a variety of other impact surfaces. Data have been collected on the forces transmitted to the body in a variety of activities, from walking to lifting. For example, in a study conducted in 2010 by Bischof et al., the researchers found that women runners produce ground reaction forces as high as 2.5 times body weight.

One area that has long been of concern in injury prevention is the study and modification of load-lifting techniques. Researchers in ergonomics (the study of work) have gathered data not only on the forces generated by lifting various loads but also on the limitations of the structures doing the lifting. A number of studies have been done to establish the loads at which the various structures of the vertebral column begin to fail. These data have been used to build general models of safe load limits and safe lifting practices.

Rehabilitation

A large amount of the work that has been done in quantitative gait analysis, electromyography, and load handling has been done by researchers in the rehabilitation field. Immediately following World War II, many hospitals and clinics began studying gait in depth, hoping to produce a model of the "normal" gait to aid in efforts to rehabilitate wounded soldiers. From the early work by researchers such as Murray and coworkers (1964, 1970), Inman, and Ralston (Rose & Gamble, 1994) came the bases for clinical rehabilitation work that is done today. In most therapeutic and rehabilitation settings, quantitative data are collected on patients on a regular basis. These data are then compared with the models of normal patterns, and from these comparisons, programs of rehabilitation and remediation are designed. The extent to which quantitative biomechanics has been used in physical therapy and rehabilitation fills volumes in most university and clinic libraries. The reading of current rehabilitation research should become a habit for any student of human movement.

Summary

This closing chapter has included a brief overview of some of the technology that is being used by those who work with human movement. As technology becomes more available, the use of once complex systems will become commonplace. Therefore, it is imperative that the student of human movement be comfortable with computer technology. As this book is being written, technology is spreading to larger and larger segments of the population. Physical therapists regularly use video-based gait analysis systems, computer-driven rehabilitation devices, and computer-based treatment plans. Teachers are using computer technology to work with physical education students throughout the school years. Middle school students are using videotape to examine their own performances. With sophisticated technology available to a large segment of the population, movement professionals are obligated to examine and search constantly for ways to use technology to further the work they do.

The student of human movement is encouraged to keep abreast of the latest in technology by reading and exploring. A perusal of the articles and books listed in the References and Selected Readings section of each chapter of this text provides a broad overview of the current state of instrumentation and technology in the area of kinesiology and biomechanics. With the ready availability of reference material online, an incredible wealth of material on the latest developments in the measurement of human motion is accessible. Carefully read the section on methodology in a number of research articles to become familiar with measurement techniques. Many of the articles listed in this chapter serve this primary purpose, the teaching of methodology.

Appendix A Classification of Joints and Their Movements

Type	Articulation	Movement
	Diarthrodial: Nonaxial	
	Shoulder girdle	
	Sternoclavicular	Limited motion of end of clavicle in all three planes
		Elevation–depression
		Forward-backward
		Rotation: forward-downward; backward-upward
	Acromioclavicular	Movements of scapula (including motion in both joints)
Irregular;		Elevation–depression
Arthrodial;		Rotation: upward-downward
Plane		Abduction–adduction
		Upward tilt—reduction of same
	Intercarpal	Slight gliding movements in cooperation with movements of wrist and metacarpals
	Intertarsal	Slight gliding movements in cooperation with movements of talonavicular and ankle joints
	Diarthrodial: Uniaxial	
	Elbow	
	Humeroulnar	Flexion–extension–hyperextension (slight)
	Knee	
	Tibiofemoral	Flexion–extension–hyperextension (slight)
Hinge;	Ankle	
Ginglymus	Talotibial and talofibular	Dorsiflexion–plantar flexion (extension)
	Fingers and thumb	Flexion–extension
	Interphalangeal	
	Toes	
	Interphalangeal	Flexion–extension
	Forearm	
	Proximal and distal radioulnar	Supination–pronation
Pivot;	Neck	
Screw;	Atlantoaxial (first and	
Trochoid	second cervical)	Rotation: right-left

Type	Articulation	Movement
	Diarthrodial: Biaxial	
	Wrist	Flexion–extension–hyperextension
	Radiocarpal	Abduction–adduction
	Fingers	
	Metacarpophalangeal	Flexion–extension
		Abduction–adduction
Condyloid;		
Ovoid;	Toes	
Ellipsoidal	Metatarsophalangeal	Flexion–extension–hyperextension
		Abduction–adduction (limited)
	Head	
	Occipitoatlantal	Flexion–extension–hyperextension
		Lateral flexion: right-left
Saddle;		
Seller;	Thumb	
Reciprocal	Carpometacarpal	Flexion–extension–hyperextension
reception		Abduction–adduction
		Opposition (combination of abduction, hyperflexion, and possibly slight inward rotation)*
	Diarthrodial: Triaxial	
	Shoulder	Flexion–extension–hyperextension
	Glenohumeral	Abduction–adduction
		Rotation: outward-inward
Ball-and-socket;		Horizontal adduction (from abduction)
Enarthrodial		Horizontal abduction (from flexion)
	Hip	
	Femoroacetabular	Flexion–extension–hyperextension
		Abduction–adduction
		Rotation: outward-inward
		Horizontal adduction (from abduction)
		Horizontal abduction (from flexion)
Shallow	Foot	
ball-and-socket	Talonavicular	Dorsiflexion–plantar flexion (very slight)
		Abduction–adduction (slight)
		Inversion–eversion (very slight)
	Combination Diarthrodial Nonaxial and Fibrocartilaginous Synarthrodial	
Triaxial simulated	Vertebral bodies	
ball-and-socket	Intervertebral cartilages	Flexion
		Extension
		Hyperextension
Nonaxial irregular	Vertebral arches	Lateral flexion: right-left
		Rotation: right-left

*Opinions differ with respect to inward rotation.

Appendix B Joint Range of Motion

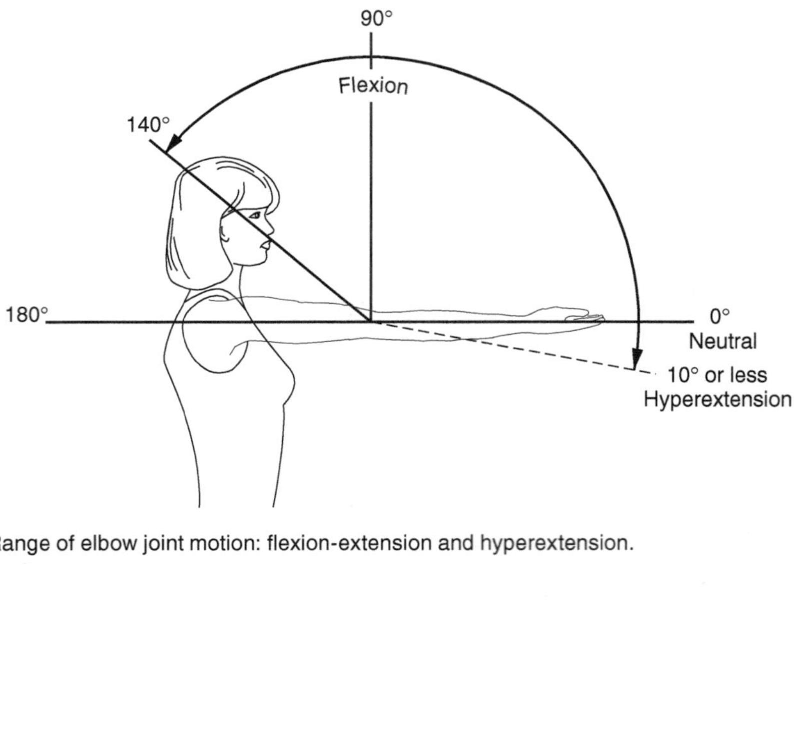

Figure B.1 Range of elbow joint motion: flexion-extension and hyperextension.

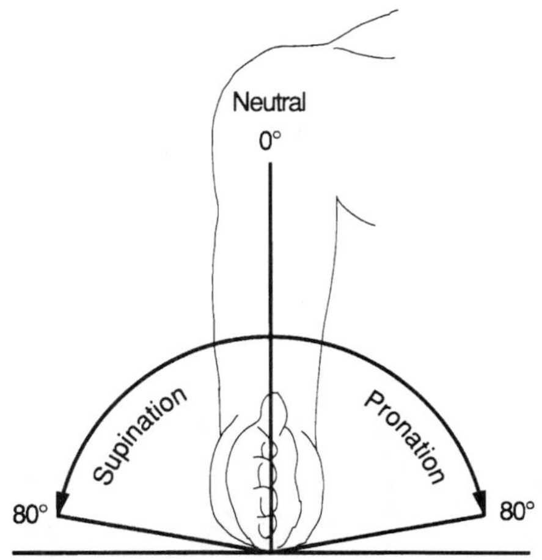

Figure B.2 Range of forearm motion: pronation and supination.

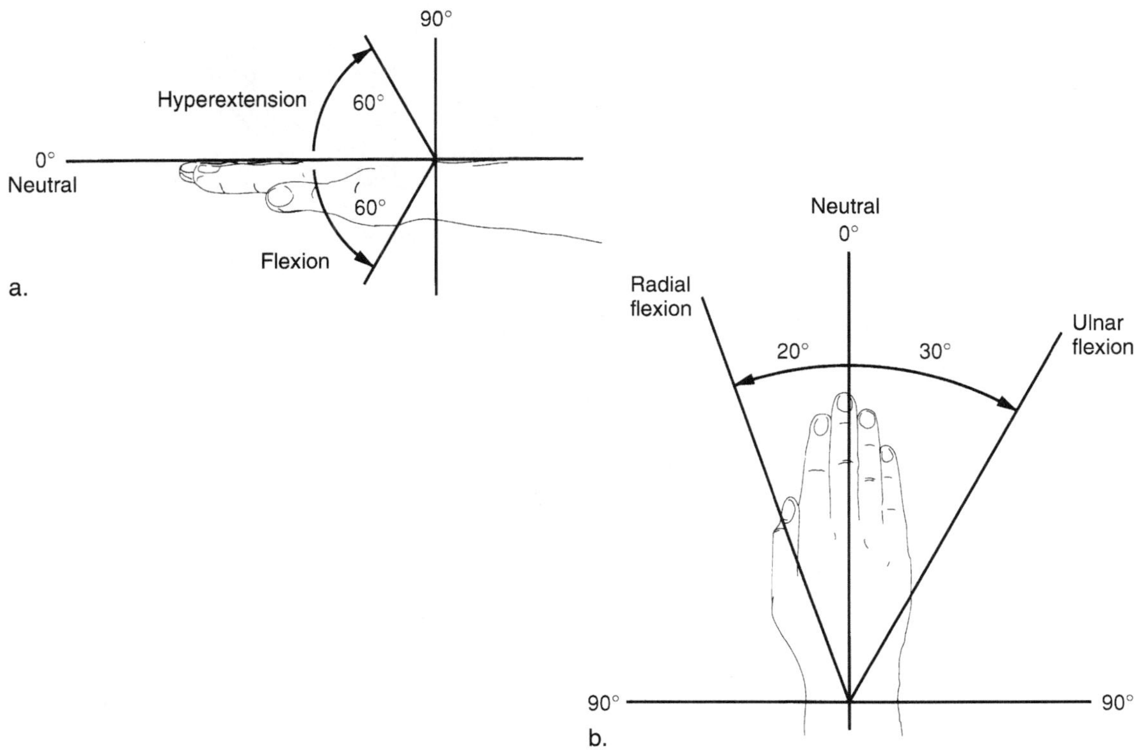

Figure B.3 Range of wrist joint movement: (a) flexion-extension and hyperextension; (b) radial and ulnar flexion.

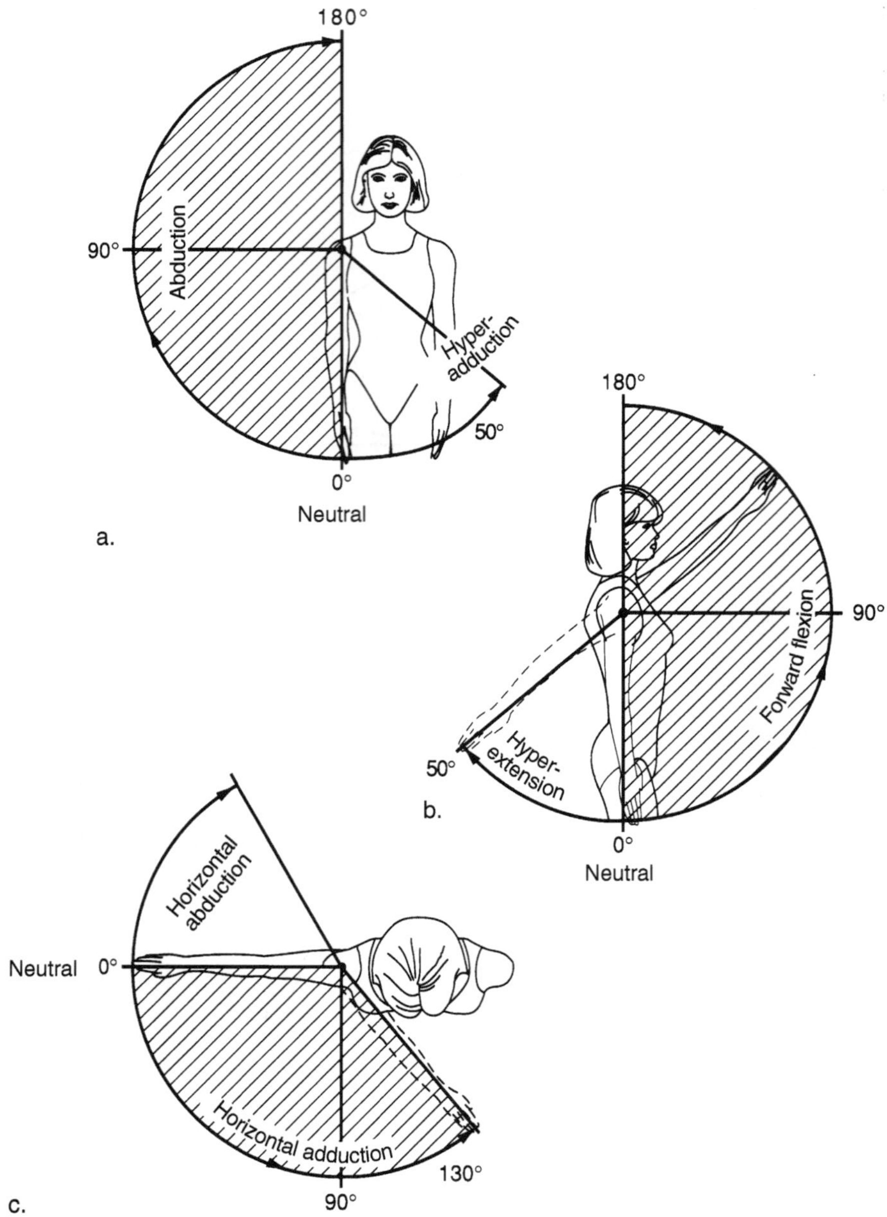

Figure B.4 Range of arm movement on trunk (involving both shoulder joint and shoulder girdle): (a) abduction and adduction; (b) flexion and hyperextension; (c) horizontal adduction and abduction.

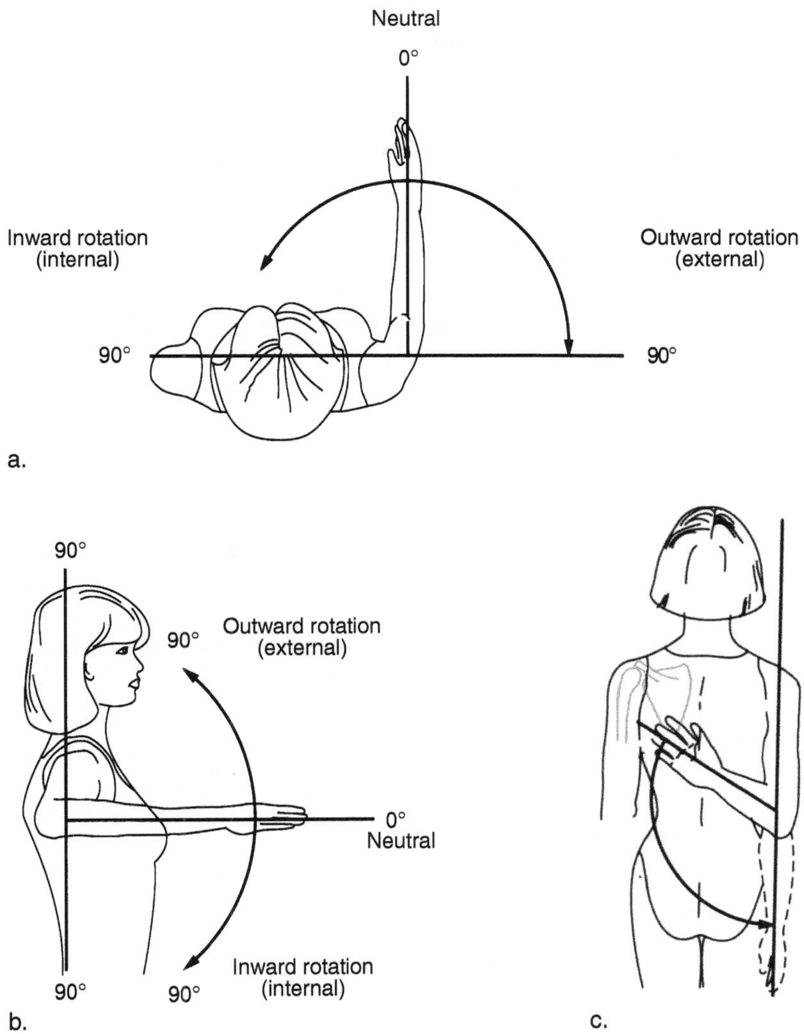

Figure B.5 Range of arm movement on trunk (involving both shoulder joint and shoulder girdle): (a) rotation with arm at side; (b) rotation with arm in abduction; (c) internal rotation posteriorly.

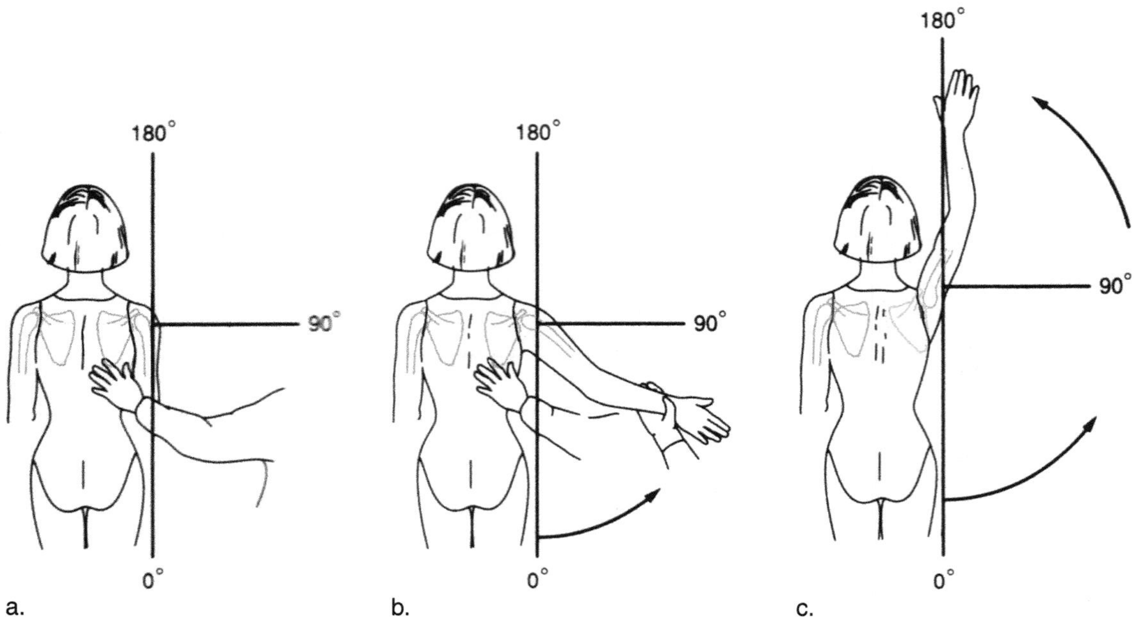

Figure B.6 Range of shoulder joint (glenohumeral) motion: (a) starting position; (b) abduction; (c) sideward-upward elevation of arm (combining abduction of arm and upward rotation of scapula).

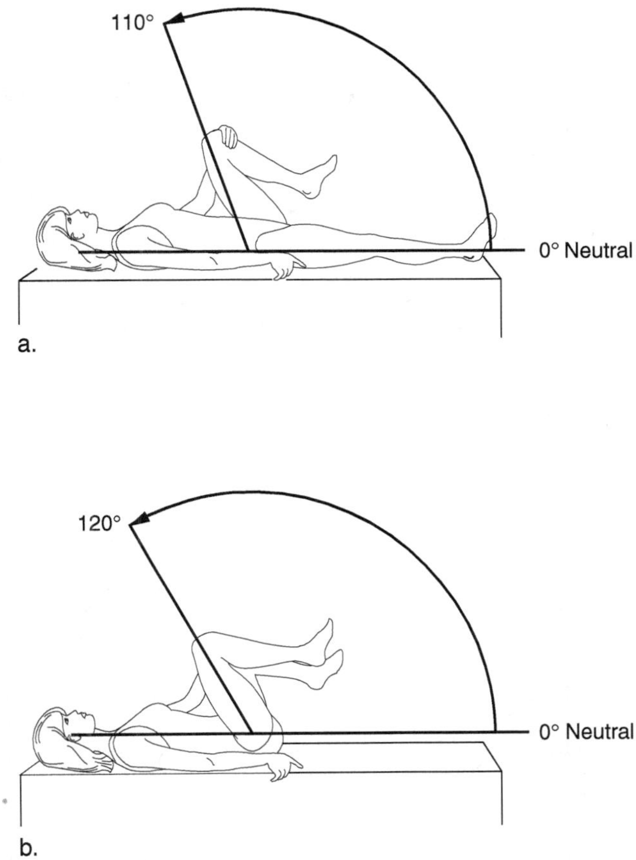

Figure B.7 Range of hip joint flexion: (a) starting position; (b) maximal flexion without rotating pelvis.

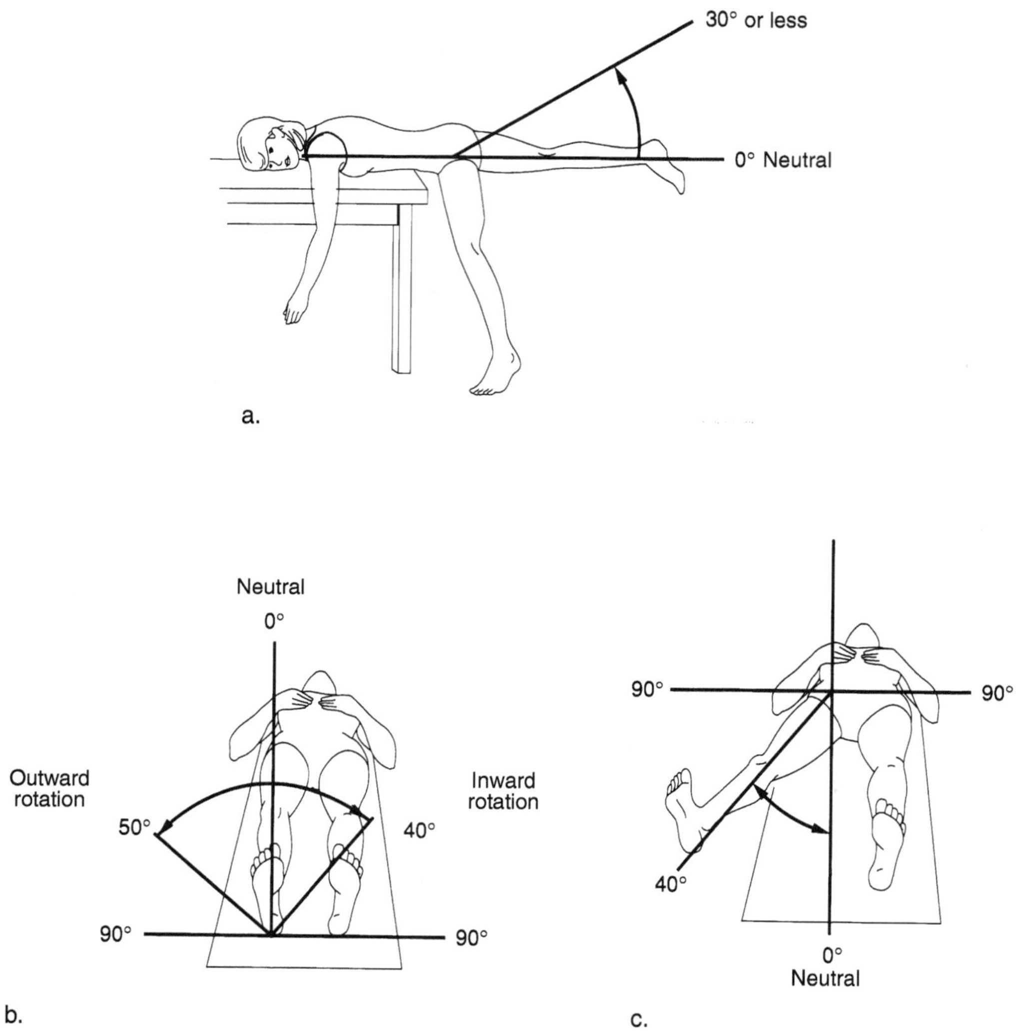

Figure B.8 Range of hip joint movement: (a) hyperextension; (b) inward and outward rotation; (c) abduction.

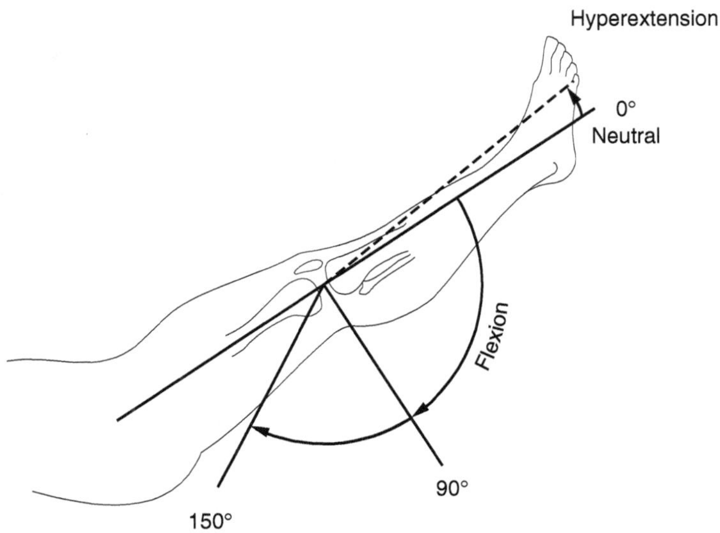

Figure B.9 Range of knee joint motion: flexion–extension and hyperextension.

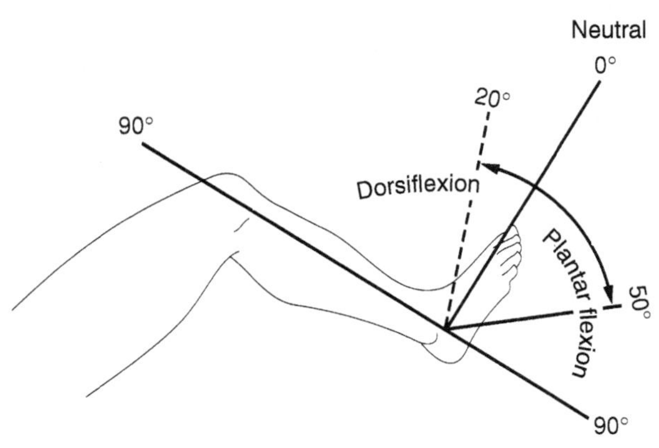

Figure B.10 Range of ankle joint dorsiflexion and plantar flexion with knee in flexed position.

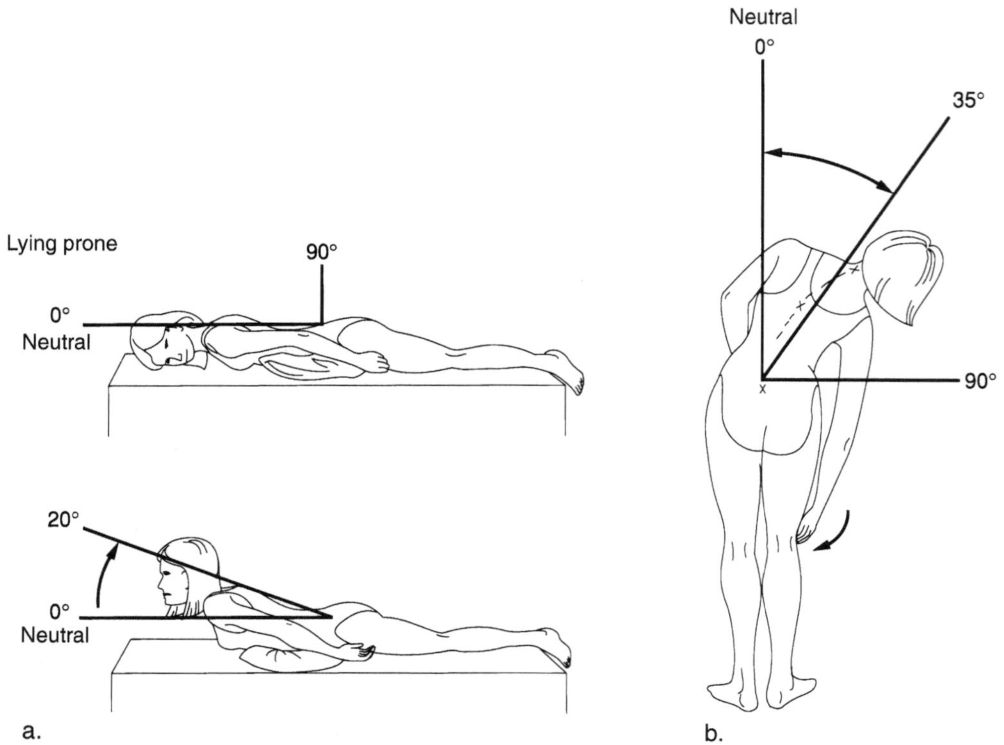

Figure B.11 Range of motion in the thoracic and lumbar spine: (a) hyperextension; (b) lateral flexion.

Muscular Attachments and Nerve Supply

Appendix C

The Upper Extremity*

Muscle	Proximal Attachments	Distal Attachments	Nerve Supply
		Shoulder Joint	
Coracobrachialis	Coracoid process of scapula	Inner surface of humerus opposite deltoid attachment	Musculocutaneous nerve
Deltoid	Anterior: anterior border of outer third of clavicle		Axillary (circumflex) nerve
	Middle: acromion process and outer end of clavicle	Lateral aspect of humerus, near midpoint	
	Posterior: lower margin of spine of scapula		
Infraspinatus and teres minor	Axillary border and posterior surface of scapula below scapular spine	Posterior aspect of greater tuberosity of humerus	Suprascapular and axillary nerves
Latissimus dorsi	Spinous processes of lower six thoracic and all lumbar vertebrae; posterior surface of sacrum; crest of ilium; lower three ribs	Anterior surface of humerus below head by flat tendon just anterior to, and parallel with, tendon of pectoralis major	Thoracodorsal (middle subscapular) nerve
Pectoralis major	Medial two-thirds of clavicle; anterior surface of sternum; cartilages of first six ribs; slip from aponeurosis of external oblique abdominal muscle	Lateral surface of humerus just below head by flat tendon 2 to 3 inches wide	Medial and lateral anterior thoracic nerves
Subscapularis	Entire anterior surface of scapula	Lesser tuberosity of humerus	Subscapular nerve
Supraspinatus	Medial two-thirds of supraspinatus fossa above scapular spine	Top of greater tuberosity of humerus	Suprascapular nerve
Teres major	Posterior surface of inferior angle of scapula	Anterior surface of humerus below head, just medial to latissimus dorsi tendon	Lower subscapular nerve

*See Chapters 5 and 6.

		Shoulder Girdle	
Coracobrachialis	Coracoid process of scapula	Inner surface of humerus opposite deltoid attachment	Musculocutaneous nerve
Levator scapulae	Transverse processes of first four cervical vertebrae	Vertebral border of scapula between medial angle and scapular spine	Dorsal scapular and branches from third and fourth cervical nerves
Pectoralis minor	Anterior surface of third, fourth, and fifth ribs near cartilages	Tip of coracoid processes of scapula	Medial anterior thoracic nerve
Rhomboids: major and minor	Spinous processes of seventh cervical and first five thoracic vertebrae	Vertebral border of scapula from spine to inferior angle	Dorsal scapular nerve
Serratus anterior	Outer surface of upper nine ribs at side of chest	Anterior surface of vertebral border and inferior angle of scapula	Long thoracic nerve
Trapezius	Occipital bone; ligamentum nuchae; spinous processes of seventh cervical and all thoracic vertebrae	Part I: posterior border of lateral third of clavicle Part II: top of acromium process Part III: upper border of scapular spine Part IV: root of scapular spine	Spinal accessory and branches from third and fourth cervical nerves
		Elbow and Forearm	
Anconeus	Posterior surface of lateral epicondyle of humerus	Lateral side of olecranon process and posterior surface of upper part of ulna	Branch from radial nerve
Biceps brachii	Long head: upper margin of glenoid fossa Short head: apex of coracoid process of scapula	Bicipital tuberosity of radius	Musculocutaneous nerve
Brachialis humerus	Anterior surface of lower half of humerus	Anterior surface of coronoid process of ulna	Musculocutaneous and branch from radial nerves
Brachioradialis	Upper two-thirds of lateral supracondylar ridge of humerus	Lateral side of base of styloid process of radius	Radial nerve
Pronator teres	Medial epicondyle of humerus and medial side of coronoid process of ulna	Lateral surface of radius near middle	Medial nerve

The Upper Extremity *(continued)*

Pronator quadratus	Anterior surface of lower one-fourth of ulna	Anterior surface of lower one-fourth of radius	Branch from median nerve
Supinator	Lateral condyle of humerus; adjacent portion of ulna; radial collateral and annular ligaments	Lateral surface of upper third of radius	Branch from deep radial nerve
Triceps brachii	Long head: infraglenoid tuberosity Lateral head: posterior surface of upper half of humerus Medial head: posterior surface of lower two-thirds of humerus	Olecranon process of ulna	Radial nerve
		Wrist	
Extensor carpi radialis brevis	Lateral epicondyle of humerus	Posterior surface of base of third metacarpal	Radial nerve
Extensor carpi radialis longus	Lateral epicondyle of humerus and supracondylar ridge above	Posterior surface of base of second metacarpal	Radial nerve
Extensor carpi ulnaris	By two heads from lateral epicondyle of humerus and middle third of posterior ridge of ulna	Posterior surface of base of fifth metacarpal	Deep radial nerve
Flexor carpi radialis	Medial epicondyle of humerus	Anterior surface of base of second metacarpal	Median nerve
Flexor carpi ulnaris	By two heads from medial condyle of humerus and medial border of olecranon process of ulna	Palmar surface of pisiform and hamate carpal bones, and base of fifth metacarpal	Ulnar nerve
Palmaris longus	Medial epicondyle of humerus	Transverse carpal ligament and palmar aponeurosis	Median nerve
		Thumb and Fingers	
Abductor pollicis longus	Dorsolateral surface of ulna below anconeus, dorsal surface of radius near center, and intervening interosseous membrane	Lateral surface of base of first metacarpal	Deep radial nerve
Extensor digiti minimi	Proximal tendon of extensor digitorum	Fifth finger's extensor digitorum tendon	Deep radial nerve

Extensor digitorum	Lateral epicondyle of humerus	By four tendons, one to each finger, each tendon dividing into three slips, the middle one attaching to dorsal surface of second phalanx and the other two uniting to attach to dorsal surface of base of distal phalanx	Deep radial nerve
Extensor indicis	Dorsal surface of lower half of ulna	Index finger's extensor digitorum tendon	Deep radial nerve
Extensor pollicis brevis	Dorsal surface of radius below abductor pollicis longus	Dorsal surface of base of first phalanx	Deep radial nerve
Extensor pollicis longus	Dorsal surface of middle third of ulna	Dorsal surface of base of distal phalanx	Deep radial nerve
Flexor digitorum profundus	Upper two-thirds of anterior and medial surfaces of ulna	By four tendons (one to each finger) to base of distal phalanx, after passing through tendon of flexor digitorum superficialis	Interosseous branch of median nerve
Flexor digitorum superficialis	Humeroulnar head: medial epicondyle of humerus, ulnar collateral ligament, medial margin of coronoid process Radial head: oblique line on anterior surface of radial shaft	By four tendons to the four fingers, each tendon splitting to attach to either side of base of middle phalanx	Median nerve
Flexor pollicis longus	Anterior surface of middle half of radius	Anterior surface of base of distal phalanx of thumb	Volar interosseous branch of median nerve
Abductor digiti minimi	Pisiform bone and tendon of flexor carpi ulnaris	Ulnar side of base of first phalanx of fifth finger and ulnar border of aponeurosis of extensor digiti minimi	Ulnar nerve
Abductor pollicis brevis	Anterior surface of transverse carpal ligament and greater multangular and navicular bones	Radial side of base of first phalanx of thumb	Median nerve
Adductor pollicis	Carpal (oblique) head: deep carpal ligaments, capitate bone, and bases of second and third metacarpals Metacarpal (transverse) head: lower two-thirds of anterior surface of third metacarpal	Ulnar side of base of proximal phalanx of thumb	Deep palmar branch of ulnar nerve

The Upper Extremity *(continued)*

Flexor digiti minimi brevis	Hook of hamate bone and adjacent parts of transverse carpal ligament	Ulnar side of base of first phalanx of fifth finger	Palmar division of ulnar nerve
Flexor pollicis brevis	Superficial head: greater multangular bone and adjacent part of transverse carpal ligament	Superficial head: radial side of base of first phalanx of thumb	Median nerve
	Deep head: ulnar side of first metacarpal	Deep head: ulnar side of base of first phalanx of thumb	
Interossei dorsales	By two heads from adjacent sides of metacarpals in each interspace	Base of proximal phalanx and aponeurosis of extensor muscles on each side of middle finger, on thumb side of index finger, and on ulnar side of fourth finger	Palmar branch of ulnar nerve
Interossei palmares	First: ulnar side of second metacarpal	First: ulnar side of base of first phalanx of index finger and expansion of extensor digitorum tendon	Ulnar nerve
	Second: radial side of fourth metacarpal	Second: radial side of base of first phalanx of fourth finger and expansion of extensor digitorum tendon	
	Third: radial side of fifth metacarpal	Third: radial side of base of first phalanx of fifth finger and expansion of extensor digitorum tendon	
Lumbricales	Tendons of flexor digitorum profundus in center of palm	Extensor aponeuroses on radial side of proximal phalanges	First and second: median nerve; third and fourth: ulnar nerve
Opponens digiti minimi	Hook of hamate bone and adjacent parts of transverse carpal ligament	Entire length of ulnar border of fifth metacarpal	Deep palmar branch of ulnar nerve
Opponens pollicis	Anterior surface of greater multangular bone and transverse carpal ligament	Entire radial border of anterior surface of first metacarpal	Median nerve

The Lower Extremity*

Muscle	Proximal Attachments	Distal Attachments	Nerve Supply
		Hip Joint	
Adductor brevis	Outer surface of body and inferior ramus of pubis	Line from lesser trochanter to linea aspera and upper fourth of linea aspera	Obdurator and accessory obdurator nerves
Adductor longus	Anterior surface of pubis	Medial lip of middle half of linea aspera	Obdurator nerve
Adductor magnus	Inferior rami of pubis and ischium and lateral border of inferior surface of ischial tuberosity	Linea aspera, medial supracondylar line, and adductor tubercle on medial condyle of femur	Obdurator nerve
Biceps femoris, long head	Lower and medial impression on tuberosity of ischium	Lateral side of head of fibula and lateral condyle of tibia	Sciatic nerve
Gluteus maximus	Posterior gluteal line of ilium and adjacent portion of crest; posterior surface of lower part of sacrum and side of coccyx	Posterior surface of femur on ridge below greater trochanter; iliotibial tract of fascia lata	Inferior gluteal nerve
Gluteus medius	Posterior surface of ilium between crest, posterior gluteal line, and anterior gluteal line	Oblique ridge on lateral surface of greater trochanter	Superior gluteal nerve
Gluteus minimus	Posterior surface of ilium between anterior and inferior gluteal lines	Anterior border to greater trochanter	Superior gluteal nerve
Gracilis	Anterior aspect of lower half of symphysis pubis and upper half of pubic arch	Medial surface of tibia just below condyle	Obturator
Iliopsoas	Psoas major: sides of bodies and intervertebral cartilages of last thoracic and all lumbar vertebrae; front and lower borders of transverse processes of lumbar vertebrae Iliacus: anterior surface of ilium and base of sacrum	Both: lesser trochanter of femur and for a short distance below along medial border of shaft	Femoral nerve

*See Chapters 7 and 8.

The Lower Extremity *(continued)*			
Pectineus	Pectineal line between iliopectineal eminence and tubercle of pubis	Pectineal line of femur, between lesser trochanter and linea aspera	Femoral nerve
Rectus femoris	Anterior inferior iliac spine and groove above brim of acetabulum	Base of patella, as part of quadriceps femoris tendon; by means of patellar ligament it attaches to the tibial tuberosity	Femoral nerve
Sartorius	Anterior superior iliac spine and upper half of notch below it	Anterior and medial surface of tibia just below condyle	Femoral nerve
Semimembranosus	Upper and lateral impression on tuberosity of ischium	Horizontal groove on posterior surface of medial condyle of tibia	Sciatic nerve
Semitendinosus	Lower and medial impression on tuberosity of ischium with biceps femoris	Upper part of medial surface of shaft of tibia	Sciatic nerve
Six deep outward rotators	Outer and inner surfaces of sacrum and of pelvis in region of obturator foramen	Posterior and medial aspects of greater trochanter	Third, fourth, and fifth lumbar and first and second sacral nerves
Tensor fasciae latae	Anterior part of outer lip of iliac crest and outer surface of anterior superior iliac spine	Iliotibial tract of fascia lata on lateroanterior aspect of thigh, about one-third of the way down	Superior gluteal nerve
		Knee Joint	
Biceps femoris	Long head: lower and medial impression on tuberosity of ischium Short head: lateral lip of linea aspera	Lateral side of head of fibula and lateral condyle of tibia	Sciatic nerve
Gracilis	See hip joint		
Popliteus	Lateral surface of lateral condyle of femur	Posterior surface of tibia, above popliteal line	Tibial nerve
Rectus femoris sartorius, semimembranosus, semitendinosus	See hip joint		

The three vasti	V. lateralis: upper part of intertrochanteric line; anterior and lower borders of greater trochanter; lateral lip of gluteal tuberosity; upper half of linea aspera V. intermedius: anterior and lateral surface of upper two-thirds of shaft of femur V. medialis: lower half of intertrochanteric line; medial lip of linea aspera; upper part of medial supracondylar line	The tendons of the three vasti muscles unite with that of rectus femoris to form the quadriceps femoris tendon; this attaches to the base of the patella and, indirectly, by means of the patellar ligament, to the tuberosity of the tibia	Femoral nerve
	Ankle Joint, Foot, and Toes		
Extensor digitorum longus	Lateral condyle of tibia and upper three-fourths of anterior surface of fibula	Dorsal surface of second and third phalanges of four lesser toes	Deep peroneal nerve
Extensor hallucis longus	Middle half of anterior surface of fibula	Dorsal surface of base of distal phalanx of hallux (great toe)	Deep peroneal nerve
Flexor digitorum longus	Posterior surface of middle three-fifths of tibia	Plantar surface of base of distal phalanx of each of the four lesser toes	Tibial nerve
Flexor hallucis longus	Posterior surface of lower two-thirds of fibula	Plantar surface of base of distal phalanx of hallux (great toe)	Tibial nerve
Gastrocnemius	Posterior surface of each femoral condyle and adjacent parts by two separate heads	Posterior surface by calcaneus by means of calcaneal tendon (tendon of Achilles)	Tibial nerve
Peroneus brevis	Lateral surface of lateral two-thirds of fibula	Tuberosity on lateral side of base of fifth metatarsal	Superficial peroneal nerve
Peroneus longus	Lateral condyle of tibia; lateral surface of head and upper two-thirds of fibula	Lateral margin of plantar surface of first cuneiform and base of first metatarsal	Superficial peroneal nerve

The Lower Extremity *(continued)*

Peroneus tertius	Anterior surface of lower third of fibula	Dorsal surface of base of fifth metatarsal	Deep peroneal nerve
Soleus	Posterior surface of head of fibula and upper two-thirds of shaft; popliteal line and medial border of middle third of tibia	Posterior surface of calcaneus by means of calcaneal tendon (tendon of Achilles)	
Tibialis anterior	Lateral condyle and upper two-thirds of lateral surface of tibia	Plantar surface of base of first metatarsal and medial surface of first cuneiform	Deep peroneal nerve
Tibialis posterior	Posterior surface of upper two-thirds of tibia beginning at popliteal line; medial surface of upper two-thirds of fibula	Tuberosity of navicular bone with branches to sustentaculum tali of calcaneus, to three cuneiforms, to cuboid, and to bases of three middle metatarsal bones	Tibial nerve

The Spinal Column*

Muscle	Proximal Attachments	Distal Attachments	Nerve Supply
Deep posterior spinal muscles	Posterior surface of sacrum and posterior processes of all the vertebrae	Spinous and transverse processes and laminae of vertebrae slightly higher than lower attachments	Branches of spinal nerves for all but levatores costarum, which is innervated by intercostal and eighth cervical nerves
Erector spinae	Thoracolumbar fascia; posterior portions of lumbar, thoracic and lower cervical vertebrae; angles of ribs	Angles of ribs; posterior portions of cervical and thoracic vertebrae; mastoid process of temporal bone	Posterior branches of spinal nerves
Hyoid muscles	Suprahyoid: hyoid bone Infrahyoid: sternum, clavicle, and scapula	Temporal bone and mandible Hyoid bone	Facial, inferior alveolar, hypoglossi, and ansa hyperglossi
Levator scapula	See shoulder girdle		
Obliquus externus abdominis	Anterior half of crest of ilium; aponeurosis from ribs to crest of pubis	Lower border of lower eight ribs by tendinous slips that interdigitate with those of serratus anterior	Lower seven intercostal nerves and iliohypogastric nerves

*See Chapter 9.

Muscle	Proximal Attachments	Distal Attachments	Nerve Supply
Obliquus internus abdominis	Inguinal ligament; crest of ilium; thoracolumbar fascia	Anterior and middle fibers into crest of pubis, linea alba, and aponeurosis on front of body; posterior fibers, by three separate slips, into cartilages of lower three ribs	Lower three intercostal nerves, the iliohypogastric and the ilioinguinal nerves
Prevertebral muscles	Anterior surfaces of various parts of cervical vertebrae and of upper three thoracic vertebrae		Anterior portions of occipital bone and of cervical vertebrae
Psoas	See hip joint		
Quadratus lumborum	Crest of ilium and iliolumbar ligament	Lower border of twelfth rib and tips of transverse processes of upper four lumbar vertebrae	Branches from the upper three or four lumbar nerves
Rectus abdominis	Crest of pubis	Cartilages of fifth, sixth, and seventh ribs	Anterior branches of lower six intercostal nerves
Scalenes (three)	First two ribs	Transverse processes of cervical vertebrae	Branches from second to seventh cervical nerves inclusive
Semispinalis thoracis, cervicis, and capitis	Transverse processes of all thoracic and seventh cervical vertebrae; articular processes of lower four cervical vertebrae	Spinous process of upper four thoracic and lower five cervical vertebrae; occipital bone	Posterior branches of cervical and upper six thoracic nerves
Splenius capitis and cervicis	Lower half of ligamentum nuchae; spinous processes of seventh cervical and upper six thoracic vertebrae	Mastoid process of temporal bone and adjacent part of occipital bone; transverse processes of upper three cervical vertebrae	Branches from second, third, and fourth cervical nerves
Sternocleidomastoid	By two heads from top of sternum and medial third of clavicle	Mastoid process of temporal bone and adjacent portion of occipital bone	Accessory and branches from the second and third cervical nerves
Suboccipitals	Posterior portions of atlas and axis	Occipital bone and transverse process of atlas	Branches from the first two cervical nerves

Major Respiratory Muscles*

Muscle	Proximal Attachment	Central Attachment	Nerve Supply
Diaphragm	Circumference of thoracic outlet	Central tendon, a cloverleaf-shaped aponeurosis	Phrenic nerve
	Upper Attachments	**Lower Attachments**	
Intercostales externi	Lower border of each rib but last	Upper border of rib immediately below	Branches from corresponding intercostal nerves
Intercostales interni	Inner surface and costal cartilage of each rib but last	Upper border of rib immediately below	Branches from corresponding intercostal nerves
Levatores costarum	Transverse processes of seventh cervical and upper eleven thoracic vertebrae	Upper eight: each to rib immediately below, between tubercle and angle Lower four: by two bands each, one to rib immediately below and other to second rib below	Branches from corresponding intercostal nerves
Serratus posterior inferior	Lower borders of lower four ribs	Spinous processes and ligaments of lower two thoracic and upper two or three lumbar vertebrae	Branches from ninth, tenth, and eleventh intercostal nerves
Serratus posterior superior	Upper borders of second, third, fourth, and fifth ribs	Spinous processes and ligaments of lower two or three cervical and upper two thoracic vertebrae	Branches from the first four intercostal nerver
Transversus abdominis	Linea alba and crest of pubis	Inguinal ligament, crest of ilium, thoracolumbar fascia, and cartilages of lower six ribs	Branches of lower six intercostal nerves, iliohypogastric, and ilioinguinal nerves
Transversus thoracis	Lower half of inner surface of sternum and adjoining costal cartilages	Lower borders and inner surfaces of costal cartilages of second, third, fourth, fifth, and sixth ribs	Branches from upper six thoracic intercostal nerves

Additional Muscles That Participate in Respiration

Muscles of shoulder joint or shoulder girdle	Muscles of the spinal column
Pectoralis major	Quadratus lumborum
Pectoralis minor	Scalenes: anterior, posterior, medialis
Trapezius I and II	Sternocleidomastoid

*See Chapter 9

Mathematics Review

Appendix D

1. **Order of Arithmetic Operations**

Certain arithmetic operations take precedence over others. In completing problems with a series of operations the following guidelines apply:

a. Addition or subtraction may occur in any order.

Example: $4 + 8 - 7 + 3 = 8$ or $8 + 3 + 4 - 7 = 8$

b. Multiplication or division must be completed before addition or subtraction.

Example: $48 \div 6 + 2 = 10$

Example: $4 + (2/3)(1/2) = 4\ 1/3$

c. Any quantity above a division line, under a division line or a radical sign ($\sqrt{000}$), or within parentheses or brackets must be treated as one number.

Example: $\sqrt{32 - 25} = \sqrt{11}$

Example: $2(5 + 3 - 4) = 8$

Example: $\dfrac{9 + 2}{3} = \dfrac{11}{3}$

2. **Fractions, Decimals, and Percents**

a. To add (or subtract) fractions, the denominator in each term must be the same. (Choose the lowest common denominator for each term. Multiply each term by the common denominator and then add [or subtract].)

Example: $\dfrac{3}{4} + \dfrac{5}{3} = \dfrac{29}{12} = 2\dfrac{5}{12}$

(lowest common denominator = 12)

Solution:

$$\left(\frac{\frac{3}{4} \times 12}{12}\right) + \left(\frac{\frac{5}{3} \times 12}{12}\right) = \frac{9}{12} + \frac{20}{12} = \frac{29}{12} = 2\frac{5}{12}$$

Example: $\dfrac{cd}{x} + \dfrac{x}{c} = \dfrac{c^2d + x^2}{xc}$

(lowest common denominator = xc)

Solution:

$$\left(\frac{\frac{cd}{x} \cdot xc}{xc}\right) + \left(\frac{\frac{x}{c} \cdot xc}{xc}\right) = \frac{c^2d}{xc} + \frac{x^2}{xc} = \frac{c^2d + x^2}{xc}$$

b. To multiply fractions, multiply the numerators by each other and the denominators by each other.

Example: $\dfrac{3}{8} \cdot \dfrac{2}{3} = \dfrac{6}{24} = \dfrac{1}{4}$

Example: $pq\left(\dfrac{p}{q}\right) = \dfrac{p^2}{q} = p^2$

c. To divide fractions, invert the divisor and multiply.

Example: $\dfrac{3}{8} \div \dfrac{9}{2} = \dfrac{3}{8} \times \dfrac{2}{9} = \dfrac{6}{72} = \dfrac{1}{12}$

Example: $\dfrac{n}{r} \div \dfrac{s}{t} = \dfrac{n}{r} \times \dfrac{t}{s} = \dfrac{nt}{rs}$

Example: $\left(\dfrac{1}{a} + \dfrac{1}{b}\right) \div \left(\dfrac{1}{a} - \dfrac{1}{b}\right)$

$$= \frac{b + a}{\cancel{ab}} \cdot \frac{\cancel{ab}}{b - a} = \frac{b + a}{b - a}$$

d. To convert a fraction to a percentage divide the numerator by the denominator and multiply by 100.

Example: $\dfrac{3}{8} = 0.375 \times 100 = 37.5\%$

Note: To convert a percentage to a decimal, move the decimal point two places to the left.

e. When *dividing* by a decimal, divide by the integer and add sufficient zeros to move the decimal point the appropriate number of digits to the *right*.

Example: $36 \div 0.04 = 900$ or
$36 \div 4 = 9$ plus $00 = 900$

(appropriate number of digits to right = 2)

When *multiplying* by a decimal, multiply the integer and add enough zeros to move the decimal point the appropriate number of digits to the *left*.

Example: $6 \times 0.012 = 0.072$ or
$6 \times 12 = 72$ plus 0 to left 0.072
(appropriate number of digits to left = 3)

f. Decimals may be expressed as positive or negative powers of 10:

$$10^0 = 1$$
$$10^1 = 10$$
$$10^2 = 100$$
$$10^3 = 1000$$

Example: $5{,}624 = 56.24 \times 10^2 = 5.624 \times 10^3 = .5624 \times 10^4$

$$10^{-1} = 0.1$$
$$10^{-2} = 0.01$$
$$10^{-3} = 0.001$$
$$10^{-4} = 0.0001$$

Example: $0.0379 = 3.79 \times 10^{-2} = 37.9 \times 10^{-3} = 379 \times 10^{-4}$

3. Proportions, Formulas, and Equations

The location of values in proportions, equations, or formulas may be shifted provided that whatever addition, subtraction, multiplication, or division is performed on one side of the equation is also performed on the other side.

Example: $\dfrac{a}{b} = \dfrac{c}{d}$

Solve for d: $d \cdot \dfrac{a}{b} = \dfrac{c}{\cancel{d}} \cdot \cancel{d}$

$$d \cdot \frac{\cancel{a}}{\cancel{b}} \cdot \frac{\cancel{b}}{\cancel{a}} = c \cdot \frac{b}{a}$$

$$d = c \cdot \frac{b}{a}$$

Example: $v^2 = u^2 + 2as$

Solve for s: $2as = v^2 - u^2$

$$s = \frac{v^2 - u^2}{2a}$$

4. Right Triangles and Trigonometric Equations

a. In a right triangle, one angle always equals 90°. The other two angles will always be acute angles, and the sum of these two angles will be 90° since the sum of the angles in any triangle is 180°.

b. In a right triangle the *sides* are related to each other so that the square of the longest side or *hypotenuse* (*c*) is equal to the sum of the squares of the two sides: $c^2 = a^2 + b^2$. This is the Pythagorean theorem.

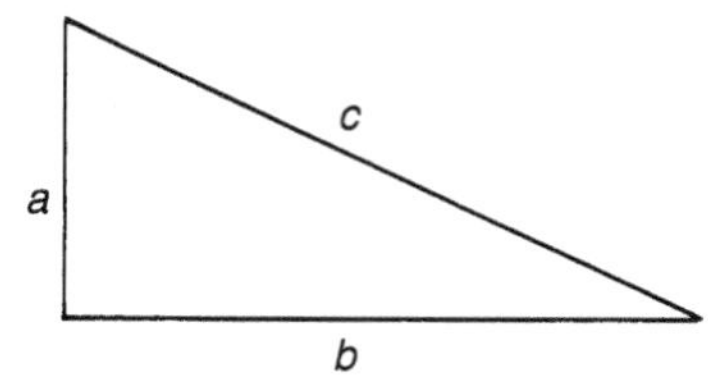

c. In triangle *ABC,* side *a* is called the side opposite angle *A*, side *b* is opposite angle *B,* and the hypotenuse, *c,* is opposite the right angle. Side *b* is named the side *adjacent* to angle *A* and side *a* is the side adjacent to angle *B*.

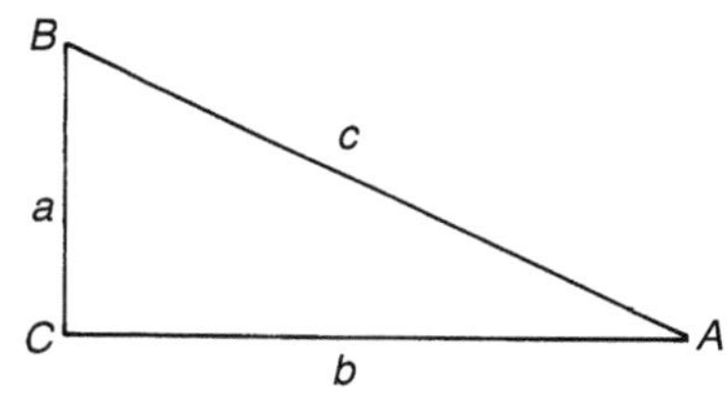

d. *Trigonometric functions* are ratios between the sides of a right triangle and are determined by the value of one of the acute angles. There are six trigonometric functions—the sine, cosine, tangent, cotangent, secant, and cosecant—but it will be necessary to consider only the first four here.

In $\triangle ABC$ the ratio between the side opposite one of the acute angles and the hypotenuse is called the *sine* of the angle. For angle *A* it would be written as

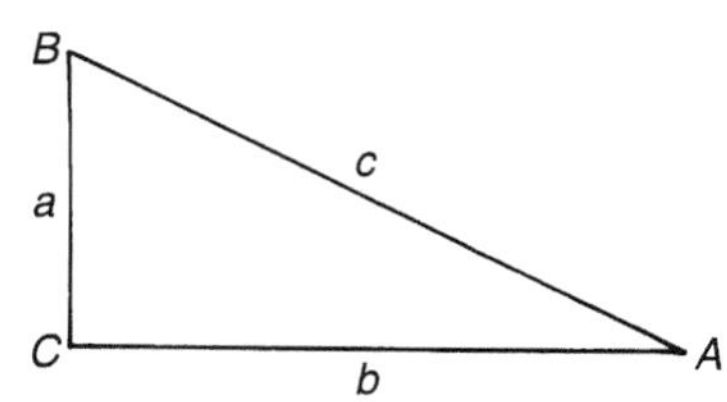

the sine $\angle A = \dfrac{a}{c}$, or $\sin A = \dfrac{a}{c}$;

the sine $\angle B = \frac{b}{c}$, or $\sin B = \frac{b}{c}$.

The *cosine* expresses the ratio between the side adjacent and the hypotenuse. For angle

A, $\cos A = \frac{b}{c}$; for angle B, $\cos B = \frac{a}{c}$.

The *tangent* and *cotangent* represent ratios between the two sides of the

triangle. For A, $\tan A = \frac{a}{b}$ and $\cot A = \frac{b}{a}$; for angle B, $\tan B = \frac{b}{a}$ and $\cot B = \frac{a}{b}$.

A glance at these values shows that $\sin A = \cos B$, and that $\tan A = \cot B$.

As can be seen from studying these ratios, two functions may have the same ratio. For instance, the $\sin A = \cos B$ and the $\tan A = \cot B$.

In general terms these trigonometric functions are expressed as follows:

$$\sin \theta^* = \frac{\text{side opposite}}{\text{hypotenuse}} \quad \text{or} \quad \sin \theta = \frac{\text{opp}}{\text{hyp}}$$

$$\cos \theta = \frac{\text{side adjacent}}{\text{hypotenuse}} \quad \text{or} \quad \cos \theta = \frac{\text{adj}}{\text{hyp}}$$

$$\tan \theta = \frac{\text{side opposite}}{\text{side adjacent}} \quad \text{or} \quad \tan \theta = \frac{\text{opp}}{\text{adj}}$$

$$\cot \theta = \frac{\text{side adjacent}}{\text{side opposite}} \quad \text{or} \quad \cot \theta = \frac{\text{adj}}{\text{opp}}$$

e. Value of trigonometric functions may be obtained from tables of trigonometric functions (see Appendix E) or from handheld calculators with trigonometric function capability.
Example: $\sin 60° = 0.8660$
$\cos 30° = 0.8660$
$\tan 22° = 0.4040$
$\cot 68° = 0.4040$

Tables of trigonometric functions usually go up to 90°. Angles greater than 90° may be handled as follows:

(1) Functions of angles greater than 90° but less than 180° are the same as functions of an angle equal to 180° minus the angle in question. All functions of angles in this range are negative except the sine.
Example: $\sin 120° = \sin 60°$
$\tan 150° = -\tan 30°$

(2) Functions of angles greater than 180° but less than 270° are the same as functions of an angle equal to 270° minus the angle in question. Functions of angles in this range are negative except for the tan and cot.
Example: $\cos 220° = -\cos = 50°$
$\tan 195° = \tan 75°$

(3) Functions of angles greater than 270° but less than 360° are the same as functions of an angle equal to 360° minus the angle in question. All functions of angles in this range are negative except the cosine.
Example: $\cot 300° = -\cot 60°$
$\sin 330° = -\sin 30°$

f. Through the use of trigonometric functions, it is possible to determine the values of all components of a triangle when the values of *one side and one angle* or the values of *two sides* are known.
Example 1: In triangle ABC, angle $A = 25°$ and the length of the hypotenuse is 15 m. Find the length of the other two sides.

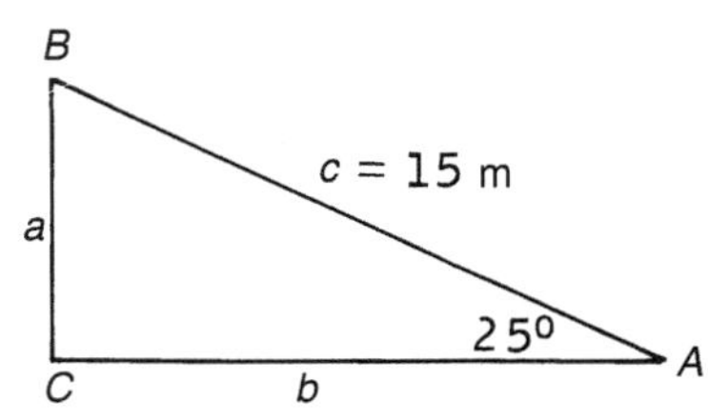

Solution:

(1) $\sin 25° = \frac{a}{c} = \frac{a}{15}$

$a = 15 \sin 25°$

$a = (15)(0.4226)$

$\boxed{a = 6.34 \text{ m}}$

*θ (Greek letter, theta) is the symbol for angle.

(2) $\cos 25° = \frac{b}{c} = \frac{b}{15}$

$b = 15 \cos 25°$

$b = (15)(0.9063)$

$\boxed{b = 13.59 \text{ m}}$

Example 2: In triangle *ABC* the lengths of the sides are 3 cm and 5 cm. What is the length of the hypotenuse and the size of both acute angles?

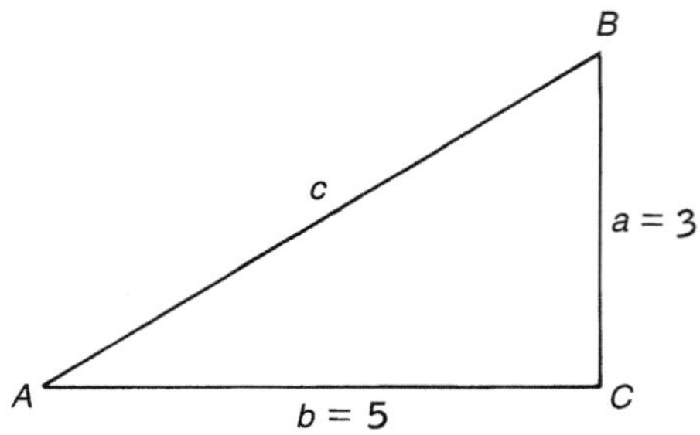

Solution:

(1) $\tan A = \frac{a}{b} = \frac{3}{5}$

$A = \arctan 0.600$

(*i.e.*, A = angle whose tan is 0.600)

$\boxed{A = 31°}$

(2) $B = 90 - A$; $\boxed{B = 59°}$

(3) $\sin A = \frac{a}{c} = \frac{3}{c}$

$c = \frac{3}{\sin A} = \frac{3}{\sin 31°}$

$c = \frac{3}{0.5150} = \boxed{5.83 \text{ cm}}$

Note: c may also be found using the Pythagorean theorem: $C^2 = a^2 + b^2$

5. **Geometry of Circles**
   a. The circumference of a circle is calculated using the formula $C = 2\pi r$, where C is the circumference, r is the radius, and π (pi) is a constant value of 3.1416. Pi is the ratio that exists between the diameter of a circle and its circumference.
   b. In making one complete turn about a circle, the radius goes through one revolution, 360° or 2π radians. A radian is the angle subtended by an arc of a circle equal in length to the radius. One radian equals $\frac{360°}{2\pi}$ or 57.3°. Some equivalents for these angular units of measure are as follows:

Revolutions	Radians			Degrees
1	2π	or	6.28	360°
0.5	1π	or	3.14	180°
0.25	0.5π	or	1.57	90°
2	4π	or	12.56	720°

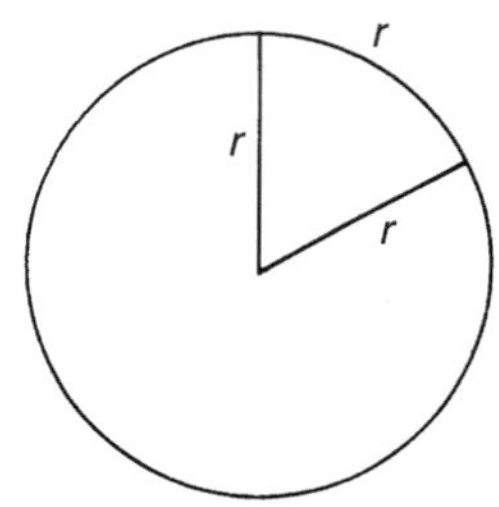

(1) To convert degrees to revolutions, divide by 360.
Example: 1260° = 3.50 rev

(2) To convert radians to revolutions, divide by 6.28.
Example: 15.75 radians = 2.51 rev

(3) To convert degrees to radians, divide by 57.3.
Example: 360° = 6.28 radians

(4) To convert revolutions to radians, multiply by 6.28.
Example: 2.3 rev = 14.44 radians

(5) To convert revolutions to degrees, multiply by 360.
Example: 2.3 rev = 828°

(6) To convert radians to degrees, multiply by 57.3.
Example: 7.6 radians = 435.5°

Appendix E

Table of Trigonometric Functions*

Degrees	Sines	Cosines	Tangents	Cotangents	
0	0.0000	1.0000	0.0000		90
1	0.0175	0.9998	0.0175	57.290	89
2	0.0349	0.9994	0.0349	28.636	88
3	0.0523	0.9986	0.0524	19.081	87
4	0.0698	0.9976	0.0699	14.301	86
5	0.0872	0.9962	0.0875	11.430	85
6	0.1045	0.9945	0.1051	9.5144	84
7	0.1219	0.9925	0.1228	8.1443	83
8	0.1392	0.9903	0.1405	7.1154	82
9	0.1564	0.9877	0.1584	6.3138	81
10	0.1736	0.9848	0.1763	5.6713	80
11	0.1908	0.9816	0.1944	5.1446	79
12	0.2079	0.9781	0.2126	4.7046	78
13	0.2250	0.9744	0.2309	4.3315	77
14	0.2419	0.9703	0.2493	4.0108	76
15	0.2588	0.9659	0.2679	3.7321	75
16	0.2756	0.9613	0.2867	3.4874	74
17	0.2924	0.9563	0.3057	3.2709	73
18	0.3090	0.9511	0.3249	3.0777	72
19	0.3256	0.9455	0.3443	2.9042	71
20	0.3420	0.9397	0.3640	2.7475	70
21	0.3584	0.9336	0.3839	2.6051	69
22	0.3746	0.9272	0.4040	2.4751	68
23	0.3907	0.9205	0.4245	2.3559	67
24	0.4067	0.9135	0.4452	2.2460	66
25	0.4226	0.9063	0.4663	2.1445	65
26	0.4384	0.8988	0.4877	2.0503	64
27	0.4540	0.8910	0.5095	1.9626	63
28	0.4695	0.8829	0.5317	1.8807	62
29	0.4848	0.8746	0.5543	1.8040	61
30	0.5000	0.8660	0.5774	1.7321	60
31	0.5150	0.8572	0.6009	1.6643	59
32	0.5299	0.8480	0.6249	1.6003	58
33	0.5446	0.8387	0.6494	1.5399	57
34	0.5592	0.8290	0.6745	1.4826	56
35	0.5736	0.8192	0.7002	1.4281	55
36	0.5878	0.8090	0.7265	1.3765	54
37	0.6018	0.7986	0.7536	1.3270	53
38	0.6157	0.7880	0.7813	1.2799	52
39	0.6293	0.7771	0.8098	1.2349	51
40	0.6428	0.7660	0.8391	1.1918	50
41	0.6561	0.7547	0.8693	1.1504	49
42	0.6691	0.7431	0.9004	1.1106	48
43	0.6820	0.7314	0.9325	1.0724	47
44	0.6947	0.7193	0.9657	1.0355	46
45	0.7071	0.7071	1.0000	1.0000	45
	Cosines	**Sines**	**Cotangents**	**Tangents**	

*Note: With angles above 45° be sure to use the headings that appear at the bottom of the columns.

U.S.–Metric Equivalents

Appendix F

To Convert from	To	Multiply by
Inches	Centimeters	2.54
Centimeters	Inches	0.39
Feet	Meters	0.305
Meters	Feet	3.28
Yards	Meters	0.91
Meters	Yards	1.09
Miles	Kilometers	1.61
Kilometers	Miles	0.62
Pounds	Kilograms	0.45
Kilograms	Pounds	2.21
Pounds	Newtons	4.45
Newtons	Pounds	0.225
Slugs	Kilograms	14.59
Kilograms	Slugs	0.068
Ft · lb	Joules	1.36
Joules	Ft · lb	0.735
Ft · lb/sec (power)	Watts	1.36
Watts	Ft · lb/sec	0.735

Appendix G Exercises for Kinesiological Analysis

These exercises and techniques, intended as laboratory material for the student, are presented for analysis (major joint and muscle action) of movements. Many are commonly used to develop strength, increase flexibility, and improve posture. In most instances they are organized according to the major body segments (the upper and lower extremities and the trunk–head–neck). Many of the exercises are illustrated by three views: (1) the starting position, (2) the movement, and (3) the return to the starting position. The various exercises were selected on the basis of their use in (1) physical fitness and posture programs, (2) conditioning programs for improving athletic performance, and (3) tests for assessing strength and muscular endurance. The sports and gymnastics techniques are representative of movements involving the imparting of motion to one's own body and to external objects. The exercises are organized in the following series:

- Series 1 Weight-Training Exercises (barbells and weights)
- Series 2 Isometric Tension Exercises (singly and with partners)
- Series 3 Flexibility Exercises
- Series 4 Core Exercises
- Series 5 Selected Sports and Gymnastics Techniques

The exercises within each series are numbered consecutively in the following manner: The first exercise in Series 1 is numbered 1.1, the second, 1.2. The first exercise in Series 2 is numbered 2.1, followed by 2.2, and so on in similar fashion.

Series 1. Weight-Training Exercises
The Upper Extremity

Starting Position	Movement	Return to Starting Position

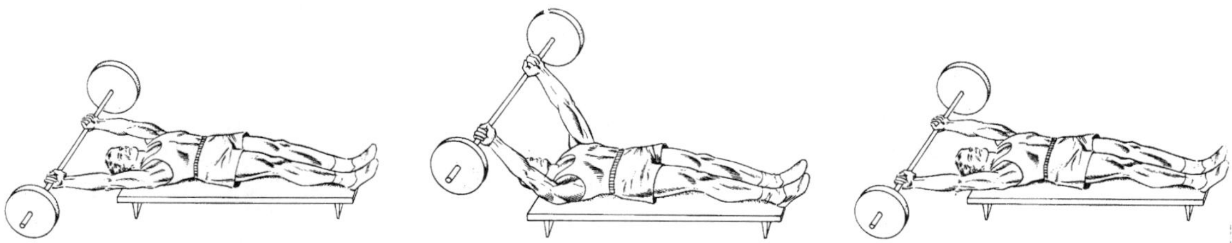

Exercise 1.1

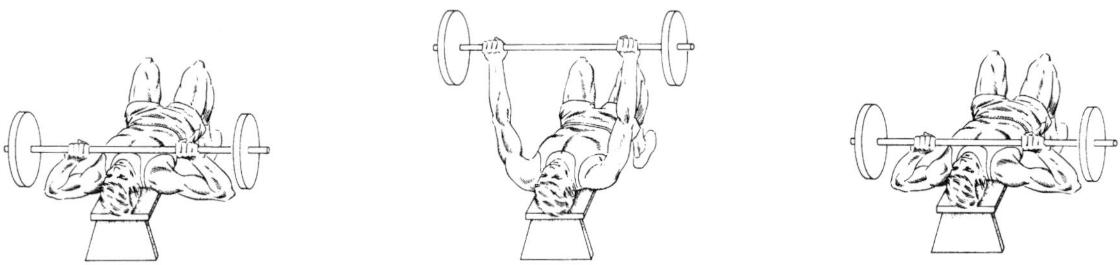

Exercise 1.2

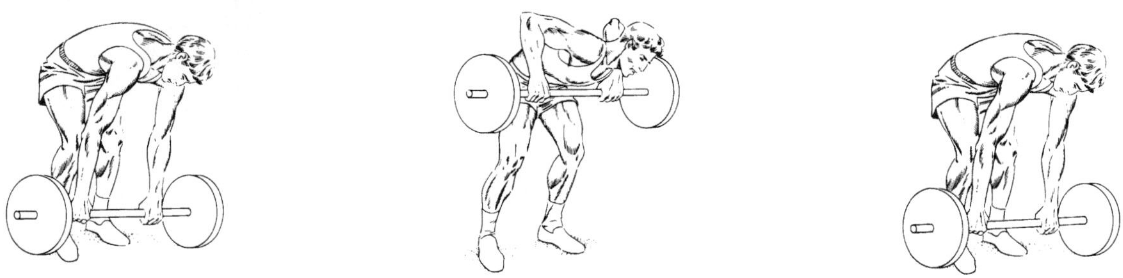

Exercise 1.3

Series 1. Weight-Training Exercises
The Upper Extremity

Starting Position **Movement** **Return to Starting Position**

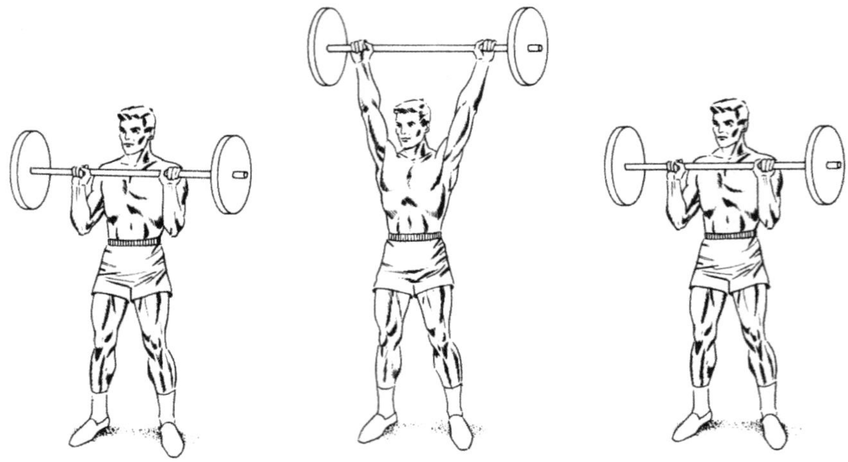

Exercise 1.4

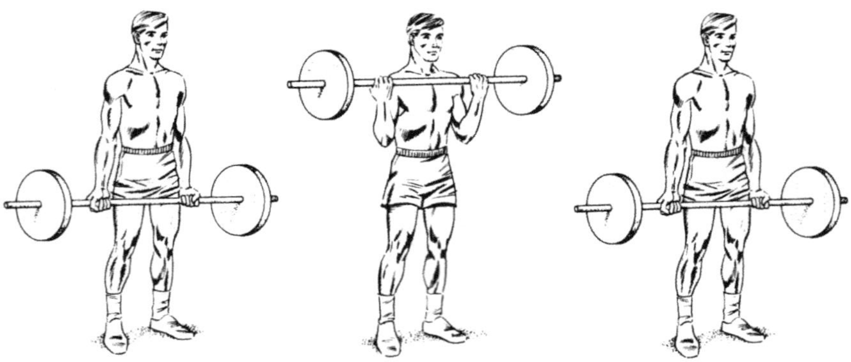

Exercise 1.5

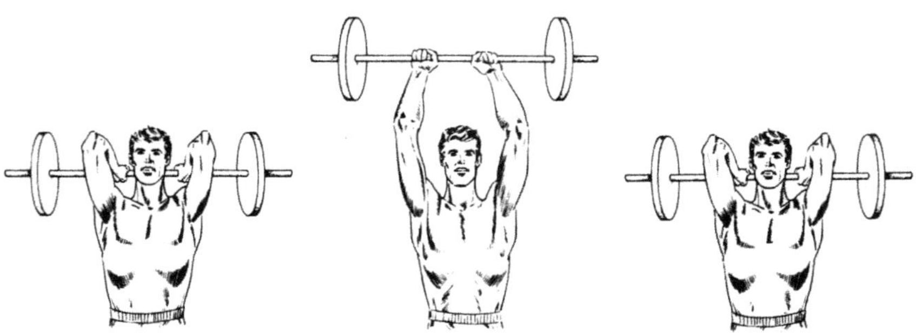

Exercise 1.6

Series 1. Weight-Training Exercises
The Upper Extremity

Starting Position | **Movement** | **Return to Starting Position**

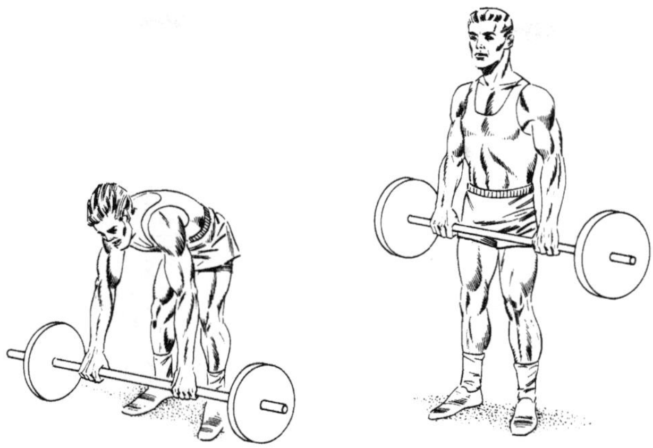

Exercise 1.7

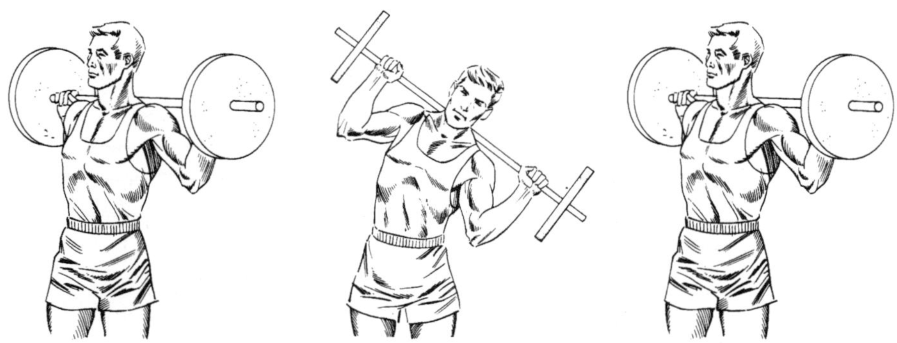

Exercise 1.8

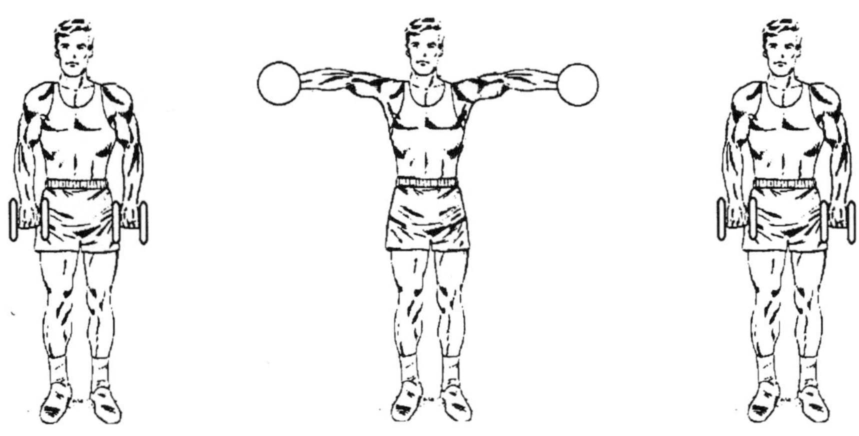

Exercise 1.9

Series 1. Weight-Training Exercises
The Upper Extremity

Starting Position	Movement	Return to Starting Position

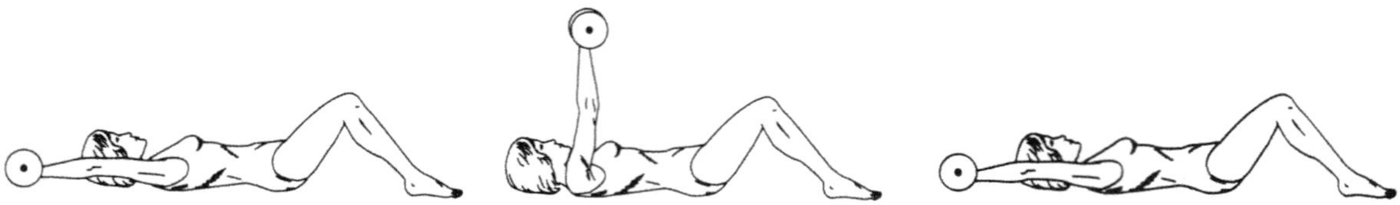

Exercise 1.10

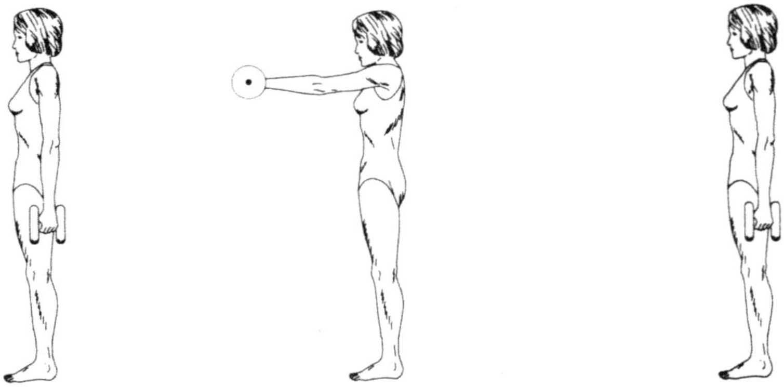

Exercise 1.11

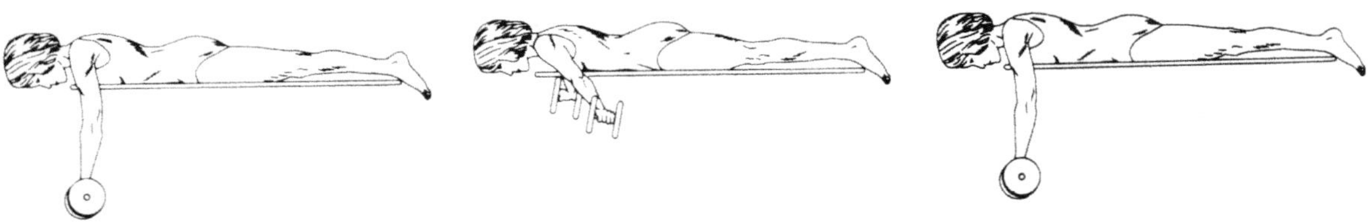

Exercise 1.12

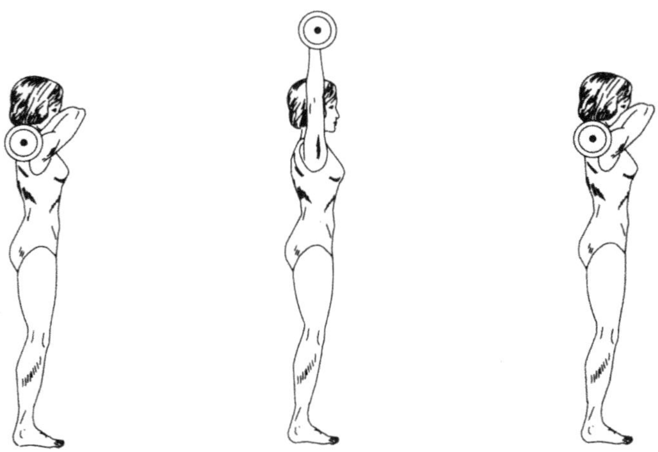

Exercise 1.13

Series 1. Weight-Training Exercises
The Lower Extremity

Starting Position **Movement** **Return to Starting Position**

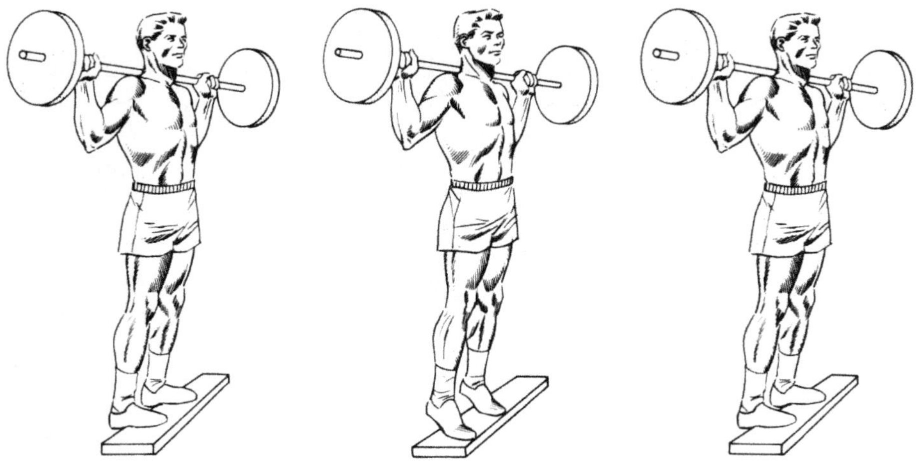

Exercise 1.14

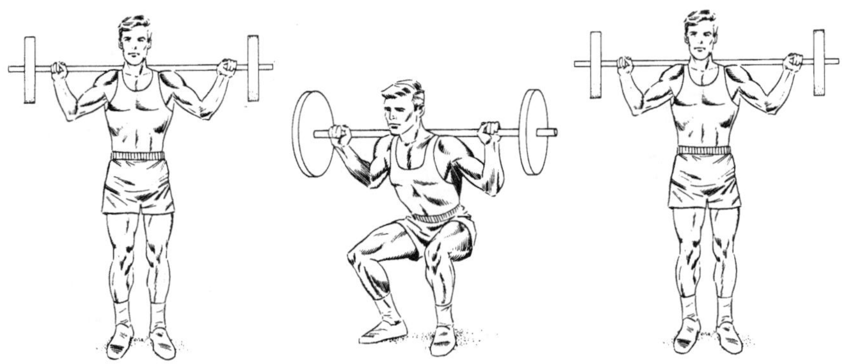

Exercise 1.15

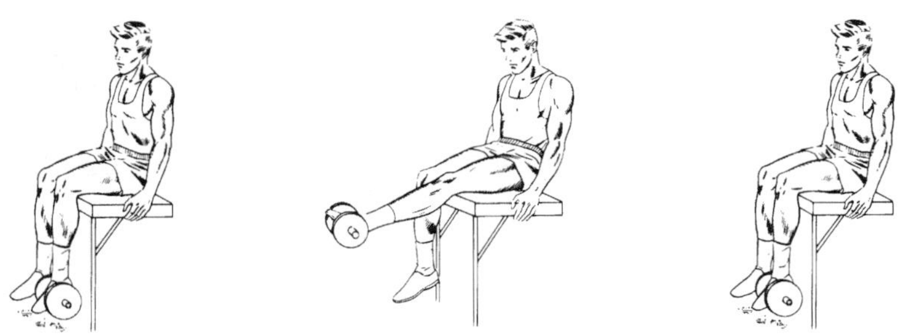

Exercise 1.16

Series 2. Isometric Tension Exercises
The Upper Extremity

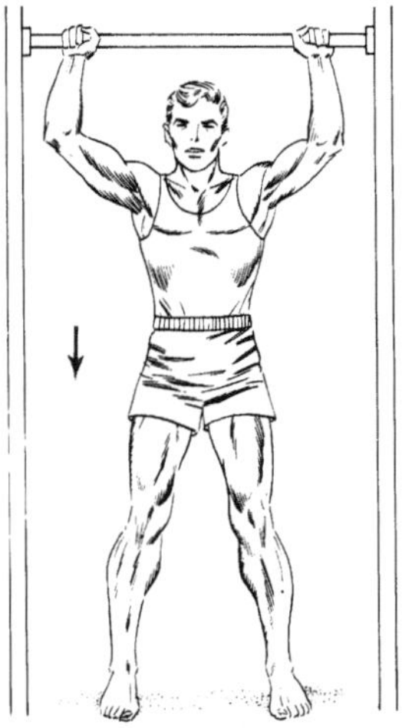

Exercise 2.1 Pull down.

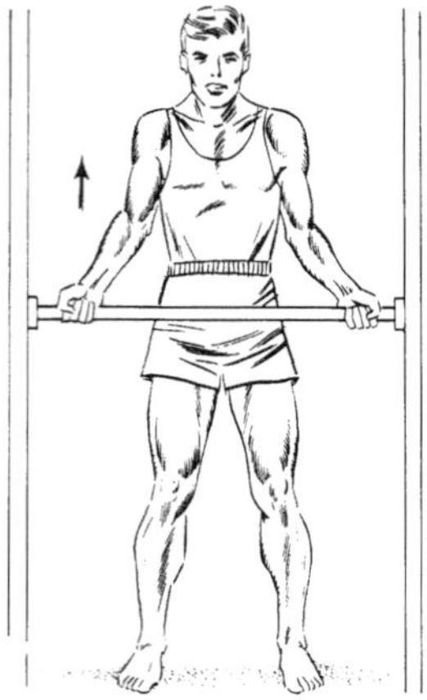

Exercise 2.2 Pull up.

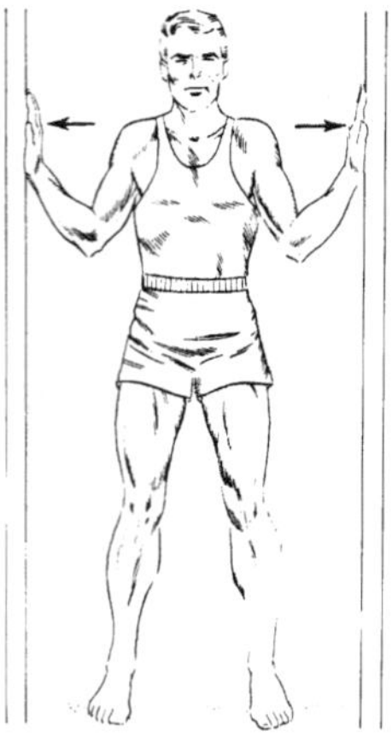

Exercise 2.3 Push out.

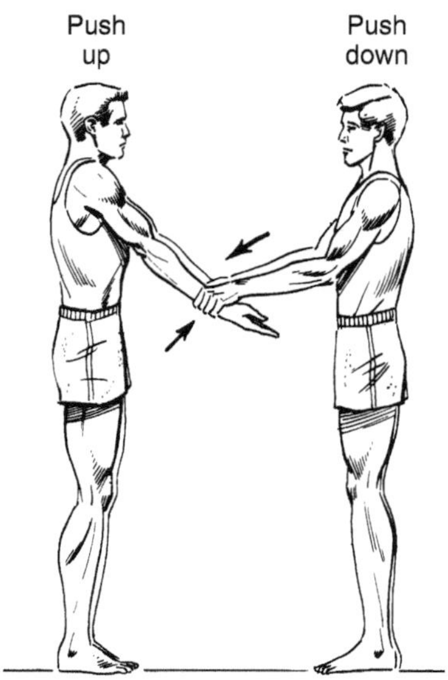

Exercise 2.4

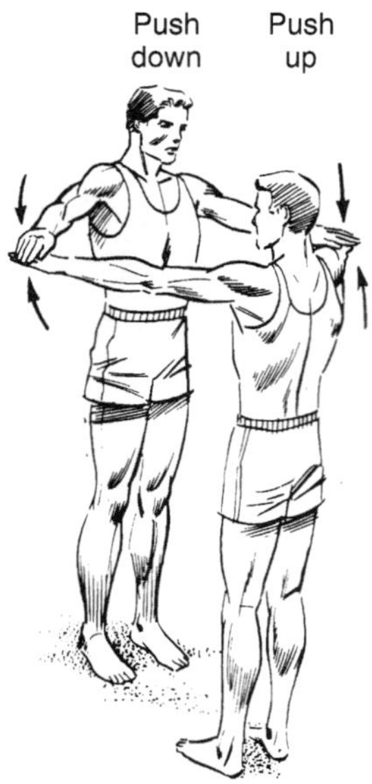

Exercise 2.5

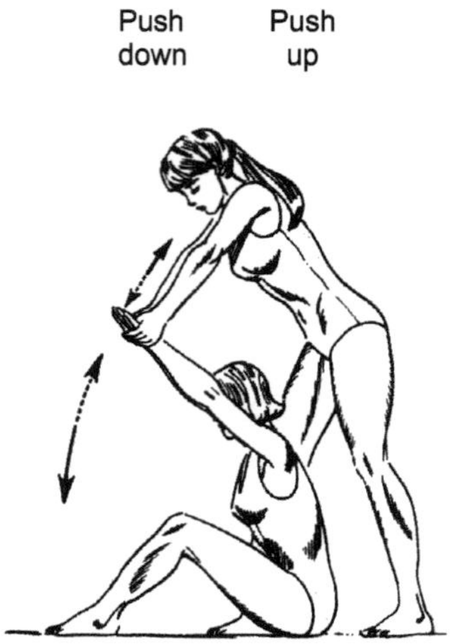

Exercise 2.6

Series 2. Isometric Tension Exercises
The Lower Extremity and Trunk

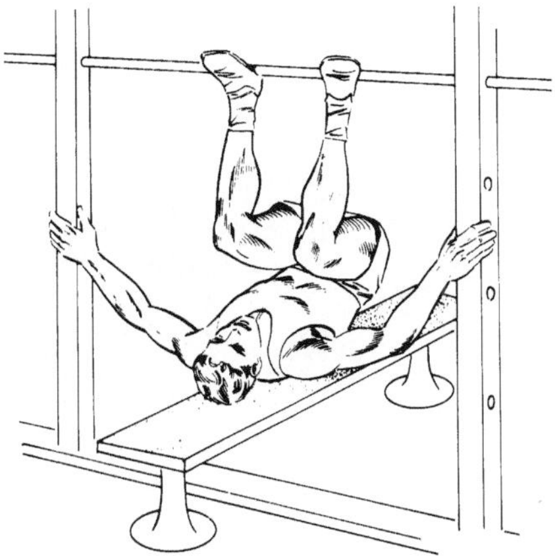

Exercise 2.7

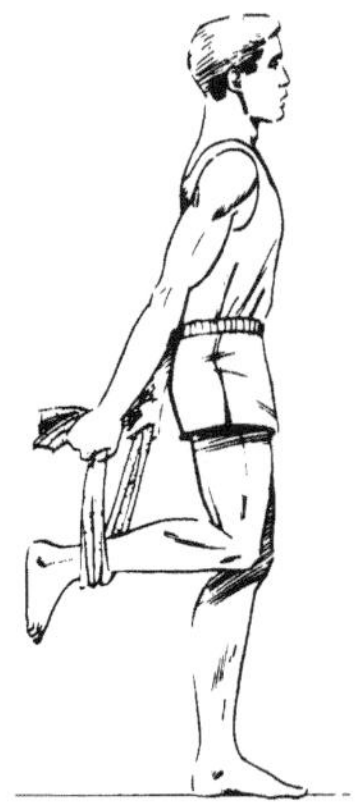

Exercise 2.8

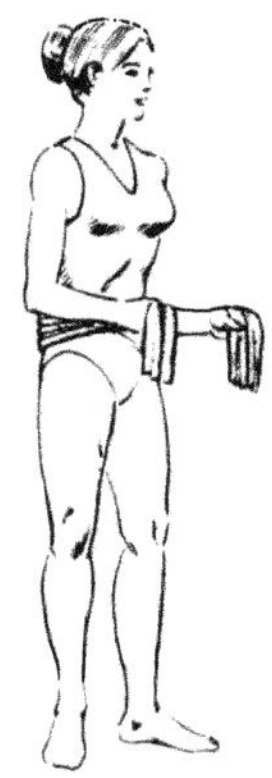

Exercise 2.9

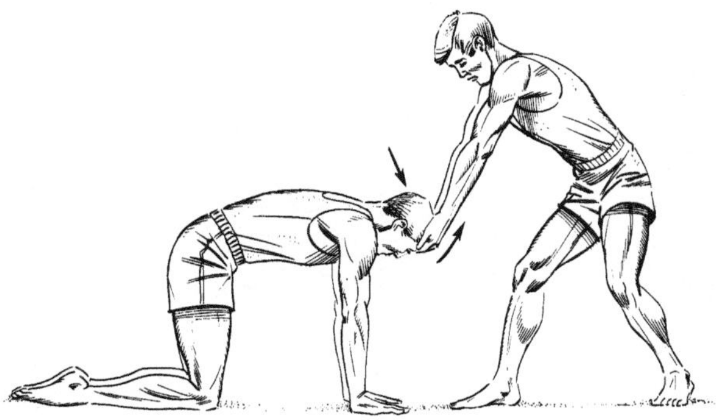

Exercise 2.10 Push down, pull up.

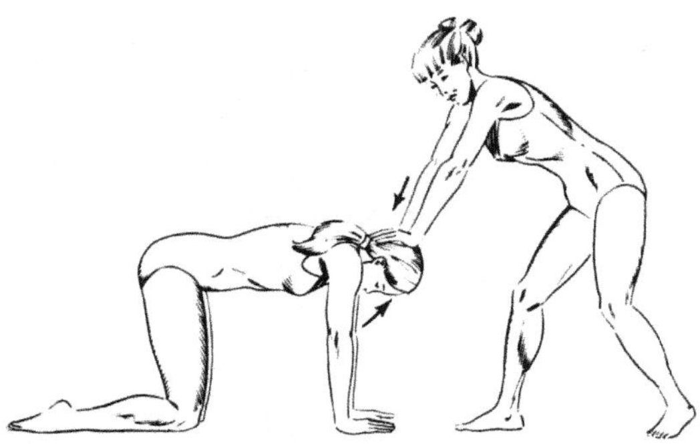

Exercise 2.11 Pull up, push down.

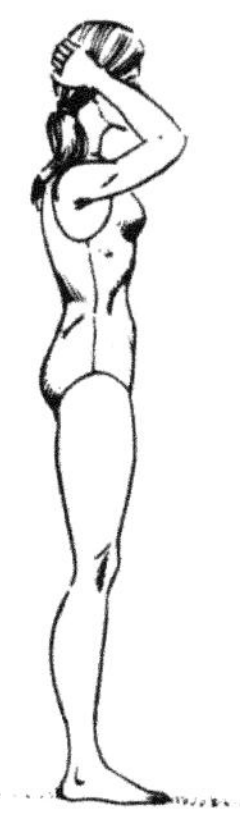

Exercise 2.12 Pull neck backward.

Series 3. Flexibility Exercises for Major Joints

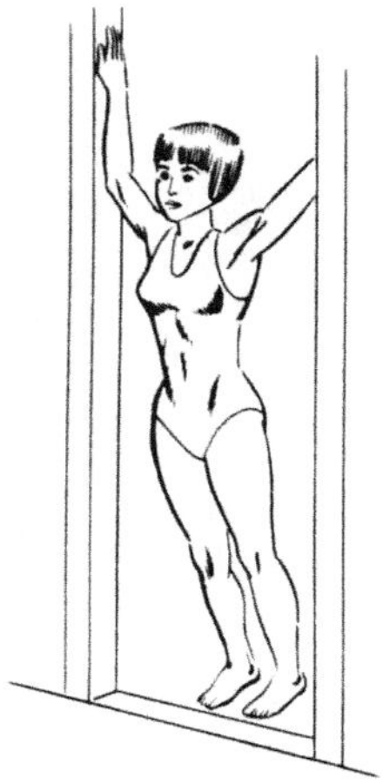

Exercise 3.1

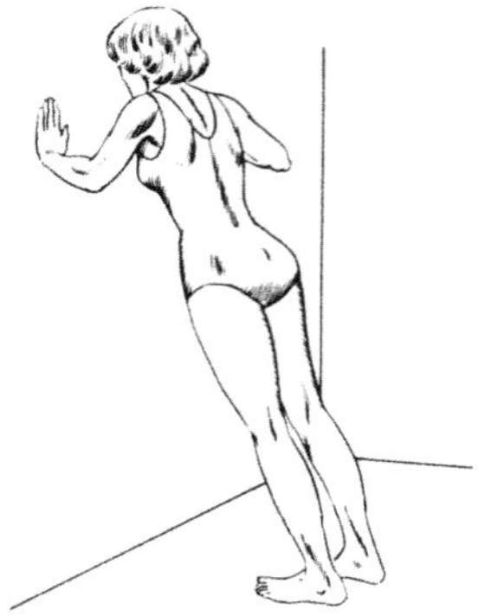

Exercise 3.2

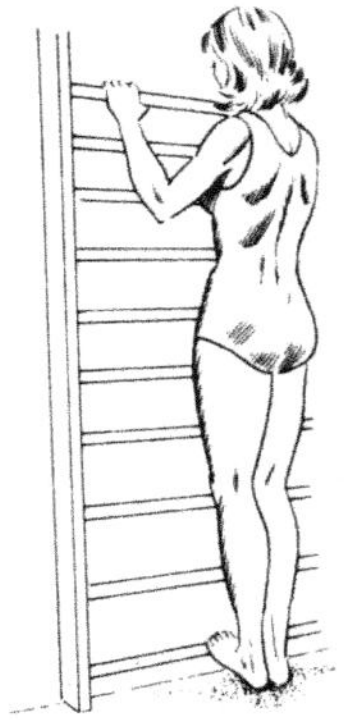

Exercise 3.3

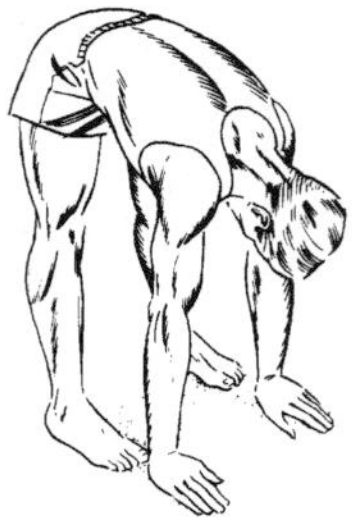

Exercise 3.4

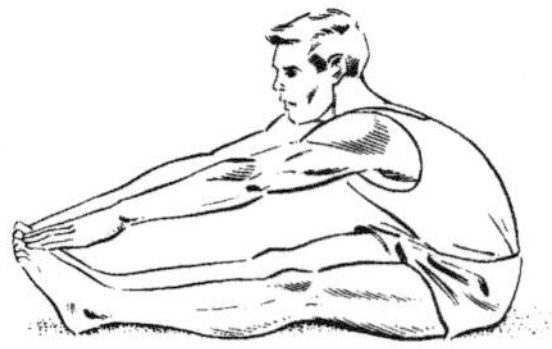

Exercise 3.5

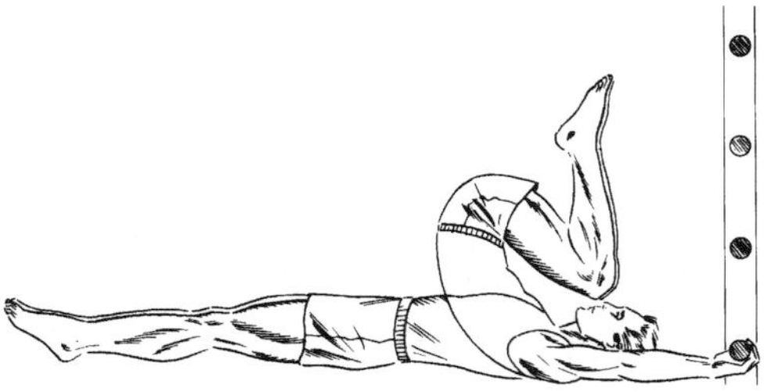

Exercise 3.6

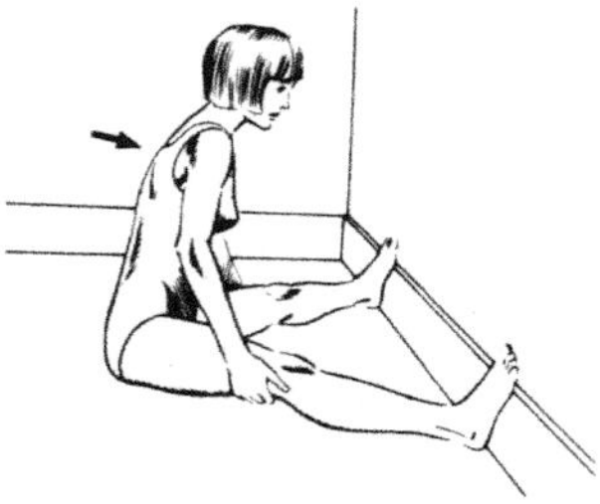

Exercise 3.7

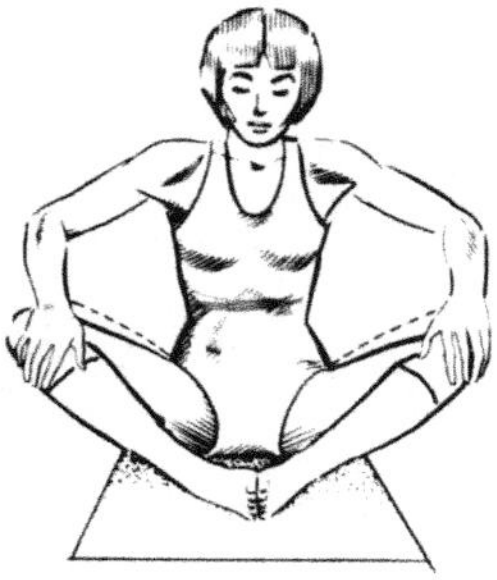

Exercise 3.8

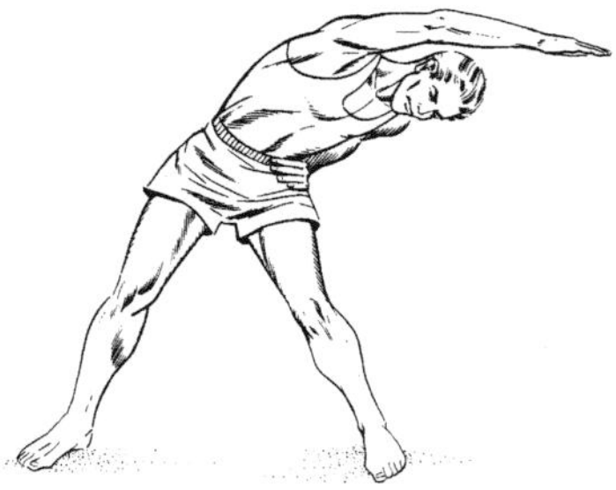

Exercise 3.9

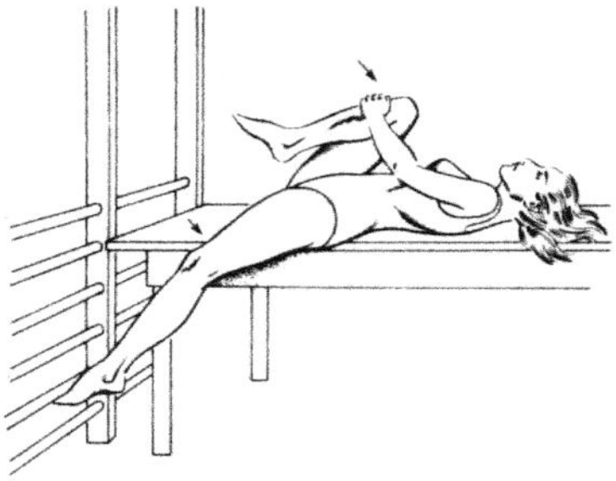

Exercise 3.10

Series 4. Core Exercises

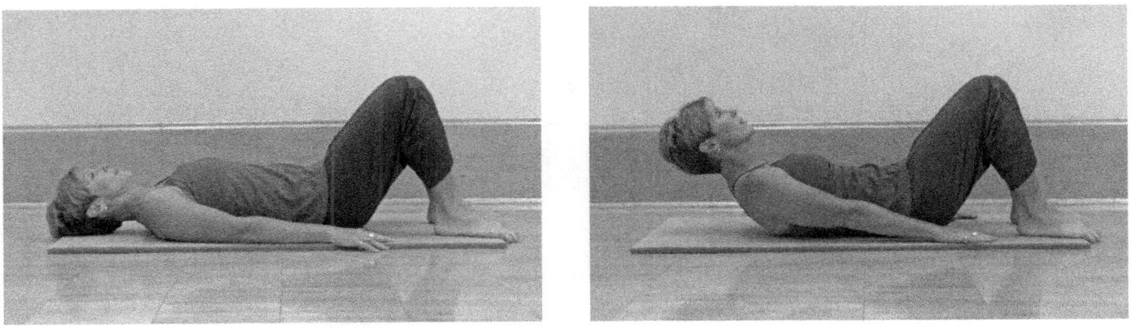

Exercise 4.1 Crunch.

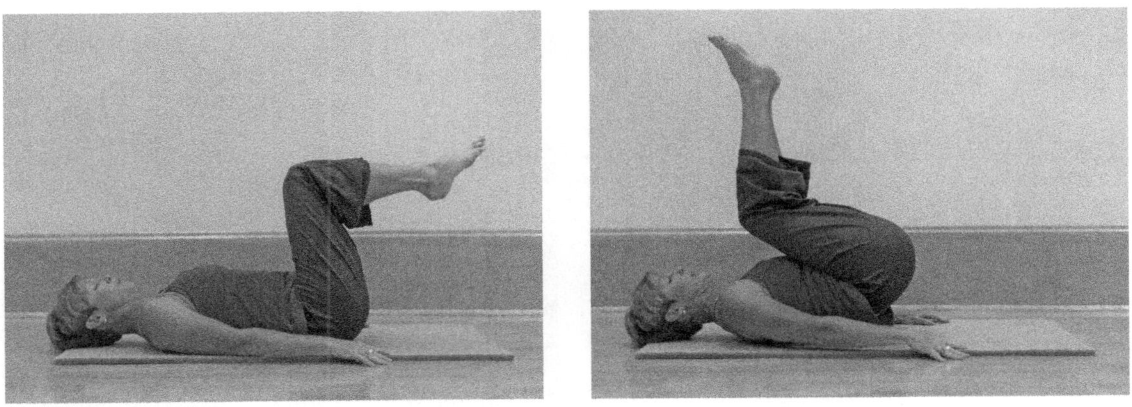

Exercise 4.2 Reverse Crunch.

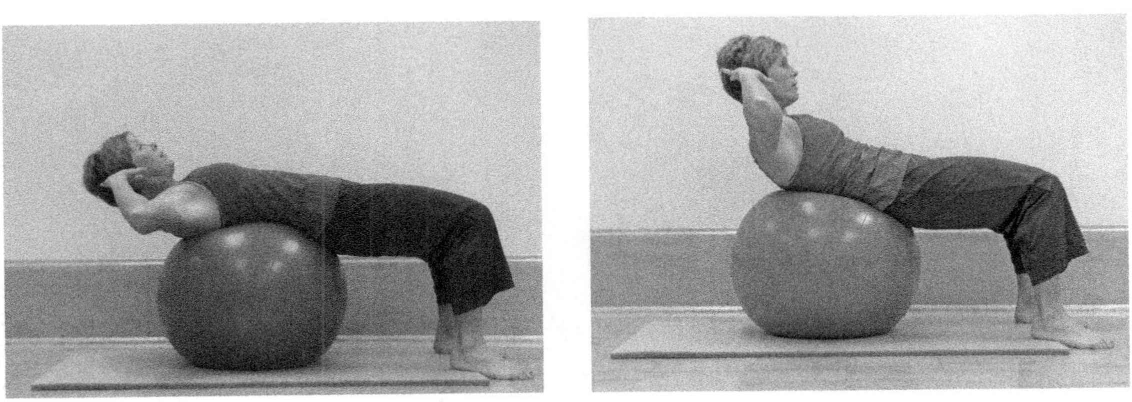

Exercise 4.3 Crunch on Stability Ball.

Series 4. Core Exercises

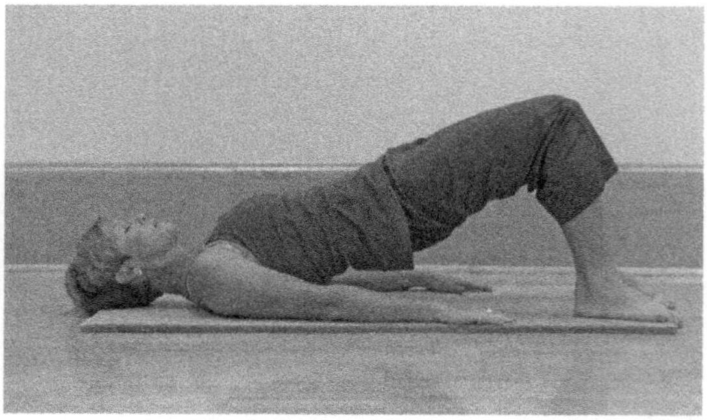

Exercise 4.4 Bridge.

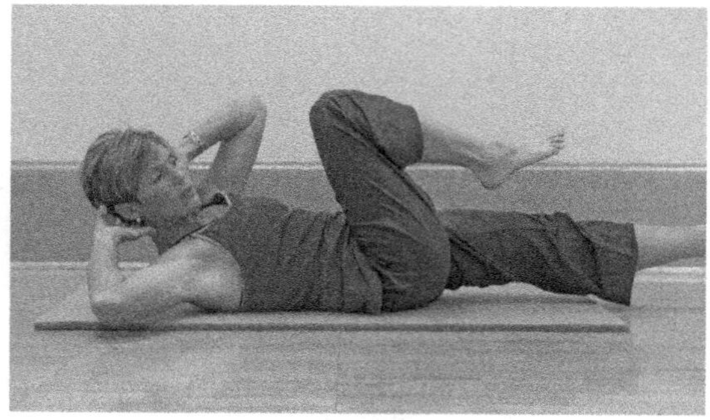

Exercise 4.5 Bicycle.

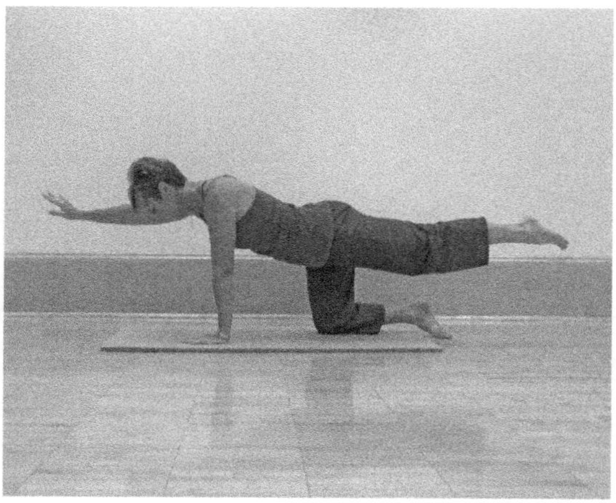

Exercise 4.6 Spinal Balance.

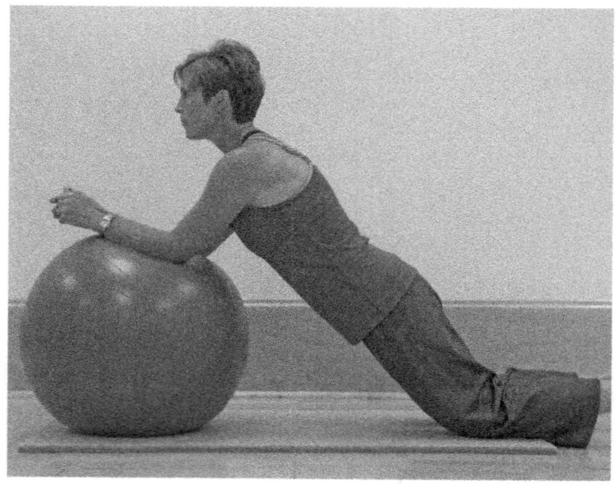

Exercise 4.7 Roll Out.

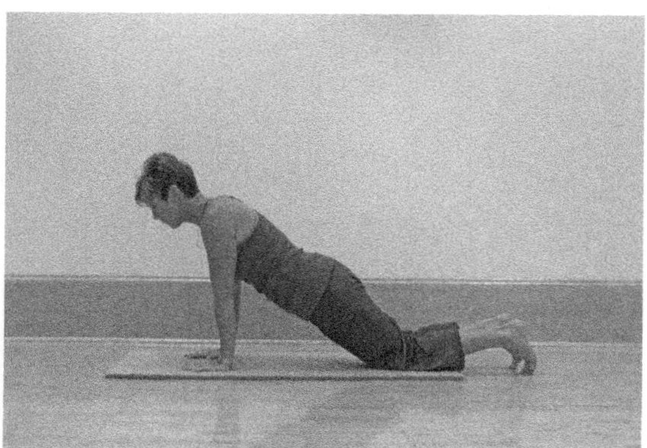

Exercise 4.8 Modified Plank.

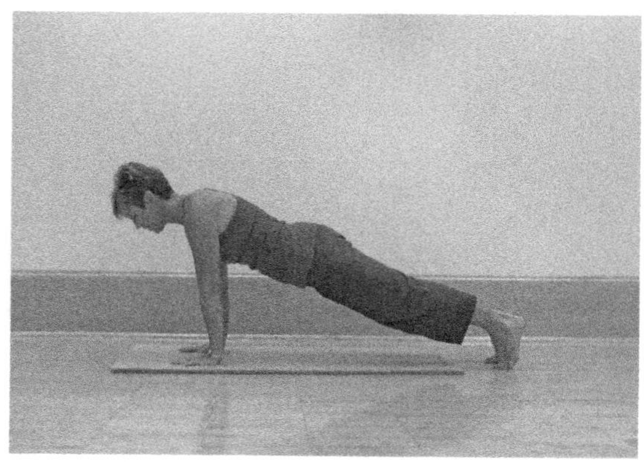

Exercise 4.9 Full Plank.

Series 5. Sports Techniques

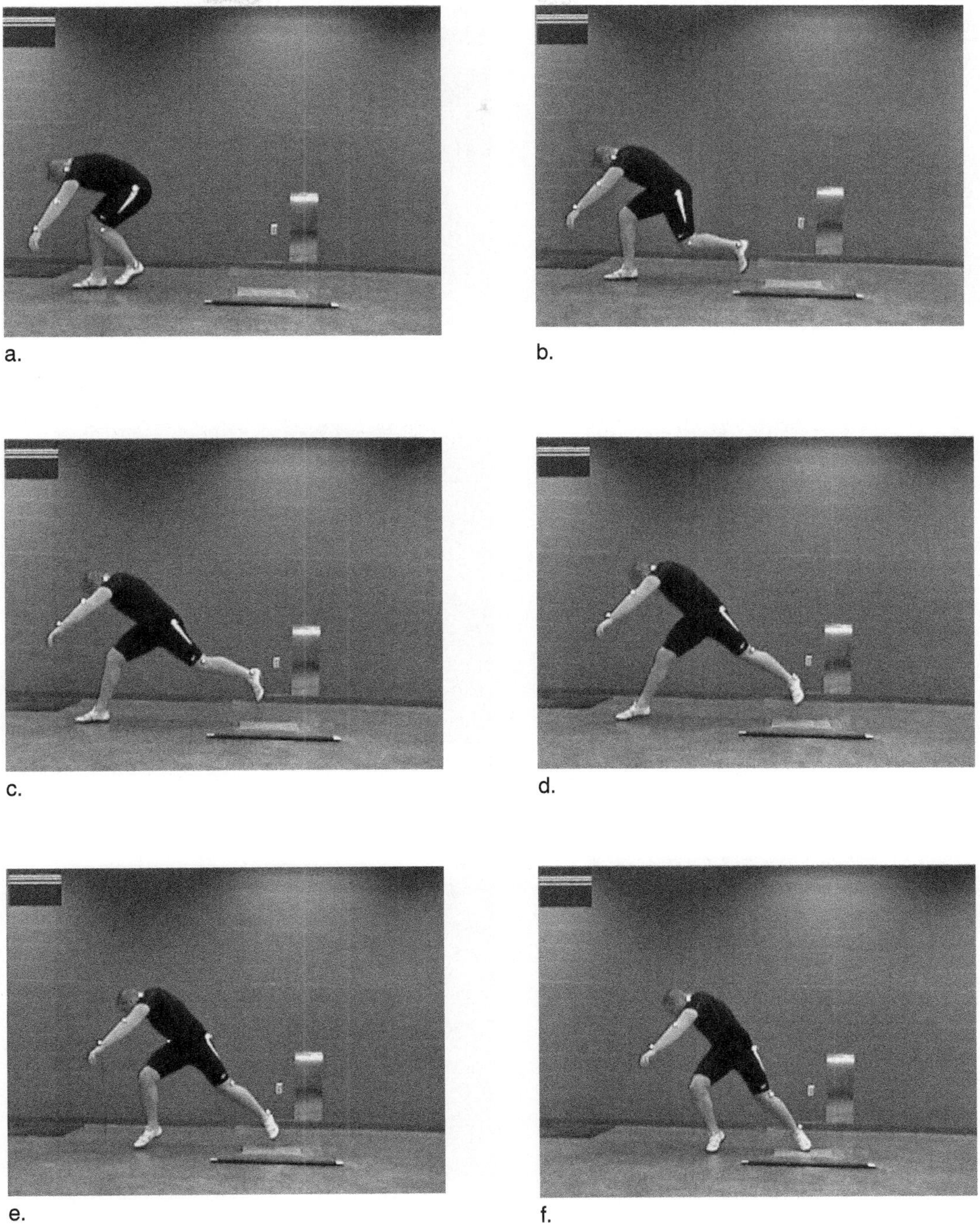

Exercise 5.1 Shot put. (Time between frames is 0.10 seconds.)

Series 5. Sports Techniques

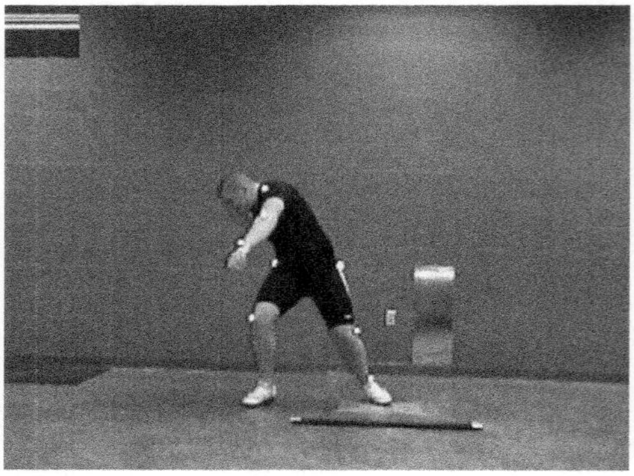

g.

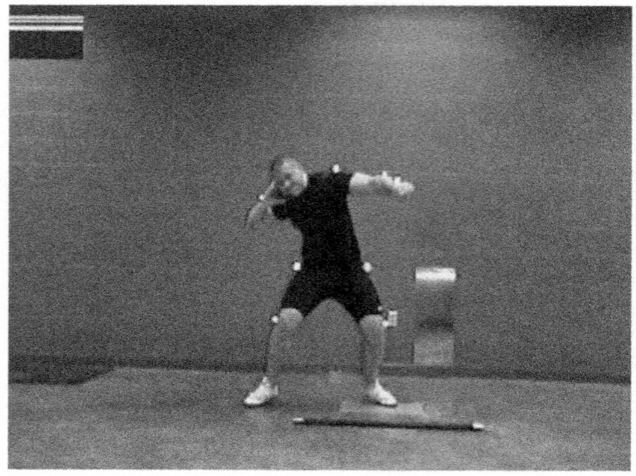

h.

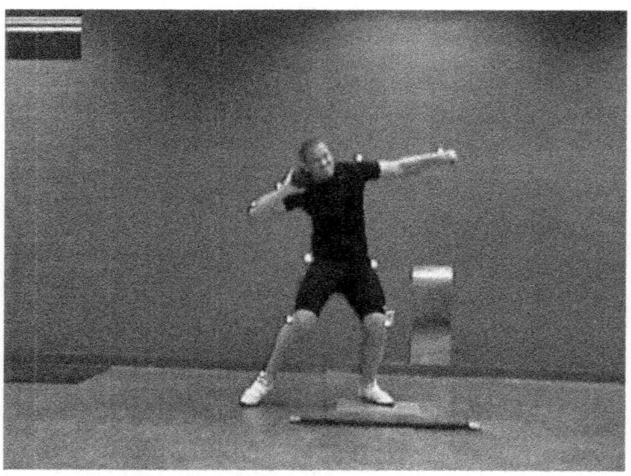

i.

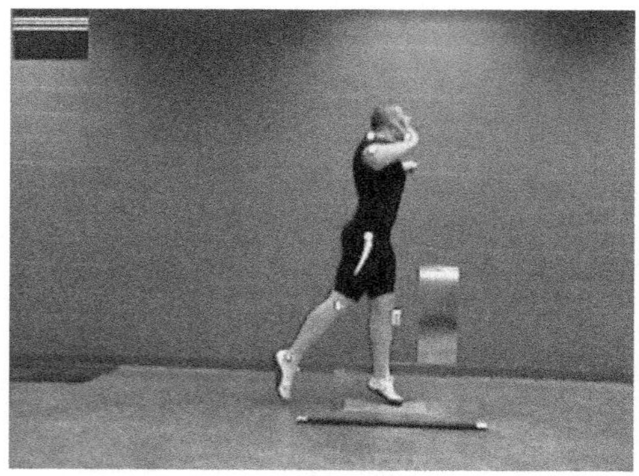

j.

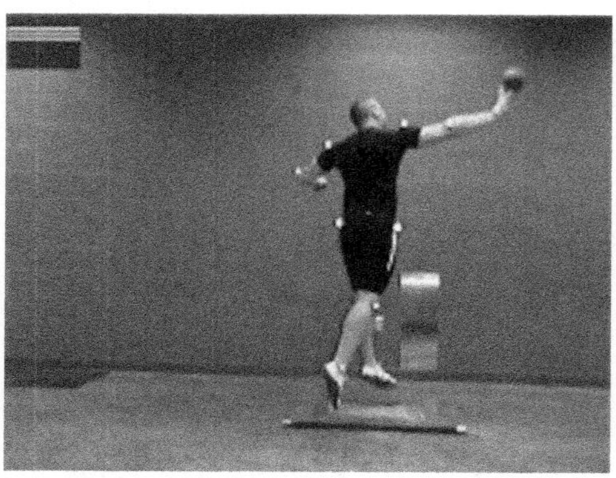

k.

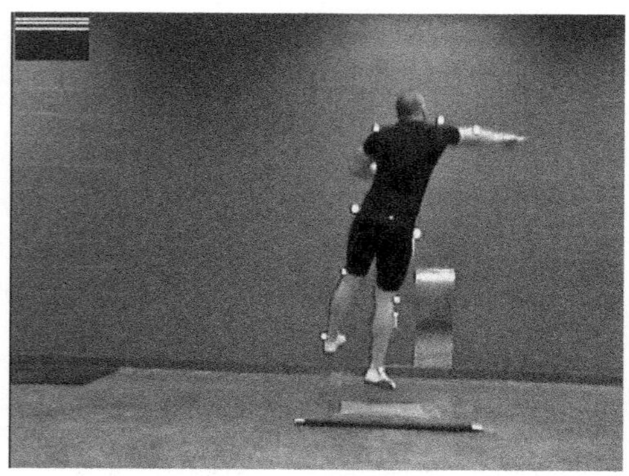

l.

Exercise 5.1 (continued)

Series 5. Sports and Gymnastics Techniques

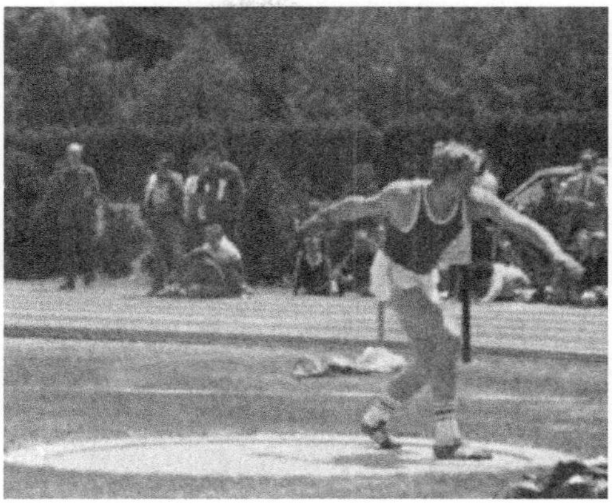

a.

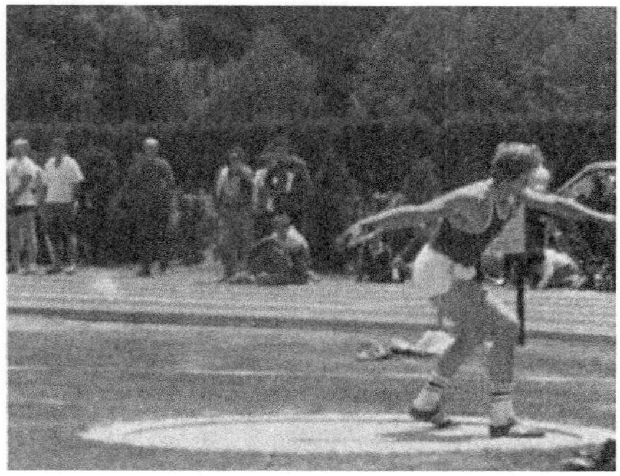

b.

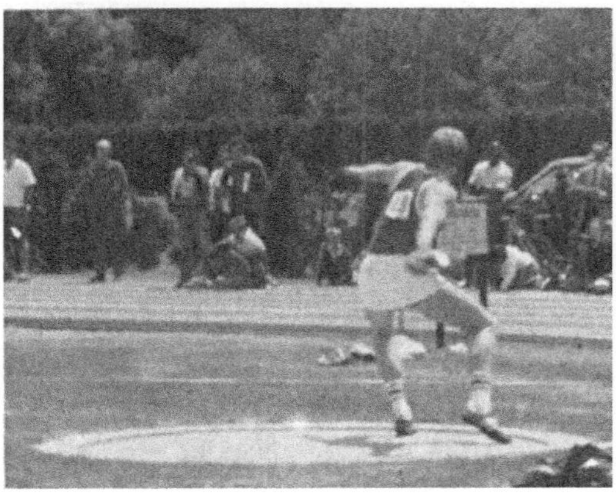

c.

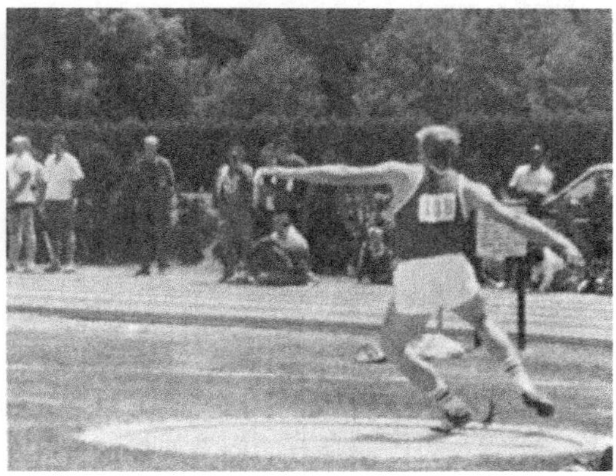

d.

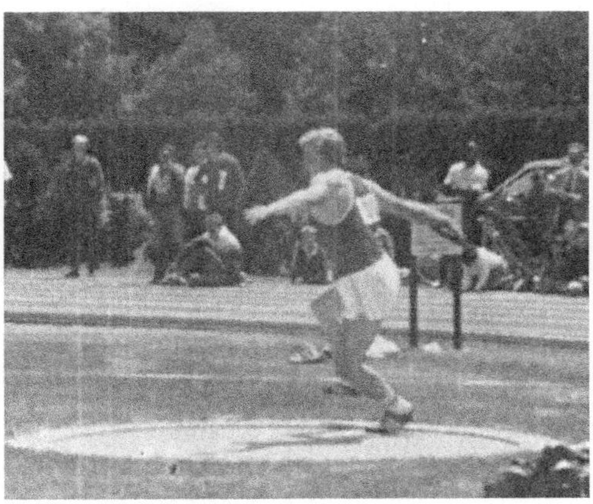

e.

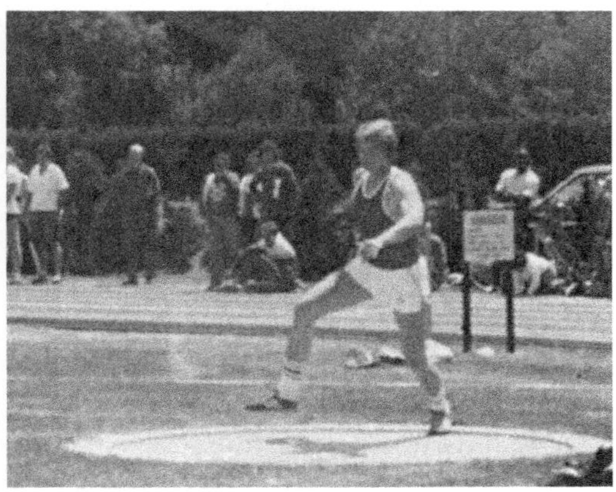

f.

Exercise 5.2 Discus throw. (Time between each frame is 0.125 sec.)

Series 5. Sports and Gymnastics Techniques

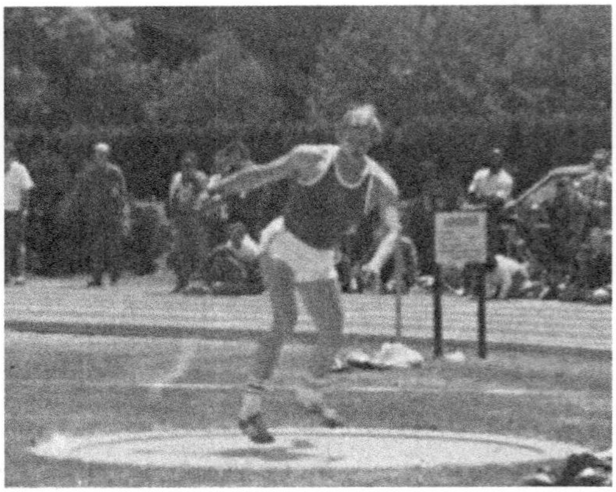

g.

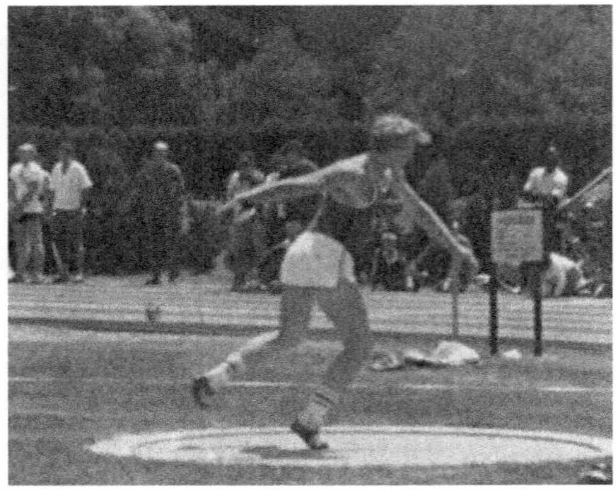

h.

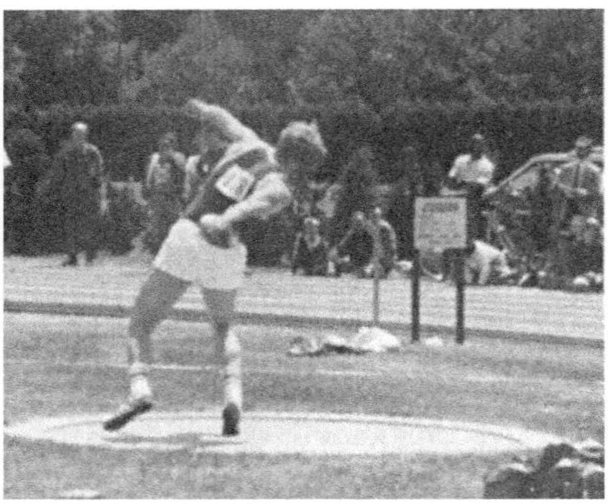

i.

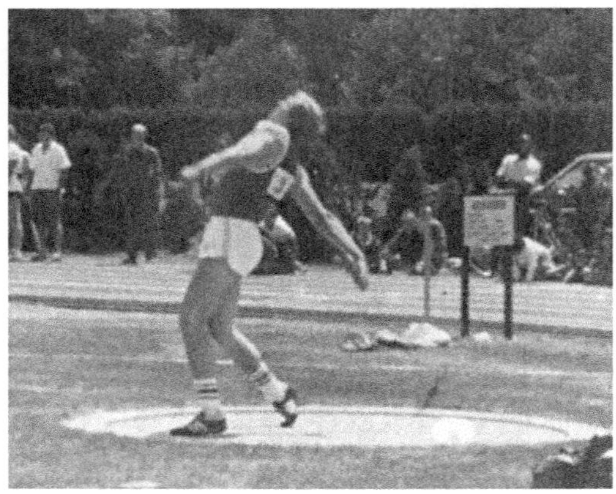

j.

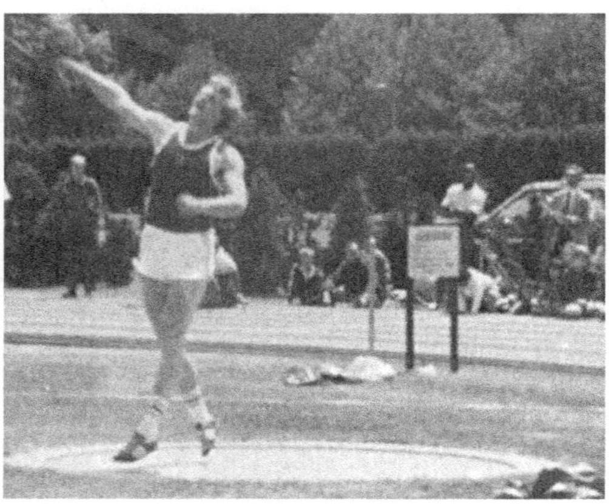

k.

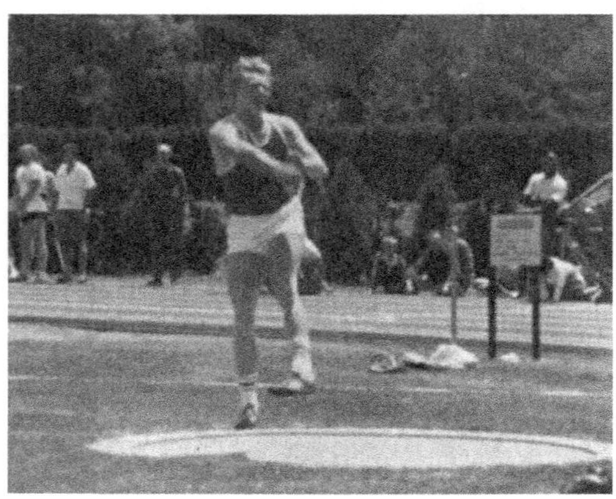

l.

Exercise 5.2 (continued)

Series 5. Sports and Gymnastics Techniques

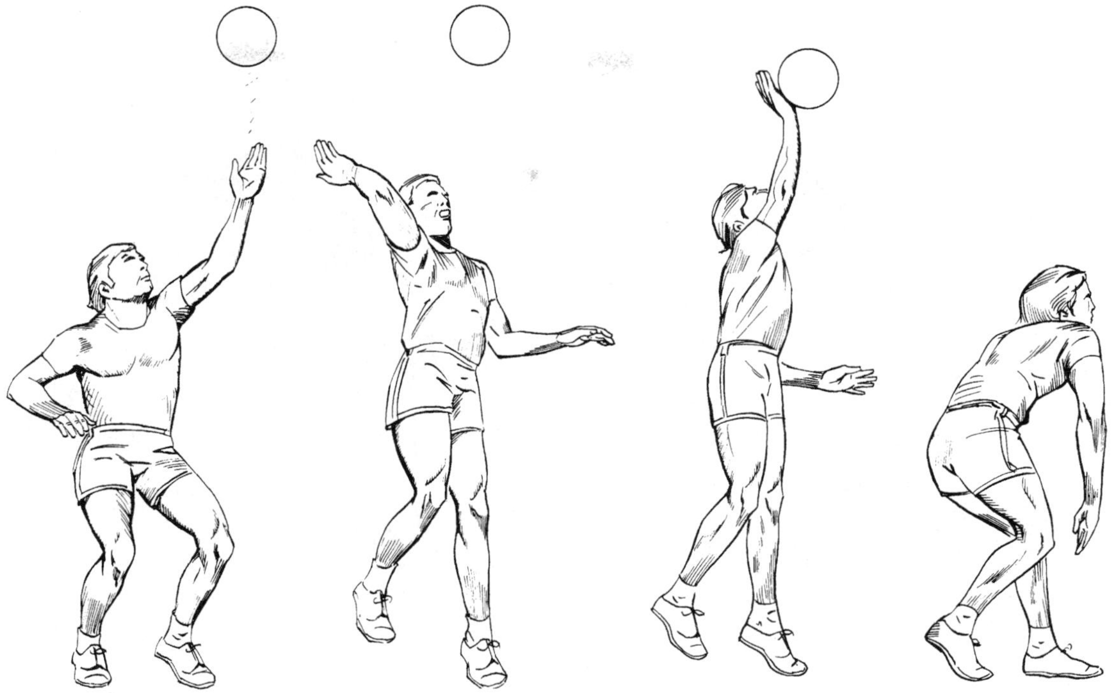

a. b. c. d.

Exercise 5.3 Volleyball serve.

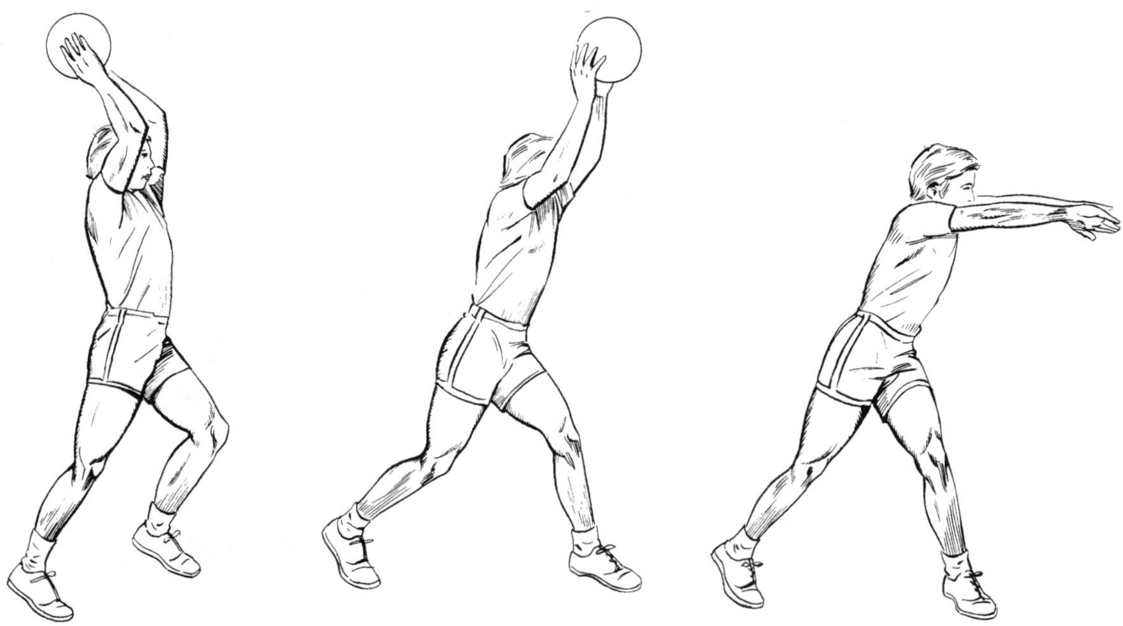

e. f. g.

Exercise 5.4 Soccer throw-in.

Series 5. Sports and Gymnastics Techniques

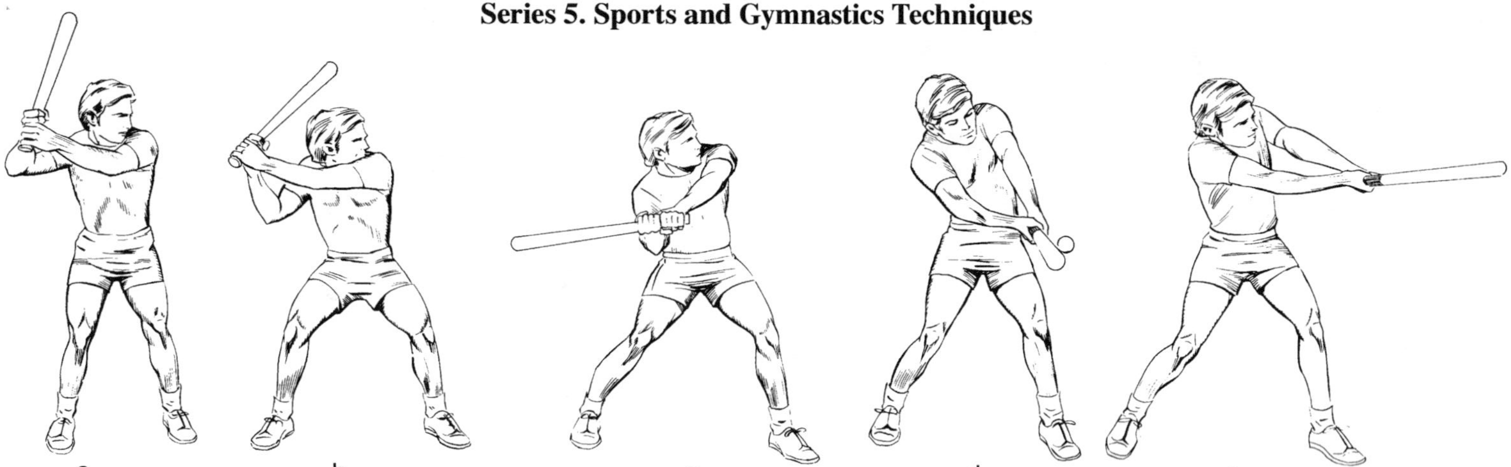

a. b. c. d. e.

Exercise 5.5 Baseball swing.

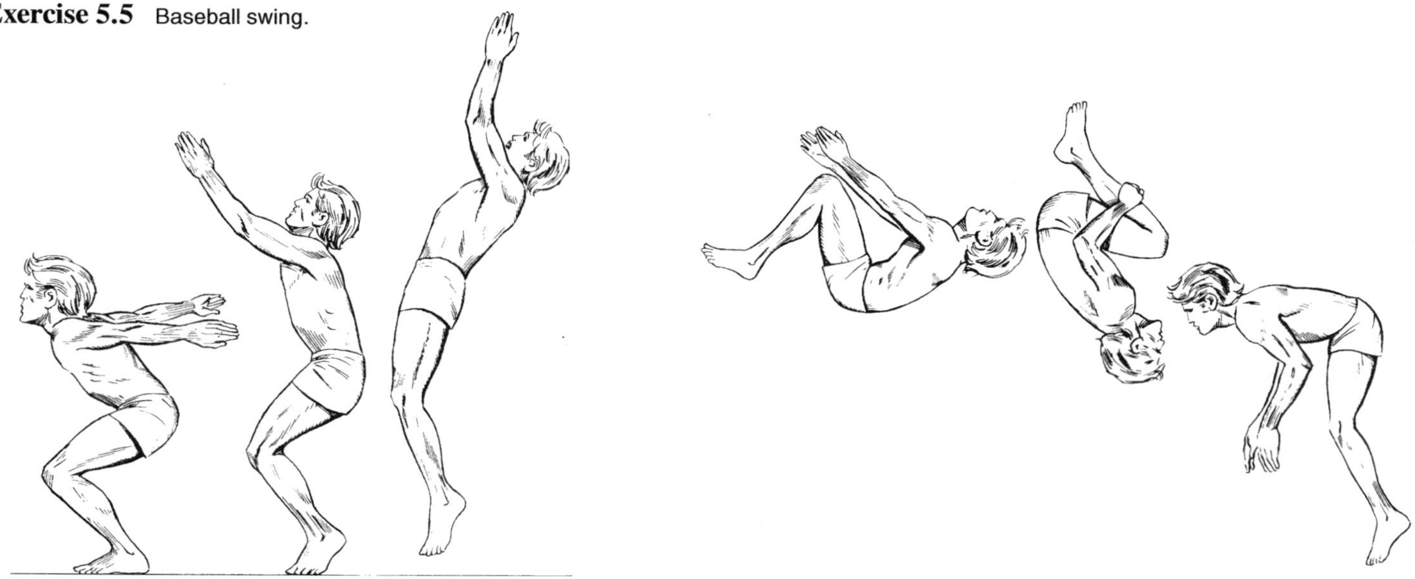

a. b. c. d. e. f.

Exercise 5.6 Backward somersault.

Series 5. Sports and Gymnastics Techniques

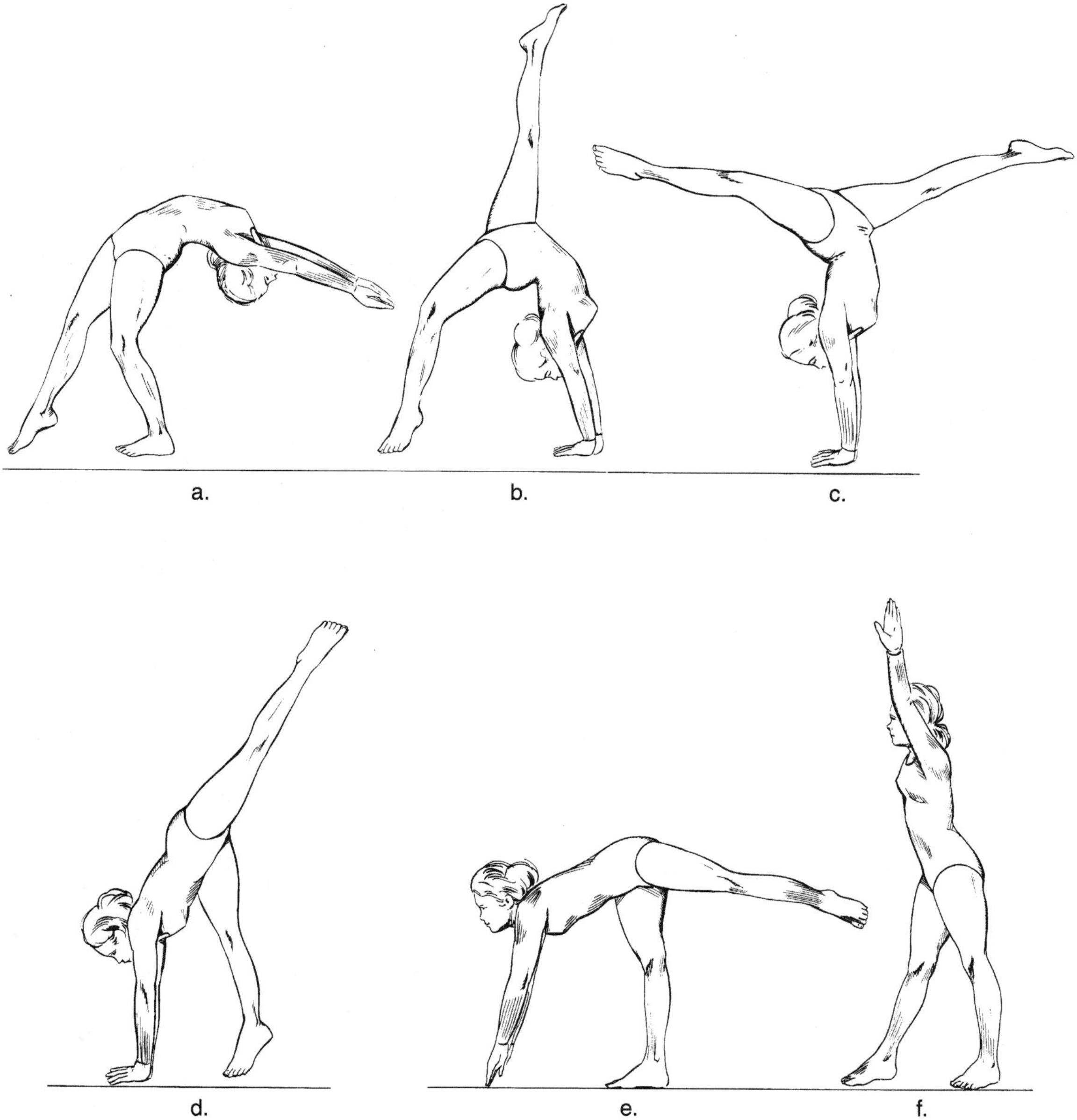

Exercise 5.7 Back walkover.

Appendix H Answers to Problems in Part II

Chapter 10

2. a. 111.25 N
   b. 73 kg
   c. 27.94 cm
   d. 6.1 m/s
   e. 2.84 liters
3. a. 50 cm
   b. 22.4 cm
   c. 54 cm
   d. 71.7 cm
4. a. $x = 40.78$ m/s; $y = 19.02$ m/s
   b. $x = -60.1$ N; $y = 60.1$ N
   c. $x = 75.85$ kg; $y = -90.39$ kg
   d. $x = -21.65$ m/s^2; $y = -12.5$ m/s^2
5. $s = 28$ m; $d = 12$ m
6. $x = 627.8$ N; $y = 168.2$ N
7. $V = 28.65$ m/s; $v = 93.98$ ft/s;
   $\theta = 29.25$ degrees or .51 radians
8. Horizontal (x) = 103.4 N;
   vertical (y) = 37.6 N
9. b. 1992 m at 106°
   c. Rectangular = −535 m, 1919 m
      Polar = 1992 m, −74 degrees or
      106 degrees from start
10. $x = 112.5$ lb; $y = 51$ lb; $R = 123.5$ lb;
    $\theta = 24°$
11. b. x (stabilizing) ≈ 834.5 N;
       y (rotary) ≈ 337 N
12. 1359 N; $\theta = 20$ degrees

Chapter 11

3. 1,500 m = 12.19 m/s
   5,000 m = 11.27 m/s
   10,000 m = 11.09 m/s
5. $t = 0.177$ sec
7. $t = 3.9$ sec up; total = 7.8 s
   $y = 38.2$ m/s
11. $t = 3.46$ sec; $s = 58.7$ m
    $t = 2.4$ sec; $s = 49.88$ m
12. Start of force: $\omega = 1{,}089.7$ deg/sec
    (19 rad/sec)
    Contact: $\omega = 1{,}153.8$ deg/sec (20 rad/sec)
    $v = 7$ m/s

Chapter 13

4. x (stabilizing) = 77.6 N; y (rotary) = 289.8 N
9. $E = 6.7$ N
10. $EA = 1.6$ m; $RA = 0.4$ m
14. $E = 287.5$ N
15. 3 cm: $T = 16.5$ Nm
    15 cm: $T = 82.4$ Nm

GLOSSARY

A

abduction Movement of a segment in the frontal plane away from the midline of the body

acceleration The rate at which velocity changes

adduction Movement of a segment in the frontal plane toward the midline of the body

afferent neuron Neuron that carries impulse toward the central nervous system; sensory neuron

agonist Muscle primarily responsible for motion; prime mover

angle of attack The angle between the long axis of a projected object and the direction of airflow

angle of incidence The angle at which an object strikes a hard surface

angle of projection The angle between the horizontal and the initial velocity vector of a projectile

angle of pull The angle between the mechanical axis of bone and the line of pull of a muscle

angle of reflection The angle at which an object will leave a hard surface after striking it

angular acceleration The rate at which angular velocity changes

angular displacement Any change in angle

angular impulse A torque applied over some period of time

angular momentum The quantity of angular motion a lever possesses, equal to the product of the moment of inertia and the angular velocity

angular velocity The rate at which angular displacement takes place

anteroposterior (AP) axis The axis that passes horizontally from front to back, perpendicular to the frontal plane

Archimedes' Principle Law governing buoyancy, which states that a body immersed in water is buoyed up by a force equal to the weight of the fluid displaced by the body

B

backward tilt Pelvic motion in which the posterior surface moves somewhat backward and downward

base of support Any part of the body in contact with the supporting surface and the intervening area

Bernoulli's Principle Law governing fluid forces, which states that when flow velocity is high, fluid pressure is low, and when flow velocity is low, fluid pressure is high

bilateral axis The axis that passes horizontally from side to side, perpendicular to the sagittal plane

biomechanics The study of the mechanics of biological systems

boundary layer A layer of fluid that is immediately adjacent to the surface of an object

buoyancy An upward force that acts to support a body immersed in water

C

cardinal plane A primary plane, one that passes through the center of gravity

center of buoyancy That point in the body at which the upward force of buoyancy acts

center of gravity The "balance point" of the body; the center of mass; the intersection of the three cardinal planes

centrifugal force The "center-fleeing" force acting on an object undergoing circular motion; a reaction force to centripetal force

centripetal force The "center-seeking" force constraining an object to a circular path

coefficient of elasticity A number that represents the ability of a material to resist deformation and to return to its original state

coefficient of friction A number that represents the resistance to rolling or sliding motion that exists between any two surfaces

coefficient of restitution See **coefficient of elasticity**

compression Force that acts to press or compact

concentric muscle contraction Contraction in which the muscle fibers shorten

concurrent forces Forces acting at the same time and point of application but at different angles

concurrent muscle action Action in which a biarticular muscle loses tension at one attachment while increasing tension at the other, producing no net change in muscle tension

conservation of angular momentum In the absence of any angular impulse, angular momentum remains constant

conservation of momentum In the absence of an impulse, momentum remains constant

countercurrent muscle action One biarticular muscle shortens at both joints while the antagonist lengthens at both joints

curvilinear motion Motion that follows a curved path

D

deceleration The rate at which velocity decreases

density The amount of mass per unit of volume

diagonal planes Infinite number of planes of motion lying on the diagonal between the cardinal planes

displacement A vector quantity that reflects any change in position

distance A scalar quantity that reflects the amount of space moved

drag A fluid force that acts to resist motion

dynamics The study of objects or systems subject to acceleration

E

eccentric contraction A lengthening muscle contraction

eccentric force An "off-center" force, one that is not in line with the center of gravity or the axis and therefore tends to cause rotation

efferent neurons Neurons that carry impulses away from the central nervous system; motor neurons

effort arm (EA) The perpendicular distance between the applied effort force and the axis of a lever

elasticity The ability to resist deformation and to return to the original shape

energy The ability to do work, based on either position or motion

equilibrium A state of balance

extension The return from flexion

F

first-class lever One in which the effort and the resistance are on opposite sides of the axis

flexion A reduction in joint angle

force A push or a pull

force couple Parallel forces on either side of the axis acting in opposite directions

form drag Fluid resistance to forward motion based on the cross-sectional area of a body

forward tilt Movement of the pelvic girdle in the sagittal plane so that the symphysis pubis moves forward and downward

free-body diagram A schematic representation of all the forces and levers that make up a defined system

friction A resistance to rolling or sliding, based on the nature of the two interacting surfaces

frontal plane Vertical plane passing through the body from side to side, dividing it into anterior and posterior halves

fulcrum An axis; the point about which rotation occurs

G

gravity An acceleration toward the center of the earth

ground reaction force Equal and opposite reaction produced by the supporting surface

H

horizontal abduction Movement of a segment in the transverse plane away from the midline of the body

horizontal adduction Movement of a segment in the transverse plane toward the midline of the body

I

impulse The product of a force and the amount of time over which it is applied

inertia A resistance to motion based on the mass of an object

isokinetic Exercise done with a constant rate of motion

isometric Exercise involving no motion and no change in muscle length

isotonic Exercise done with constant muscle tension

K

kinematics The "measurement of motion"; those variables that describe motion with respect to time

kinesiology The study of human movement.

kinetic energy Energy based on motion; a product of mass and velocity

kinetics The study of the forces that act to produce motion

L

laminar flow Smooth, unbroken fluid flow

Law of Acceleration The law states that the acceleration of an object is directly proportional to the force causing it , is in the same direction as the force, and is inversely proportional to the mass of the object

Law of Inertia The law of motion states that a body continues in its state of rest or of uniform motion unless an unbalanced force acts on it

Law of Reaction The law of motion that states that for every action, there will be an equal and opposite reaction

lever A rigid bar that is fixed at a single point, about which it may be made to rotate

lift A fluid force that acts in response to the pressure differential produced by differing flow velocities around an aerodynamic shape; acts perpendicular to fluid flow

line of gravity A line that extends from the center of gravity of an object toward the center of the earth

linear forces Forces applied in the same direction and along the same line of action

linear motion Motion in a line, in which all parts of the object move in the same direction and at the same speed

M

Magnus effect An explanation of the lift forces that cause a spinning object to curve in the direction of the spin

mass The quantity of matter an object contains

mechanical advantage The ratio of effort arm to resistance arm, or the ratio of resistance to effort in a lever

mechanical axis of bone A line drawn from the proximal joint center to distal joint center

moment arm The perpendicular distance from any force to an axis in a lever system

moment of inertia The quantity of a rotating mass and its distribution around the axis of rotation

momentum The amount of motion an object possesses; the product of mass and velocity

motor unit A single motor neuron and all the muscle fibers it innervates

P

parallel forces Forces that act parallel to each other

plyometric Exercise using an eccentric muscle contraction immediately followed by an explosive concentric muscle contraction

potential energy Energy based on the position of an object, usually its height from the surface

power The rate at which work is done

principle of levers For a lever to be in equilibrium, the clockwise torques must equal the counterclockwise torques; $E \times EA = R \times RA$

projectile An object that is given some initial velocity and then is released

R

radian A unit of angular measure, 57.3°

reciprocating motion Repetitive motion

relative motion Motion with respect to some reference object

resistance arm (RA) Perpendicular distance between the resistance force vector and the axis of a lever

resultant The combined effect of two or more vector quantities

rotary component That vector component of force which acts perpendicular to a lever

S

sagittal plane Vertical plane passing through the body from front to back, dividing it into right and left halves

scalar A single quantity, measuring only amount

second-class lever One in which the resistance is closer to the axis than is the effort

specific gravity Ratio between the density of an object and that of water

speed Scalar quantity specifying the rate of motion

stability The ability to remain in or return to a state of equilibrium

stabilizing component That vector component of force which acts parallel to a lever

statics The study of the mechanics of systems or objects in equilibrium

strain The amount of deformation experienced by an object when stressed

stress The force applied per unit of area

surface drag Resistance to forward motion produced by the interaction of a fluid with a surface

T

tension A form of stress that involves pulling forces

third-class lever One in which the effort is closer to the axis than is the resistance

torque The tendency for rotation; turning effect

torsion A form of stress that involves twisting

transverse plane Horizontal plane that passes through the body, dividing it into upper and lower halves

turbulence Chaotic fluid motion at the trailing edge of a moving object

V

vector A double quantity; one that specifies both magnitude and direction

velocity A vector quantity describing the rate of displacement

vertical axis The axis that is perpendicular to the ground

W

weight The product of the mass of an object and the acceleration that is due to gravity

work The product of a force and the distance over which that force produces motion

PHOTO CREDITS

All photos author provided unless otherwise noted.
Page 446: ©John G. Zimmerman Archive;
471: ©Robert Daly/age fotostock;
474: (bottom) ©Karl Weatherly/Getty Images;
476: ©spotpoint74/123RF;
502: Digital Vision/Getty Images;
510: ©Graham Oliver/123RF;
511: ©Bike Rider London/Shutterstock.com;
523: Comstock Images;
536: JASON CONNOLLY/AFP/Getty Images

INDEX

A

B

C

D

E

G

H

I

J

K

L

M

N

O

P

Q

R

S

T

U

V

W

X

Y

Z